ADVANCES IN NEUROLOGY

Volume 87

Advances in Neurology

INTERNATIONAL ADVISORY BOARD

Advances in Neurology
Volume 87

Gait Disorders

Editors

Evžen Růžička, M.D., Ph.D.
Movement Disorder Center
Department of Neurology
Charles University
Prague, Czech Republic

Mark Hallett, M.D.
National Institute of Neurological Disorders and Stroke
National Institutes of Health
Bethesda, Maryland, U.S.A.

Joseph Jankovic, M.D.
Director
Parkinson's Disease and Movement Disorders Clinic
Department of Neurology
Baylor College of Medicine
Houston, Texas, U.S.A.

LIPPINCOTT WILLIAMS & WILKINS
A **Wolters Kluwer** Company
Philadelphia • Baltimore • New York • London
Buenos Aires • Hong Kong • Sydney • Tokyo

Acquisitions Editor: Anne M. Sydor
Developmental Editor: Mildred G. Ramos
Production Editor: Jonathan Geffner
Manufacturing Manager: Benjamin Rivera
Compositor: TechBooks
Printer: Maple Press

530 Walnut Street
Philadelphia, PA 19106 USA
LWW.com

Printed in the USA

Library of Congress Cataloging-in-Publication Data
ISBN: 0-7817-2123-7
ISSN: 0091-3952

Care has been taken to confirm the accuracy of the information presented and to describe generally accepted practices. However, the authors, editors, and publisher are not responsible for errors or omissions or for any consequences from application of the information in this book and make no warranty, expressed or implied, with respect to the currency, completeness, or accuracy of the contents of the publication. Application of this information in a particular situation remains the professional responsibility of the practitioner.

The authors, editors, and publisher have exerted every effort to ensure that drug selection and dosage set forth in this text are in accordance with current recommendations and practice at the time of publication. However, in view of ongoing research, changes in government regulations, and the constant flow of information relating to drug therapy and drug reactions, the reader is urged to check the package insert for each drug for any change in indications and dosage and for added warnings and precautions. This is particularly important when the recommended agent is a new or infrequently employed drug.

Some drugs and medical devices presented in this publication have Food and Drug Administration (FDA) clearance for limited use in restricted research settings. It is the responsibility of the health care provider to ascertain the FDA status of each drug or device planned for use in their clinical practice.

10 9 8 7 6 5 4 3 2 1

Advances in Neurology Series

Vol. 86: Parkinson's Disease: *D. Calne and S. M. Calne, editors.* 512 pp., 2001.
Vol. 85: Tourette Syndrome: *D. J. Cohen, J. Jankovic, and C. G. Goetz, editors.* 432 pp., 2001.
Vol. 84: Neocortical Epilepsies: *P. D. Williamson, A. M. Siegel, D. W. Roberts, V. M. Thadani, and M. S. Gazzaniga, editors.* 688 pp., 2000.
Vol. 83: Functional Imaging in the Epilepsies: *T. R. Henry, J. S. Duncan, and S. F. Berkovic, editors.* 352 pp., 2000.
Vol. 82: Corticobasal Degeneration and Related Disorders: *I. Litvan, C. G. Goetz, and A. E. Lang, editors.* 284 pp., 2000.
Vol. 81: Plasticity and Epilepsy: Aspects of Brain Function: *H. Stefan, P. Chauvel, F. Anderman, S. D. Sharvon, editors.* 416 pp., 1999.
Vol. 80: Parkinson's Disease: *Gerald M. Stern, editor.* 704 pp., 1999.
Vol. 79: Jasper's Basic Mechanisms of the Epilepsies. Third Edition: *A. Delgado-Escueta, W. Wilson, R. Olsen, R. Porter, editors.* 1104 pp., 1999.
Vol. 78: Dystonia 3: *S. Fahn, C. D. Marsden, M. R. DeLong, editors.* 400 pp., 1998.
Vol. 77: Consciousness: At the Frontiers of Neuroscience: *H. H. Jasper, L. Descarries, V. F. Castellucci, S. Rossignol, editors.* 320 pp., 1998.
Vol. 76: Antiepileptic Drug Development: *J. A. French, I. E. Leppik, M. A. Dichter, editors.* 304 pp., 1998.
Vol. 75: Reflex Epilepsies and Reflex Seizures: *B. G. Zifkin, F. Andermann, A. Beaumanoir, A. J. Rowan, editors.* 336 pp., 1998.
Vol. 74: Basal Ganglia and New Surgical Approaches for Parkinson's Disease: *J. A. Obeso, M. R. DeLong, C. Ohye, and C. D. Marsden, editors.* 304 pp., 1997.
Vol. 73: Brain Plasticity: *H.-J. Freund, B. A. Sabel, and O. W. Witte, editors.* 448 pp., 1997.
Vol. 72: Neuronal Regeneration, Reorganization, and Repair: *F. J. Seil, editor.* 416 pp., 1996.
Vol. 71: Cellular and Molecular Mechanisms of Ischemic Brain Damage: *B. K. Siesjö and T. Wieloch, editors.* 560 pp., 1996.
Vol. 70: Supplementary Sensorimotor Area: *H. O. Lüders, editor.* 544 pp., 1996.
Vol. 69: Parkinson's Disease: *L. Battistin, G. Scarlato, T. Caraceni, and S. Ruggieri, editors.* 752 pp., 1996.
Vol. 68: Pathogenesis and Therapy of Amyotrophic Lateral Sclerosis: *G. Serratrice and T. L. Munsat, editors.* 352 pp., 1995.
Vol. 67: Negative Motor Phenomena: *S. Fahn, M. Hallett, H. O. Lüders, and C. D. Marsden, editors.* 416 pp., 1995.
Vol. 66: Epilepsy and the Functional Anatomy of the Frontal Lobe: *H. H. Jasper, S. Riggio, and P. S. Goldman-Rakic, editors.* 400 pp., 1995.
Vol. 65: Behavioral Neurology of Movement Disorders: *W. J. Weiner and A. E. Lang, editors.* 368 pp., 1995.
Vol. 64: Neurological Complications of Pregnancy: *O. Devinsky, E. Feldmann, and B. Hainline, editors.* 288 pp., 1994.
Vol. 63: Electrical and Magnetic Stimulation of the Brain and Spinal Cord: *O. Devinsky, A. Beric, and M. Dogali, editors.* 352 pp., 1993.
Vol. 62: Cerebral Small Artery Disease: *P. M. Pullicino, L. R. Caplan, and M. Hommel, editors.* 256 pp., 1993.
Vol. 61: Inherited Ataxias: *A. E. Harding and T. Deufel, editors.* 240 pp., 1993.
Vol. 60: Parkinson's Disease: From Basic Research to Treatment: *H. Narabayashi, T. Nagatsu, N. Yanagisawa, and Y. Mizuno, editors.* 800 pp., 1993.
Vol. 59: Neural Injury and Regeneration: *F. J. Seil, editor.* 384 pp., 1993.
Vol. 58: Tourette Syndrome: Genetics, Neurobiology, and Treatment: *T. N. Chase, A. J. Friedhoff, and D. J. Cohen, editors.* 400 pp., 1992.
Vol. 57: Frontal Lobe Seizures and Epilepsies: *P. Chauvel, A. V. Delgado-Escueta, E. Halgren, and J. Bancaud, editors.* 752 pp., 1992.
Vol. 56: Amyotrophic Lateral Sclerosis and Other Motor Neuron Diseases: *L. P. Rowland, editor.* 592 pp., 1991.
Vol. 55: Neurobehavioral Problems in Epilepsy: *D. B. Smith, D. Treiman, and M. Trimble, editors.* 512 pp., 1990.
Vol. 54: Magnetoencephalography: *S. Sato, editor.* 1990.
Vol. 53: Parkinson's Disease: Anatomy, Pathology, and Therapy: *M. B. Streifler, A. D. Korczyn, E. Melamed, and M. B. H. Youdim, editors.* 640 pp., 1990.
Vol. 52: Brain Edema: Pathogenesis, Imaging, and Therapy: *D. Long, editor.* 640 pp., 1990.
Vol. 51: Alzheimer's Disease: *R. J. Wurtman, S. Corkin, J. H. Growdon, and E. Ritter-Walker, editors.* 1990.

Contents

Principles of Gait Disorders

Edited by Joseph Jankovic

Disorders of Sensory Systems, Balance, and Coordination

Edited by Mark Hallett

Gait in Parkinson's and Related Disorders

Edited by Joseph Jankovic

Higher-Level Gait Disorders

Edited by Joseph Jankovic

Pharmacotherapy

Edited by Evžen Růžička

Surgery

Edited by Joseph Jankovic

Transdisciplinary Approach to Gait Disorders in Craniocerebral Trauma, Brain Injury, and Stroke

Edited by Evžen Růžička

Gait Rehabilitation in Parkinson's Disease, Gait Apraxia, and Huntington's Disease

Edited by Evžen Růžička

Contributing Authors

Yves Agid, M.D.
Professor
Federation of Neurology
Salpêtrière Hospital
47 Boulevard de l'Hôpital
75013 Paris
France

Isabelle Arnulf, M.D.
Neurologist
Service of Functional Pneumological Explorations
Salpêtrière Hospital
Paris 75013
France

Dennis J. Beckley, M.D.
Director, Human Balance Laboratory
Department of Neurology Services—127
Veteran's Administration—Northern California System of Clinics
150 Muir Road
Martinez, California 94553
U.S.A.

Boulos-Paul Bejjani, M.D.
Chief of Clinic
Department of Neurology
Faculty of Medicine
University of Saint Joseph
Rue Dumas
Beirut, Lebanon
Director
Parkinson & Movement Disorders Center
Notre Dame des Secours Hospital
Byblos-Jbeil
Lebanon

Judy Benson, M.A.
Team Assistant
Neurological Research Center
Ludwig-Maximilians University
Marchioninistrasse 23
81377 Munich
Germany

Francesco Benvenuti, M.D.
Diregente 1 Livello
Department of Geriatric Medicine
Italian National Research Institute on Aging
41 Viale Michelangiolo
Florence 50125
Italy

Wiltrud Berger, M.D., Ph.D.
Associate Professor
Department of Neurology
University of Freiburg
Breisacherstasse 64
D-79106 Freiburg
Germany

Kailash P. Bhatia, M.D.
Senior Lecturer
Department of Clinical Neurology
Institute of Neurology
Honorable Consultant Neurologist
National Hospital for Neurology
Queen Square
London WC1N 3BG
United Kingdom

Olivier Blin, M.D., Ph.D.
Professor
Department of Clinical Pharmacology
UMR CNRS Université Mediterranée
Chief, CPCET
Timone University Hospital
F-13385 Marseille Cedex 5
France

Baastian R. Bloem, M.D., Ph.D.
Assistant Professor
Department of Neurology
University Hospital Nijmegen
P.O. Box 9101
6500 HB Nijmegen
The Netherlands

Anne-Marie Bonnet, M.D.
Neurologist
Federation of Neurology
Salpêtrière Hospital
Paris 75013
France

Jan J. Borremans, M.D.
Wissenschaftlicher Assistant
Department of Neurosurgery
Albert-Ludwigs University
Neurozentrum–Uniklinik Freiburg
Breisacherstrasse 64
D-79106 Freiburg
Germany

Thomas Brandt, M.D.
Professor
Director, Neurology Clinic
Ludwig-Maximilians University
Grosshadern Clinic
Marchioninistrasse 15
81377 Munich
Germany

Christine Brefel-Courbon, M.D.
Associate Professor
Department of Pharmacology
Toulouse University
37 Allés Jules Guesde
31073 Toulouse, France
Hospital Physician
Department of Pharmacology
Toulouse Hospital
Place du Docteur Baylac
31059 Toulouse
France

Margaret Bruce, Diploma of Physiotherapy
Physiotherapist
Movement Disorder Program
Southern Health
Kingston Centre
Warrigal Road
Cheltenham, Victoria 3192
Australia

Robert E. Burke, M.D.
Chief
Laboratory of Neural Control
National Institute of Neurological Disorders and Stroke
National Institutes of Health
Bethesda, Maryland 20892-4455
U.S.A.

Edmond Chiu, A.M., M.B.B.S., D.P.M.
Academic Unit of Psychiatry of Old Age
University of Melbourne
Director, Huntington's Disease Clinic
St. George's Health Service
283 Cotham Road
Kew, Victoria 3101
Australia

Andrew J. Churchyard, M.B.B.S., Ph.D.
Honorary Lecturer
Department of Medicine
Monash University
Monash Medical Center
Clayton Road
Clayton, Victoria 3168
Australia
Consultant Neurologist
Movement Disorders Unit
Kingston Centre
Warrigal Road
Cheltenham, Victoria 3192
Australia

Randall Cooper, Bachelor of Physiotherapy
Research Fellow
School of Physiotherapy
Faculty of Health Science
La Trobe University
Bundoora, Victoria 3083
Australia

Philippe Damier, M.D., Ph.D.
Professor
Department of Neurology
Faculty of Medicine
University Hospital of Nantes
1, Rue Gaston Veil
Nantes F-44035
Chief
Department of Neurology
Laennec Hospital
CHU Nantes
Nantes F-44093
France

Axel Darmon, Ph.D.
UMR–CNRS–FRE–DPM
Timone University Hospital Researcher
CPCET
Timone Hospital
F-13385 Marseille
France

Marianne Dieterich, M.D.
Full Professor
Department of Neurology
Ludwig-Maximilians University
Senior Physician
Department of Neurology
Grosshadern Clinic
Marchioninistrasse 15
81377 Munich
Germany

Volker Dietz, M.D.
Professor
Department of Paraplegiology
University of Zurich
Director
Swiss Paraplegic Centre
University Hospital Balgrist
Forchstrasse 340
CH-8008 Zurich
Switzerland

Georg Ebersbach, M.D.
Chief
Movement Disorders Clinic
Movement Disorders and Parkinson's Clinic
Strass nach Fichtenwalde 16
14547 Beelitz-Heilstätten
Germany

Alberto Esquenazi, M.D.
Associate Professor
Department of Physical Medicine and Rehabilitation
Thomas Jefferson School of Medicine
Director
Gait and Motion Analysis Laboratory
MossRehab Hospital
1200 West Tabor Road
Philadelphia, Pennsylvania 19141
U.S.A.

Nelly Fabre, M.D.
Associate Professor
Department of Neurology
Toulouse University
37 Route de Narbonne
Physician
Department of Neurology
Toulouse University Hospital
Avenue J Poulhes
31 Toulouse
France

Michael Faist, M.D.
Resident
Department of Neurology
University of Freiburg
Breisacherstrasse 64
D-79106 Freiburg
Germany

Nellie Georgiou, Ph.D.
Lecturer
Department of Psychology
Monash University
Wellington Road
Clayton, Victoria 3168
Australia

Nir Giladi, M.D.
Department of Neurology
Tel-Aviv University
Director
Movement Disorders Unit
Department of Neurology
Tel-Aviv Medical Center
6 Weizmann Street
Tel-Aviv 64239
Israel

Robert G. Grossman, M.D.
Professor
Department of Neurosurgery
Baylor College of Medicine
6550 Fannin, Suite 944
Houston, Texas 77030
Chief
Neurosurgical Service
The Methodist Hospital
6565 Fannin, M.S. 409, Room 417
Houston, Texas 77030-2707
U.S.A.

Mark Hallett, M.D.
Chief, Human Motor Control Section
National Institute of Neurological Disorders and Stroke
National Institutes of Health
Building 10, Room 5N226
10 Center Drive, MSC 1428
Bethesda, Maryland 20892-1428
U.S.A.

Ryoichi Hayashi, M.D., Ph.D.
Professor
Division of Clinical Neurophysiology
School of Allied Medical Sciences
Shinsu University
Asahi 3-1-1
Matsumoto, Nagano 390-8621
Japan

Fay B. Horak, Ph.D., P.T.
Senior Scientist and Professor
Neurological Sciences Institute
Departments of Neurology and Physiology and Pharmacology
Oregon Health Sciences University
505 Northwest 185th Avenue
Beaverton, Oregon 97006
U.S.A.

Jean-Luc Houeto, M.D.
Assistant
Department of Neurology
Clinical Investigation Center
Salpêtrière Hospital
47 Boulevard de l'Hospital
Paris 75013
France

Frances E. Huxham, Grad Dip (HRM)
Senior Research Physiotherapist
Geriatric Research Unit
Kingston Centre
Southern Health
Warrigal Road
Cheltenham, Victoria 3192
Australia

Robert Iansek, Ph.D.
Professor
Department of Medicine
Monash University
Wellington Road
Clayton, Victoria 3168
Director
Department of Geriatric Neurology
Kingston Centre
Warrigal Road
Cheltenham, Victoria 3192
Australia

Páll E. Ingvarsson, M.D.
Department of Neurology
Göteborg University
41674 Göteborg
Sweden

Noor H. Ismail, M.B.B.S., F.A.M.S.
Consultant
Department of Geriatric Medicine
Tan Tock Seng Hospital
11 Jalan Tan Tock Seng
Singapore 308433

Joseph Jankovic, M.D.
Professor
Department of Neurology
Baylor College of Medicine
Director of Parkinson's Disease Center and Movement Disorders Clinic
6550 Fannin, Suite 1801
Senior Attending Neurologist
The Methodist Hospital
Houston, Texas 77030
U.S.A.

Bo Johnels, M.D., Ph.D.
Associate Professor
Department of Neurology
Göteborg University
Sahlgrenska University Hospital
SE 41345 Göteborg
Sweden

Kenton R. Kaufman, Ph.D., P.E.
Associate Professor of Bioengineering
Department of Orthopaedic Surgery
Mayo Clinic and Foundation
200 First Street Southwest
Director
Orthopedic Biomechanics Laboratory
128 Guggenheim Building
Rochester, Minnesota 55905
U.S.A.

Mary Ann E. Keenan, M.D.
Professor
Department of Orthopaedic Surgery
Thomas Jefferson University School of Medicine
1020 Chestnut Street
Philadelphia, Pennsylvania 19107
Director
Neuro-orthopaedic Program
Department of Orthopedic Surgery
Albert Einstein Medical Center
5501 Old York Road
Philadelphia, Pennsylvania 19141
U.S.A.

Siegbert Krafczyk, Ph.D.
Department of Neurology
Ludwig-Maximilians University
Chief Engineer
Department of Neurology
Grosshadern Clinic
Marchioninistrasse 15
81366 Munich
Germany

Joachim K. Krauss, M.D.
Professor and Vice Chairman
Department of Neurosurgery
University Hospital Mannheim
Ruprecht-Karls-University Heidelberg
Theodor-Kutzer-Ufer 1-3
68167 Mannheim
Germany

Vilém Kuthan, M.D., Ph.D.
Assistant Professor
Institute of Physiology
Charles University
Albertov 5
Prague 2
Czech Republic CZ-128 00

Eugene C. Lai, M.D., Ph.D.
Associate Professor
Department of Neurology
Baylor College of Medicine
6550 Fannin, Suite 1801
Houston, Texas 77030
Active Staff
Neurology Service
The Methodist Hospital
6565 Fannin Street
Houston, Texas 77030-2707
U.S.A.

Carl H. Lücking, M.D.
Professor
Department of Neurology
Albert-Ludwigs University
Head
Department of Neurology
University Clinic
Breisacherstrasse 64
D-79106 Freiburg
Germany

Joseph C. Masdeu, M.D., Ph.D.
Professor and Director
Department of Neurology
University of Navarre
Director
Department of Neurology
University Hospital of Navarre
Avda Pio XII, 26
Pamplona 31008
Spain

Kiyoji Matsuyama, M.D., Ph.D.
Associate Professor
Department of Physiology
Sapporo Medical University School of Medicine
South-1, West-17 Chuo-ku
Sapporo, Hokkaido 060-8556
Japan

Nathaniel H. Mayer, M.D.
Emeritus Professor
Department of Rehabilitation Medicine
Temple University
3401 North Broad Street
Philadelphia, Pennsylvania 19140
Director
Motor Control Analysis Center
MossRehab
1200 West Tabor Road
Philadelphia, Pennsylvania 19141
U.S.A.

Jennifer McGinley, B.App.Sci. (PT)
Senior Research Physiotherapist
Geriatric Research Unit
Southern Health–Kingston Centre
Warrigal Road
Cheltenham, Victoria 3195
Australia

Serge Mesure, Ph.D.
UPRES EA 2991
Montpellier
Department of Neurology
Timone University Hospital
13385 Marseille
France

Malika Miloudy, M.D.
Resident
Federation of Neurology
Salpêtrière Hospital
Paris 75013
France

Hiroshi Mitoma, M.D., Ph.D.
Chief
Mitoma Neurological Clinic
1-2-10 Minami-ikebukuro
Toshima, Tokyo 171-0022
Japan

José L. Molinuevo, M.D.
Consultant
Department of Neurology
Hospital de Palamos
c/Hospital 36
Palamos, 17230 Girona
Spain

Jean-Louis Montastruc, M.D., Ph.D.
Professor
Department of Clinical Pharmacology
Toulouse University
37 Allés Jules Guesde
31073 Toulouse
Chief
Department of Pharmacology
Toulouse University Hospital
Place dr Bayloc
31059 Toulouse
France

Futoshi Mori, M.D., Ph.D.
Research Associate
Department of Biological Control System
National Institute of Physiological Sciences
38 Nishigo-naka Myodaiji
Okazaki, Aichi 444-8585
Japan

Shigemi Mori, M.D., Ph.D.
Professor
Department of Biological Control System
National Institute of Physiological Sciences
Myodaiji cho
Okazaki 444-8585
Japan

Meg E. Morris, Ph.D.
Professor
School of Physiotherapy
La Trobe University
Bundoora, Victoria 3086
Australia

Katsumi Nakajima, M.D., Ph.D.
Research Associate
Department of Biological Control System
National Institute for Physiological Sciences
38 Nishigonaka Myodaiji
Okazaki 444-8585
Japan

John H. Noseworthy, M.D.
Professor and Chairman
Department of Neurology
Mayo Medical School
Mayo Clinic
200 First Street Southwest
Rochester, Minnesota 55905
U.S.A.

John G. Nutt, M.D.
Professor
Department of Neurology
Oregon Health Sciences University
L-226, 3181 Southwest Sam Jackson Park Road
Portland, Oregon 97201
U.S.A.

Christopher F. O'Brien, M.D.
Vice President
Department of Medical Affairs
Elan Pharmaceuticals
700 Gateway Boulevard
South San Francisco, California 94080
U.S.A.

Sharon L. Olson, Ph.D., P.T.
Associate Professor
School of Physical Therapy
Texas Woman's University
1130 MD Anderson Boulevard
Houston, Texas 77030
U.S.A.

Torsten Olsson, Ph.D.
Professor of Medical Electronics
Department of Signals and Systems
Chalmers University of Technology
SE-41296 Göteborg
Sweden

William G. Ondo, M.D.
Assistant Professor
Department of Neurology
Baylor College of Medicine
6550 Fannin, Suite 1801
Active Staff
Department of Neurology
The Methodist Hospital
6565 Fannin Street
Houston, Texas 77030
U.S.A.

Werner Poewe, M.D.
Chairman
Department of Neurology
University of Innsbruck
Anichstrasse 35
A-6020 Innsbruck
Germany

Veronika Querner, M.D.
Department of Neurology
Grosshadern Clinic
University of Munich
Marchioninistrasse 15
D-81377 Munich
Germany

Olivier Rascol, M.D., Ph.D.
Professor
Department of Clinical Pharmacology
Toulouse Faculty of Medicine
37 Allés J. Guesde
Toulouse 31073
France
Coordinator
Clinical Investigation Center
Toulouse Hospital
Place Dr Baylac
Toulouse 31059
France

Deborah Roberts-Warrior, P.T., Ph.D.
Assistant Professor
Department of Rehabilitation Sciences
University of Oklahoma
Health Sciences Center
801 Northeast 13th Street
Oklahoma City, Oklahoma 73190
U.S.A.

Evžen Růžička, M.D., Ph.D.
Associate Professor
Department of Neurology
Charles University
1st Medical Faculty
Director, Movement Disorder Center
General Faculty Hospital
Kateřinská 30
Prague 2
Czech Republic 120 00

Martin Schubert, M.D.
Departments of Neurology and Neurophysiology
Albert-Ludwigs University
Breisacherstrasse 64
D-79106 Freiburg
Germany

William J. Shaughnessy, M.D.
Assistant Professor
Department of Orthopedics
Mayo Medical School
Chair, Division of Pediatric Orthopedics
Department of Orthopedics
Mayo Clinic
200 First Street Southwest
Rochester, Minnesota 55905
U.S.A.

Göran Steg, M.D.
Professor Emeritus
Department of Neurology
Göteborg University
SE-41345 Göteborg
Sweden

Michael Strupp, M.D.
Lecturer
Department of Neurology
Ludwig-Maximilians University
Senior Physician
Department of Neurology
Grosshadern Clinic
Marchioninistrasse 15
D-81377 Munich
Germany

Lewis R. Sudarsky, M.D.
Associate Professor
Department of Neurology
Harvard Medical School
Director of Movement Disorders
Department of Neurology
Brigham & Women's Hospital
75 Francis Street
Boston, Massachusetts 02115
U.S.A.

Philip D. Thompson, M.B.B.S., Ph.D.
Professor of Neurology
Department of Medicine
University of Adelaide
Director
Department of Neurology
Royal Adelaide Hospital
North Terrace
Adelaide, South Australia 5000

Francesc Valldeoriola, M.D.
Staff Physician
Department of Neurology
Hospital Clinic
Villarroel 170
08036 Barcelona
Spain

Josep Valls-Solé, M.D.
Associate Professor
Department of Medicine
University of Barcelona
Casanova, 143
Consultant
Department of Neurology
Hospital Clinic
Villarroel, 170
08036 Barcelona
Spain

Jeroen P. P. van Vugt, M.D.
Assistant in Neurology
Department of Neurology
Leiden University Medical Centre
P.O. Box 9600
2300 RC Leiden
The Netherlands

Nobuo Yanagisawa, M.D., Ph.D.
Professor Emeritus
Department of Medicine
Shinshu University School of Medicine
3-1-1 Asahi
Matsumoto, 390-8621 Japan
President
Chubu National Hospital
36-3 Gengo, Morioka
Obu, Aichi 474-8511
Japan

Preface

Locomotion is a fundamental function of most animals, but its importance for humans should not be undervalued. From the moment a person becomes capable of automatic bipedal gait, he or she is hardly aware of its crucial importance until the ability to walk is lost. Physicians need to understand this complex motor action in order to help patients.

Gait problems represent one of the most common manifestations of developmental disorders, different neurological illnesses, and trauma. Falls as a consequence of unstable gait are one of the most important causes of morbidity and mortality in elderly people. Neurologists, neurosurgeons, orthopedic surgeons, physiotherapists, and other specialists are trying to establish a classification of gait disorders in order to improve diagnosis. New techniques make detailed laboratory analysis of gait possible and new therapeutic approaches help in some conditions that used to be untreatable.

The present volume represents the proceedings of the International Symposium on Gait Disorders that took place in Prague, Czech Republic, in September 1999. Both scientists devoted to the study of locomotion and medical specialists dealing with gait problems gathered to present the contemporary state of knowledge in the field of gait disorders and their treatment. The first part of the volume is dedicated to basic science, followed by chapters on diagnostic methods, classification of gait disorders, and the clinical characteristics of individual gait disorders. The last section of the book describes latest advances in pharmacological, surgical, and rehabilitation therapies of gait disorders.

Despite the progress that has been made in our understanding of human gait, there is more work to be done. We hope that this volume will stimulate further research and will increase clinical interest in this field.

Evžen Růžička
Mark Hallett
Joseph Jankovic

Acknowledgments

The Symposium was organized with the kind support of the Movement Disorder Society. The scientific program was prepared with the invaluable help of the members of the International Advisory Board and Organization Committees:

International Advisory Board

T. Brandt (*Munich, Germany*)
D. Dressler (*Rostock, Germany*)
A. Esquenazi (*Philadelphia,U.S.A.*)
N. Giladi (*Tel Aviv, Israel*)
M. Hallett (*Bethesda, U.S.A.*)
S. Hesse (*Berlin, Germany*)
F. Horak (*Portland, U.S.A.*)
R. Iansek (*Melbourne, Australia*)
J. Jankovic (*Houston, U.S.A.*)
B. Johnels (*Göteborg, Sweden*)
L. Lisý (*Bratislava, Slovakia*)
C. Lücking (*Freiburg, Germany*)
† C. D. Marsden (*London, U.K.*)
J. C. Masdeu (*New York, U.S.A.*)
M. Morris (*Melbourne, Australia*)
J. G. Nutt (*Portland, U.S.A.*)
C. F. O'Brien (*Denver, U.S.A.*)
W. Poewe (*Innsbruck, Austria*)
L. R. Sudarsky (*Boston, U.S.A.*)
P. D. Thompson (*Adelaide, Australia*)
E. Tolosa (*Barcelona, Spain*)
F. Viallet (*Aix-en-Provence, France*)

International and Local Organization Committees

J. Blazer (*New York, U.S.A.*)
C. Colosimo (*Rome, Italy*)
A. Friedman (*Warsaw, Poland*)
P. Kaňovský (*Brno, Czech Republic*)
A. Kurfürstová (*Prague, Czech Republic*)
Z. Pirtošek (*Ljubljana, Slovenia*)
J. Roth (*Prague, Czech Republic*)
E. Růžička, Chairman (*Prague, Czech Republic*)
K. Štěpánková (*Prague, Czech Republic*)
D. Urgošík (*Prague, Czech Republic*)

†, deceased.

ADVANCES IN NEUROLOGY

Volume 87

Gait Disorders. Advances in Neurology, Vol. 87,
edited by E. Růžička, M. Hallett, and J. Jankovic.
Lippincott Williams & Wilkins, Philadelphia © 2001.

1

Jan Evangelista Purkyně and His Contributions to Neurosciences, Analysis of Eye Movements, and Postural Mechanisms

*Vilém Kuthan and †Evžen Růžička

**Institute of Physiology, Charles University, 1st Medical Faculty, Prague, Czech Republic 12800; and*
†Department of Neurology, Charles University, 1st Medical Faculty and Movement Disorders Center, General Faculty Hospital, Prague, Czech Republic 12000

The International Symposium on Gait Disorders, held in Prague in September 1999, became an opportunity to remember and celebrate the seminal scientific contributions of Jan Evangelista Purkyně (also spelled Purkinje), a giant figure in the fields of neurology and neurophysiology, who lived and worked in Prague. Although most recognized for his description of the ganglion cells in the cerebellum, this is only one of his many discoveries that contributed to a better understanding of motor control. Purkyně was the first to describe the presence of pigment in the substantia nigra cells. He was also deeply interested in the analysis of vertigo, nystagmus, and the perception of motion. Most of Purkyně's original notions are still valid today, more than a century and a half later. Much of the information on balance and gait presented in this volume is based on the original observations and scientific foundations established by Purkyně; therefore, it is fitting to begin this book with a tribute to the influential Czech neurophysiologist and neuropathologist.

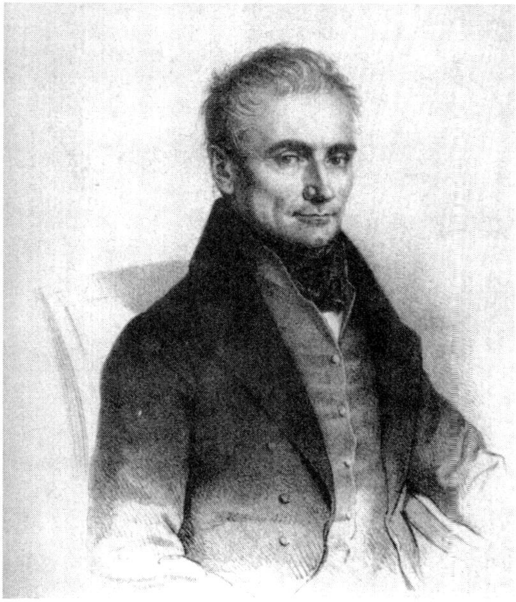

FIG. 1.1. Jan Evangelista Purkyně (Purkinje), original lithography by F. Šír, 1837.

Jan Evangelista Purkyně (1787–1869), was born in Libochovice in northern Bohemia and completed his medical studies at Charles University in Prague in 1818. In 1823 he was appointed Professor of Physiology and Pathology at the University in Wroclaw (Breslau), where he worked for 27 years and founded the world's first Institute of Physiology in 1836 (Fig. 1.1). He returned to Prague in 1850 and opened the Physiological Institute at Charles University in 1851.

Purkyně's research concerned two main areas, physiology/pharmacology and morphology. Purkyně was deeply interested in the structure and function of the nervous system. Today, we admire Purkyně's brilliant ability to make exact

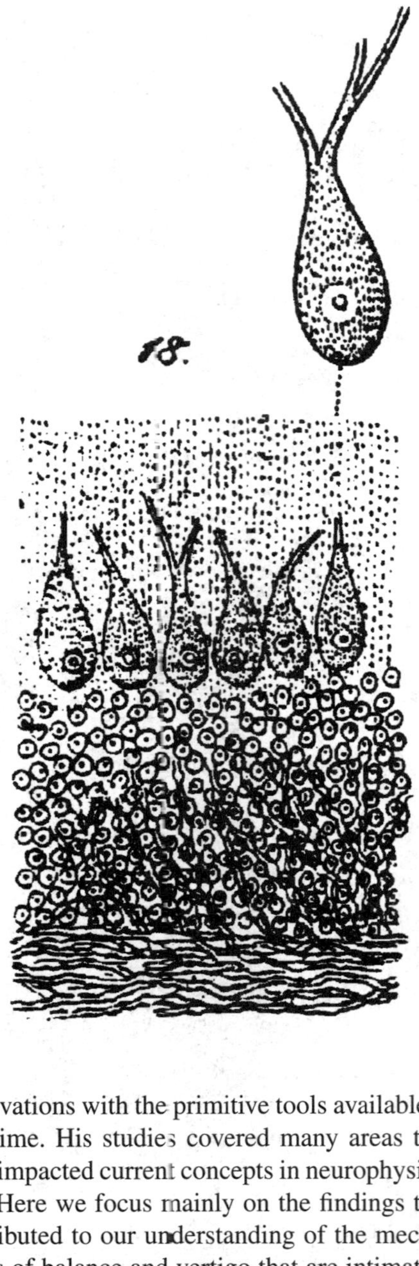

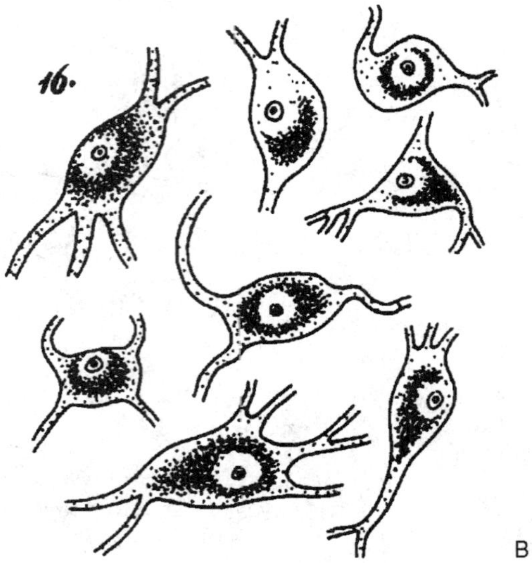

FIG. 1.2. Purkyně's original drawings of (**A**) structure of cerebellar cortex (probably the first known figure of a brain section) with large (Purkinje) cells and (**B**) pigment containing cells from substantia nigra, pars compacta. (From Purkyně JE. *Neueste Untersuchungen aus der Nervenund Hirnanatomie.* In: Sternberg K, von Krombholz JV, eds. *Bericht über die Versammlung Deutscher Naturforscher und Aerzte in Prag im September 1837. Prag* 1838: 177–180.)

observations with the primitive tools available at that time. His studies covered many areas that have impacted current concepts in neurophysiology. Here we focus mainly on the findings that contributed to our understanding of the mechanisms of balance and vertigo that are intimately connected with the study of posture and gait.

NEUROMORPHOLOGICAL STUDIES

Some of Purkyně's fundamental discoveries in the field of neurohistology are briefly mentioned here. He described the structure of the nerve fiber, with the central *Nervencylinder* or *Achsencylinder,* i.e. axon, enveloped within two sheets (1). He demonstrated the ganglion cells in various areas of the brain for the first time, although he is best known for cerebellar *Purkinje cells.* According to Purkyně, these cells branch into the molecular layer of the cerebellar cortex and contain a nucleus and nucleolus (1,2). He visualized the laminated structure (three of four laminae) of the cerebellar cortex for the first time (Fig. 1.2A).

According to Purkyně, neurons are mutually connected by means of their appendages (foreshadowing the concept of neuronal theory), and they represent elements that function as collectors, producers, and distributors of energy. It was Purkyně's idea that the function of neurons depends on their position at certain levels of the hierarchy of the central nervous system (3).

It is important to note that Purkyně was the first to describe the presence of pigment granules—today known as neuromelanin—in the perinuclear zone of neurons in the substantia nigra pars compacta and in some other regions of the brain (Fig. 1.2B) (2). Purkyně also observed the Brownian movement of pigment granules.

STUDIES OF VISION AND OCULAR MOVEMENTS

Purkyně devoted great effort to the study of the physiology of the sensory organs, in addition to his neuromorphological work. He had a major interest in visual phenomena, including the analysis of eye movements and the investigation of vertigo, as acknowledged by Grüsser (4) and Brandt (5).

Vision

There are three Purkyně monographs concerning vision: (a) his Prague doctoral dissertation, (b) his Breslauer professorial dissertation, and (c) his next book on the subject (6–8). These pioneering studies were performed mainly by subjective observation (Heautognosia). Reflecting on the results of Purkyně's work, Tschermak-Seysenegg called him a "founder of exact subjectivism" (9).

Some of Purkyně's discoveries in visual physiology are well known, for example, Purkyně's phenomenon (the shift of visual spectral sensitivity at different levels of illumination) and Purkyně's images (catoptric light reflexes from the cornea and lens) (7,8). It is not so well known, however, that Purkyně designed the construction of the perimeter for clinical examination of the visual field in different planes (7). This device did not come into common use until the mid-19th century, when von Graefe reintroduced it (10). Similarly important are Purkyně's observations on binocular vision, where he demonstrated the function of corresponding retinal areas by overlapping phosphenes elicited by pressure of homonymous parts of the eyeballs and by demonstrating the fusion of images in foveal regions of the retina (11).

Ocular Movements

Purkyně's work on ocular movements concerned the analysis of their significance in pattern vision, different states of vigilance, ocular activity in the perception of motion, and vertigo.

Purkyně described in his doctoral dissertation that "the center of the visual field, where the vision is the most distinct, shifts to and fro along the boundaries of planes and lines of external objects." This mechanism has been confirmed by finer examination methods (12) which also verified another of Purkyně's observations, 'that in complete vision, the point moves through all important spots and lines of an object, but in superficial vision only through single points and lines. . ." (6). His statement that, "among straight lines, the ones that can be followed the best are horizontal, and, in particular, vertical lines, thus demonstrating that the influence of habit and practice is by no means small, since these lines we see more frequently in everyday life" is correct and recently has been confirmed. These lines can be detected faster and easier than oblique lines, a fact that might be correlated, for example, with preferential perception of orientation of a visual stimulus in the receptive fields of some neurons in the visual cortex of higher primates (13).

Perception of Motion

Purkyně also studied the role of indirect (peripheral) vision in the perception of motion. He stressed that complicated movements could not be seen without being "caught up" at the periphery of the visual field (14). The stimulus projecting onto the periphery of the retina elicits ocular saccades, which provide a progressive stepwise shift of the retinal image to the fixation point with highest visual acuity or greatest discrimination capacity. Gould and Dill, for instance, found—quite in line with Purkyně—that this capacity depended on the interest or the information content of the object perceived at the periphery of the visual field (15).

Further, according to Purkyně, "The perception and pursuing of the objective movement of a defined object requires a system of relatively stabilized visible loci, in regard to which the moving body changes its spatial relations, direction and distance in every movement. This simultaneously in space existing system, in which the movement will be perceived like in a stationary body, is given only by the extent of indirect vision" (14). Thus was outlined the existence of retinal and extrapersonal space coordinates. Purkyně was aware that the process of recalibration between these two systems of coordinates during the saccadic eye movement was slower than the duration of this movement. Purkyně's progressive concepts about the perception of movement were recently acknowledged (16).

Purkyně also studied the differences of motion perception (apparent and real motion), depending on whether the eye itself is moving or is motionless, or whether it moves actively or passively (e.g., by pressure by the finger from one side) (14). Purkyně anticipated the later approaches of Helmholtz and came very close to the modern cybernetic formulations of von Holst and von Mittelstaedt as well as Sperry in answering the question of why involuntary (saccadic) movements of the eye are not perceived when the place of the image projecting on the retina changes (17–19). "Its explanation presupposes a general spatial sense, which controls all the special senses and incorporates their individual sensations and observations in itself. Sensations received by the conscious mind are abolished by this function, and the movement of the percept in the sensory organ is thus compensated . . . . On the other hand, if the eye moves too fast . . . this compensation between subjective movement and localization activity of the spatial sense cannot be complete . . . whereby the result is the perception of apparent movement" (20,21).

In modern terminology, this mechanism is referred to as a reafference principle, which can be briefly described as follows. At the same time that the command for movement of the eye (efference) is sent via higher centers to the nuclei of oculomotor nerves, another signal (corollary discharge), which is a kind of copy of the above efference (efference copy) is formed in the brain and is transmitted to the places where the movement is perceived. When the eye moves and thereby causes a change of visual input, the subsequent change in signal (reafference) to higher centers of the visual system produced by the shift of image on the retina is compared with the copy of the efference signal (corollary discharge). During saccadic movements the signals compensate each other and the shift of the retinal image is not perceived. In smooth pursuit eye movements, however, when a relatively slowly moving object is registered in the foveal region and the shift of the retinal image is practically nil, a reafference signal is not formed and the efference copy (corollary discharge) induces visual perception of motion. It has been suggested that the reafference principle does not provide visual stability in the presence of saccadic eye movements (at least not by itself). MacKay concluded that this feedback circuit participated in the control of eye movements rather than in maintaining visual stability (22). This feedback mechanism is assumed also to work in other circuits controlling motor activities (23), as Purkyně recognized (14).

It seems probable that at least some of Purkyně's further research on eye movements was based on the general concept that apparent movement resulted when the function of hypothesized feedback circuits was altered, and concentrated on testing its validity. For example, when stationary objects are observed and rapid voluntary eye movements to the left and right are performed, the objects are perceived as moving in opposite directions (14). Another example is the apparent movement observed when the eye is deflected with a finger, and a motionless object is seen to move to the contralateral side. In this case—explained in terms of reafference principle—corollary discharge is absent and only a noncompensated signal for a change in the position of the image on the retina comes into play. On the other hand, if the eyeball is prevented from moving by finger pressure, corollary discharge occurs, but reafference concerned with the change in the position of the retinal image is blocked; this results in the perception of movement of the image in the intended direction of the eye movement.

STUDIES OF VERTIGO AND NYSTAGMUS

Purkyně was interested in the coordination of movements of eyes, head, and whole body that occur particularly during vertigo (8,11,24,25).

Purkyně defined vertigo two times. In the first preliminary definition he stated "vertigo is the apparent movement of sensual phenomena, which is caused by subjective states and transferred by illusion to the external objects" (11). However, in 1827, Purkyně emphasized the involvement of the motor system: "Vertigo is a disturbance of the dynamic relationship between the brain and motor actions of the body, which manifests itself as an excitement of one side (of the body). In the inner sense, vertigo is a collision of (real) spatial visual sensations with apparent ones, that do not correspond to the movement of real objects, outwardly (objectively) vertigo becomes evident by involuntary muscular actions" (25).

It is remarkable that Purkyně precisely described the vertiginous phenomena occurring during and after revolving around the longitudinal axis of the body in a rotatory chair that was used for therapy of different mental diseases at that time (Fig. 1.3). These manifestations of vertigo were dependent (according to Purkyně's law of vertigo) on the direction of rotation and the position of head (vertical, bent forward and backward, tilted toward the shoulder). Interestingly, the positions of head used by Purkyně correspond to the planes of respective semicircular canals, the role of which was completely unknown in the regulation of balance in his time.

Flourens, who was unacquainted with Purkyně's research, first dissected semicircular canals in animals, but he could not properly explain their function in balance regulation (26,27). He ascribed only a modulatory role to them, whereas according to his former lesional studies, the main "regulatory effects" were exerted from the cerebellum (28). The correct explanation of these early Flourens' experiments was impeded by the fact pointed out by Barány that the manifestation of vertigo in animals is different to that in humans (29,30). Animals circle, tilt their heads (nystagmus of the head), and perform somersaults; similar behavioral effects are not seen in humans. Goltz initiated a great step in the recognition of function of semicircular canals when he repeated Flourens' experiments and cut the individual canals in pigeons (26,27,31). He showed that immediately after cutting the loss of balance was present and the form of behavioral manifestation differed, depending on which canal was lesioned. Then, Breuer was successful in the demonstration of functioning of semicircular canals in balance regulation (32,33). For the first time, he revolved the animals on a rotating platform, and compared the results of these observations with the results attained on the canal-lesioned animals. In this way, he correctly concluded that the semicircular canals were really the receptor organs for the perception of rotation of the head. Almost at the same time, Ernst Mach performed experiments with exclusion of other sources of excitation coming from different organs (e.g., skin, muscles, blood circulation). Based on his findings, he suggested angular acceleration as the adequate stimulus for the excitation of semicircular canals (34). Interestingly, Mach, working in Prague, was in touch with Purkyně, and asked

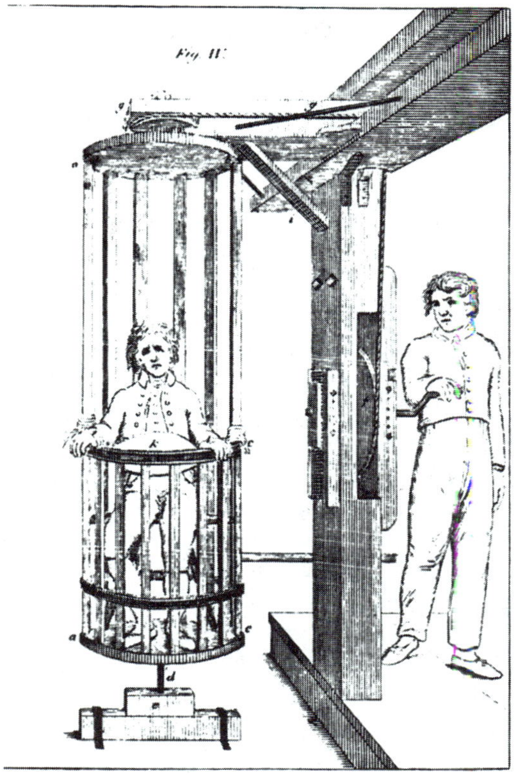

FIG. 1.3. Rotating chair used by Purkyně in his experiments on vertigo. (From Hayner CAF. *Über einige mechanische Vorrichtungen, welche in Irrenanstalten mit Nutzen gebraucht werden können. Z. Psychische Ärtzte* 1818;1:339–366.)

him for a loan of his model of the inner ear structures in a letter dated June 14, 1867.

Purkyně analyzed per-rotational and postrotational nystagmus, with eyes closed or open, described its "voluntary" (fast, central) and "involuntary" (slow, vestibular) components, and classified its forms (horizontal, rotatory, vertical, and oblique) by direct observation or by palpation through the eyelids (11). It was then known that rotation of the body around its own axis and gazing at moving objects evoked eye movements (35,36). These were rarely described objectively, however, and only subjectively perceived apparent movements of seen objects were usually studied.

Purkyně presented a detailed description of nystagmus and its components. During the slow ("involuntary") component, when the body rotates around its own axis, we try to fixate objects that are apparently moving in the opposite direction. The retinal image also moves in the course of the fast ("voluntary") component, but we do not perceive this movement. Purkyně likewise discovered that nystagmus might be stopped by fixation of a near object.

He distinguished optokinetic and vestibular nystagmus; however, he regarded them as a manifestation of "visual" (Gesichtsschwindel) or "ocular" (Augenschwindel) vertigo. In "visual" nystagmus, the only effective stimulation was with eyes following the moving objects (nystagmic slow or "involuntary" component). On the other hand, "ocular" nystagmus also could be induced with eyes closed, and in this case, the excitation of brain structures was probably in play, according to Purkyně.

He explained vestibular vertigo as a result of action of mechanical, centrifugal, or shearing forces on different body organs that produce vegetative disorders (e.g., tachycardia, nausea, and particularly the cerebellum). Although this hypothesis proved to be incorrect, it is noteworthy that Purkyně's explanation of presupposed changes in the brain tissue may be perfectly applied, *mutatis mutandis,* to the demonstration of endolymph flow in the semicircular canals: "When we are moving a vessel with water in horizontal plane, so the water will delay in opposite direction, exerting pressure on the wall of the vessel, which is opposite to the direction of this movement" (25). Von Campenhausen presents the same model, including the demonstration of Coriolis acceleration force impact on endolymph of semicircular canals, which was phenomenologically recognized by Purkyně, and thereafter studied in aviation medicine (37).

Purkyně, in agreement with Flourens (28), suspected that the cerebellum is the primary structure—the receptor—in which vertiginous phenomena are perceived. Reference was made in the dissertation of his doctorate student Krauss to similarities between the manifestation of vertigo and the reactions of animals with cerebellar lesions (38). These reactions (e.g., rotation around the longitudinal axis of the body toward the side operated on, transverse rolling, impaired motor coordination, muscular tonic deviations, falls) depend in their form and degree on the localization of lesion. Foreshadowing of the topical organization of function in the cerebellum might be seen in these experiments.

Purkyně's observations on persons revolving in a rotatory chair also involved the muscular tonic deviation (the vestibulospinal reflex), which he classified as a manifestation of "tactile vertigo" (*Tastschwindel*). When one leans a hand or foot against a wall after rotation has been stopped, "it seems that this obstacle is moving against these limbs." The direction of these tonic deviations depend also on the direction of previous rotation and head position. According to Purkyně's observation: "When we rotate . . . with the head tilted to the right shoulder, and afterwards we stop, and . . . holding an immobile object with both hands without changing the head position, . . . so it seems, that the object in our hands is moving round the vertical axis . . . . When we change the position of the head to the vertical, in the case that the vertigo is still present—it seems, . . . that the object falls against us, and the floor declines backwards" (11).

Purkyně found that the contours and colors of the images fused and eye movements stopped when optokinetic stimulation exceeded a certain velocity. He also discovered rhythmic eye movements that persisted after the visual stimulation had ended (i.e., optokinetic afternystagmus). During a horse parade he observed that his eyes moved involuntarily in the same direction (the slow component of optokinetic nystagmus) when he fixated the individual riders in succession (11). On this occasion he described a type of "movement aftereffect," in which the houses in the background of the scene appeared to move in the opposite direction to that of the previously marching cavalry unit. This adaptation phenomenon, which is often called "the waterfall illusion," might be associated with the activity changes in neurons at different levels of the visual system, which are selectively sensitive to the direction of the movement of a structured image moving in one direction.

Purkyně's research on vertigo differentiated phenomena resulting from rotation (angular acceleration) from those noticeable in straightforward movement (linear acceleration). As we know today, this is caused by stimulation of the maculae utriculi and sacculi. The first step in Purkyně's study of the perception of verticality occurred when he stood on the circumference of a large carousel and, facing in the direction of the rotation, he perceived the apparent inclination of the carousel and had a feeling that he would fall off. Ernst Mach, who followed Purkyně in these studies and analyzed his observations in detail, remarked: "These experiments were in part carried out by Purkyně, and I would have saved much of my effort in the beginning of my work, if I had been acquainted with Purkyně's work" (34). The phenomenon in which the activity of otoliths and impulses coming from tactile, visual, and other receptors participate, is called "oculogravic illusion" today (39).

Purkyně also studied galvanic vertigo using the passage of electric current with electrodes attached to the earlobes (11,25). Before him, only Ritter and Augustin had very briefly mentioned that vertigo could be observed under these circumstances (40–42). Purkyně, on the other hand, described vertiginous phenomena and the tonic inclination of the head and its dependence on the direction of the passing current. This tonic movement was directed to the site of anode. The opposite tonic effect appeared after stopping the stimulation. In addition, Purkyně was the first to observe galvanic nystagmus, although he wrote about it only briefly: "At the end, the galvanic stimulation induces similar oscillating eye and object movements" (14). It was Eduard Hitzig who accomplished the analysis of this effect of the electrical stimulation of vestibular system in detail and recognized the original contribution of Purkyně (42). Barány doubted whether this kind of stimulation could be employed in clinical examination (29). However, recent studies suggest that galvanic vestibular stimulation can be very useful in the research of posture and gait and of their disorders (43–47).

Purkyně included the states that may be seen after ingestion of narcotics and poisons among the forms of vertigo (11,25). Relevant in this regard are positional alcohol nystagmus and vertigo syndrome, which are caused by diffusion of alcohol into the cupula fluid, rendering it less dense than endolymph (5,48,49). This may be manifested by nystagmus beating to the lower or upper ear, when the person lies down, depending on the time span after alcohol consumption.

REFERENCES

1. Purkyně JE. *Neueste Beobachtungen über die Struktur des Gehirns. Übersicht d. Arb. u. Veränderungen der Schles. Gesell. f. vaterl. Kultur* 1837:87–88.
2. Purkyně JE. *Neueste Untersuchungen aus der Nerven- und Hirnanatomie.* In: Sternberg K, von Krombholz JV, eds. *Bericht über die Versammlung Deutscher Naturforscher und Aerzte in Prag im September 1837.* Prag 1838:177–180.
3. Purkyně JE. *Papierstreifen aus dem Portefeuille eines verstorbenen Naturforschers: Neues Planetenbuch oder Mikro- und Makrokosmos. Hypothese von Ernst.* Breslau: Verlag von JU Kern, 1847.
4. Grüsser OJ. J.E. Purkyně's contribution to the physiology of the visual, the vestibular and the oculomotor systems. *Hum Neurobiol* 1984;3:129–144.
5. Brandt T. Man in motion. Historical and clinical aspects of vestibular function. A review. *Brain* 1991;114:2159–2174.
6. Purkyně JE. *Beobachtungen und Versuche zur Physiologie der Sinne. Erstes Bändchen. Beiträge zur Kentniss des Sehens in subjectiver Hinsicht.* Prague: J. Calve, 1819, 1823.
7. Purkyně JE. *Commentatio de examine physiologico organi visus et systematis cutanei.* Vratislaviae: Typis Universitatis, 1823.
8. Purkyně JE. *Beobachtungen und Versuche zur Physiologie der Sinne. Zweites Bändchen. Neue Beiträge zur Kenntniss des Sehens in subjectiver Hinsicht.* Berlin: G. Reimer, 1825.
9. Tschermak-Seysenegg A. *Joh. Ev. Purkyně als Begründer des exacten Subjektivismus.* In: Páta F,

Psotnićková J, Studnička FK, eds. *In memoriam Joh. Ev. Purkyně 1787–1937.* Prague: Purkyně Society, 1937: 76–96.
10. von Graefe A. *Ueber die Untersuchung des Gesichtsfelds bei amblyopischen Affectionen. Archiv f Ophtalmol* 1856;2:258–298.
11. Purkyně JE. *Beiträge zur näheren Kenntniss des Schwindels aus heautognostischen Daten, Medizinische Jahrbücher des k. k. Österreichischen Staates* 1820;6:79–125.
12. Buswell GT. How people look at pictures. University of Chicago Press, Chicago 1935, quoted after Kolers PA. Buswell's discoveries. In: Monty RA, Senders JW, eds. *Eye movements and psychological processes.* Hillsdale, NJ: LEA, 1976:373–395.
13. Mansfield RJ. Neural basis of orientation perception in primate vision. *Science* 1974;186:1133–1135.
14. Purkyně JE. *Ueber die Scheinbewegungen, welche im subjectiven Umfange des Gesichtssines vorkommen. Ausserordentliche Beilage der Neuen Breslauer Zeitung No 86. Viertes Bulletin der naturwissenschaftlichen Section der schles. Gesellschaft* 2. 6. 1825.
15. Gould JD, Dill A. Eye movement parameters and pattern recognition. *Perception Psychophys* 1969;6:311–320.
16. Grüsser OJ. The effect of gaze motor signals and spatially directed attention on eye movements and visual perception. *Progr Brain Res* 1986;64:391–404.
17. von Helmholtz H. *Handbuch der Physiologischen Optik.* Hamburg: L Voss, 1896.
18. von Holst E, von Mittelstaedt H. *Das Reafferenzprinzip (Wechselwirkung zwischen Zentralnervensystem und Peripherie). Naturwissenschaften* 1950;37:464–476.
19. Sperry RW. Neural basis of the spontaneous optokinetic response produced by visual inversion. *J Comp Physiol Psychol* 1950;43:482–489.
20. Purkyně JE. *Über die Scheinbewegungen, welche im subjectiven Umfange des Gesichtssines vorkommen. Uebersicht der Arbeiten und Veränderungen der schlesischen Gesellschaft für vaterländische Cultur im Jahre 1825.* Breslau, 1826.
21. Purkyně JE. *Physiologische Versuche über den Schwindel. Uebersicht der Arbeiten und Veränderungen der schlesischen Gesellschaft für vaterländische Cultur im Jahre 1825.* Breslau, 1826.
22. MacKay H, Teuber L. *Perception.* Berlin: Springer, 1973:805–845.
23. Schmidt RF, Thews G. *Physiologie des Menschen.* Berlin: Springer, 1995
24. Purkyně JE. *Physiologische Versuche über den Schwindel. Ausserordentliche Beilage der Neuen Breslauer Zeitung No 8. Zehntes Bulletin der naturwissenschaftlichen Section der schles. Gesellschaft* 14. 1. 1826.
25. Purkyně JE. *Ueber die physiologische Bedeutung des Schwindels und die Beziehung desselben zu den neuesten Versuchen über die Hirnfunctionen. Magazin für die gesammte Heilkunde (herausgegeben von J. N. Rust),* 1827;23:284–310.
26. Flourens JMP. *Expériences sur les canaux semicirculaires de l'oreille dans les oiseaux. Mémoires de l'Académie royale des sciences de l'Institut de France* 1830a;9:455–466.
27. Flourens JMP. *Expériences sur les canaux semicirculaires de l'oreille, dans les mammiféres. Mémoires de l'Académie royale des sciences de l'Institut de France* 1830b;9:467–477.
28. Flourens JMP. *Versuche und Untersuchungen über die Eigenschaften und Verrichtungen des Nervensystems bei Thieren mit Rückenwirbeln. Aus dem Französichen (Recherches expérimentales sur les proprietés et les fonctions du systéme nerveux dans les animaux vertébrés, Paris 1824), von Becker GW.* Leipzig: Reinsche Buchhandlung, 1824.
29. Barány R. *Der Schwindel und seine Beziehungen zum Bogenapparat des inneren Ohres, Bogenapparat u. Kleinhirn. (Historische Darstellung. Eigene Untersuchungen.) Naturwissenschaften* 1913;1:396–401, 425–428.
30. Gottschick J. *Die Leistungen des Nervensystems.* Jena: Gustav Fischer, 1952.
31. Goltz F. *Über die physiologische Bedeutung der Bogengänge des Ohrlabyrinths. Archiv für die gesammte Physiologie des Menschen und der Thiere* 1870;3:172–192.
32. Breuer J. *Über die Function der Bogengänge des Ohrlabyrinths. Medizinische Jahrbücher der k. k. Gesellschaft der Ärzte* 1874:72–124.
33. Breuer J. *Beiträge zur Lehre vom statischen Sinn (Gleichgewichtsorgan, Vestibularapparat des Ohrlabyrinths). Medizinische Jahrbücher der k. k. Gesellschaft der Ärzte* 1875:87–156.
34. Mach E. *Grundlinien der lehre von de bewegungsempfindungen.* Leipzig: Wilhelm Engelmann, 1875.
35. Girtanner Ch. *Ausführliche Darstellung des Darwinischen Systemes der praktischen Heilkunde, nebst einer Kritick desselben.* 2. Göttingen: Johann Georg Rosenbusch, 1799:101–132.
36. Herz M. *Versuch über den Schwindel.* Wien: Aloys Doll, 1817.
37. von Campenhausen Ch. *Die Sinne des Menschen.* Stuttgart: Georg Thieme Verlag, 1981.
38. Krauss HCG. *De cerebri laesi ad motum voluntarium relatione, certaque vertiginis directione ex certis cerebri regionibus laesis pendente. Dissertation inauguralis.* Vratislaviae: Typis Kupferianis, 1824.
39. Lackner JR. Some mechanisms underlying sensory and postural stability in man. In: Autrum H, Jung R, Loewenstein WR, et al, eds. *Handbook of sensory physiology.* Berlin: Springer, 1973:805–845.
40. Ritter JW. *Versuche und Bemerkungen über den Galvanismus der Voltaischen Batterie. Annalen der Physik* 1801;7:431–484.
41. Augustin FL. *Versuch einer vollständigen systematischen Geschichte der galvanischen Elektrizität und ihrer medizinischen Anwendung.* Berlin, 1803, quoted after Hitzig, 1871.
42. Hitzig E. *Ueber die beim Galvanisieren des Kopfes entstehenden Störungen der Muskelinnervation und der Vorstellungen vom Verhalten im Raume. Archiv für Anatomie und Physiologie und wissenschaftliche Medicin* 1871;716–771.
43. Fitzpatrick R, Burke D, Gandevia SC. Task-dependent reflex responses and movement illusions evoked by galvanic vestibular stimulation in standing humans. *J Physiol* 1994;478:363–372.
44. Fitzpatrick RC, Wardman DL, Taylor JN. Effects of galvanic vestibular stimulation during human walking. *J Physiol* 1999;517:931–939.

45. Inglis JT, Shupert CL, Hlavacka F, et al. Effect of galvanic vestibular stimulation on human postural responses during support surface translations. *J Neurophysiol* 1995;73:896–901.
46. Day BL, Caquil AS, Bartolomei L, et al. Human body-segment tilts induced by galvanic stimulation: a vestibularly driven protection mechanism. *J Physiol* 1997;500:661–672.
47. Bent LR, Fadyen BJ, Merkley VF, et al. Magnitude effects of vestibular stimulation on the trajectory of human gait. *Neurosci Lett* 2000;279:157–160.
48. Barányi R. *Experimentelle Alkoholintoxication. Monatsschrift für Ohrenheilkunde, sowie für Kehlkopf-, Nasen-, Rachenkrankheiten* 1911;45:952–962.
49. Money KE, Myles WS, Hoffert BM. The mechanism of positional alcohol nystagmus. *Can J Otolaryngol* 1974;3:302–313.

Gait Disorders. Advances in Neurology, Vol. 87,
edited by E. Růžička, M. Hallett, and J. Jankovic.
Lippincott Williams & Wilkins, Philadelphia © 2001.

2

The Central Pattern Generator for Locomotion in Mammals

Robert E. Burke

Laboratory of Neural Control, National Institute of Neurological Disorders and Stroke, National Institutes of Health, Bethesda, Maryland 20892-4455

The central nervous system (CNS) of mammals is replete with rhythmic processes, with cycle times ranging from milliseconds to months (1). When such processes generate rhythmic movements that resemble those produced by intact animals, the underlying neuronal mechanisms offer, at least in principle, model systems by which specific behaviors can be linked to specific CNS circuits. A classic example is locomotion. Early in this century, Philippson demonstrated that coordinated hindlimb locomotion was possible in dogs with acute low spinal trans-section (2). Brown later showed that this was also true in acutely spinalized cats even after complete deafferentation (3). These and other contemporaneous results suggested that the mammalian spinal cord contains neuronal circuits, now collectively referred to as a central pattern generator (CPG), which can generate autonomously the coordinated patterns of muscle activity that result in locomotion (4).

This chapter deals with the degree to which the patterns of activity produced by the mammalian spinal CPG for locomotion resembles actual locomotion in intact, behaving animals. An important element in making this assessment is the fact that the locomotor CPG not only drives muscular activity but also modulates spinal reflexes in correspondingly predictable patterns. Because the spinal CPG is embedded in the larger CNS, interruption of the influences that control it results in degradation of its performance in relation to natural locomotion. Consideration of these factors seems important to understanding the genesis of gait disorders and in designing therapies for them.

CENTRAL PATTERN GENERATORS IN INVERTEBRATES

A CPG is loosely defined as a specialized ensemble of neurons found in the CNS that produces rhythmic, coordinated patterns of movements without external specification (5). This means that external inputs, although often required to activate the rhythmic output, need not themselves be rhythmic. In addition, the output rhythms can occur in the absence of phasic sensory feedback. The term central pattern generator was used by Donald Wilson to describe a neuronal circuit in a locust ganglion that, even when isolated *in vitro,* produces the same pattern of motoneuron activations observed during flight (6). A variety of invertebrate CPGs have since been characterized in exquisite detail (5,7,8). Some consist entirely of interconnected motoneurons (e.g., the stomatogastric ganglion of crabs and lobsters), whereas others are made up of interneurons that drive motoneurons (e.g., the ganglia that produce swimming rhythms in the leech and a variety of mollusks) (7,9,10). The internal operations of such invertebrate CPGs are remarkably complex and their outputs are the result of interactions between the intrinsic properties of the individual neurons and synapses of which they are composed, as well as the details of the interconnections between these neurons (11). Although the basic operating principles found in invertebrate CPGs may or may not be applicable to vertebrates, they nevertheless provide an important conceptual framework for ideas about locomotion control in vertebrates, including mammals.

CENTRAL PATTERN GENERATORS IN VERTEBRATES

All vertebrates, from primitive fish, through amphibians and birds, to higher mammals, have spinal CPGs that produce coordinated locomotorlike movements in the absence of rhythmic external drive or phasic afferent feedback (12–14). There is evidence that the human spinal cord also has a locomotor CPG, although its existence is much more difficult to demonstrate in primates than in quadrupeds (15–18). Much of the work on the locomotor CPG has been done in the lumbosacral spinal cord of cats. Although cats with thoracic spinal trans-section have obvious deficiencies in control of balance, the isolated lumbosacral spinal cord can produce patterns of hindlimb muscle activation that resemble those during actual locomotion in intact animals (19). Systematic training can in fact lead to quite effective propulsion in chronically spinalized cats and the same idea is now being applied to rehabilitation of humans with spinal cord injury (20,21).

In the 1960s, Shik and colleagues discovered that electrical stimulation of a localized region in the midbrain, called the mesencephalic locomotor region (MLR), can reliably produce walking movements in decerebrate cats on a treadmill. The ability to generate such "controlled locomotion" in the laboratory, even in animals immobilized with neuromuscular blocking agents (referred to as fictive locomotion), opened the way for a great number of systematic studies of the neural mechanisms that underlie walking and running (22–24). It is now possible to use drugs to activate the locomotor CPG in the isolated spinal cord of neonatal rodents *in vitro,* which permits studies at invasive levels not possible in the whole animal (25).

A vertebrate CPG includes two basic functions: (a) production of oscillatory activity to give the basic timing of the output rhythm, and (b) shaping these basic "clock" pulses into an organized spatiotemporal pattern that is then delivered to the target neurons. For simplicity, the schematic in Figure 2.1 shows these two functions embodied in different groups of interneurons, although in fact the same neurons may be involved in both functions, as is true in many invertebrate CPGs. The actual circuitry involved in the mammalian locomotor CPG is unknown but the evidence available suggests that the CPG for the hindlimb in cats and rodents involves a complex network of neurons distributed through multiple spinal segments (26,27).

How Closely Does Fictive Locomotion Resemble Actual Stepping Rhythms?

This question is critical to understanding the neuronal machinery involved in producing locomotion. The records shown in Figure 2.2 explore this issue. The top set of traces (Fig. 2.2A) are electromyographic (EMG) records from five hindlimb muscles in a normal cat walking on a treadmill, showing alternating activity in two extensor (plantaris [Plant] and flexor hallucis longus [FHL]) and three flexor muscles (flexor digitorum longus muscle [FDL], extensor digitorum longus [EDL], and tibialis anterior [TA]) (28). It is particularly important to note that the FDL exhibits little activity during the stance phase, in contrast to its mechanical synergist FHL, but rather emits a short burst of activity just before paw liftoff (oblique arrows) and is then silent throughout the rest of the swing (flexion) phase (29).

The middle set of records (Fig. 2.2B) was obtained from a curarized, decerebrate cat during spontaneous fictive locomotion (30). Motoneuron activity was in this case recorded from the muscle nerves (electroneurograms, or ENGs). The alternating pattern of activity in extensor (lateral gastrocnemius [LGS] and FHL) and flexor muscle nerves (TA and posterior biceps and semitendinosus [PBST]) was similar to those in the intact animal. More important, the signature short bursts (oblique arrows) in the FDL muscle nerve were also evident just after the extensor activity fell silent, exactly as in

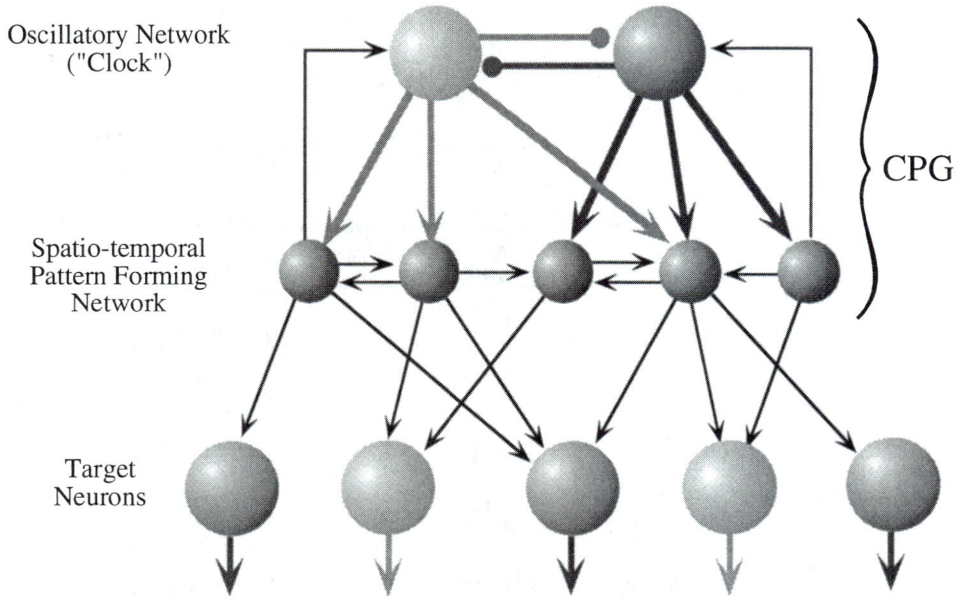

FIG. 2.1. Schematic diagram of a hypothetical central pattern generator (*CPG*) that includes neurons with reciprocal inhibitory interconnections that can produce oscillatory output that drives other neurons to generate a spatiotemporal pattern of output drive to target neurons. The neurons in the pattern-forming network presumably have complex interconnections and may feed back to the oscillatory network. Each neuron symbol is meant to denote sets of many neurons.

normal locomotion. The top trace in Figure 2.2B (FDL IC) is an intracellular record from an individual FDL motoneuron, which was technically possible only because the animal was immobile. The short ENG burst in FDL was preceded by a correspondingly brief depolarizing potential in the motoneuron, followed by a hyperpolarization through the rest of the flexion phase. These events match quite closely the EMG patterns found in the intact cat, suggesting that fictive locomotion in decerebrate animals provides a reasonably good approximation of actual stepping.

The records in Figure 2.2C were obtained in a decerebrate, paralyzed cat with acute low spinal trans-section. Fictive locomotion in this case was induced by intravenous injection of the noradrenergic precursor, L-Dopa (31). The alternation between extensor (LGS and FHL) and flexor (EDL) muscle nerves was slower than found in either the normal or decerebrate animals (note time scale) and the flexion phase was longer than extension, unlike the other examples. The FDL burst was also prolonged and much less "crisp" than in the other examples but it occurred with the same timing (i.e., in the interval between the cessation of extensor muscle activity and EDL bursting). The intracellular record from an FDL motoneuron (FDL IC) showed an almost sinusoidal pattern of depolarization that peaked during the FDL ENG bursts, rather than the sharp waves found in the decerebrate state (Fig. 2.2B; FDL IC). Thus, although the locomotion was degraded in comparison to that in the decerebrate animal, the basic timing of motoneuron activations and the synaptic drive to FDL cells were qualitatively similar. On the other hand, the quality of locomotion in chronic spinal kittens actually walking on a treadmill with afferent feedback intact is much closer to the normal situation, which indicates the critical role of afferent information in shaping the output of the spinal CPG (32).

Control of Cutaneous Reflexes by the Locomotor CPG

One approach to analysis of the structure of the mammalian locomotor CPG is to examine the range of its outputs. The spinal CPG obviously activates and deactivates motoneurons to

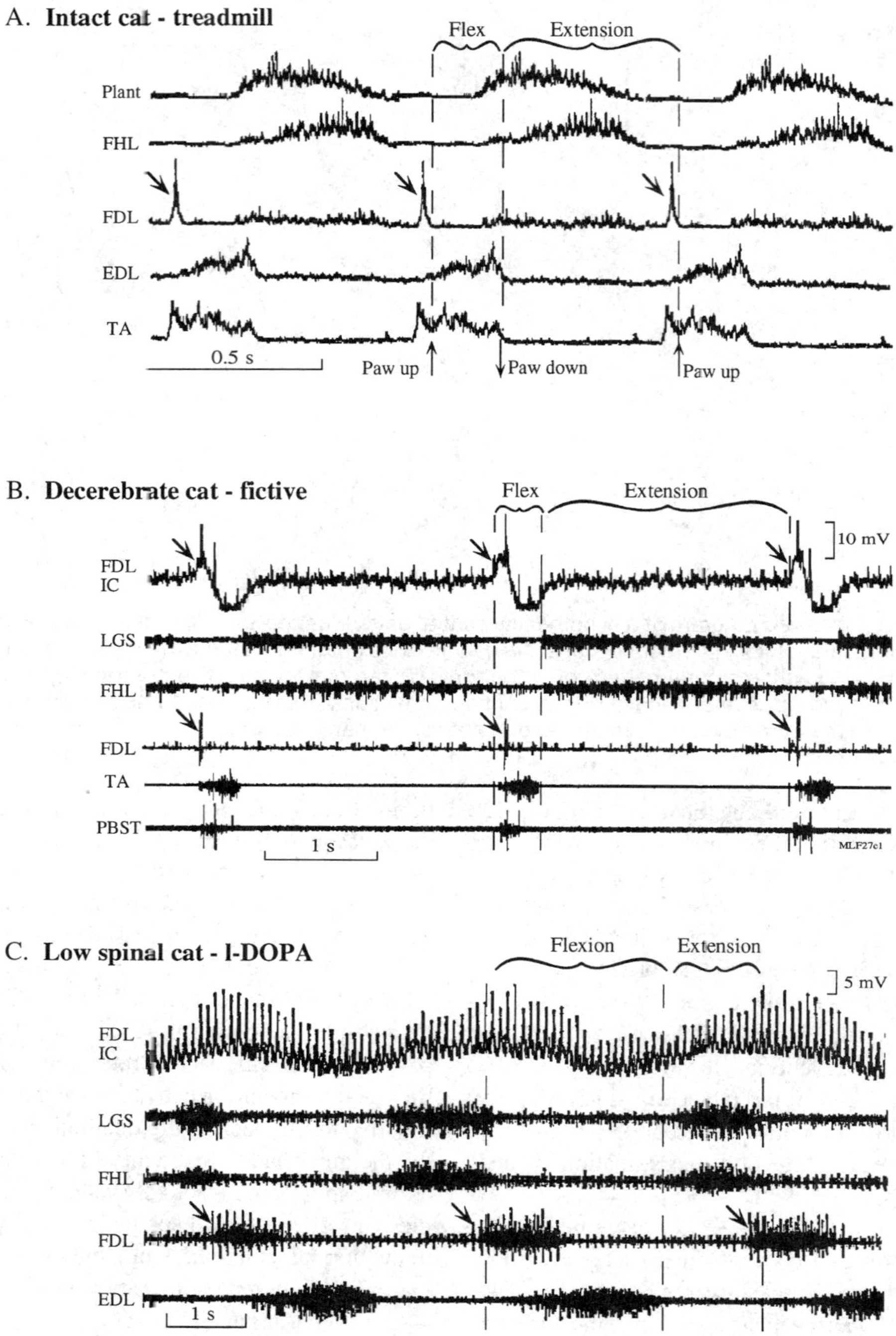

FIG. 2.2. Comparison of locomotor patterns in three different cat preparations. **A:** Normal locomotion in an intact cat. Integrated and rectified electromyographic (EMG) recordings from five hindlimb muscles, plantaris (*Plant*), flexor hallucis longus (*FHL*), flexor digitorum longus (*FDL*), extensor digitorum longus (*EDL*), and tibialis anterior (*TA*), in an intact cat walking voluntarily on a treadmill. The swing (flexion) phase begins with paw lift and ends with paw placement (*paw up and paw down arrows, respectively*). Note the brief bursts in the FDL muscle just before paw lift (*oblique arrows*). (Adapted from Carlson-Kuhta P, Trank TV, Smith JL. Forms of forward quadrupedal locomotion. II. A comparison of posture, hindlimb kinematics, and motor patterns for upslope and level walking.

produce walking movements. However, it is now clear that cutaneous reflexes in motoneuron pools can also be enhanced or suppressed during different phases of the stepping cycle (24,33,34), in patterns that have proven to be as robust as those of muscle activations (35). Although it is difficult to determine the mechanisms underlying this control from EMG observations alone, intracellular recording of synaptic potentials in motoneurons can provide direct evidence that spinal interneurons in reflex pathways are important targets for CPG control (36,37).

For example, the superficial peroneal (SP) excitatory postsynaptic potentials (EPSPs) in the FDL IC records in Figure 2.2C clearly show modulation synchronized with the step cycle; the intracellular EPSPs were largest during the FDL bursts when the FDL motoneuron was maximally depolarized. The records in Figure 2.3A show that these EPSPs exhibited early and later components (inflections at the open arrows) that were larger during early flexion as compared to midextension. The early component in both EPSPs had central latencies less than 2.0 ms, which indicates the presence of only one layer of interneurons between the afferent synapses and the motoneurons, referred to as a disynaptic pathway (31,38,39).

The shape and amplitude of SP EPSPs in the absence of fictive locomotion is virtually the same as that found during the extension phase (38). Accordingly, these observations are best explained by assuming that the interneurons that generate the SP EPSP also receive increased excitatory drive from the locomotor CPG during the early flexion phase, when FDL motoneurons are active (Fig. 2.3B) (31). The flexion half-center of the CPG is assumed to excite the premotoneuronal cells in the disynaptic pathway during early flexion, causing more of these cells to be activated by the SP afferent volley, which produces larger and earlier EPSPs in this locomotor phase. The observed shifts in central latencies can be accounted for by assuming that some interneurons in the disynaptic pathway are fired earlier in the presence of increased CPG drive. This is an example of "spatial facilitation," which can be used to investigate indirectly the organization of interneuron pathways in the spinal cord (37,40). Although presynaptic inhibition in cutaneous afferents occurs during fictive locomotion (41), it is unlikely that this mechanism accounts for the observed modulation (30,31,38).

Figure 2.4A illustrates similarly averaged records of SP EPSPs, in this case obtained from the FDL motoneuron shown in Figure 2.2B in

J Neurophysiol 1998;79:1687–1701, with permission.) **B:** Spontaneous fictive locomotion in a curarized, decerebrate cat. The lower traces are electroneurograms (ENGs) from five muscle nerves (*LGS,* lateral gastrocnemius and soleus; *PBST,* posterior biceps and semitendinosus; other abbreviations as in **A**). The locomotor rhythm was slower than in the intact animal **(A)** mainly because of the longer extension phases. However, the FDL activity (*oblique arrows*) exhibited the same brief bursts at the transition from extension to flexion as in the intact cat. The top trace (*FDL IC*) is an intracellular record from an FDL motoneuron, showing a sharp depolarizing wave preceding the muscle nerve bursts (*arrows*), followed by a hyperpolarization indicating postsynaptic inhibition. The sharp upward deflections are excitatory postsynaptic potentials (EPSPs) produced by superimposing 10-Hz stimulation of the cutaneous superficial peroneal nerve (SP) on the locomotor rhythm (shown in Fig. 2.4A). (See Degtyarenko AM, Simon ES, Norden-Krichmar T, et al. Modulation of oligosynaptic cutaneous and muscle afferent reflex pathways during fictive locomotion and scratching in the cat. *J Neurophysiol* 1998;79:447–463 for further details.) **C:** Fictive locomotion in a curarized, decerebrate cat with acute low spinal cord trans-section given intravenous L–Dopa. Format as in panel **B.** Note the slower time base. The bursts in the FDL nerve (*arrows*) were longer than during decerebrate locomotion **(B)** but their timing was similar. The intracellular record from an FDL motoneuron (*FDL IC*) showed much slower and less crisp depolarizing potentials than in **B.** As in panel **B,** the sharp upward deflections are SP EPSPs that were modulated in amplitude with step cycle phase, being largest during the FDL ENG bursts (see Fig. 2.3A). (Adapted from Figure 2 in Schmidt BJ, Meyers DE, Fleshman JW, et al. Phasic modulation of short latency cutaneous excitation in flexor digitorum longus motoneurons during fictive locomotion. *Exp Brain Res* 1988;71:568–578, with permission.)

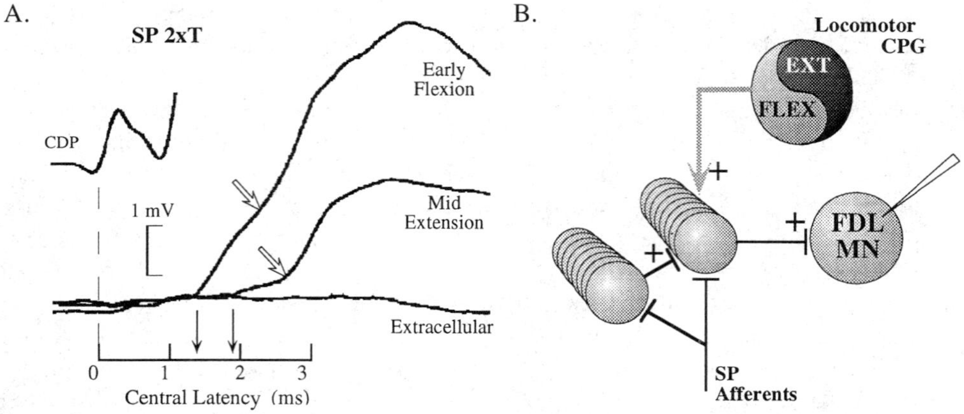

FIG. 2.3. Modulation of superficial peroneal (*SP*) excitatory postsynaptic potentials (EPSPs) during low spinal fictive locomotion (Fig. 2.2C). **A:** Averaged records of EPSPs produced in the flexor digitorum longus (*FDL*) motoneuron shown in Figure 2.2C by 10 Hz, low threshold ($2 \times T$) electrical stimulation of the SP nerve during fictive stepping. The responses were sorted by computer to average separately EPSPs during FDL bursts (*early flexion*) and midway through the extensor bursts in lateral gastrocnemius (LGS) and FHL (*midextension*). The potential at the dorsal surface of spinal cord (*CDP*) shows the entry of the volley in the most rapidly conducting SP afferents (*dashed line*). The time between this point and the onset of the EPSPs is the central latency. Open arrows denote the inflection between disynaptic and trisynaptic EPSP components (central latencies <2.0 ms and >2.0 ms, respectively). **B:** Schematic diagram showing circuit organization that can explain the records in panel **A.** The *Yin-Yang symbol* denotes the locomotor CPG, including the rhythm generating and pattern formation elements (Fig. 2.1). The output path from the flexor half-center is undefined but is assumed to excite the last-order interneurons in the SP reflex pathway.

a decerebrate cat with intact spinal cord. The same pattern of EPSP facilitation is evident as that found during the slower and less crisp locomotion in the low spinal cat (Fig. 2.3A). The disynaptic component (central latency = 1.9 ms) was evident only in F1 (oblique arrow) but the trisynaptic responses were still larger than during extension. The timing of the SP EPSP facilitation is in keeping with the "stumbling corrective response," an exaggerated flexion of the hindlimb found when the dorsal surface of the hindpaw, which is innervated by the SP nerve, encounters an obstacle during stepping in intact cats (33,42). This appears to be due mainly to cutaneous input (43). It is likely that the short latency EPSP enhancement during fictive stepping is part of an automatic mechanism that prepares the animal to respond quickly to specific external perturbations.

The medial plantar nerve (MPL) innervates the skin on the ventral surface of the cat hindpaw toes and plantar pad. Electrical stimulation of the MPL nerve also produces disynaptic EPSPs in FDL at rest and during the extension phase of fictive locomotion (Fig. 2.4B) (38). However, in sharp contrast to the findings with SP EPSPs, the disynaptic component of the cutaneous MPL EPSP is completely suppressed during the entire flexion phase (*oblique arrow,* F1–F3). Such differential modulation during fictive locomotion demonstrates that the last-order excitatory interneurons in the SP and MPL reflex pathways are completely independent of one another (38). This precise organization is particularly striking because the innervation territories of the SP and MPL nerves are immediately adjacent to one another on the distal hindpaw.

Using the same approach, a variety of distinct excitatory and inhibitory cutaneous reflex pathways, all of which are disynaptic, have been identified that project to four hindlimb motoneuron pools (30,38). These are schematically shown in Figure 2.5. There is remarkable specificity in the organization of cutaneous reflexes from the

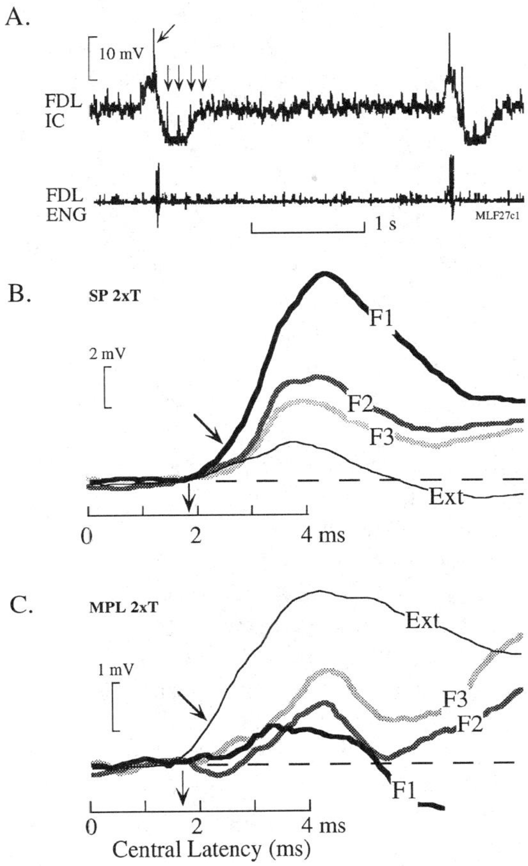

FIG. 2.4. Modulation of superficial peroneal (*SP*) excitatory postsynaptic potentials (EPSPs) during decerebrate fictive locomotion shown in Figure 2.2B. **A:** Selected records from Figure 2.2B to illustrate changes in the SP EPSPs (*small arrows*) during the step cycle. The *oblique arrow* denotes the largest EPSP coincident with maximum flexor digitorum longus (*FDL*) depolarization. **B:** Computer sorted and averaged records of SP EPSPs during the first, second and third parts of flexion (*thicker traces, F1, F2,* and *F3,* respectively) and during extension (*thin trace, Ext*). The disynaptic component (central latency <2 ms; *arrow*) was present only in F1, although the trisynaptic component was facilitated throughout flexion. **C:** As in **B,** but showing averaged EPSPs produced in the same FDL motoneuron by low threshold ($2 \times T$) afferents in the medial plantar nerve (*MPL*). MPL stimuli were delivered at 10 Hz midway between the SP stimuli but the small individual responses are not present in panel **A.** Note that the disynaptic EPSPs evident during the extension phase (*arrow*) were completely suppressed throughout flexion.

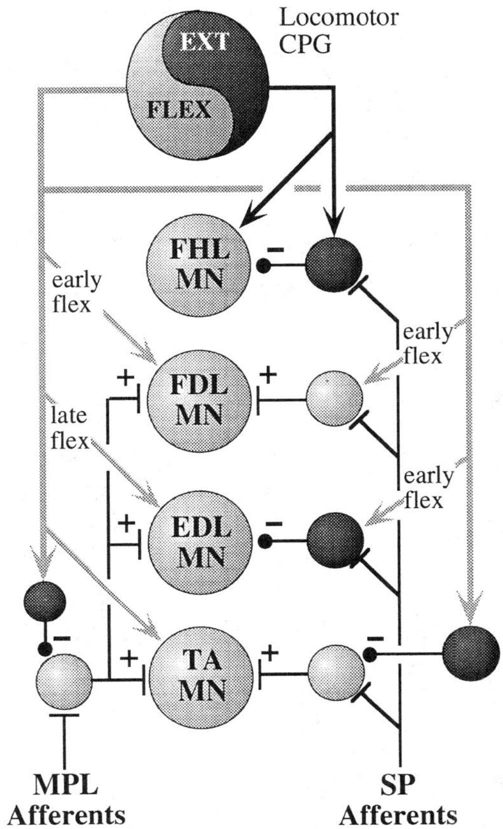

FIG. 2.5. Schematic diagram of the central pattern generator (*CPG*) control of disynaptic reflex pathways from two cutaneous nerves, superficial peroneal (*SP*) and medial plantar (*MPL*). The existence of the different sets of interneurons in the SP to motoneuron (*MN*) pathways is deduced from the patterns of differential control during locomotion and their different synaptic polarities. The disynaptic excitation from the MPL nerve is suppressed during the flexion phase in flexor digitorum longus (*FDL*), extensor digitorum longus (*EDL*), and tibialis anterior (*TA*) motoneurons, so that it is possible that the pathway to all three pools includes common interneurons that are inhibited by the flexor half-center of the locomotor CPG. The drive to interneurons and motoneurons from the flexor half-center is primarily during early flexion to FDL cells and later to EDL motoneurons. (From Degtyarenko AM, Simon ES, Burke RE. Differential modulation of disynaptic cutaneous inhibition and excitation in ankle flexor motoneurons during fictive locomotion. *J Neurophysiol* 1996;76:2972–2985, with permission.)

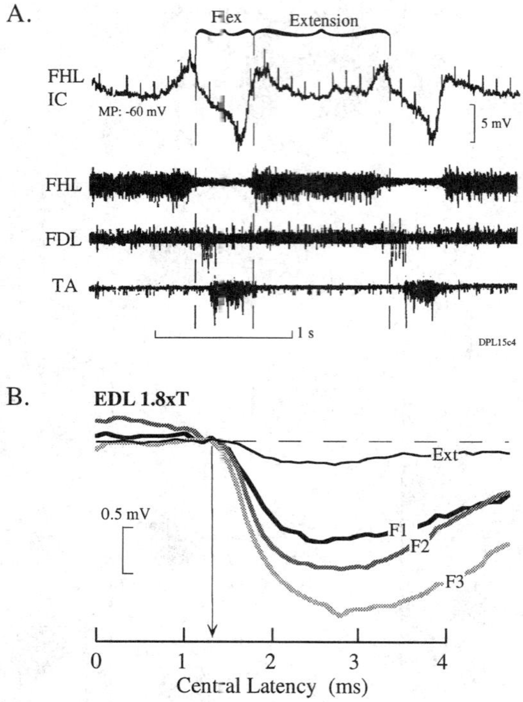

FIG. 2.6. An example of facilitation of antagonist extensor digitorum longus (*EDL*) group Ia disynaptic inhibitory postsynaptic potentials (IPSPs) in an extensor flexor hallucis longus (*FHL*) motoneuron during fictive locomotion in a decerebrate cat. (Adapted from Figure 9 in Degtyarenko AM, Simon ES, Norden-Krichmar T, et al. Modulation of oligosynaptic cutaneous and muscle afferent reflex pathways during fictive locomotion and scratching in the cat. *J Neurophysiol* 1998;79:447–463, with permission.) **A:** Sample electroneurographic and intracellular records, as in earlier figures. Note hyperpolarizing potential shifts in the FHL motoneuron during the flexion (*Flex*) phases. **B:** Averaged records of group Ia disynaptic IPSPs (central latency = 1.3 ms) produced by stimulation of the antagonist EDL nerve at 1.8 times threshold (group Ia maximum). The barely detectable IPSP during extension was markedly enhanced during the flexion phase (see *Flex* in **A**) in parallel with hyperpolarizing membrane potential shifts. Such enhancements can be explained by premotoneuronal facilitation of transmission through the reciprocal group Ia interneurons (Fig. 2.8).

SP nerve, which are transmitted through distinct sets of last-order interneurons. It is particularly interesting that the EDL muscle receives powerful disynaptic SP inhibition during early flexion, exactly the obverse of the SP excitation in the antagonist FDL, whereas some extensor FHL motoneurons receive disynaptic SP inhibition only during the *extension* phase (30). Finally, disynaptic SP excitation in many TA motoneurons is inhibited during the flexion phase, which fits with recent observations in humans (44). The only pathway that may involve common interneurons to multiple motor nuclei is that from the MPL system that delivers input from the plantar surface of the hindpaw.

The possible functional roles of these pathways are discussed in the references. What is important in the present context is that the patterns of control of these pathways by the locomotor CPG are as robust and reproducible as the patterns of motoneuron firing. This indicates that the neural machinery that makes up the spinal CPG for locomotion in the cat includes not only systems that drive motoneurons in the proper sequences but also prepares the spinal networks for cutaneous reflex responses to external perturbations at precisely timed phases of the stepping cycle.

Phase-dependent modulation of cutaneous reflexes, and even reversal of sign from excitation to inhibition, have been demonstrated during human locomotion (45). In fact, there is evidence for differential control of cutaneous reflexes from different parts of the foot during walking in normal human subjects (46). It should be noted that the latencies of such responses are relatively long and their relevance to the control of the oligosynaptic (largely disynaptic) responses described in the cat, therefore, is uncertain. Nevertheless, there is little doubt that the spinal cord of cat and humans contain neural circuits that powerfully control cutaneous reflexes in highly specific and reliable ways. It seems reasonable to suggest that the primary mechanisms responsible for such modulation are incorporated in the spinal segmental pathways that make up the locomotor CPG and its pattern-forming circuits.

Control of Muscle Afferent Reflexes by the Locomotor Central Pattern Generator

Group Ia muscle spindle afferents excite their own (homonymous) motoneurons in stretch reflexes and simultaneously inhibit motoneurons

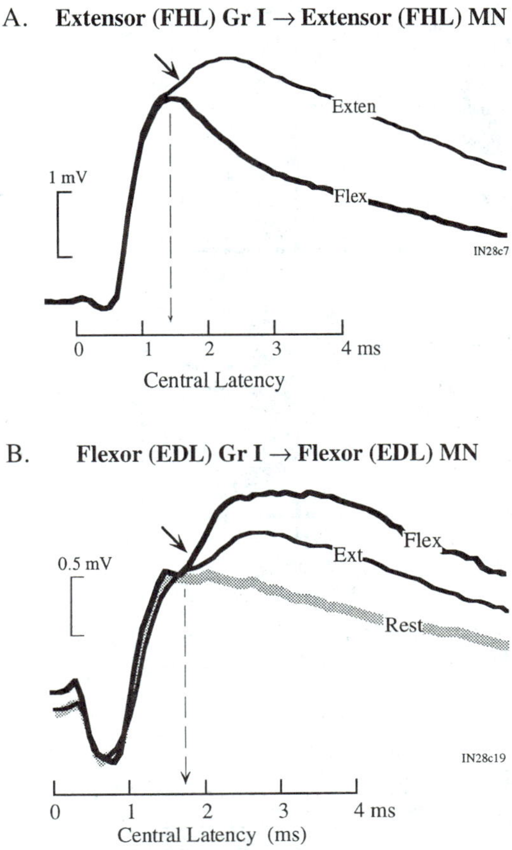

FIG. 2.7. Examples of enhancement of disynaptic group I excitatory postsynaptic potentials (EPSPs) during fictive locomotion. **A:** Homonymous group I EPSPs in an extensor flexor hallucis longus (*FHL*) motoneuron (*MN*) produced by stimulation (1.8 × T) of the FHL muscle nerve. The falling phase of the monosynaptic EPSP during the flexion phase (*Flex*) (central latency 0.7 ms) exhibited no late component. However, a disynaptic EPSP (*arrow;* central latency = 1.4 ms) appeared during extension when the FHL muscle nerve was active. (Adapted from Figure 4 in Degtyarenko AM, Simon ES, Norden-Krichmar T, et al. Modulation of oligosynaptic cutaneous and muscle afferent reflex pathways during fictive locomotion and scratching in the cat. *J Neurophysiol* 1998;79:447–463, with permission.) **B:** Group I EPSPs in a flexor extensor digitorum longus (*EDL*) motoneuron produced by stimulation (1.8 × T) of the homonymous EDL nerve. In the absence of fictive locomotion (*Rest*) the response was an uncomplicated monosynaptic EPSP. However, a disynaptic component (central latency 1.75 ms) appeared during the extension phase of fictive locomotion and grew larger during the flexion phase. The large negative deflection before the EPSP was owing to antidromic invasion of other EDL motoneurons. (Adapted from Figure 7 in Degtyarenko AM, Simon ES, Norden-Krichmar T, et al. Modulation of oligosynaptic cutaneous and muscle afferent reflex pathways during fictive locomotion and scratching in the cat. *J Neurophysiol* 1998; 79:447–463, with permission.)

of antagonist muscles (47). The powerful reciprocal inhibition is produced by inhibitory last-order interneurons that receive monosynaptic input from group Ia afferents from a given muscle and project with inhibitory synapses onto motoneurons of the antagonist motor pool (48,49). Interneurons in this pathway can be identified by the fact that they also receive recurrent inhibition from Renshaw interneurons (50). Using this feature, Feldman and Orlovsky demonstrated that inhibitory interneurons in the reciprocal group Ia pathway are phasically driven during fictive locomotion in the phase when the muscle that gives rise to their group Ia input is active (51). This implies, of course, that these interneurons can contribute to inhibition of antagonist motoneurons even without input from muscle spindles. Thus, they function as part of the neural machinery that distributes CPG inhibition to appropriate motoneuron pools, as well as transmitting group Ia information as part of the stretch reflex.

One would expect, therefore, that disynaptic group Ia inhibition of motoneurons should be enhanced during step cycle phases in which those cells are normally silent. This has been demonstrated using the spatial facilitation method during fictive locomotion (52,53). An example is shown in Figure 2.6, from an extensor FHL motoneuron. There was a remarkable parallel in this cell between the depth of flexor phase hyperpolarization and the enhancement of the disynaptic group Ia IPSP, in keeping with the idea that CPG drive to the reciprocal Ia inhibitory interneurons is an important component of the "off" phase inhibition in motoneurons.

Although the reciprocal group Ia inhibitory pathway has been known for decades, the recent demonstration of the existence of a disynaptic group Ia *excitatory* pathway was revealed only during fictive locomotion. During intracellular recording in anesthetized animals, stimulation of

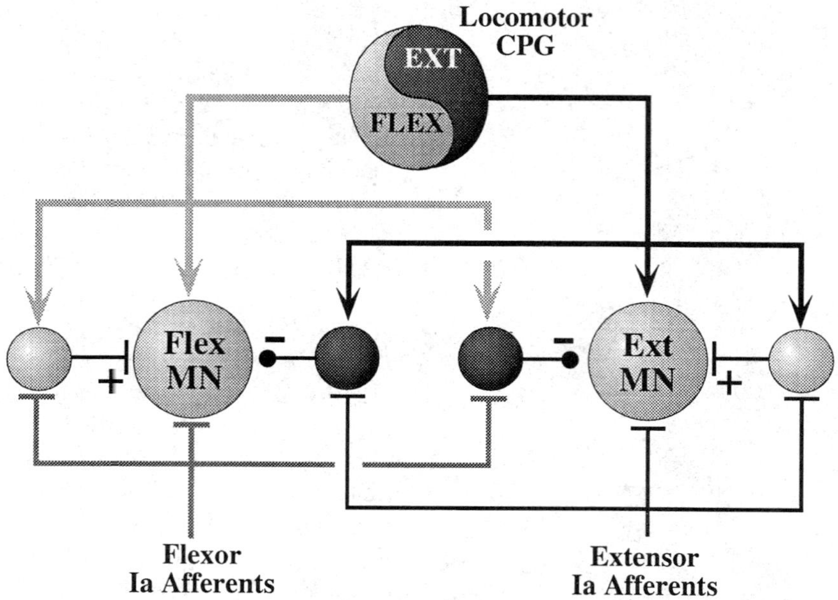

FIG. 2.8. Schematic diagram to illustrate the pattern of central pattern generator (*CPG*) control of interneurons in the disynaptic group I excitatory and inhibitory pathways found in most extensor and flexor motoneuron pools in the cat hindlimb. Symbols as in Figure 2.5.

the group Ia afferents from the same (homonymous) or synergist muscle nerve produces pure monosynaptic EPSPs in most motoneurons (central latencies less than 1.0 ms), with no evidence of later components (Fig. 2.7B). However, Schomburg and coworkers found that disynaptic group I EPSPs with longer central latencies appeared in some motoneurons during fictive locomotion during the step cycle phase in which the motoneuron was depolarized and active (54). McCrea and colleagues extended this observation to show that the disynaptic EPSPs with central latencies between 1.6 and 1.8 ms are widespread in many types of extensor motoneurons during the extension phase of fictive locomotion in the cat (55,56). They also provided evidence that stretch-sensitive group Ia afferents are largely responsible for this disynaptic excitation. Degtyarenko and coworkers later demonstrated that disynaptic group Ia EPSPs appear in many types of flexor motoneurons during fictive locomotion, with facilitation during the flexion phase (53). Figure 2.7 illustrates examples from an extensor and a flexor motoneuron.

The general schema of locomotor CPG control of the disynaptic group Ia pathways is shown in Figure 2.8. The extension half-center of the CPG enhances transmission through last-order interneurons that receive direct input from group Ia afferents from extensor muscles, resulting in enhanced disynaptic EPSPs in extensor motoneurons and disynaptic IPSPs in flexor cells. The same is true in mirror image for Ia input from flexor muscles, which is enhanced by the flexion half-center. As noted, there is evidence that last-order inhibitory interneurons in the reciprocal group Ia pathway contribute to inhibition of motoneurons during the "off" phase of stepping, even without phasic group Ia input. Whether or not this is also true of the disynaptic Ia *excitatory* interneurons is not yet known.

There is considerable evidence that the effect of stretch reflexes is modulated during locomotion in normal animals and human (24,57,58). Indeed, reversal of the sign of these reflexes, from excitation to inhibition and vice versa, has been observed during particular phases of stepping (59). Such sign reversal has also been demonstrated for polysynaptic excitation

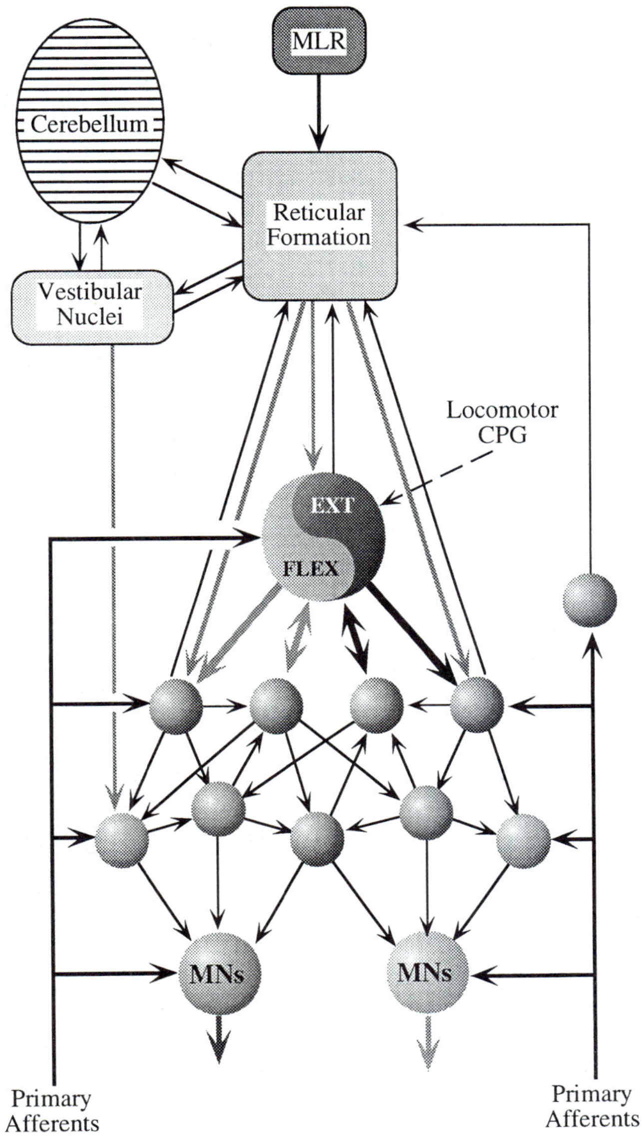

FIG. 2.9. Simplified schematic diagram to show the locomotor central pattern generator (*CPG*) embedded in the central nervous system. The CPG outputs are assumed to be transmitted to motoneurons through spinal segmental interneurons that can interact in complex ways. Some of these interneurons receive primary afferent information (i.e., are in reflex pathways) and some also send ascending information to the reticular formation, cerebellum, and other brain regions. The mesencephalic locomotor region (*MLR*) activates the locomotor CPG through links in the reticular formation. In intact animals, the spinal CPG is subject to layers of hierarchical control that ensure adaptation of stepping to the immediate situation. *EXT,* extension; *FLEX,* flexion; *MNs,* motoneurons.

versus inhibition produced by group Ib afferents from Golgi tendon organs in muscle (60). There is clear coactivation of alpha and gamma motoneurons during fictive locomotion in the spinal (61) and decerebrate (thalamic) states (62), so that muscle afferent input to the cord should be substantial during normal locomotion (58). Although it is possible that the modulation of muscle afferent reflexes during locomotion may involve presynaptic inhibition, it appears likely that CPG control of the disynaptic excitatory links is of equal, if not greater, importance (63).

CONCLUSION

The locomotor CPG located within the spinal cord is embedded in the CNS, subject to interactions with afferent information and with supraspinal commands. This notion is depicted in the schematic diagram in Figure 2.9. The outputs from the extensor and flexor half centers are assumed to drive segmental interneurons that can interact with one another and perhaps feedback to the CPG itself (double-headed arrows). Many of these cells also receive information from primary afferents as well as descending control from supraspinal centers, including rubrospinal and corticospinal axons that are not included in the diagram (49). As pictured, both afferents and descending commands also can access the CPG itself, as judged by the ability of these inputs to reset locomotor rhythms (64). As documented in the preceding sections, some of the interneurons are also in specific reflex pathways. The interactions between interneurons represented by the arrows between them are strictly schematic and do not represent particular pathways, for indeed these are mostly unknown at present.

Finally, some spinal interneurons have direct or indirect projections to the reticular formation, cerebellum, thalamus, and other structures in the brain (65). There is evidence that neurons in the reticular formation are driven into phasic activity by ascending input from the spinal cord during fictive locomotion (66), as well as during stepping in intact animals (67). The resulting reticulospinal output, especially as modulated by the cerebellum, undoubtedly shapes and regulates the activity of the spinal CPG and its attendant circuitry during locomotion in the low spinal cat (Fig. 2.2C) as compared to the decerebrate and normal situations (Fig. 2.2A,B).

In order to make sense of this highly distributed and complex system, a great deal of additional information is necessary about the organization of interneuronal circuits in the spinal cord. A large number of segmental interneurons are driven phasically during fictive locomotion (70,71) but, with the exception of a few disynaptic reflex pathways, at present we know little about their positions in the circuit hierarchy (Figs. 2.5 and 2.8) (72). Despite our present lack of detailed information, the available evidence indicates that the spinal locomotor CPG is not autonomous in the intact CNS. Disturbances in supraspinal regulation because of spinal or supraspinal lesions thus can be expected to produce abnormalities of gait, despite the degree of automatic control that has been built into the spinal circuitry over the entire history of vertebrate evolution. Changes in spinal reflex pathways that are under segmental CPG control can be expected to add importantly to the overall net effect. This aspect of locomotor CPG function is becoming clearer and that information, although admittedly incomplete, may be important to understand dysfunctions of gait in humans.

REFERENCES

1. Gray CM. Synchronous oscillations in neuronal systems: mechanisms and functions. *J Comp Neurosci* 1994;1:11–38.
2. Philippson M. L'autonomie et al. centralisation dans le systéme nervaux des animaux. *Trav Lab Physiol Inst Solvay, Bruxelles* 1905;7:1–208.
3. Brown TG. The intrinsic factor in the act of progression in the mammal. *Proc Roy Soc (Lond, Ser B)* 1911;84:308–319.
4. Grillner S. Locomotion in vertebrates: central mechanisms and reflex interactions. *Physiol Rev* 1975;55:247–304.
5. Selverston AI. Are central pattern generators understandable? *Behav Brain Sci* 1980;3:535–571.
6. Wilson DM. The central nervous control of flight in a locust. *J Exp Biol* 1961;38:471–479.
7. Selverston A, Elson R, Rabinovich M, et al. Basic principles for generating motor output in the stomatogastric ganglion. In: Kiehn O, Harris-Warrick RM, Jordan LM, et al., eds. *Neuronal mechanisms for generating locomotor activity.* New York: The New York Academy of Sciences, 1998:35–50.
8. Lukowiak K. Central pattern generators: some principles learned from invertebrates. *J Physiol (Paris)* 1991;85:63–70.
9. Stent GS, Kristan WB, Freisen WO, et al. Neural generation of the leech swimming movement. *Science* 1978;200:1348–1357.
10. Arshavsky YI, Deliagina TG, Orlovsky GN, et al. Analysis of the central pattern generator for swimming in the mollusk Clione. In: Kiehn O, Harris-Warrick RM, Jordan LM, et al., eds. *Neuronal mechanisms for generating locomotor activity.* New York: The New York Academy of Sciences, 1998:51–69.
11. Getting PA. Emerging principles governing the operation of neural networks. *Ann Rev Neurosci* 1989;12:185–204.

12. Grillner S, Parker D, El Manira A. Vertebrate locomotion: a lamprey perspective. In: Kiehn O, Harris-Warrick RM, Jordan LM, et al., eds. *Neuronal mechanisms for generating locomotor activity.* New York: The New York Academy of Sciences, 1998:1–18.
13. Wheatley M, Jovanovic K, Stein RB, et al. The activity of interneurons during locomotion in the *in vitro* Necturus spinal cord. *J Neurophysiol* 1994;71:2025–2032.
14. Sholomenko GN, Funk GD, Steeves JD. Avian locomotion activated by brainstem infusion of neurotransmitter agonists and antagonists. I. Acetylcholine, excitatory amino acids and substance P. *Exp Brain Res* 1991;85:659–673.
15. Calancie B, Needham-Shropshire B, Jacobs P, et al. Involuntary stepping after chronic spinal cord injury. *Brain* 1994;117:1143–1159.
16. Hanna JP, Frank JI. Automatic stepping in the pontomedullary stage of central herniation. *Neurology* 1996;45:985–986.
17. Dimitrijevic MR, Gerasimenko Y, Pinter MM. Evidence for a spinal central pattern generator in humans. In: Kiehn O, Harris-Warrick RM, Jordan LM, et al., eds. *Neuronal mechanisms for generating locomotor activity.* New York: The New York Academy of Sciences, 1998:360–376.
18. Eidelberg E, Walden JG, Nguyen LH. Locomotor control in macaque monkeys. *Brain* 1981;104:647–663.
19. Grillner S, Zangger P. How detailed is the central pattern generation for locomotion? *Acta Physiol Scand* 1975;88:367–371.
20. de Leon RD, Hodgson JA, Roy RR, et al. Locomotor capacity attributable to step training versus spontaneous recovery following spinalization in cats. *J Neurophysiol* 1998;79:1329–1340.
21. Barbeau H, Norman K, Fung J, et al. Does neurorehabilitation play a role in the recovery of walking in neurological populations? In: Kiehn O, Harris-Warrick RM, Jordan LM, et al., eds. *Neuronal mechanisms for generating locomotor activity*. New York: The New York Academy of Sciences, 1998:377–392.
22. Shik M, Severin F, Orlovsky G. Control of walking and running by means of electrical stimulation of the midbrain. *Biophysics* 1966;11:756–765.
23. Grillner S. Control of locomotion in bipeds, tetrapods and fish. In: Brooks VB, ed. *Handbook of physiology.* Washington, DC: American Physiological Society, 1981;1179–1236.
24. Rossignol S. Neural control of stereotypic limb movements. In: Rowell IB, Shepherd JT, eds. *Handbook of physiology.* Bethesda, MD: American Physiological Society, 1996;173–216.
25. Smith JC, Feldman JL. In vitro brainstem-spinal cord preparations for study of motor systems for mammalian respiration and locomotion. *J Neurosci Meth* 1987;21:321–333.
26. Deliagina TG, Orlovsky GN, Pavlova GA. The capacity for generation of rhythmic oscillations is distributed in the lumbosacral spinal cord of the cat. *Exp Brain Res* 1983;53:81–90.
27. Kiehn O, Kjaerulff O. Distribution of contral pattern generators for rhythmic motor outputs in the spinal cord of limbed vertebrates. In: Kiehn O, Harris-Warrick RM, Jordan LM, et al., eds. *Neuronal mechanisms for generating locomotor activity.* New York: The New York Academy of Sciences, 1998:110–129.
28. Carlson-Kuhta P, Trank TV, Smith JL. Forms of forward quadrupedal locomotion. II. A comparison of posture, hindlimb kinematics, and motor patterns for upslope and level walking. *J Neurophysiol* 1998;79:1687–1701.
29. O'Donovan MJ, Pinter MJ, Dum RP, et al. The actions of FDL and FHL muscles in intact cats: functional dissociation between anatomical synergists. *J Neurophysiol* 1982;47:1126–1143.
30. Degtyarenko AM, Simon ES, Burke RE. Differential modulation of disynaptic cutaneous inhibition and excitation in ankle flexor motoneurons during fictive locomotion. *J Neurophysiol* 1996;76:2972–2985.
31. Schmidt BJ, Meyers DE, Fleshman JW, et al. Phasic modulation of short latency cutaneous excitation in flexor digitorum longus motoneurons during fictive locomotion. *Exp Brain Res* 1988;71:568–578.
32. Forssberg H, Grillner S, Halbertsma J. The locomotion of the low spinal cat I. Coordination within a hindlimb. *Acta Physiol Scand* 1980;108:269–281.
33. Forssberg H, Grillner S, Rossignol S. Phase dependent reflex reversal during walking in chronic spinal cats. *Brain Res* 1975;85:103–107.
34. Abraham L, Marks W, Loeb G. The distal hindlimb musculature of the cat: cutaneous reflexes during locomotion. *Exp Brain Res* 1985;58:594–603.
35. Loeb GE. The distal hindlimb musculature of the cat: interanimal variability of locomotor activity and cutaneous reflexes. *Exp Brain Res* 1993;96:125–140.
36. Schomburg ED, Behrends HB. Phasic control of the transmission in the excitatory and inhibitory reflex pathways from cutaneous afferents to a-motoneurones during fictive locomotion in cats. *Neurosci Letts* 1978;8:277–282.
37. Burke RE, Fleshman JW. Strategies to identify interneurons involved in locomotor pattern generation in the mammalian spinal cord. In: Grillner S, Stein PSG, Stuart DG, et al., eds. *Neurobiology of vertebrate locomotion.* London: Macmillan, 1986:245–268.
38. Moschovakis AK, Sholomenko GN, Burke RE. Differential control of short latency cutaneous excitation in cat FDL motoneurons during fictive locomotion. *Exp Brain Res* 1991;83:489–501.
39. Moschovakis AK, Solodkin M, Burke RE. Anatomical and physiological study of interneurons in an oligosynaptic cutaneous reflex pathway in the cat hindlimb. *Brain Res* 1992;586:311–318.
40. Lundberg A. Control of spinal mechanisms from the brain. In: Brady RO, ed. *The nervous system.* New York: Raven Press, 1975:253–265.
41. Gossard J-P, Cabelguen JM, Rossignol S. Intra-axonal recordings of cutaneous primary afferents during fictive locomotion in the cat. *J Neurophysiol* 1989;62:1177–1188.
42. Forssberg H. Stumbling corrective reaction: a phase-dependent compensatory reaction during locomotion. *J Neurophysiol* 1979;42:936–953.
43. Wand P, Prochazka A, Sontag KH. Neuromuscular responses to gait perturbations in freely moving cats. *Exp Brain Res* 1980;38:109–114.
44. Zehr EP, Komiyama T, Stein RB. Cutaneous reflexes during human gait: electromyographic and kinematic responses to electrical stimulation. *J Neurophysiol* 1997;77:3311–3325.
45. Duysens J, Trippel M, Horstmann GA, et al. Gating and

reversal of reflexes in ankle muscles during human walking. *Exp Brain Res* 1990;82:351–358.
46. Van Wezel BMH, Ottenhoff FAM, Duysens J. Dynamic control of location-specific information in tactile cutaneous reflexes from the foot during human walking. *J Neurosci* 1997;17:3804–3814.
47. Sherrington CS. Note on the knee-jerk and the correlation of action of antagonistic muscles. *Proc Roy Soc (Lond)* 1893;52:556–564.
48. Eccles JC, Fatt P, Landgren S. The central pathway for the direct inhibitory action of impulses in the largest afferent fibers to muscle. *J Neurophysiol* 1956;19:75–98.
49. Baldissera F, Hultborn H, Illert M. Integration in spinal neuronal systems. In: Brooks VB, ed. *Handbook of physiology.* Bethesda, MD: American Physiological Society, 1981:509–595.
50. Hultborn H, Jankowska E, Lindstrom S. Recurrent inhibition of interneurones monosynaptically activated from group Ia afferents. *J Physiol* 1971;215:613–636.
51. Feldman A, Orlovsky G. Activity of interneurons mediating reciprocal Ia inhibition during locomotion. *Brain Res* 1975;84:181–194.
52. Pratt CA, Jordan L. Ia inhibitory interneurons and Renshaw cells as contributors to the spinal mechanisms of fictive locomotion. *J Neurophysiol* 1987;57:56–71.
53. Degtyarenko AM, Simon ES, Norden-Krichmar T, et al. Modulation of oligosynaptic cutaneous and muscle afferent reflex pathways during fictive locomotion and scratching in the cat. *J Neurophysiol* 1998;79:447–463.
54. Schomburg ED, Behrends HB. The possibility of phase-dependent monosynaptic and polysynaptic Ia excitation to homonymous motoneurones during fictive locomotion. *Brain Res* 1978;143:533–537.
55. McCrea DA, Shefchyk SJ, Stephens NJ, et al. Disynaptic group I excitation of synergist ankle extensor motoneurones during fictive locomotion in the cat. *J Physiol* 1995;487:527–539.
56. Angel MJ, Guertin P, Jimenez I, et al. Group I extensor afferents evoke disynaptic EPSPs in cat hindlimb extensor motorneurones during fictive locomotion. *J Physiol* 1996;494:851–861.
57. Stein RB, Capaday C. The modulation of human reflexes during functional tasks. *Trends Neurosci* 1988;11:21–36.
58. Whelan PJ. Control of locomotion in the decerebrate cat. *Prog Neurobiol* 1996;49:481–515.
59. Yang JF, Stein RB. Phase-dependent reflex reversal in human leg muscles during walking. *J Neurophysiol* 1990;63:1109–1117.
60. Gossard J-P, Brownstone RM, Barajon I, et al. Transmission in a locomotor-related group Ib pathway from hindlimb extensor muscles in the cat. *Exp Brain Res* 1994;98:213–228.
61. Sjostrom A, Zangger P. Muscle spindle control during locomotor movements generated by the deafferentate spinal cord. *Acta Physiol Scand* 1976;97:281–291.
62. Cabelguen J-M. Static and dynamic fusimotor controls in various hindlimb muscles during locomotor activity in the decorticate cat. *Brain Res* 1981;213:83–97.
63. Stein RB. Presynaptic inhibition in humans. *Prog Neurobiol* 1995;47:533–544.
64. Hultborn H, Conway BA, Gossard J-P, et al. How do we approach the locomotor network in the mammalian spinal cord? In: Kiehn O, Harris-Warrick RM, Jordan LM, et al., eds. *Neuronal mechanisms for generating locomotor activity.* New York: The New York Academy of Sciences, 1998:70–82.
65. Lundberg A. Function of the ventral spinocerebellar tract, a new hypothesis. *Exp Brain Res* 1971;12:317–330.
66. Perrault MC, Drew T, Rossignol S. Activity of medullary reticulospinal neurons during fictive locomotion. *J Neurophysiol* 1993;69:2232–2247.
67. Drew T, Cabana T, Rossignol S. Responses of medullary reticulospinal neurones to stimulation of cutaneous limb nerves during locomotion in intact cats. *Exp Brain Res* 1996;111:153–168.
68. Armstrong DM. The supraspinal control of mammalian locomotion. *J Physiol (Lond)* 1988;405:1–37.
69. Orsal D, Perret C, Cabelguen J-M. Comparison between ventral spinocerebellar and rubrospinal activities during locomotion in the cat. *Behav Brain Res* 1988;28:159–162.
70. Orlovskii G, Fel'dman A. Classification of lumbosacral neurons by their discharge patterns during evoked locomotion. *Neirofiziologiya* 1972;4:410–417.
71. Edgerton VR, Grillner S, Sjostrom A, et al. Central generation of locomotion in vertebrates. In: Herman RM, Grillner S, Stein PSG, et al., eds. *Neural control of locomotion.* New York: Plenum Press, 1976:439–464.
72. Shefchyk S, McCrea D, Kriellaars D, et al. Activity of interneurons within the L4 spinal segment of the cat during brainstem-evoked fictive locomotion. *Exp Brain Res* 1990;80:290–295.

Gait Disorders. Advances in Neurology, Vol. 87,
edited by E. Růžička, M. Hallett, and J. Jankovic.
Lippincott Williams & Wilkins, Philadelphia © 2001.

3

Supraspinal Sites That Induce Locomotion in the Vertebrate Central Nervous System

*Shigemi Mori, †Kiyoji Matsuyama, *Futoshi Mori, and *Katsumi Nakajima

**Departments of Biological Control System, National Institute for Physiological Sciences, Okazaki, 444-8585 Japan; and †Department of Physiology, Sapporo Medical University School of Medicine, Sapporo, Hokkaido, 060-8356 Japan*

Supraspinal sites whose activation produces locomotion have been identified within the vertebrate central nervous system (CNS) of surgically reduced experimental animals from the lamprey to the nonhuman primate (1–4). Such a site is defined operationally as one whose repetitive (nonrhythmic) electrical and/or chemical stimulation *alone* is sufficient to produce locomotion. Shik and coworkers were the first to identify such an area in the cat (5). Their preparation was the unanesthetized high-decerebrate cat. They demonstrated that quadrupedal locomotion could be produced in this preparation by unilateral, punctate electrical stimulation (microstimulation) of a site located approximately 4 mm lateral from the midline and approximately 6 mm ventral from the surface of the inferior colliculus (Horsley-Clarke coordinates, P 2.0, L/R 4.0, H0) (Fig. 3.1). In addition, contiguity with the brainstem was required of reticular core rostral to the site of stimulation. This core had to extend rostrally to the plane of a section from the anterior margin of the superior colliculus dorsally to the anterior margin of the exit of the third nerve ventrally. Presumably, this latter core of reticular substance is required to set an appropriate level of overall brainstem excitability upon which the superimposition of mesencephalic locomotor region (MLR) stimulation is sufficient to set in motion the lower brainstem/spinal cord (SC) circuitry that produces locomotion.

Particularly noteworthy were the simplicity and relatively broad range of stimulus parameters used by Shik and coworkers to induce locomotion (5). These involved a wide array of stimulus pulses (square to sinusoidal, 0.1 to 1.0 ms duration), frequency (greater than 10 to 1,000 Hz), and duration (10 to 100 seconds at 3-min intervals). Furthermore, by changing either the stimulus intensity or the treadmill speed, it was possible to produce a transition in gait from a walk to a trot and then to a gallop, or vice versa. The original locomotion-inducing site of Shik et al. (5) corresponded to the caudal portion of the cuneiform nucleus (CNF) and was subsequently termed the "mesencephalic locomotor region" (MLR). The evoked locomotion became widely known as "controlled locomotion" (i.e., regulated by the strength of the stimulus) (6,7). Several years later, Garcia-Rill and coworkers produced virtually identical locomotion in the same preparation by a focal injection of provisional excitatory neurotransmitters into the electrically identified MLR (8). They also showed that infusions of inhibitory neurotransmitters into the MLR blocked chemically induced locomotion. In the same animal, chemically induced locomotion was more 'natural' than electrically elicited stepping. In macaque monkeys *(M. fascicularis)* decerebrated at the midthalamic level, Eidelberg et al. also evoked "controlled quadrupedal locomotion" with electrical stimulation of the posterior thalamic region in the

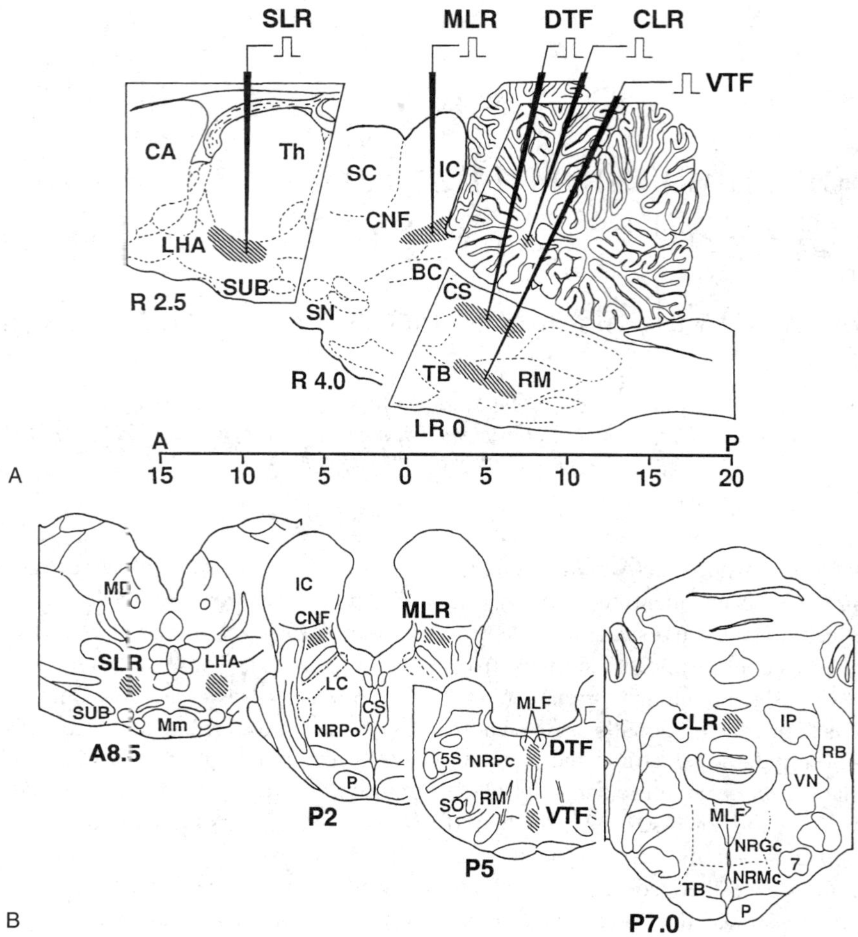

FIG. 3.1. Location of the subthalamic locomotor region (*SLR*), mesencephalic locomotor region (*MLR*), dorsal tegmental field (*DTF*), ventral tegmental field (*VTF*), and cerebellar locomotor region (*CLR*) on the parasagittal planes along *R2.5*, *R4.0*, and *LR0* **(A)** and frontal planes at *A8.5* (SLR), *P2* (MLR), *P5* (DTF, VTF), and *P7.0* (CLR) of the brainstem and the cerebellum **(B)**. The horizontal axis under the parasagittal plane in **A** represents the rostrocaudal Horsley-Clarke coordinates. *5S*, spinal trigeminal nucleus; 7, facial nucleus; *BC*, brachium conjunctivum; *CA*, caudate nucleus; *CNF*, cuneiform nucleus; *CS*, nucleus centralis superior; *IC*, inferior colliculus; *IP*, nucleus interpositus; LHA, lateral hypothalamic area; LC, nucleus locus caeruleus; *MD*, mediodorsal nucleus of the thalamus; *MLF*, medial longitudinal fasciculus; *Mm*, mammillary body; *NRGc*, nucleus reticularis gigantocellularis; *NRMc*, nucleus reticularis magnocellularis; *NRPc*, nucleus reticularis pontis caudalis; *NRPo*, nucleus reticularis pontis oralis; *P*, pyramidal tract; *RB*, restiform body; *RM*, nucleus raphe magnus; *SUB*, subthalamic nucleus; *SC*, superior colliculus; *SO*, superior olive; *SN*, substantia nigra; *TB*, trapezoid body; *Th*, thalamus; *VN*, vestibular nuclei.

vicinity of the CNF and the superior cerebellar peduncle (3).

Clearly, the preceding results demonstrated that a group of cells in and around the CNF in both cats and monkeys must be involved in triggering brainstem and SC neural circuitry involved in the initiation and control of locomotion (2–5). For the identification and characterization of a specific neural substrate as a locomotion-inducing site in the CNS, both electrical and chemical stimulation techniques have been extensively employed, but they have advantages and disadvantages, as is discussed in the following. The circuitry of such a site and the neuronal constituent of the positive-site itself should be delineated by multifaceted analyses, which include the site's afferent input and efferent output (9,10). Also important, but not addressed subsequent to the original Shik et al. report, is delineation of the *rostral* extent of the core of reticular substance that must remain in contiguity with the lower brainstem for stimulation of a locomotion-inducing site to bring about the desired effect (5).

To emphasize the functional significance of controlled locomotion, the present report addresses five major aspects of suprasegmental locomotion-inducing sites in the high-decerebrate cat: (a) technical aspects of their delineation, (b) previously identified sites within the hypothalamus and brainstem, (c) a newly identified cerebellar locomotor region (CLR), (d) the role of the pontomedullary reticular formation (PMRF) in mediating locomotor command signals to the SC, (e) and the lower-order and higher-order control of posture and locomotion.

FOUR BASIC METHODS FOR IDENTIFYING LOCOMOTION-INDUCING SITES

Stein and Glickstein have emphasized that the multiplicity of techniques used to study the CNS can, in reality, be reduced to four: (a) tracing neural connections, (b) noting effects of electrical stimulation, (c) recording CNS activity (by use of electrophysiologic, optic, blood flow measurements, etc.), and (d) noting the effects of ablating CNS tissue (11). All four of these techniques have a pharmacological counterpart, that is, respectively: (a) histochemistry, (b) local application of provisional neurotransmitter agonists or antagonists (chemical microstimulation), (c) measurements of extracellular level of transmitter release by microdialysis, and (d) application of permanent (e.g., kainic acid) or temporary (muscimol, procaine) blocking agents.

Electrical stimulation, using appropriate intracellular and extracellular recording methods, can be used to confirm the anatomic and synaptic connections of a given CNS site, and thereby electrophysiologically delineate it. The other use of stimulation is to evoke a neural system, or sequence of systems, into operation in a controlled (graded) manner. This strategy has been used to identify, among others, the subthalamic locomotor region (SLR), the MLR, and the ponto-bulbar locomotor region (P-BLR) (5,12–14). A key pitfall of both electrical and chemical stimulation, however, is the danger of stimulating unintentionally nearby (nonrelevant) neurons, or *fibers of passage.* Ablation techniques have the same limitation. Often, stimulation and ablation studies have provided controversial results, and thereby made it difficult to attribute the observed motor effects to a specific site within the CNS (15).

In the case of cerebellar nuclei such as the fastigial nucleus (FN), the inhibitory output of the Purkinje cell confounds the interpretation of the effects of stimulation and ablation. For example, axons of the Purkinje cells of the vermal cerebellar cortex, which project to the vestibular nucleus, pass through the fastigial nucleus (Fig. 3.2C) (16). Resolution of such an issue necessitates the combination of stimulation and ablation techniques with anterograde and/or retrograde tracing methods (17–19). This need is underscored by our recent discovery that selective electrical stimulation of the hook bundle of Russel, through which pass crossed fastigioreticular, fastigiovestibular, fastigiotectal, and fastigiospinal fibers, produces controlled locomotion in the high-decerebrate cat; in sharp contrast, stimulation of the fastigial nucleus itself failed to produce such locomotion (20,21).

SUPRASPINAL LOCOMOTION-INDUCING AND SUPPRESSING SITES

Induction Sites

Within the hypothalamus and brainstem, four sites have been shown to play a role in the initiation and control of posture and locomotion in both lightly anesthetized and high-decerebrate cats (Fig. 3.1) (15). Proceeding rostrocaudally, these (and the necessary stimulus strengths) are: the SLR (30 to 50 μA) in the lateral

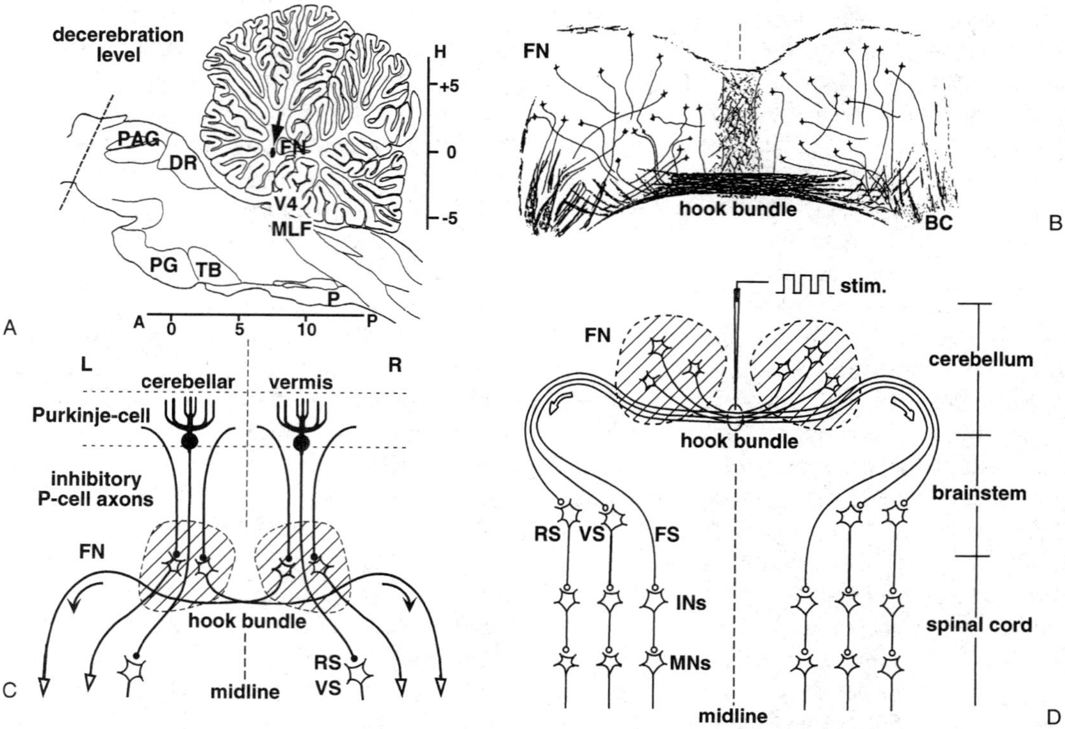

FIG. 3.2. Location of the cerebellar locomotor region (CLR), and anatomic and functional projection patterns of fastigiofugal fibers. Location of the CLR on the midsagittal plane of the cerebellum **(A)**, cells in the fastigial nuclei and hook bundle of Russel **(B)**, *fibers of passage* coursing through the fastigial nucleus **(C)**, trajectory of crossed fastigioreticular, fastigiovestibular, and fastigiospinal fibers **(D)**. Hatched areas in **C** and **D** indicate the fastigial nucleus (*FN*). Abbreviations: *L*, left side; *R*, right side; *BC*, brachium conjunctivum; *DR*, dorsal nucleus of the raphe; *PAG*, periaquaductal gray; *PG*, pontine gray; *TB*, trapezoid body; *FS*, fastigiospinal fibers; *INs*, interneurons; *MLF*, medial longitudinal fasciculus; *MNs*, motoneurons; *RS*, reticulospinal fibers; *VS*, vestibulospinal fibers; V4, fourth ventricle; *stim*, pulse-train microstimulation. (See the text for further details.)

hypothalamic area (LHA); the MLR (10 to 30 μA), which corresponds to the CNF and probably the pedunculopontine nucleus (PPN) in the posterior midbrain (22); the P-BLR (20 to 40 μA), which is presumed to be a multi-synaptic system descending from the MLR (14); and, the ventral tegmental field (VTF; 10 to 20 μA) of the caudal pons along its midline, which corresponds to the rostral portion of the nucleus raphe magnus (23). The latter includes *fibers of passage* from the CNF (10,24). Interestingly, stimulation of the VTF *alone* with a *subthreshold* stimulus intensity for evoking locomotion results in a general augmentation of postural muscle tone (25). When its stimulation is combined with that of the MLR, both at a *subthreshold* level for evoking locomotion, the result is full-blown locomotion (23).

A Suppression Site

The dorsal tegmental field (DTF) of caudal pons has been identified as a locomotion-suppressing site (Fig 3.1). Stimulation of this structure *alone* along its midline (at 10 to 30 μA) results in a general suppression of postural muscle tone. During MLR-evoked locomotion, the concomitant stimulation of this DTF site reduces postural muscle tone and *stops locomotion* (23).

Anatomically, the DTF corresponds to the caudal portion of the nucleus centralis superior, where few cell bodies are located (23,25). This suggests that the locomotor-suppressive effects of DTF result from activation of *fibers of passage.* We have shown that a focal microinjection of the neural tracer, horseradish peroxidase (HRP), into the microlesioned DTF results in a bilateral retrograde labeling of cells mainly in the nuclei reticularis pontis oralis (NRPo) and nuclei reticularis pontis caudalis (NRPc) (15,26). This demonstrated that fibers descending from the pontine reticular formation (PRF) pass through the DTF area. Subsequently, we found that ipsilateral or bilateral stimulation of the dorsomedial regions of NRPo resulted in a bilateral, simultaneous suppression of tonic electromyographic activity in the extensor muscles of the neck, back, forelimb, and hindlimb (27). Descending fibers from the NRPo have been shown to excite a group of reticulospinal (RS) cells in the nucleus reticularis gigantocellularis (NRGc). These RS cells, in turn, were shown to exert nonreciprocal inhibitory effects on α-motoneurons innervating extensor and flexor muscles of the hindlimb (28).

Responses of the Unrestrained, Intact Cat

We have shown that the separate electrical microstimulation of the SLR, MLR, and the VTF in the intact, unrestrained, conscious cat produces stimulus site-specific changes in posture and locomotion. These are combined always with behavioral arousal/orienting reactions such as "searching" and "looking around" behavior (15,29). The more rostral versus caudal the preceding stimulation sites (e.g., SLR versus VTF), the more natural versus "robotic" the evoked postural and locomotor movements. These results suggested that the control mechanisms (subprograms) for posture and locomotor movements form a distributed system within the CNS. They appear to be structured hierarchically within the rostrocaudal axis of the midbrain and lower brainstem (15).

When the same unrestrained, conscious preparation is walking spontaneously along the floor, DTF stimulation evokes a series of postural changes. A few seconds after beginning DTF stimulation, the cat stops walking and remains standing with a posture "primed" for locomotion. As DTF stimulation continues, the animal exhibits a progressive sequence of coordinated relaxing maneuvers, first by squatting, and then laying down on the floor by use of a stereotyped sequence of movements (29). The cat maintains the latter position (posture) for several minutes, even after termination of DTF stimulation. An identical DTF effect is evident during locomotion, as brought on by stimulation of the SLR, MLR, or VTF.

Taken together, the described effects of DTF stimulation on natural and controlled locomotion show that an essential prerequisite for the initiation and maintenance of locomotion is the development of an appropriate amount of postural muscle tone (postural preparation), and further suggest that neural mechanisms involved in postural and locomotor control are shared, partly, in common in both the brainstem and the spinal cord (9,15,23).

THE CEREBELLAR LOCOMOTOR REGION

We have recently identified a cerebellar locomotor region (CLR), using criteria identical to those described in the preceding, for previously established locomotion-inducing sites (21). Four illustrations in Figure 3.2 show the location of the CLR (A), functional anatomy of the fastigial nucleus and crossed fastigiofugal fibers (Hook bundle) (B), axons of the Purkinje cells of the vermal cortex which pass through the fastigial nucleus (C), and multiple and parallel pathways descending, bilaterally, to the spinal interneurons (INs) and motoneurons (MNs) in the SC (D). As shown in Figure 3.2A, the CLR is located at the midline of the cerebellar white matter, rostral to the most rostral pole of the fastigial nuclei, where a decussation of fastigiofugal fibers occurs (16,18). The optimal locus for evoking locomotion is at Horsley-Clarke coordinates H0 and P 7.0. In the midsagittal plane, the CLR stimulus sites were within a disklike region (diameter approximately 0.5 mm) (Fig. 3.2A).

It is most noteworthy that the lowest effective stimulus intensity at the optimal site was 5 to 8 μA; that is, much *less* than that required at the MLR. During the period in which the high-decerebrate cat maintained a reflexively

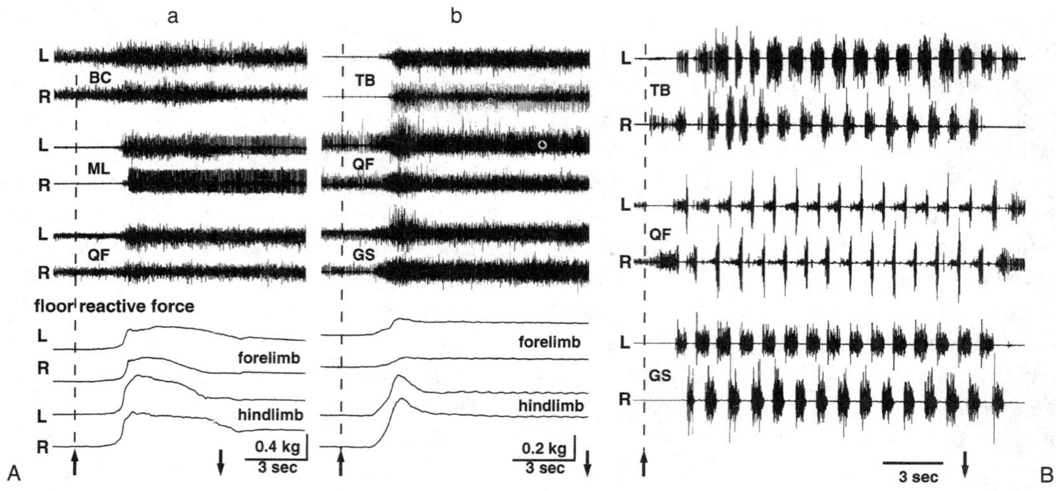

FIG. 3.3. Cerebellar-evoked augmentation of postural muscle tone and initiation of locomotion. Electromyographies (EMGs) and forelimb and hindlimb ground-reaction forces recorded during cerebellar-evoked augmentation of postural muscle tone in two animals (*a* and *b* in **[A]**). EMGs recorded during CLR-evoked locomotion **(B).** In each set of the records, upward and downward arrows represent the beginning and termination of the period of CLR stimulation, respectively. Abbreviations: *L*, left side; *R*, right side; *BC*, biventer cervicis; *GS*, gastrocnemius-soleus; *ML*, multifidus lumbaris; *QF*, quadriceps femoris; *TB*, triceps brachii. (See the text for further details.)

activated standing posture on a still treadmill surface, we also found that CLR stimulation, with the stimulus strength subthreshold for evoking locomotion, provoked general augmentation of electromyographic activity of neck, forelimb and hindlimb extensor muscles, bilaterally, with an increase in the ground reaction force (Fig. 3.3A). With a slight increase in the stimulus strength, air-stepping was evoked. On a moving treadmill, stimulation of the optimal site in the CLR evoked well-coordinated quadrupedal locomotion (Fig. 3.3B). At the same stimulus strength, stimulation of sites located dorsally or ventrally from the best loci provoked locomotion with slower frequencies of forelimb and hindlimb movements. Stimulation of sites located rostrally or caudally from the best loci occasionally provoked locomotion with slightly different frequencies of forelimb and hindlimb movements (21).

Concomitant stimulation of the optimal foci in the CLR and the MLR, each at a subthreshold strength, produces locomotor movements identical to those seen with suprathreshold stimulation of each site alone. Stimulation to left or right of the CLR midline can produce locomotion, but this requires stronger stimulus intensity, and the locomotor movement patterns are no longer symmetric. Rather, they are shifted to emphasize movements of the forelimbs and hindlimbs contralateral to the site of stimulation. Controlled locomotion can still be evoked by stimulating the remaining intact site at the original stimulus strength after making tiny, unilateral or bilateral ablative lesions at either the CLR or MLR (21).

Anatomic Features

We have found that the cells of origin of fibers, which project to and through the CLR, are located exclusively in the bilateral fastigial nuclei (18,19). This was established by use of a retrograde tracing method. It employed a cholera-toxin b subunit conjugated HRP (CTb-HRP) as the neural tracer. CTb-HRP was focally injected into the lesioned site of the CLR by use of a double-barreled pipette composed of a stimulating microelectrode and an injection glass pipette. The former was used to evoke locomotion and subsequently sever the fibers *en passage* that coursed through the effective stimulus site. The attached pipette was used for microinjection of

CTb-HRP into the lesioned stimulus site so that CTb-HRP can be transported both retrogradely and anterogradely. All CTb-HRP-stained sections of the cerebellum were examined under a light microscope to locate the retrogradely labeled cells and trace the trajectory of fibers of passage (18).

Most of the labeled cells were multipolar-shaped, with a somal diameter of 15 to 40 μm. These cells were distributed exclusively throughout the extent of the left and right fastigial nuclei. The trajectory of descending fibers coursing through the CLR was essentially the same as that identified by injecting an anterograde neural tracer, *Phaseolus vulgaris* leukoagglutinin (PHA-L), into the fastigial nucleus (30). We showed further that PHA-L–labeled efferent fibers coursed through the hook bundle and projected caudally to the pontomedullary reticular formation (PMRF) and the vestibular complex. In both of these structures, terminal boutons of the descending labeled fibers were apposed closely to a number of large-sized cells. These latter cells were considered to be the cells of origin of long descending RS and vestibulospinal (VS) fibers, respectively (31).

The preceding results revealed that the CLR corresponds to the hook bundle of Russel at the midline of the cerebellum (Fig. 3.2A,B). At this site, crossed fastigioreticular and fastigiovestibular fibers decussate, together with other fastigiospinal fibers that terminate in the upper cervical segments and fastigiotectal fibers that terminate in the superior colliculus (32–38).

Physiologic Features

We have shown that CLR stimulation activates a majority of RS cells by a monosynaptic connection (39,40). The excited RS cells were located mainly in the bilateral, gigantocellar tegmental field (FTG) of the medullary reticular formation (MRF), which corresponds to the NRGc. Descending fibers of these RS cells were shown to project through the ventral and ventrolateral funiculi to the lumbar segments. The conduction velocity of the majority of these RS fibers was greater than 55 m/s. In contrast, MLR stimulation activated such RS cells by largely a polysynaptic connection. Furthermore, we showed that the synaptic efficacy (responsiveness) of RS cells to CLR stimulation is much higher than that to MLR stimulation. In a preliminary study, we found also that CLR stimulation resulted in a monosynaptic activation of VS cells, in agreement with our anatomic findings (40). During CLR-evoked locomotion, the RS cells in NRGc exhibited a major increase in discharge frequency with some phasic, locomotor-rhythm modulation. In selected instances, the action potentials (APs) of tonically firing RS cells were time-locked to each stimulus pulse of the CLR stimulus pulse-train, and the different RS cells had peak firing rates at different times throughout the hindlimb step cycles. In contrast, no time-locked discharges of RS cells were found during MLR-evoked locomotion. These results indicate that locomotor command signals evoked by stimulating the CLR are relayed directly to medullary RS cells, and thence to the SC.

The elaboration of well-coordinated locomotion requires integrated control of head, neck, body, and limb movements including orienting of the eyes, head, and neck to the moving object in the environment, in addition to balance control. The described findings make it attractive to speculate that the command signals for this integration are conveyed by fastigiospinal, fastigioreticular, and fastigiovestibular fibers, in addition to fastigiotectal fibers, which terminate in the superior colliculus. Such commands seem to concern the maintenance of balance, coordination of head-neck movements, fixation of the body's axis, and activation of the overall central pattern generator (CPG) for locomotion (41). It is important to note that the vermis of the cerebellum integrates exteroceptive, proprioceptive, vestibular, and visual afferent information that originates from a wide variety of sources (42–45).

In summary on the CLR, it is clear that the fastigial nucleus is one of the key supraspinal locomotion-inducing sites. It receives and integrates multimodal afferent signals. On the output side, it exerts simultaneously a particularly strong excitatory effect on selected cells of origin of the bilateral RS and VS tracts. Thus, the fastigial nuclei can independently and simultaneously trigger brainstem and spinal locomotor subprograms, which were formerly believed to

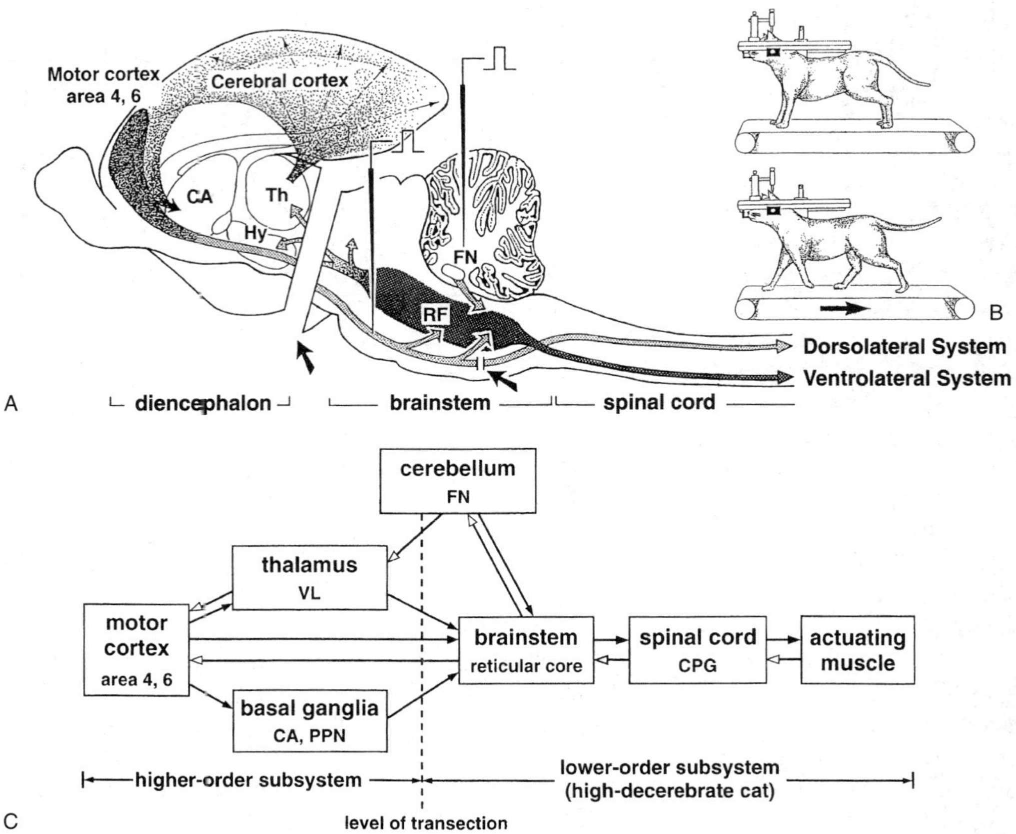

FIG. 3.4. Schematic illustration of stimulus sites in the pyramidal tract (PT) and fastigial nucleus (*FN*) in relation to the pontomedullary reticular formation (*RF*) in a high-decerebrate cat **(A).** *Two upward arrows* indicate the transection levels of the brainstem and the pyramidal tracts, respectively. Reflexively activated posture and locomotor figure of the cat on a still **(top)** and moving treadmill surface **(bottom) (B).** An *arrow* inside the treadmill indicates the direction of a moving treadmill surface. A block diagram of higher-order and lower-order control systems **(C).** *Arrows* with open and closed heads indicate ascending and descending connections, respectively. A broken line between the thalamus/basal ganglia and brainstem represents the transection level. Abbreviations: *CA*, caudate nucleus; *CPG*, central pattern generator; *Hy*, hypothalamus; *PPN*, pedunculopontine nucleus; *Th*, thalamus; *VL*, ventrolateral nucleus. (See the text for further details.)

be the sole domain of various brainstem regions, including the MLR and the SLR (21,41).

PATHWAYS MEDIATING LOCOMOTOR COMMAND SIGNALS TO THE SPINAL CORD

Electrophysiologic Findings

Shik and coworkers were the first to propose that the PMRF is implicated in the initiation of locomotion (46). They showed in the high-decerebrate cat that stimulation of the rostral pyramidal tract (PT) produced controlled locomotion, provided that the PTs were sectioned bilaterally at the medullary level, immediately caudal to the site of stimulation (Fig. 3.4A). Such stimulation evoked only walking or trotting, and, in general, PT-evoked locomotion was much less stable than its MLR-evoked counterpart. Concomitant MLR/PT stimulation, each at subthreshold strength, produced well-coordinated locomotion. After PT-section and ablative bilateral MLR lesions, rostral PT stimulation still evoked locomotion. They proposed that PT-evoked locomotion resulted from the stimulus activating corticoreticular fibers and collaterals of corticospinal fibers, such as to provide a synaptic activation of RS cells in the PMRF. This proposal implied that locomotor command signals could originate in the motor cortex, as was shown two decades later by Armstrong (42), with its clear-cut anatomical basis provided a further decade later (47). All these results suggest that the locomotor control system, as a whole, is composed of higher-order and lower-order control subsystems (Fig. 3.4B).

Several studies subsequent to that of Shik et al. (46) showed that locomotor command signals originating from the SLR, MLR, and the P-BLR are conveyed by RS cells to the locomotor CPG circuitry of the SC (1,2,4,5,12). Particularly noteworthy was Orlovsky's demonstration that electrical stimulation of the SLR and MLR in the high-decerebrate cat evoked monosynaptic and polysynaptic EPSPs in RS cells of the medial PMRF (48). Garcia-Rill and Skinner also demonstrated the bilateral monosynaptic and polysynaptic activation of RS cells in the MRF by stimulation of the MLR (49).

Anatomy of the Mesencephalic Locomotor Region and Its Descending Projections

The physiologically identified MLR is localized within a large circular area centered in the posterior CNF. It includes and/or contacts several neighboring areas, including the inferior colliculus, brachium conjunctivum, mesencephalic trigeminal nucleus, and PPN (22,50). Garcia-Rill showed that microstimulation of the *pars compacta* of the PPN in the high-decerebrate cat produced controlled locomotion (50). The MLR–PPN complex has a particularly complex anatomy; therefore, the appeal of its physiologic definition on the basis of the locomotor responses to its electrical and chemical activation has not been well settled. Garcia-Rill suggested that it would be preferable to label a locomotion-inducing site solely on the basis of what specific anatomic structure(s) was stimulated, because *precise* neuronal substrate of the MLR is not yet established (51). His well-considered viewpoint has not yet gained support, however. Rather, the focus has been on the anatomic projections of the *physiologically identified* MLR. For example, by use of autoradiographic tracing, Steeves and Jordan showed that the MLR projects to the FTG and magnocellular tegmental fields (FTM) of the medial MRF (24). There were clearly *no direct projections to the SC.* Garcia-Rill and coworkers also found that efferent fibers from the PPN–MLR project to the transition zone between FTM and FTG of the MRF (10). These medullary projection areas of the MLR correspond to those whose electrical stimulation produces locomotion and an augmentation of postural muscle tone in the decerebrate cat (12,21).

Descending Projections of Reticulospinal and Vestibulospinal Axons

By use of the PHA-L anterograde tracing method in the cats with different survival periods (4 to 8 weeks), Matsuyama found recently that about 80% of single RS axons, which descend from the pontine reticular formation (PRF), give off multiple, mainly unilateral axon collaterals at each of the cervical and lumbar enlargements (Fig. 3.5A) (52–54). Remaining axons innervated the gray matter bilaterally. These axon collaterals terminate mainly in Rexed's laminae VII–VIII, and the medial portion of lamina IX: that is, where INs and MNs innervating proximal muscles are located, respectively. We found also that like RS axons, single VS axons (survival periods of the animals: 4 to 12 weeks), which descend from the lateral vestibular nucleus, give off multiple, unilateral axon collaterals, and in a segment-specific manner (55). Terminal VS fiber endings were distributed in laminae VII–VIII at the similar regions where terminal RS fiber endings were distributed (Fig. 3.5B).

Such a multiple collateralization of RS and VS axons throughout the whole length of spinal neuraxis seems particularly suited to controlling columns of INs and MNs that innervate postural muscles contributing to fixation of the body's axis. Some RS cells may contribute also to the activation of a group of INs implicated in the CPG for locomotion. In contrast to the multisegmental innervation by RS and VS axons, we found that

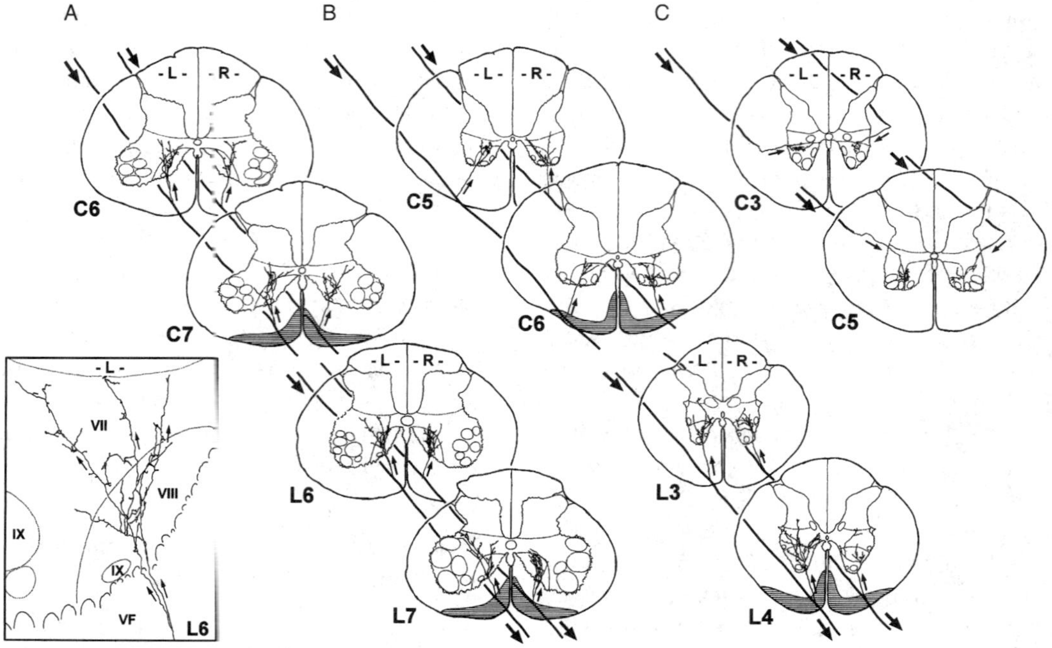

FIG. 3.5. Representative collateral branching patterns of reticulospinal **(A),** vestibulospinal **(B),** and fastigiospinal axons **(C).** The sketches of branching patterns at cervical and lumbar segments were made in animals with different survival periods. The **inset** sketch in the left bottom corner shows the detailed branching patterns at *L6* segment in **(A).** *Arrows* indicate descending trajectory of single axons. Axon collaterals were given off tangentially from the stem axons. The results in **(C)** have not been published. *VII*, *VIII*, and *IX* in the inset sketch represent Rexed's laminae VII, VIII, and IX. Abbreviations: *L*, left side; *R*, right side; *VF*, ventral funiculus.

single fastigiospinal axons *did not exhibit collateralization.* Rather, each fastigiospinal axon terminated directly in a specific region of laminae VII–VIII at one of the upper cervical segments, probably activating a single neck muscle (Fig. 3.5C).

Pontomedullary Reticular Formation Activated Lumbar Spinal Interneurons and Their Fine Morphology

During MLR-evoked fictive locomotion in the immobilized high-decerebrate cat, Matsuyama and Mori have succeeded in making intra-axonal recordings from L4-7 lumbar INs in the ventral funiculus (VF) (56). Axons were defined as interneuronal if they were activated monosynaptically by stimulation of the NRPo and/or NRGc. Following characterization of the axon's rhythmic (locomotor-related) firing pattern, neurobiotin (NB) was injected intra-axonally at the recording site. This allowed the subsequent visualization of the axon's anterograde arborization pattern, together with the location and fine morphology of the retrogradely labeled soma. Most of the somas of the INs, which discharged rhythmically, were located in lamina VIII, contralateral to the stimulus side of the NRPo and NRGc. The stem axon of *all* of these INs crossed the midline ventral to the central canal, indicating that rhythmically discharging INs are commissural. The stem axon then ascended or descended for two to four segments in the contralateral VF. Fine terminal fibers originating from the main collaterals of the commissural INs on the right side were distributed mainly in laminae VII–VIII on the left side, where spinal INs are located. Some axon collaterals directly innervated the

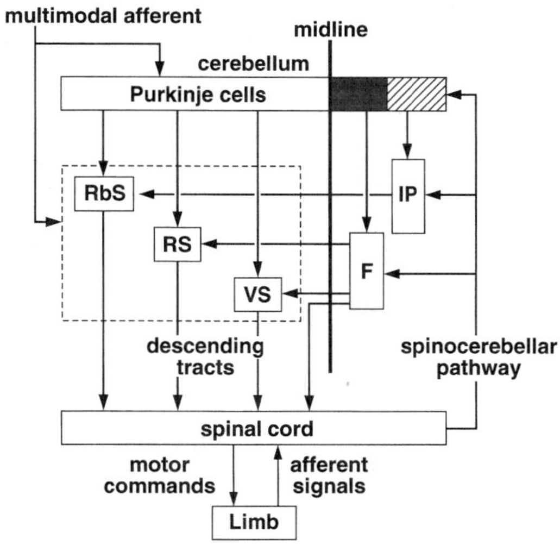

FIG. 3.6. The "closed," multisynaptic cerebellospinal loop. *Dark and hatched areas* of the cerebellar cortex along right of the midline represent its vermal and intermediate portions, respectively. Abbreviations: *F*, fastigial nucleus; *IP*, interpositus nucleus; *RbS*, *RS*, and *VS*, cells of origin of rubrospinal, reticulospinal, and vestibulospinal tracts, respectively. (See the text for further details.)

contralateral lamina IX, where motoneurons (MNs) are located that supply hindlimb muscles.

The preceding results are all in keeping with the recorded commissural INs having been potential components of the CPG circuitry for locomotion. Thus, evidence is now on hand to support our proposition that RS axons are involved in activation of spinal INs that play a role in generation of the locomotor rhythm.

HIGHER-ORDER CONTROL OF POSTURE AND LOCOMOTION

In humans and other mammals, it is well established that midline cerebellar injuries and atrophies produce mainly instabilities of posture (truncal ataxia) and locomotor movements (57). For the treadmill locomotion of both the intact and high-decerebrate cat Udo and coworkers found that temporary cooling of the intermediate cerebellar cortex and closely adjacent areas induced hyperflexed locomotor movements in the ipsilateral forelimb (58). An acute lesion of the intermediate cortex also produced changes in locomotor movements that were similar to those produced by cooling. In cats, Yu and Eidelberg found that bilateral fastigial lesions produced severe, ataxic locomotor movements with hyperflexion of all four limbs (59). During the first week after these lesions, the animals were incapable of standing and walking.

Descending Fastigial Projections and the Spinocerebellar Loop

In mammals, and probably nonmammalian vertebrates, as well, a functionally complex "closed" spinocerebellar or cerebellospinal loop is formed by motor pathways descending from the brainstem to the SC, the SC, the ascending spinocerebellar pathways, and the cerebellofugal fibers back to the brainstem and the SC (Fig. 3.6) (44,45). Spinocerebellar fibers project not only to the cerebellar cortex, but also, collaterals of spinocerebellar mossy fiber afferents project to all the deep cerebellar nuclei, including the fastigial nucleus and interpositus nucleus. Cerebellofugal fibers include both those originating from Purkinje cells and those arising from the deep cerebellar nuclei (16,43,44). The interpositus nucleus projects to the cells of origin of the rubrospinal tract, whereas the fastigial nucleus project to those of the reticulospinal and vestibulospinal tracts (43,45). These three descending motor tracts originate from the brainstem (31).

The various effects of fastigial lesions on posture and locomotion have been attributed to an "abnormal" state of brainstem and spinal reflexes, and, in addition, to the absence of cyclic ascending inflow of feedback signals related to ongoing locomotion (43). The cerebellar vermal cortex integrates proprioceptive, exteroceptive, visual, and vestibular afferent information that originates from a wide variety of sources. Therefore, it is likely that the cerebellar vermis and the fastigial nucleus (to which project efferent fibers from the vermis) are concerned with the maintenance of posture, and with elaborating and coordinating associated body and neck movements. Interestingly, Chambers and Sprague suggested this arrangement over four decades ago (60,61).

Ascending Fastigial Projections and the Thalamocortical Loop

There are ascending as well as descending fastigiofugal projections, which include fastigiothalamic fibers (62,63) Fastigiothalamic fibers terminate in the nucleus ventralis medialis (VM) and the adjacent medial part of the nucleus ventralis lateralis (VL) in cat and monkey (38,64). These are the main conduits for the cerebellocortical pathway (Fig. 3.4). Rispal-Padel and Massion showed mediolateral topography within the cat's VL by use of electrophysiology, with medial VL neurons projecting to area 6 of the cerebral cortex, and more lateral neurons to area 4 (65). By stimulation of the precruciate cortex, they also demonstrated topographically organized corticothalamic projections. These electrophysiologic results, together with the degeneration study of the corticothalamic projection, suggest the presence of a positive feedback system between the medial VL and cortical area 6 (66). Taken together, all of the preceding results suggest that the control of posture and locomotion exerted by the fastigial nucleus has the potential to include an ascending pathway by way of VL to the motor (area 4) and supplementary areas (area 6) of the cerebral cortex. As has been well demonstrated, cortical cells in area 6 and 4 influence mainly axial and proximal, and distal musculatures, respectively (67).

Corticoreticular and Corticopontine Projections

Projection patterns of corticoreticular and corticopontine fibers, which originate from cortical areas 4 and 6, have been studied in detail by use of the PHA-L tracing method by Matsuyama and Drew (47). PHA-L-labeled corticoreticular fibers were found to descend in the ipsilateral PT and distribute their terminal endings bilaterally within *all regions* of the PMRF. (Recall that long descending RS fibers originate in the PMRF) (31). On the basis of their quantitative analysis of PHA-L labeling, they were able to identify clear-cut differences in the density and distribution of terminal endings in the PMRF for fibers descending from area 4 versus 6. Throughout the *full* pontomedullary extent of the PMRF, the corticoreticular projection was more numerous and dense from area 6 versus 4. Dense corticopontine projections, mainly ipsilateral, were also found from area 4 and a part of area 6. The pontine nuclei are the most massive of all precerebellar nuclei that give off most of their efferents to the cerebellar hemisphere, contralaterally, and also to the vermis, bilaterally, although the projection to the vermis is smaller than to the hemisphere (68).

Based on the finding of extremely fine and delicate corticoreticular and RS projections patterns, we suggested that the corticoreticulospinal pathway superimposes a fine control on the brainstem's repertoire of control mechanisms for the elaboration of posture and locomotion (41,69). This more phylogenetically recent pathway provides the ability to execute relatively independent movements of the limbs, and especially their distal components. This particular property of the cortico-reticulospinal system, together with cortico-ponto-cerebellar system projecting to the fastigial nucleus, seems to add flexibility and maneuverability to the ability of higher brain structures to initiate, coordinate and maintain the automatic and voluntary control of posture and movement.

CONCLUSION

Integration of Lower-order and Higher-order Control Mechanisms

To initiate and terminate locomotor movements of both the biped and quadruped, a smooth transition is required from and to a standing (upright) posture. Bipedal standing and the upright posture of the quadruped are both *active* motor programs, with CNS control mechanisms that have more similarities than differences (15). The transition from locomotion to standing, and vice versa, appears to be accomplished by two different control mechanisms. One is an *automatic*, lower-order control process, and the other is a *volitional*, higher-order process (Fig. 3.4) (70).

The lower-order process is composed of a number of posture-related and locomotor-related subprograms. These are distributed within the brainstem and the SC, and they permit the high-decerebrate cat to walk automatically in a straight line. The higher-order process involves mechanisms that appear to reside within the cerebellum, basal ganglia, and the cerebral cortex (22,43,45, 49,71,72). It should be mentioned here that some crossed fastigiofugal fibers terminate in the superior colliculus from which tectoreticular fibers originate (38). Tectoreticular fibers influence reticulospinal cells, which project to cervical, thoracic, and lumbar segments, and have been shown to be involved in orienting of eyes, head, and body toward the moving object in the environment (73). Locomotor-driving signals descending through the fastigio-tecto-reticulospinal pathway, together with those descending through other fastigiofugal pathways, will allow an intact conscious animal to control, on a moment-to-moment basis, the speed and direction of locomotion, and to circumvent all obstacles.

By combining and/or integrating the automatic and voluntary control processes, the animal can adjust its posture and locomotion even to the most complex, rapid and unexpected of perturbations. For such mastery, adaptive and anticipatory control mechanisms also are required. All of the preceding mechanisms have been provided in a relatively large number of previous empirical studies on experimental animals and humans (2,4,6,7,15,43,57,72). The experimental data so provided are now sufficient to permit the modeling and simulation of the control of posture and movement (74).

Centralized and Parallel Control of Body Segments

One of the most striking features of studies on high-decerebrate cats is that pulse-train microstimulation of selected areas within the CNS, such as the CLR and the MLR, can produce controlled locomotion by coordinating and/or integrating the individual movements of a sufficient number of body segments that reasonably normal locomotion can ensue. To achieve such overall control, each locomotion-inducing site in the CNS must be able to act as a "centralized control center," capable of ensuring that subprograms controlling the movements of individual body segments are activated in parallel, and in a highly coordinated manner. The available evidence suggests that such a control center can recruit postural and locomotor synergisms, which reside within the brainstem and the SC, while activating a number of subprograms and motor systems, which descend in parallel from the brainstem to the SC. Among these control centers, it is noteworthy that the neuroanatomical characteristics and afferent/efferent organization of the most recently discovered one, the CLR, are far better delineated than the corresponding properties of the originally described MLR (18,19,21).

The fastigial nucleus is located at a particularly strategic level in the CNS for exerting an integrated control over locomotion (19,41). It is optimally situated for uniting the activity of the cerebello-brainstem-spinal loop, and the cerebello-thalamo-cerebral loop (Fig. 3.4C). These loops are major components of lower-order and higher-order control processes, respectively, for the automatic including adaptive or reflexive, and volitional including anticipatory control of posture and locomotion. As such, it is most likely that the fastigial nucleus is the most critical of the locomotion-inducing sites delineated to this point. For locomotion, the cerebellum has been conventionally considered not to be directly involved in its initiation, but, rather, in the coordination of its ongoing locomotor movements (2,43–45). We think that our results provided a new opening in the study of the functional role of the cerebellum and its fastigial nucleus in the initiation and modulation of posture and locomotion.

ACKNOWLEDGMENTS

The authors express sincere appreciation to Dr. Douglas G. Stuart, Department of Physiology, The University of Arizona School of Medicine, for his critical review and editing of the final version of the manuscript, and thanks to Miss C. Takasu for preparation of the illustrations. This study was supported by the Ministry of Health of Japan Grant in Aid on Comprehensive Research on Aging and Health; by a grant from Uehara Memorial Foundation to S. Mori; by the Ministry of Education, Science, Sports and Culture of Japan Grant in Aid for Encouragement of Young Scientists to F. Mori; and by the Ministry of Education, Science, Sports, and Culture of Japan Grant in Aid for Scientific Research on Priority Areas (C) to K. Nakajima.

REFERENCES

1. Grillner S. Locomotion in vertebrates: central mechanisms and reflex interaction. *Physiol Rev* 1975;55:247–304.
2. Grillner S. Control of locomotion in bipeds, tetrapods, and fish. In: Brooks VB, ed. *Handbook of physiology: the nervous system.* Bethesda, MD: American Physiology Society, 1981:1179–1236.
3. Eidelberg E, Walden JG, Nguyen LH. Locomotor control in macaque monkeys. *Brain* 1981;104:647–663.
4. Mori S, Matsuyama K, Miyashita E, Nakajima K. Basic neurophysiology of primate locomotion. *Folia Primatol* 1996;66:192–203.
5. Shik ML, Severin FV, Orlovsky GN. Control of walking and running by means of stimulation of the mid-brain. *Biophysics* 1966;11:756–765.
6. Orlovsky GN, Shik ML. Control of locomotion: A neurophysiological analysis of the cat locomotor system. *International Rev Physiol Neurophysiol* II. 1976;10:281–317.
7. Shik ML, Orlovsky GN. Neurophysiology of locomotor automatism. *Physiol Rev* 1976;56:465–501.
8. Garcia-Rill E, Skinner RD, Fitzgerald JA. Chemical activation of the mesencephalic locomotor region. *Brain Res* 1985;330:43–54.
9. Mori S. Contribution of postural muscle tone to full expression of posture and locomotor movements: multifaceted analyses of its setting brainstem-spinal cord mechanisms in the cat. *Jpn J Physiol* 1989;39:785–809.
10. Garcia-Rill E, Skinner RD, Gilmore SA, et al. Connections of the mesencephalic locomotor region (MLR). II. Afferents and efferents. *Brain Res Bull* 1983;10:63–71.
11. Stein JF, Glickstein M. Role of the cerebellum in visual guidance of movement. *Physiol Rev* 1992;72:967–1017.
12. Waller WH. Progression movements elicited by subthalamic stimulation. *J Neurophysiol* 1940;3:300–307.
13. Grossman RG. Effects of stimulation of nonspecific thalamic system on locomotor movements in cat. *J Neurophysiol* 1958;21:85–93.
14. Mori S, Shik ML, Yagodnitsyn AS. Role of pontine tegmentum for locomotor control in mesencephalic cat. *J Neurophysiol* 1977;40:284–295.
15. Mori S. Integration of posture and locomotion in acute decerebrate cats and in awake, freely moving cats. *Prog Neurobiol* 1987;28:161–195.
16. Ito M. *The cerebellum and neural control.* New York: Raven Press, 1984.
17. Ohta Y, Mori S, Kimura H. Neuronal structures of the brainstem participating in postural suppression in cats. *Neurosci Res* 1988;5:181–202.
18. Asanome M, Matsuyama K, Mori S. Augmentation of postural muscle tone induced by the stimulation of the decussating fibers in the midline of the cerebellar white matter in the acute decerebrate cat. *Neurosci Res* 1998;30:257–269.
19. Mori S, Matsui T, Kuze B, et al. Cerebellar induced locomotion: Reticulospinal control of spinal rhythm generating mechanisms in cats. *Ann NY Acad Sci* 1998:94–105.
20. Rasmussen AT. Origin and course of the fasciculus uncinatus (Russell) in the cat, with observations on other fiber tracts arising from the cerebellar nuclei. *J Comp Neurol* 1933;57:165–197.
21. Mori S, Matsui T, Kuze B, et al. Stimulation of a restricted region in the midline cerebellar white matter evokes coordinated quadrupedal locomotion in the decerebrate cat. *J Neurophysiol* 1999;82:290–300.
22. Garcia-Rill E, Houser CR, Skinner RD, et al. Locomotion-inducing sites in the vicinity of the pedunculopontine nucleus. *Brain Res Bull* 1987;18:731–738.
23. Mori S, Nishimura H, Kurakami C, et al. Controlled locomotion in the mesencephalic cat: distribution of facilitatory and inhibitory regions within pontine tegmentum. *J Neurophyiol* 1978;41:1580–1591.
24. Steeves JD, Jordan LM. Autoradographic demonstration of the projections from the mesencephalic locomotor region. *Brain Res* 1984;307:263–276.
25. Mori S, Kawahara K, Sakamoto T, et al. Setting and resetting of postural muscle tone in decerebrate cat by stimulation of the brain stem. *J Neurophysiol* 1982;48:737–748.
26. Mori S, Ohta Y, Matsuyama K, et al. The setting of postural muscle tone: Its importance for behavior in freely moving, intact cats. In: Oomura Y, ed. *Emotions, neuronal and chemical control.* Tokyo: Japan Science Soc. Press, 1986:231–239.
27. Oka T, Iwakiri H, Mori S. Pontine-induced generalized suppression of postural muscle tone in a reflexively standing acute decerebrate cat. *Neurosci Res* 1993;17:127–140.
28. Takakusaki K, Ohta Y, Mori S. Single medullary reticulospinal neurons exert postsynaptic inhibitory effects via inhibitory interneurons upon alpha-motoneurons innervating cat hindlimb muscles. *Exp Brain Res* 1989;74:11–23.

29. Mori S, Sakamoto T, Ohta Y, et al. Site specific postural and locomotor changes evoked in awake, freely moving intact cats by stimulating the brainstem. *Brain Res* 1989;505:66–74.
30. Homma Y, Nonaka S, Matsuyama K, et al. Fastigiofugal projection to the brainstem nuclei in the cat: an anterograde PHA-L tracing study. *Neurosci Res* 1995;23:89–102.
31. Kuypers HGJM. Anatomy of descending pathways. In: Brookhart JM, Mountcastle VB, eds. *Handbook of physiology.* Bethesda, MD: American Physiology Society, 1981:597–666.
32. Jansen J, Jansen J Jr. On the efferent fibers of the cerebellar nuclei in the cats. *J Comp Neurol* 1955;102:607–632.
33. Matsushita M, Iwahori N. Structural organization of the fastigial nucleus. I. Dendrites and axons. *Brain Res* 1971;25:597–610.
34. Matsushita M, Iwahori N. Structural organization of the fastigial nucleus. II. Afferent fiber systems, dendrites and axons. *Brain Res* 1971;25:5611–624.
35. Walberg F, Pompeiano O, Brodal A, et al. The fastigiovestibular projection in the cat. An experimental study with silver impregnation methods. *J Comp Neurol* 1962;118:49–769.
36. Walberg F, Pompeiano O, Westrum LE, et al. Fastigioreticular fibers in the cat. An experimental study with silver methods. *J Comp Neurol* 1962;119:187–199.
37. Wilson VJ, Uchino Y, Maunz RA, et al. Properties and connections of cat fastigiospinal neurons. *Exp Brain Res* 1978;41:1–17.
38. Anguat P, Bowsher D. Ascending projections of the medial cerebellar (fastigial) nucleus: an experimental study in the cat. *Brain Res* 1970;24:49–68.
39. Matsui T, Kuze B, Asanome M, et al. Stimulus effects of cerebellum and mesencephalic locomotor region (MLR) on the reticulo- and vestibulospinal neurons in decerebrate cats. *Jpn J Physiol* 1997;47:S169.
40. Matsui T, Kuze B, Matsuyama K, et al. Response properties of pontomedullary reticulospinal cells to the stimulation of the locomotor inducing regions in the mesencephalon and cerebellum in decerebrate cats. *Abstracts Soc Neurosci* 1997;23:1043.
41. Mori S, Matsuyama K, Kuze B, et al. Features of the fastigio-reticulo-spinal system involved in the control of posture and locomotion in the cat. In: Gantchev G, Mori S, Massion J, eds. *Motor control today and tomorrow.* Sofia, Bulgaria: "Prof. Marin Drinov" Academic Publishing House, 1999:31–44.
42. Armstrong DM. The mammalian cerebellum and its contribution to movement control. *International review of physiology. Neurophysiology* III 1978;17:239–294.
43. Armstrong DM. Supraspinal contribution to the initiation and control of locomotion in the cat. *Prog Neurobiol* 1986;26:273–361.
44. Armstrong DM, Apps R, Marple-Horvat DE. Aspects of cerebellar function in relation to locomotor movements. *Prog Brain Res* 1997;114:401–421.
45. Arshavsky Yu I, Gelfand IM, et al. *Cerebellum and rhythmical movements.* Berlin: Springer-Verlag, 1986.
46. Shik ML, Orlovsky GN, Severin FV. Locomotion of the mesencephalic cat elicited by stimulation of the pyramids. *Biophysics* 1968;13:143–152.
47. Matsuyama K, Drew T. Organization of the projections from the pericruciate cortex to the pontomedullary brainstem of the cat: a study using the anterograde tracer phaseolus vulgaris-leucoaggulutinin. *J Comp Neurol* 1997;389:617–641.
48. Orlovsky GN. Work of the neurones of the cerebellar nuclei during locomotion. *Biophysics* 1972;17:1177–1185.
49. Garcia-Rill E, Skinner RD. The mesencephalic locomotor region. II. Projections to reticulospinal neurons. *Brain Res* 1987;411:13–20.
50. Garcia-Rill E. The pedunculopontine nucleus. *Prog Neurobiol* 1991;36: 363–389.
51. Garcia-Rill E. The basal ganglia and the locomotor regions. *Brain Res Rev* 1986;11:47–63.
52. Matsuyama K, Ohta Y, Mori S. Ascending and descending projections of the nucleus reticularis gigantocellularis in the cat demonstrated by the anterograde neural tracer, *phaseolus vulgaris* leucoagglutinin (PHA-L). *Brain Res* 1988;460:124–141.
53. Matsuyama K, Takakusaki K, Nakajima K, et al. Multisegmental innervation of single pontine reticulospinal axons in the cervico-thoracic region of the cat: anterograde PHA-L tracing study. *J Comp Neurol* 1997;377:234–250.
54. Matsuyama K, Mori F, Kuze B, et al. Morphology of single pontine reticulospinal axons in the lumbar enlargement of the cat: a study using the anterograde tracer PHA-L. *J Comp Neurol* 1999;410:413–430.
55. Kuze B, Matsuyama K, Matsui T, et al. Segment specific branching pattern of single vestibulospinal tract axons arising from the lateral vestibular nucleus in the cervical, thoracic and lumbar segments of the cats: a PHA-L tracing study. *J Comp Neurol* 1999;414:80–96.
56. Matsuyama K, Mori S. Lumbar interneurons involved in generation of fictive locomotion in cats. *Ann NY Acad Sci* 1998;860:441–443.
57. Dow RS, Moruzzi G. *The physiology and pathology of the cerebellum.* Minneapolis: University of Minnesota Press, 1958.
58. Udo M, Matsukawa K, Kamei H, et al. Cerebellar control of locomotion: effects of cooling cerebellar intermediate cortex in high decerebrate and awake walking cats. *J Neurophysiol* 1980;44:119–134.
59. Yu J, Eidelberg E. Recovery of locomotor function in cats after localized cerebellar lesions. *Brain Res* 1983;273:121–131.
60. Chambers WW, Sprague JM. Functional localization in the cerebellum. I. Organization in longitudinal corticonuclear zones and their contribution to the control of posture, both pyramidal and extrapyramidal. *J Comp Neurol* 1955;103:105–1312.
61. Chambers WW, Sprague JM. Functional localization in the cerebellum. II. Somatotopic organization in cortex and nuclei. *Arch Neurol Psychiatr* 1955;74:653–680.
62. Asanuma C, Thach WT, Jones FG. Brainstem and spinal projections of the deep cerebellar nuclei in the monkey. *Brain Res Rev* 1983;5:237–265.
63. Cohen D, Chambers WW, Sprague JM. Experimental study of the efferent projections from the cerebellar nuclei to the brain stem of the cat. *J Comp Neurol* 1958;109:233–257.
64. Asanuma C, Thach WT, Jones FG. Distribution of cerebellar terminations and their relation to other afferent terminations in the ventral thalamic region of the monkey. *Brain Res Rev* 1983;5:237–265.
65. Rispal-Padel L, Massion J. Relations between the ventrolateral nucleus and the motor cortex in the cat. *Exp Brain Res* 1970;10:331–339.

66. Rinvik E. The corticothalamic projection from the pericruciate and coronal gyri in the cat: an experimental study with silver-impregnation methods. *Brain Res* 1968;10:79–119.
67. Kuypers HGJM. The descending pathways to the spinal cord, their anatomy and function. In: Eccles JC, Schade JP, eds. *Organization of the spinal cord.* Amsterdam: Elsevier, 1964:178–202.
68. Brodal A. *Neurological anatomy in relation to clinical medicine,* 3rd ed. Oxford: Oxford University Press, 1981.
69. Matsuyama K, Drew T, Mori F, et al. The cortico-reticulospinal system: Organization of the corticoreticular projection and fine architecture of the reticulospinal pathway in the cat. In: Gantchev G, Mori S, Massion J, eds. *Motor control today and tomorrow.* Sofia, Bulgaria: "Prof. Marin Drinov" Academic Publishing House, 1999:45–56.
70. Mori S. Integration of posture and locomotion. In: Amblard B, Berthoz A, Clarac F, eds. *Posture and gait.* Amsterdam: Excerpta Medica, 1988, 341–354.
71. Brooks VB, Thach WT. Cerebellar control of posture and movement. In: Brooks VB, ed. *Handbook of physiology.* Bethesda, MD: American Physiology Society, 1981:877–946.
72. Kably B, Drew T. Corticoreticular pathways in the cat. II. Discharge activity of neurons in area 4 during voluntary gait modifications. *J Neurophysiol* 1998;80:406–424.
73. Isa T, Sasaki S. Neural mechanisms for the control of visually guided orienting movements of the head. In: Gantchev G, Mori S, and Massion J, eds. *Motor control today and tomorrow.* Sofia, Bulgaria: "Prof. Marin Drinov" Academic Publishing House, 1999:57–69.
74. Massion J. Movement, posture and equilibrium: interactions and coordination. *Prog Neurobiol* 1993;38:35–56.

Gait Disorders. Advances in Neurology, Vol. 87,
edited by E. Růžička, M. Hallett, and J. Jankovic.
Lippincott Williams & Wilkins, Philadelphia © 2001.

4

Physiology of Human Balance

Francesco Benvenuti

Department of Geriatric Medicine, Italian National Research Institute on Aging, Florence 50125, Italy

Postural control refers to a human's ability to maintain standing balance in response to forces that threaten body equilibrium. Such control has several different aspects: maintenance of body alignment and stability in a gravitational field (quiet standing), reaction to external perturbations (pulls, pushes, variations of the base of support), and mechanical support for action (throwing, lifting, walking, running, etc.) (1,2). This distinction, although artificial, has oriented different experimental paradigms that have helped to improve understanding of balance control. This chapter focuses on the control of maintenance of body alignment and stability because new findings in recent years have improved our understanding of this aspect of the problem.

In spite of the intrinsic instability caused by the high position of the center of gravity maintained over a relatively small base of support, humans have, in terms of muscle energy, one of the most economical antigravitary mechanisms among mammals once the upright posture is attained. The *ideal* erect posture is one in which the body segments are aligned vertically and the line of gravity passes through all joint axes (3). Normal body structure makes such an *ideal* posture quite impossible to achieve, but it is possible to attain a posture that is close to the *ideal*. In normal *optimal* standing posture the line of gravity falls close to, but not through, most joint axes. The body segments are nearly vertical, the compression forces are optimally distributed over the weight-bearing surfaces of the joint, and no excessive tension is exerted on ligaments and muscles. Therefore, in normal *optimal* standing posture countertorques generated by passive ligamentous tension may balance gravitational forces and minimal muscle activity is required (4). In the sagittal plane, when the knees are in full extension and the spine assumes its natural curve through the action of its long muscles and ligaments, minimal muscle activity is recorded, in particular in triceps surae and iliopsoas muscles. In the frontal plane, given the symmetrical characteristics of the body, the gravitational torques acting on one half of the body are opposed by gravitational torques acting on the other half. Again, minimal muscle activity is recorded, in particular in gluteus medius and tensor fasciae latae muscles.

During quiet standing, even if a subject stands as still as possible, some residual sway motion occurs because the force of gravity is constantly acting on the body and joints are not rigid structures. It continuously changes the position of the line of gravity relative to individual joint axes. This sway motion needs to be limited to maintain balance. In recent years several lines of published evidence have allowed better insights into both motor strategies and the central neural mechanisms involved in the control of balance.

MOTOR STRATEGIES

Quiet standing is a voluntary task with the apparent goal of minimizing body sway over the base

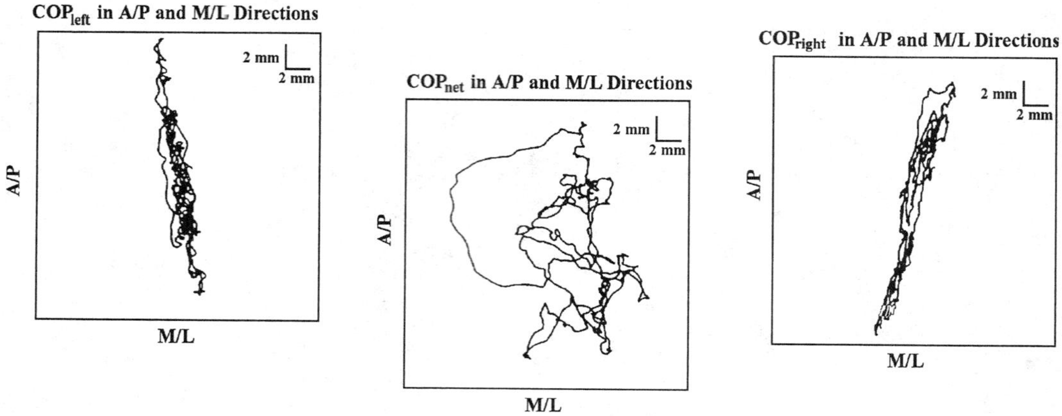

FIG. 4.1. Displacements of the left, right, and whole-body center of pressure (COP_{left}, COP_{right}, and COP_{net}, respectively) in the anterior–posterior (*A/P*) and mediolateral (*M/L*) directions in the same subject. COP_{left} and COP_{right} move back and forth but very little side to side as compared to COP_{net}. (From Winter DA. *A.B.C. (anatomy, biomechanics and control) of balance during standing and walking.* Waterloo, Canada: Waterloo Biomechanics, 1995, with permission.)

of support. Within the physiologic and biomechanical limits of the human body this goal can be achieved by using different strategies to cope with instructional and environmental demands. Subjects can adapt the position of the feet relative to each other (stance position), the distance between the feet (stance width), postural alignment, the position of the body center of mass (COM) relative to the base of support (BOS) limits, and the motor coordination between the trunk and lower limbs.

When standing, and knees are locked in a hyperextended position, four joints are below the COM of the body and may be involved for adjusting its position: the two hips and the two ankles. Ankles can either dorsiflex and plantaflex, or invert and evert. The hips can either flex and extend, or abduct and adduct. Winter et al. demonstrated that ankles and hips work through different mechanisms (5,6). The ankle mechanism generates plantar moments directly against the support surface. The hip mechanism acts by a loading/unloading mechanism on the two lower limbs. Depending on the stance position taken, many combinations of ankle mechanism and hip mechanism are used.

These two mechanisms can be evaluated by recording the center-of-pressure (COP) changes in the anterior–posterior and mediolateral direction by force platforms. The COP is the point location of the vertical ground reaction force vector (6). It represents a weighted average of all the pressure over the surface of the area in contact with the ground. If one foot is on the ground the net COP lies within that footprint. If both feet are in contact with the ground there are two COPs, one under each foot. The net COP lies somewhere between the two feet. The exact location depends on the relative weight supported by each foot. If a subject stands with both feet on a single platform the net COP is recorded. When using two force platforms it is possible to quantify COP motion within each foot (Fig. 4.1).

In the anterior–posterior direction, right and left COPs move in phase and also in phase with the net COP of the whole body (Fig. 4.2A). This does not occur in the mediolateral direction (Fig. 4.2B). Right and left COPs move out of phase and there is no relationship between them and the net COP movements. This indicates that when the feet are side-by-side ankle plantaflexor muscles dominate the anterior control of the COP, whereas ankle invertors/evertors play very little role, if any, in the control of balance in the mediolateral direction.

Figure 4.3 shows the vertical reaction force in the same subject standing with feet side-by-side. The right and left vertical reaction forces

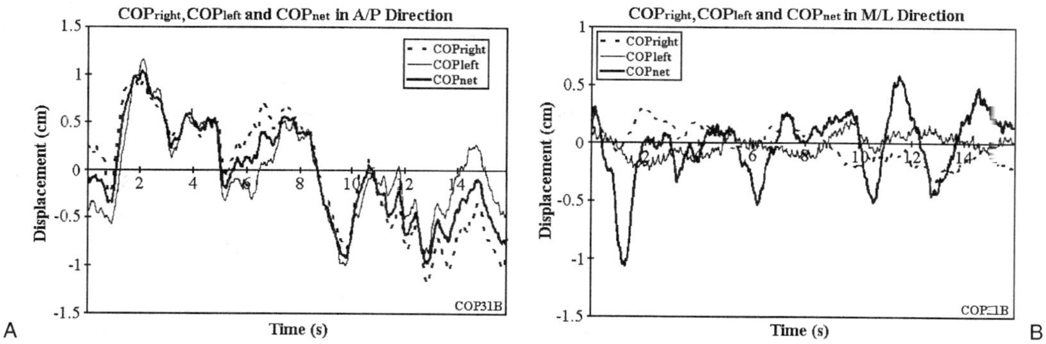

FIG. 4.2. Left, right, and whole-body center of pressure (*COP_{left}*, *COP_{right}*, and *COP_{net}*, respectively) displacements in the anterior–posterior (*A/P*) **(A)** and mediolateral (*M/L*) **(B)** directions in the same subject as Figure 4.1. In the A/P direction COP_{left} and COP_{right} move almost perfectly in phase such that COP_{net} lies almost in the middle. In the M/L direction COP_{left} and COP_{right} are almost completely out of phase and bear no relationship to COP_{net}. (For explanatory details see Figure 4.1.) (From Winter DA. *A.B.C. (anatomy, biomechanics and control) of balance during standing and walking.* Waterloo, Canada: Waterloo Biomechanics, 1995, with permission.)

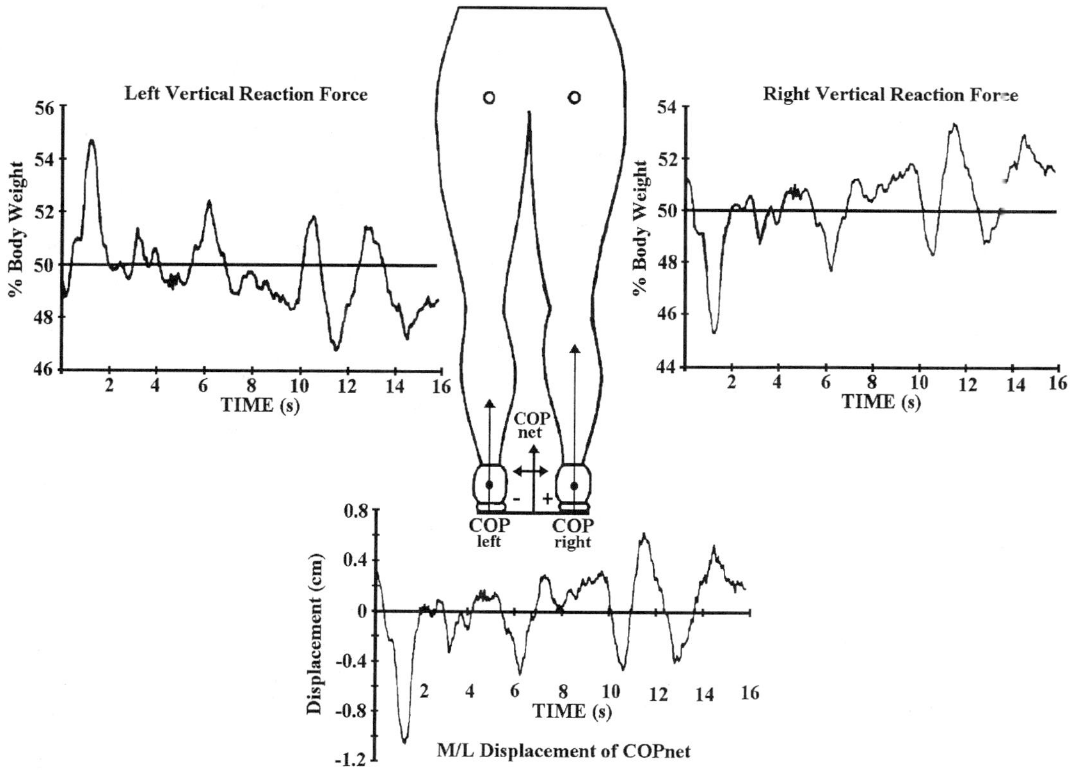

FIG. 4.3. Dynamic changes in left and right vertical ground reaction force and whole-body center of pressure (*COP_{net}*) during quiet standing in the same subject of Figure 4.1. The signals of right and left vertical ground reaction force oscillate out of phase. The mediolateral (*M/L*) displacement of COP_{net} is in phase with the right vertical reaction force. For explanatory details see Figure 4.1. (From Winter DA. *A.B.C. (anatomy, biomechanics and control) of balance during standing and walking.* Waterloo, Canada: Waterloo Biomechanics, 1995, with permission.)

are completely out of phase, which indicate a perfect mechanical coupling between the two lower limbs: When one is loaded, the other is instantaneously unloaded and vice versa. The motion of the COP of the whole body was in phase with the right vertical reaction force because the subject loaded the right side more.

The role and direction in which the two joint mechanisms act in balance control depend on the position of the feet (Fig. 4.4). As observed in the preceding, when standing with the feet side-by-side, the hip and ankle mechanisms work independently for the control of balance in the anterior–posterior and mediolateral direction. The ankle-mechanism controls the anterior–posterior sway by plantar/dorsiflexor muscles, whereas the hip mechanism controls the mediolateral sway by a loading/unloading mechanism generated by the abductor–adductor muscles. The situation changes when feet are in a tandem (heel–toe) position. The anterior–posterior balance is dominated by the hip mechanism with mixed or sometimes small or negligible contributions by the ankle plantar/dorsiflexors. For mediolateral balance the reverse is evident. Ankle invertors/evertors dominate with mixed and small contributions from the hip joint load/unload mechanism. The two mechanisms work in combination in an intermediate 45-degree stance. In the mediolateral plane the two strategies reinforce, whereas in the anterior–posterior plane the ankle mechanism must overcome and cancel most of the inappropriate contribution of the load/unload mechanism.

One of the strategies normally adopted to increase stability is to increase stance width. Day et al. studied how body segments move relative to each other in the frontal and sagittal plane and how this motion was affected by the distance between the feet (7). They found that the increase of stance width had a great effect on reducing body sway, mostly in the mediolateral plane, both with eyes open or closed. The large reduction in lateral body sway with increasing stance was mainly caused by a disproportionate reduction of angular joint motion about the ankles in the mediolateral plane.

Day et al. provided two explanations, the first being based on a mechanical model of the skeletal structure (7). If it were possible to stand with both ankle joints coincident, the lower limbs would be locked in a triangular position, which is mechanically not deformable. The only muscles able to prevent lateral rotation would be invertors/evertors of the ankle. Increasing the lateral distance between the feet allows the hip muscles to play a part in stabilizing lateral sway in addition to those of the ankles. The structure is made stiffer when feet are moved apart because more muscles are involved. The second reason

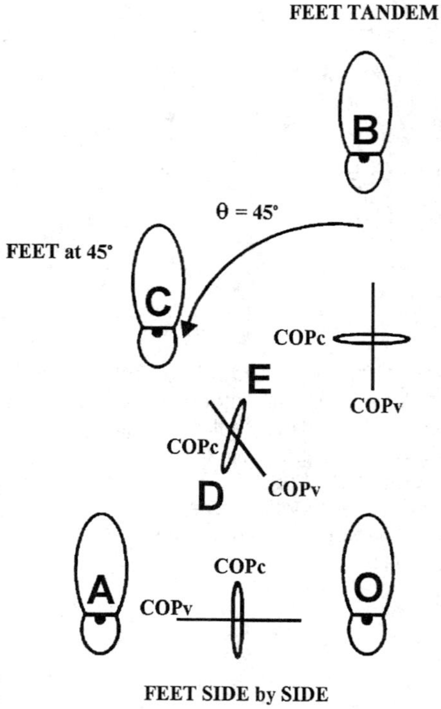

FIG. 4.4. Summary of the trajectories of the two separate mechanisms in three stance positions. The center of pressure hip load/unload mechanism (*COPV*) always acts along a line joining the individual *COPs* under each foot, whereas the center of pressure ankle mechanism (*COPC*) acts at 90 degrees (side-by-side and tandem) or at an angle less than 90 degrees in the intermediate positions. In the side-by-side and tandem positions the two mechanisms are independent; in the intermediate positions there is collaboration between hip and ankle mechanisms. (From Winter DA. *A.B.C. (anatomy, biomechanics and control) of balance during standing and walking.* Waterloo, Canada: Waterloo Biomechanics, 1995, with permission.)

TABLE 4.1. *List of variables in the posturographic protocol*

Variable	Definition
Postural motion	
COM-AREA	[COM sway area (mm^2)/base of support (mm^2)] · 100
COM-VEL	COM mean velocity ($mm \cdot sec^{-1}$)/COM height (m)
COP-VEL	COP mean velocity ($mm \cdot sec^{-1}$)/COM height (m)
Direction of postural movements	
DPM	Ratio of anterior–posterior and medio-lateral COP maximum excursions
Postural alignment (sagittal plane)	
HI-AN	Mean hip joint angle in the sagittal plane (degrees)
KN-AN	Mean knee joint angle in the sagittal plane (degrees)
AN-AN	Mean ankle joint angle in the sagittal plane (degrees)
Body position	
COP-AP	[COP distance from ankles (mm) in the sagittal plane/length of base of support (mm)] · 100.
COP-ML	[COP distance from left foot (mm) in the frontal plane/width of base of support (mm)] · 100.
COM-HEIGHT	[COM vertical position (m)/maximum theoretical height of cephalic end of the trunk (m)] · 100.
Motor coordination	
COO-AP	Correlation coefficient between the positions of the COMs of the trunk and the lower limbs in the sagittal plane.
COO-ML	Correlation coefficient between the positions of the COMs of the trunk and the lower limbs in the frontal plane.

AN-AN, ankle angle; AP, anterior–posterior; COM, center of mass; COM-AREA, COM sway area; COM-VEL, COM mean velocity; COO, correlation coefficient; COP, center of pressure; DPM, direction of postural movements; HI-AN, hip angle; KN-AN, knee angle; ML, medio-lateral.

for stabilization of lateral sway with wider bases of support could be that the more muscles are involved in the control of standing posture, the more proprioceptive input on which the central nervous system (CNS) can base reflex corrective adjustments.

During quiet standing humans behave not as a rigid but as a flexible inverted pendulum (5,7,8). Maintaining postural stability requires control of both position and momentum of the center-of-mass (COM), which is achieved by small postural movements at the level of different joints (9,10).

The problem arises how humans modify postural control strategies during quiet standing in response to changes in visual information, support surface size, and compliance characteristics. To answer this question we studied 30 healthy young subjects (age 27 ± 5 years, 16 men, and 14 women) by using a posturographic protocol designed to quantify the characteristics of balance control (11). The validity and reliability of the fundamental variables of the protocol have been determined (12). Subjects stood "as still as possible" for 20 seconds during eight separate postural tasks designed to evaluate the effects of three independent factors: vision [eyes open (EO) or closed (EC)], support surface compliance [solid surface (SS), or compliant (CS)], and base of support size (BOS) [large base (LB) or narrow (NB)]. Whole-body and segmental positions were measured using a video based ELITE movement analysis system. A single force platform provided a combined center of pressure (COP) measurement for both feet.

The main variables of the protocol are summarized in Table 4.1. COM sway area (COM-AREA), COM mean velocity (COM-VEL) in the horizontal plane, and COP mean velocity (COP-VEL) are used to describe *postural sway*. The *direction of postural movements* (DPM) is determined using a ratio of anterior–posterior and mediolateral COP maximum excursions. *Body alignment* is determined from mean hip, knee, and ankle angles in the sagittal plane (HI-AN, KN-AN, AN-AN). COP average position with respect to the anterior–posterior (COP-AP) and mediolateral (COP-ML) limits of the base of support indicated *body position*. Finally, *motor*

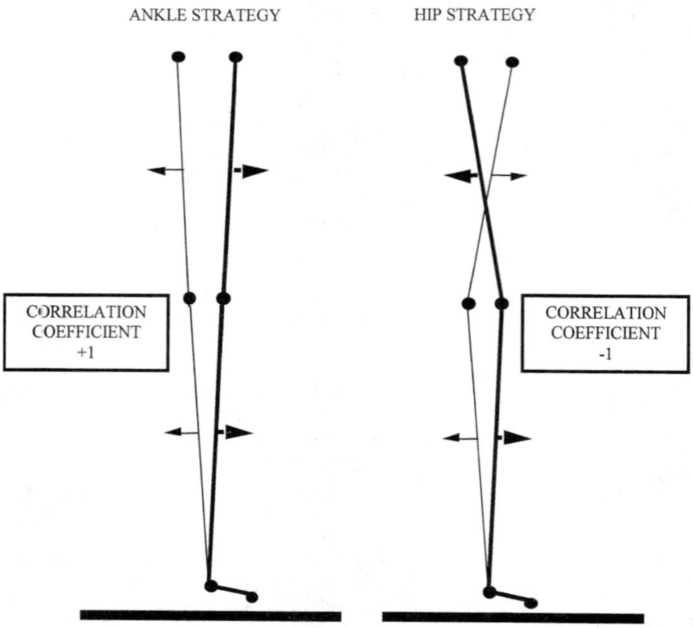

FIG. 4.5. Schematic figure representing hip and ankle postural strategies in the sagittal plane. In a pure ankle strategy, the center of mass COMs of the trunk and the lower limbs move in phase. Thus, the correlation coefficient between the positions of the two COMs is +1. In the hip strategy the forward acceleration of the trunk during hip flexion passively assists the extension of the ankles and vice versa. Thus, the two COMs move in opposite directions and the correlation coefficient is −1.

coordination between the trunk and lower limbs is indicated by correlating the anterior–posterior (COO-AP) and mediolateral (COO-ML) trunk and combined lower limb COM positions (Fig. 4.5). Repeated measures ANOVAs were used for comparison. The level of statistical significance was $P < 0.05$.

Means of the variables that showed statistically significant differences across the eight conditions are summarized in Fig. 4.6. Postural sway (COM-AREA, COM-VEL, and COP-VEL) was greatest in the EC, CS, and NB conditions. The three independent factors had an interaction effect on all postural sway measures. The DPM was influenced only by the BOS factor (increase in the mediolateral motion in the NB condition). Body position was influenced by support surface compliance. COP-AP was more anterior in the CS condition. There was an interaction effect between surface compliance and BOS on the ankle joint angles. There was greater dorsiflexion in the CS than the NB condition. Closing the eyes increased hip flexion slightly. Finally, COO-AP was higher in CS conditions, whereas COO-ML was higher in both CS and NB conditions with an interaction effect between BOS and surface compliance.

Body sway and postural motor strategies were differently influenced by the modification of the three independent factors. Eliminating vision alone resulted in a decreased effectiveness of the normal balance strategy. Decreasing the BOS size and introducing a compliant surface both resulted in a decreased control of sway and more interestingly in an alteration of the postural control strategy as determined by changes in postural alignment, body position, and motor coordination. We concluded that in normal subjects perturbation of vision alone has little effect on balance control strategies, possibly given the great redundancy of afferent information. However, decreasing the physical limits of stability (by decreasing the BOS size) and the dynamics of ankle joint moments

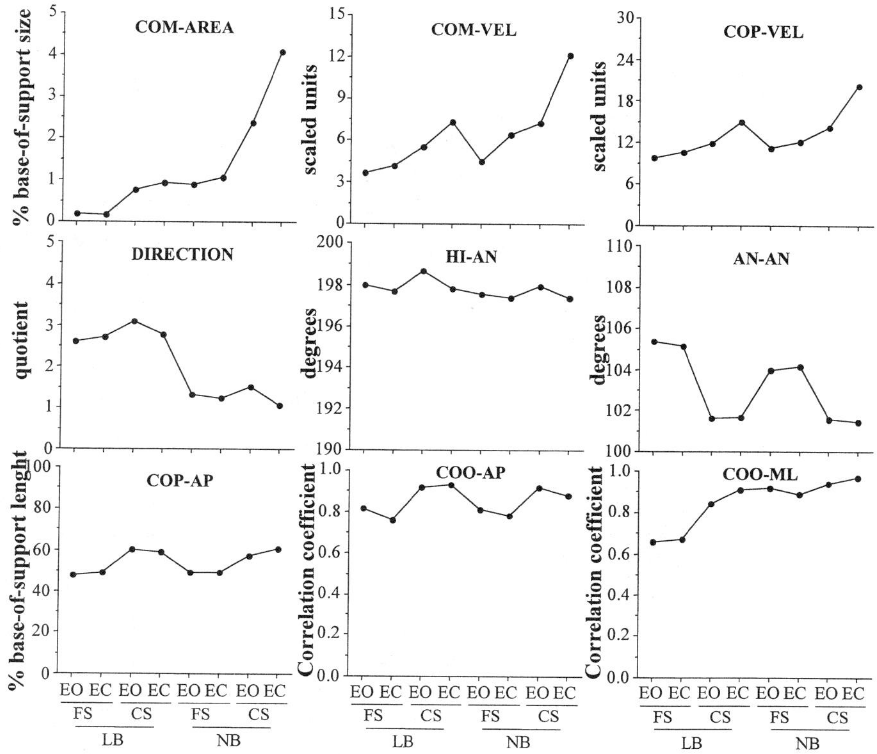

FIG. 4.6. Means of the variables that showed statistically significant differences across the eight postural tasks that were designed to evaluate the effects of vision [eyes open (*EO*) or closed (*EC*)], support surface compliance [solid surface (SS), or compliant (*CS*)], and BOS size [large base (*LB*) or narrow (*NB*)]. For definitions of variables see Table 4.1.

(by introducing a compliant surface) produces adaptive motor strategies that are less effective in the performance of this quiet standing task.

Cutaneous foot sole sensors and foot muscle proprioceptors monitor the amplitude and direction of the contact forces exerted by the body onto the ground (13–16). Replacing a firm support surface by a compliant support surface results in postural instability. This disturbs not only the dynamics of ankle joint moments but also impairs afferent inputs from the feet (13,14). In this connection, the more anterior position of the COM and the more flexed ankle position that we observed in the CS conditions could be aimed at adjusting the level of ankle stiffness, because it depends on the moment carried on the joint (17). The choice could be based on the trade-off between the accuracy of measurements and the requirement of minimal loading or minimal expenditure of energy (8). The finding of forward body inclination during space flights, when significant diminution of loading of ankle extensors challenged load estimation and measurements, supports this hypothesis (18).

As stated in the preceding, during quiet standing the body behaves not as a rigid but as a flexible inverted pendulum because small but significant motion occurs at the level of different joints and in particular of the hip joint (5,7,8). We found that the COMs of trunk and lower limbs tended to move in phase because the correlation coefficients were always high both in the frontal and sagittal plane. Further, the coordination was increased in the most demanding CS and/or NB conditions. This indicates that motion of the upper part of the body is not stochastic but differently checked by the neural control system to cope with balance demands of the different postural tasks.

CENTRAL NEURAL MECHANISMS

The intrinsic instability of human quiet standing posture requires continuous corrections to maintain the position of the COM within narrow limits. This depends on the integrity of the CNS, which receives and processes sensory information (visual, vestibular, proprioceptive) and gives these different inputs a different weight on the basis of the specific circumstances to map the position of COM in space. The CNS then sets the appropriate motor outputs to maintain body position or correct it, if needed.

Hellembrand introduced the concept of the stretch reflex strategy where the shift of the COM constantly stimulates stretch afferents of postural muscles that then contract reflexively (19). This strategy was questioned because the angular motion at the ankle during quiet standing was less than necessary to elicit stretch reflex (20). Gurfinkel and colleagues performed extensive experiments on the contributions of central neural mechanisms to posture during quiet standing (21,22). They proved that the excitability level of the monosynaptic stretch reflex decreased during stance, compared to less demanding postural tasks such as lying down, sitting, or standing with support. They also found that a mechanism by which the CNS controls balance could be that of setting a certain muscle tone (23). Then the viscoelastic properties of muscles would do the rest according to their length-tension characteristics. They studied subjects standing on a platform that could be tilted at a very low speed (0.6 deg/sec) for very small amplitudes (0.1–0.2 deg), thus causing very little dorsiflexion of the ankle joint and gentle stretch of triceps surae. They observed periods of considerable changes of ankle movements and of relatively calm portions during standing conditions. They performed their experiments during the calm periods.

They observed that during these calm periods, variations of ankle joint angle and moments were not accompanied by significant variations in the electromyographic (EMG) activity in lateral gastrocnemius muscles both during unperturbed standing and when the platform was gently rotated. Nevertheless, the magnitude of torques generated at the ankle were the same or slightly greater than those required to maintain balance. Finally, although the perturbations applied by tilting the force platform exceeded the threshold of muscle receptors, no active reaction to stretching was observed. They concluded that in conditions of vertical stance supraspinal influences raise the threshold of the stretch reflex and that the intrinsic stiffness of the ankle muscles, because of their length-tension characteristics, could be sufficient to passively maintain quiet standing balance in humans. However, standing while relying on the visco-elastic properties of the muscles, although possible, seems dangerous, because relatively minor perturbations might cause a fall. Indeed, they also found that about 350 ms after the onset of ankle movement, the activity in triceps surae EMG fell. Thus it seems likely that viscoelastic properties of muscles could represent a sort of first-aid intervention for restoring balance when COM acceleration is very little. However, in the long-term and/or for greater disturbances, adjustment of joint muscle stiffness is necessary. This implies an ongoing control of the CNS.

Visual, vestibular, and somatosensory inputs contribute to stabilization of posture (1,24). The use of varied sensory information is needed because the different types of balance disturbance do not stimulate the whole set of sensors and the sensitivity range of each category of sensors is different. Thus, the remarkable redundancy of afferent information allows phenomena of adaptation to an extreme variety of environmental demands as well as phenomena of compensation in response to pathological damage. When they are all removed it is impossible to stand unassisted as shown in a classical experiment of Horak et al. (25).

Fitzpatrick and coworkers provided evidence on the role of visual, vestibular, and somatosensory inputs in the reflex control of ankle stiffness in response to slow and gentle postural disturbances of quiet stance (26). Subjects stood on rigid platforms. Angle and torques were measured at the right ankle. They stood either unperturbed or imperceptibly perturbed by a servomotor. The perturbations caused sway similar in magnitude and rate to the sway of normal stance (imperceptible). To modify the intentional set, subjects were requested to stand either at ease or still. They were also studied in an "equivalent task" designed to simulate standing but to exclude changes in visual or vestibular inputs. To exclude changes in visual or vestibular inputs subjects were strapped to a rigid post both at their head and waist. Using their feet they had to balance a load similar to the load on their ankles when standing. They found that ankles stiffness increased when posture was imperceptibly perturbed and even more when subjects where asked to stand still. Further, ankle stiffness, as compared to the conditions when all types of inputs were available, decreased with eyes closed, and even more when both vestibular and visual inputs were removed. Thus, they provided evidence that visual, vestibular, and somatosensory sensorimotor reflexes contribute to ankle stiffness and that ankles stiffness can be altered according to the intentional set.

Collins and De Luca used a "random walk" model to study center of pressure excursions (27). Their stabilogram-diffusion plots (mean square of COP displacement versus time interval) showed two regions: one short-term and one long-term region. They hypothesized that at least two control mechanisms were operating during quiet standing. Over short-term intervals (up to about 1 second) open-loop control schemes are utilized by the postural control system. Over longer intervals, closed loop mechanisms are called into play. Because skeletal muscles are incapable of producing purely constant forces, these open-loop activation signals result in small mechanical fluctuations at various joints of the body (28). These fluctuations would be left unchecked by the postural control system until they exceed some systematic threshold, after which corrective feedback mechanisms are called into play. Within this conceptual model, the CNS still continually receives afferent information from peripheral sensory organs. However, such information is not used to modulate the efferent signals transmitted to the postural muscles unless a certain threshold value is exceeded. This open-loop/closed-loop control strategy, which allows certain sloppiness in balance control, may have evolved to take into account the inherent time delays of feedback

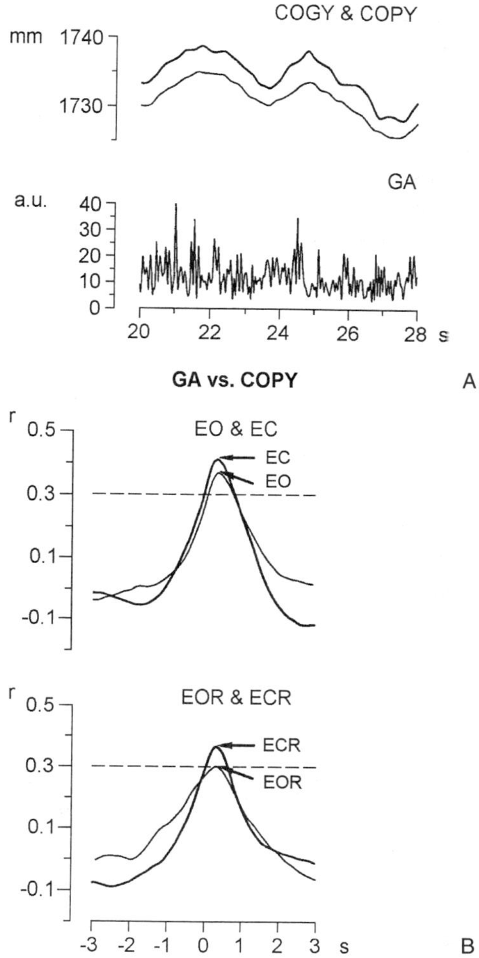

FIG. 4.7. A: Data from an epoch form 20th to 28th second of a single trial in one subject during standing with normal stance width and eyes closed. From top to bottom: anterior–posterior motion of center of gravity (*COGY*) and center of pressure (*COPY*) and lateral gastrocnemius muscle activity (*GA*) [*a.u.*, arbitrary units]. **B:** Cross-correlation function aggregated for the whole group of subjects between the right gastrocnemius muscle activity and the anterior–posterior motion of the center of pressure (GA versus COPY). **Top:** during standing with normal stance width with eyes open (*EO*) or closed (*EC*); **bottom:** during standing with narrow stance width (Romberg stance) and eyes open (*EOR*) or closed (*ECR*). (From Gatev P, Thomas S, Kepple T, et al. Feedforward ankle strategy of balance during quiet stance in adults. *J Physiol* 1999;514:915–928, with permission.)

loops and to simplify the task of integrating vast amounts of sensory information when the system is not in jeopardy of instability.

Recently, Gatev et al. found direct evidence for a feedforward control mechanism in the control of quiet standing by using cross-correlation techniques between kinematic, kinetic, and EMG data (8). They found that the EMG activity of the lateral gastrocnemius increases when the center of gravity (COG) moves forward and conversely decreases when the COG moves backward (Fig. 4.7). Further, they found that gastrocnemius muscle activity precedes the pattern of COG and COP excursions in sagittal plane. The cross-correlation function showed a positive correlation with time lags of the maximum of 250 to 300 ms.

Because of the position of the COG in front of the ankles, the forward movement of the COG leads to increased forward bending force and loading of ankle plantar flexors. The opposite occurs when the COG moves backward. This association with a positive sense agrees with the tensionlike servo control hypothesis for balance maintenance in which a muscle contracts when loaded and stays contracted until unloaded (29). However, their findings indicate that muscle activity changes are predictive of loading and not responsive to loading as in the case of a simple servo system.

In conclusion, it seems likely that quiet standing balance might be controlled by motor output signals generated by two parallel processors. A "continuous processor" works continuously to provide feedback compensation. A "stimulus-response processor" uses sensory information and/or internal commands to trigger preprogrammed responses. It seems likely, in particular when standing in dangerous conditions, that the adaptive control might arise mainly from a flexible "stimulus-response processor" rather than from alteration of the gain of a continuous feedback mechanism (8).

ACKNOWLEDGMENTS

The author wishes to thank Tito Pantaleo, Steven J. Stanhope, and Mark Hallett for reading and commenting on the manuscript.

REFERENCES

1. Massion J, Woollacott MH. Posture and equilibrium. In: Bronstein AM, Brandt T, Woollacott MH, eds. *Clinical disorders of balance posture and gait.* London: Arnold, 1996:1–18.
2. Nashner LM. Physiology of balance, with special reference to healthy aging. In: Masdeu JC, Sudarsky L, Wolfson L, eds. *Gait disorders of aging: falls and therapeutic strategies.* Philadephia: Lippincott-Raven, 1997:37–53.
3. Norkin CC, Lavangie PK. *Joint structure and function: a comprehensive analysis*, 2nd ed. Philadelphia: F.A. Davis, 1992.
4. Basmajian JV, De Luca C. *Muscle alive. Their function revealed by electromyography*. Baltimore: Williams & Wilkins, 1985.
5. Winter DA, Prince F, Frank JS, et al. Unified theory regarding A/P and M/L balance in quiet stance. *J Neurophysiol* 1996;75:2334–2343.
6. Winter DA. *A.B.C. (anatomy, biomechanics and control) of balance during standing and walking.* Waterloo, Canada: Waterloo Biomechanics, 1995.
7. Day BL, Steiger MJ, Thompson PD, et al. Effect of vision and stance width on human body motion when standing: implications for afferent control of lateral sway. *J Physiol* 1993;469:479–499.
8. Gatev P, Thomas S, Kepple T, et al. Feedforward ankle strategy of balance during quiet stance in adults. *J Physiol* 1999;514:915–928.
9. Riley PO, Benda BJ, Gill-Body KM, et al. Phase plane analysis of stability in quiet standing. *J Rehabil Res Dev* 1995;32:227–235.
10. Jeka J, Oie K, Schoner G, et al. Position and velocity coupling of postural sway to somatosensory drive. *J Neurophysiol* 1998;79:1661–1674.
11. Benvenuti F, Mecacci R, Landini L, et al. Balance control during quiet standing: adaptation to changes in base of support and absent vision. *Gait Posture* 1999;9:147.
12. Benvenuti F, Mecacci R, Gineprari I, et al. Kinematic characteristics of standing disequilibrium: reliability and validity of a posturographic protocol. *Arch Phys Med Rehabil* 1999;80:278–287.
13. Di Fabio RP, Badke MB, McEvoy A, et al. Influence of local sensory afference in the calibration of human balance responses. *Exp Brain Res* 1990;80:591–599.
14. Teasdale N, Stelmach GE, Breunig A. Postural sway characteristics of the elderly under normal and altered visual and support surface conditions. *J Gerontol Biol Sci* 1991;46:B238–244.
15. Wu G, Chiang JH. The significance of somatosensory stimulations to the human foot in the control of postural reflexes. *Exp Brain Res* 1997;114:163–169.
16. Kavounoudias A, Roll R, Roll JP. The plantar sole is a 'dynamometric map' for human balance control. *Neuroreport* 1998;9:3247–3252.
17. Bergmark, A. Stability of the lumbar spine. A study in mechanical engineering. *Acta Orthop Scand* 1989;230:1–54.
18. Clement G, Gurfinkel VS, Lestienne F, et al. Adaptation of postural control to weightlessness. *Exp Brain Res* 1984;57:61–72.
19. Hellebrandt FA. Standing as a geotropic reflex. The mechanism of the asynchronous rotation of motor units. *Am J Physiol* 1938;121:471–474.

20. Kelton IW, Wright RD. The mechanisms of easy standing by man. *Aust J Exp Biol Med* 1949;27:505–516.
21. Elner AM, Gurfinkel VS, Lipshits MI. Facilitation of stretch reflex by additional support during quiet stance. *Agressologie* 1976;17:15–20.
22. Gurfinkel VS, Lipshits MI, Popov KY. Kinestetic threshold in orthograde posture. Facilitation of stretch reflex by additional support during quiet stance. *Agressologie* 1979;20:133–134.
23. Gurfinkel VS, Lipshits MI, Popov KY. Is the stretch reflex the main mechanism in the system of regulation of the vertical posture of man? *Biofizika* 1974;4:744–748.
24. Horak FB, Shupert CL, Mirka A. Components of postural dyscontrol in the elderly. *Neurobiol Aging* 1989;10:727–738.
25. Horak FB, Nashner LM, Diener HC. Postural strategies associated with somatosensory and vestibular loss. *Exp Brain Res* 1990;82:167–177.
26. Fitzpatrick RC, Taylor JL, McCloskey DI. Ankle stiffness of standing humans in response to imperceptible perturbation: reflex and task-dependent components. *J Physiol* 1992;454:533–547.
27. Collins JJ, De Luca CJ. Open-loop and closed-loop control of posture: a random walk analysis of center-of-pressure trajectories. *Exp Brain Res* 1993;95:308–318.
28. De Luca CJ, LeFever RS, McCue MP, et al. Control scheme governing concurrently active human motor units during voluntary contractions. *J Physiol* 1982;329:129–142.
29. Walsh EG. Possible factors in postural sway. In: Walsh EG, ed. *Cerebellum, posture and cerebral palsy*. London: Little Club Clinics N.3, Heinemann, 1963:31–37.

Gait Disorders. Advances in Neurology, Vol. 87,
edited by E. Růžička, M. Hallett, and J. Jankovic.
Lippincott Williams & Wilkins, Philadelphia © 2001.

5

Physiology of Human Gait

Neural Processes

Volker Dietz

Department of Paraplegiology, University of Zurich; and Swiss Paraplegic Center, University Hospital Balgrist, CH-8008 Zurich, Switzerland

In the 18th century, the investigation of movement was grounded on the perception that upright stance and gait, in association with the differentiation of hand movements, represented a basic requirement for human cultural development (1). The consequence of this specific human behavior is that the nervous system automatically has to balance the body's center of mass over the feet during all motor activities performed in a bipedal posture: Every movement necessarily begins and ends with a postural adjustment.

In physiology, the methodical analysis of human gait began at the end of the 19th century with the development of photographic recordings of running movements by Marey (2). Later Bernstein resumed gait analysis using biomechanical recordings (3). Electrophysiological recordings during locomotion were first performed in cats (4,5).

Regulation of *human bipedal stance and gait* is in some aspects fundamentally different from that of quadrupedal locomotion as specific neuronal mechanisms are required to maintain the body in an upright position. The spinal stretch reflex has been suggested as functioning so as to adapt the preprogrammed leg muscle motor patterns to the terrain encountered and to compensate for unexpected changes in ground level (6,7). Although this neuronal mechanism explains quick unilateral patterns of reflex activity in leg extensor muscles, a more complex, bilateral coordination of leg muscle activation is needed to maintain the body equilibrium when an obstacle disturbs gait.

Discussions of the relative significance of reflexes on central rhythms and programming in locomotion were presented from the beginning of these investigations. Hoffmann described the monosynaptic pathway as the simplest spinal feedback system (8). Hoffmann emphasized that in humans the *Eigenreflexapparat* is responsible for the adaptation of the muscle innervation to unexpected strains. Foerster suggested that slow stretch reflexes and "adaptational reflexes" made an essential contribution to motor coordination (9). In cats, the locomotor pattern, however, is preserved after complete deafferentation; therefore, the theory of a "reflex chain" as the basis for the generation of the rhythmic alternating movements and, consequently, for locomotion, has been discarded (10,11). Instead, it was suggested that a spinal generator is responsible for locomotion (12). Grillner proposed that the spinal locomotor center [central pattern generator (CPG)] is activated and controlled by the brainstem and is also influenced by peripheral feedback mechanisms (13).

Central generators and programs interacting with peripheral reflexes represent, however, only a portion of the mechanisms involved in the control of locomotion: The control of human locomotion utilizes afferent information from a variety of sources within the visual, vestibular, and proprioceptive systems. The convergence of spinal reflex pathways and descending tracts on common spinal interneurons is the rule and plays an integrative role (14). The shortcomings of human studies in this field reflect the fact that the function of human motor control mechanisms usually can be gathered only by indirect methods and must be interpreted, to a large part, on the basis of knowledge gained from animal experiments. Although there are obviously some common features between the pattern of activity and the underlying neuronal mechanisms during quadripedal locomotion in cats and that seen during bipedal gait of humans, distinct differences exist and are, indeed, a requirement of the bipedal condition (13,15,16).

Irrespective of the conditions under which gait is investigated, the neuronal pattern evoked during a particular task is always directed to hold the body's center of mass over the base of support. One consequence is that the selection of afferent input by central mechanisms must correspond to the actual requirements for body stabilization. Furthermore, the neuronal signals of muscle stretch or length alone are insufficient for the control of upright posture. All control mechanisms must, therefore, be considered and discussed in this respect. Only a combination of afferent input can provide information needed to control the body equilibrium.

There is a general agreement that locomotor movements in mammals depend primarily on neuronal mechanisms in the spinal cord that can act in the absence of any afferent input (13). Afferent information is, nevertheless, essential for the execution of locomotion to adjust the spinal pattern to the external requirements (13,17–19). Both the spinal locomotor centers and the reflex mechanisms are under the control of the brainstem and supraspinal motor centers (Fig. 5.1) (20). Further refinement is achieved by a supraspinal contribution namely via cerebellum (21).

In several aspects the neurophysiology of normal human gait has again to rely on the knowledge of the neuronal basis of animal locomotion. For more detailed information about this field the reader is referred to Grillner (13) and Baldissera and coworkers (22). Biomechanical aspects of posture and gait are discussed only with respect to corresponding neuronal events, although it is obvious that neuronal mechanisms are part of biomechanical strategies as well as constrained by biomechanics (23). The neurophysiology of human gait will be centered on central programming and reflex behavior during locomotion.

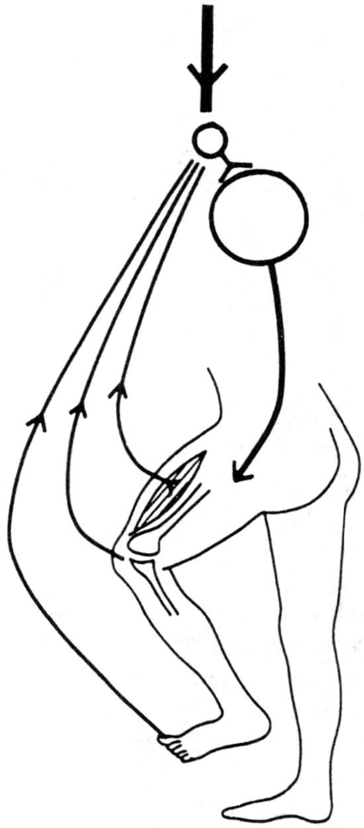

FIG. 5.1. Schematic drawing of the neuronal mechanisms involved in human gait. Leg muscles become activated by a programmed pattern generated within spinal interneuronal circuits. This pattern is modulated by a multisensory afferent input that adapts the pattern to the actual requirements. Both the programmed pattern and the reflex mechanisms are under supraspinal control. (From Jankowska E, Lundberg A. Interneurones in the spinal cord. *Trends Neurosci* 1981;4:230–233, with permission.)

CENTRAL PROGRAMMING

A motor program has been variously defined in the literature as "communications in the CNS that are based on past experience and that can generate postural adjustments and movements" or as "a set of muscle commands that are structured before a movement sequence begins and that allows entire sequence to be carried out uninfluenced by peripheral feedback" (24,25). For human gait, both definitions must be expanded in that, concerning the first definition, programs are not only based on experience but are also innate: Steplike movements are present at birth, spontaneously initiated, or triggered by peripheral stimuli. The central origin of these movements may be assumed, because the electromyographic (EMG) bursts precede the actual mechanical events (26).

With regard to the second definition of central programming, it has to be considered that "programmed" movements can be influenced by sensory input under some circumstances (24). This is illustrated by infant stepping. Although a central generator coordinates rhythmic alternating-leg movements, the infant is unable to maintain body equilibrium. In these children appropriate afferent information and integration in the programmed leg muscle EMG to achieve modulation and adaptation to the actual needs is absent in the immature state.

For a purposeful movement it is reasonable to assume that afferent information influences the central pattern and, conversely, that the central pattern generator selects the appropriate afferent information. In addition, the programmed motor response in humans can be altered by instruction or expectation. This "set"-dependent aspect of muscle response is thought to depend on cerebellar integrity (27,28). Furthermore, voluntary commands have to interact with the spinal locomotor generator in order, for example, to change the direction of gait or to avoid a visually recognized obstacle.

Recently the significance of corticospinal input on the gait pattern was investigated by transcranial magnetic stimulation of the motor cortex during locomotion (29). Only in the tibialis anterior an extrafacilitation of the evoked motor response was present prior to and in the middle of the swing phase of the stride cycle. This phase-linked facilitation was suggested to ensure postural stability in the case of a corticospinal intervention during locomotion. Furthermore, it could be shown that visual or volitional control of stepping has a conditioning effect on the motor responses (30).

A characteristic of human standing posture and gait is a high center of gravity being maintained over a relatively small base of support at the feet. To maintain constant vertical stance, postural adjustments are required. For the investigation of the mechanisms underlying the equilibrium control, perturbations have been elicited, for example, by backward or forward translation of the base of support or obstruction of the swinging leg. Directionally specific compensatory responses are induced in synergistic muscles of both legs after these perturbations.

The activity pattern to such perturbations is thought to be in large part programmed, although a reflex contribution affecting the duration of the first burst of the pattern has been demonstrated (31). The muscle response to a given displacement differs according to the actual conditions of gait: For example, an obstruction is introduced at the beginning or the end of the swing phase or displacement of the feet is induced during stance on a narrow support (32,33). For the selection of the appropriate postural movement strategy, studies performed on subjects with somatosensory or vestibular loss indicate that both modes of sensory information can play an important role (34).

The assumption that the various response patterns to perturbations of stance and gait are programmed in their basic structure (presumably on a spinal level) and appropriately selected (i.e., triggered) is based on the complexity of the patterns that cannot be explained by local afferent inputs and the dependence of the response pattern on the actual conditions (i.e., phase of the step cycle).

Furthermore, regulation of human locomotion is based on the finely tuned *coordination of muscle activation between the two legs*. The usual automatic coordination of the movement of both legs requires that adequate neuronal mechanisms exist to achieve task-directed coupling of bilateral leg muscle activation. The interlimb coordination is necessary to keep the body's center of gravity over the feet. Bilateral activation of corresponding leg muscles occurs during unilateral displacement (35). The rapid automatic cocontraction of the nondisplaced leg provides a base from which to compensate for the perturbation and to keep the body's center of gravity over the feet. During bilateral perturbation, the destabilization of body equilibrium is greater than during unilateral perturbation. The mutual enhancement of the response amplitude seen during the latter condition allows more effective contractile force to compensate the perturbation. A displacement of the legs in opposite directions requires a reduced level of compensatory responses to regain body equilibrium in that condition (35). Also unilateral tactile stimuli evoke a bilateral response pattern, which is modulated in a phase-dependent manner (36).

It is thought that interlimb coordination is based on a central mechanism, and in view of the short latencies of the bilateral responses, mediated at a spinal level (35–38). A cerebellar contribution to interlimb coordination, via reticulospinal neurons, can be assumed (39). A close interaction exists between the spinal interneuronal circuits responsible for interlimb coordination and the peripheral afferent input. When displacements of different velocity are induced unilaterally, reflex responses in synergistic muscles of both legs are graded according to the size of the proprioceptive input from the primarily displaced joint (35). The spinal coordination is assumed to be under supraspinal control, as the bilateral EMG pattern is disrupted in patients with spasticity (38).

The question arises about the localization of the locomotor pattern generator within the spinal cord. To answer this question stepping movements were induced in patients with complete paraplegia or tetraplegia and their locomotor pattern was analyzed (40).

It was found that the higher the level of spinal cord lesion the more "normal" the locomotor pattern. This suggests that neuronal circuits underlying locomotor "pattern generation" in humans are not restricted to any specific level(s) of the spinal cord, but that an intricate neuronal network contributing to bipedal locomotion extends from thoraco-lumbar to cervical levels.

REFLEX MECHANISMS

There exists a body of evidence, for example, from the postural instability (41–43) and gait impairment (44) seen in deafferented humans or subjects after loss of proprioceptive input from the legs owing to ischemic nerve blockade (45,46), that the contribution of proprioceptive input to the regulation of stance and locomotion is not "mild," as suggested by Sherrington (47). Feedback information from muscles, joints, and associated tissues mediated by proprioceptive reflex systems is required to adjust the motor program to irregularities of the ground during walking or respond if the leg encounters resistance. This proprioceptive input modulates muscle EMG activity in the legs during locomotion in connection with changes in tension that closely correlate with the level of EMG activity during different speeds of locomotion (48). Although proprioceptive information may be used to achieve servoregulation of, for example, muscle length during stabilization of posture, this represents only a restricted part of the way in which the nervous system utilizes proprioceptive input. Spinal reflex responses are not stereotyped to a given sensory input, but, depending on the descending and segmental conditions, different available pathways are utilized (14). This part of the review is centered on the action and possible significance of monosynaptic and polysynaptic spinal reflexes.

Significance of Monosynaptic Reflexes

The potential significance of the group I afferent reflex system for locomotion is based on the fact that its gain can be modulated by presynaptic inhibition and by changes of muscle spindle sensitivity through the fusimotor system (49–51). In the last few years modulation of presynaptic inhibition of group I afferents has been investigated by indirect methods in humans during gait (52–54). Both peripheral afferent inputs and supraspinal influences have been implicated in the modulation of presynaptic inhibition of transmission from primary afferents (22). This modulation of reflex gain might take place on common spinal interneurons where a convergence of descending tracts and several different afferent systems occurs (12,22,55). For spinal motor systems, presynaptic inhibition provides a way to modulate the relative contribution of afferents to a reflex.

During locomotion, the threshold and amplitude of the soleus/gastrocnemius H-reflex is modulated over the entire step cycle, with a maximal facilitation during the end of the stance phase and maximal inhibition during the swing and the beginning of stance (52,56). Over the entire step cycle, however, the H-reflex amplitude of the leg extensor muscles is considerably smaller than during stance (52–54,57).

Earlier studies have indicated that monosynaptic stretch reflexes are inhibited in much the same way as the H-reflex during gait, which also implies that there is no dramatic change in the gamma drive to soleus/gastrocnemius muscle spindles (37,58–60). Recent experiments in humans indicate that a modulation of short latency stretch reflex takes place during the step cycle with a significant reflex contribution during transition from stance to swing and at the early stance phase (61). In the latter experiments a foot dorsiflexing rotational displacement was applied during different phases of the step cycle. However, a qualitatively different response pattern with a small or lacking short-latency stretch reflex response was obtained for similar stretches of the triceps surae, when a backward translation is induced during stance and gait (37,62–64). The discrepancy between the different experiments investigating the contribution of short latency stretch reflexes to the leg muscle activation during gait may be owing to the mode of displacement with the consequence that a different contribution of extensor load receptor input occurs between translational and rotational displacements (65). This may be responsible for the different strength of monosynaptic stretch reflex activity in the two conditions of perturbations (see also Significance of Load Receptor Input).

The functional implications of the modulation of group I afferent input during locomotion has been suggested to be as follows: (a) gastrocnemius/soleus stretch reflex facilitation at the end of the stance phase contributes to the compensation for ground irregularities and assists during the push-off phase, and (b) the depression of leg extensor I a input during the swing phase prevents the occurrence of the extensor stretch reflex during ankle dorsiflexion (52,53,61).

The functional significance of monosynaptic stretch reflexes during gait remains obscure, to some extent, and should be limited for the following reasons: (a) According to the properties of the monosynaptic stretch reflex with a high sensitivity for small inputs its use during gait should be restricted to compensation for ground irregularities (41,50). During fast and large translational perturbations (e.g., slipping) monosynaptic reflexes are absent, and compensation is achieved by polysynaptic spinal reflex responses (most probably not mediated by group I afferent). (b) During postural tasks only polysynaptic EMG responses show direction-specific effects; this is not the case for short-latency EMG responses (66).

Significance of Polysynaptic Reflexes

Although the triceps surae becomes stretched with a high velocity during translational perturbations of gait, no significant EMG responses are elicited within the range of a monosynaptic transmission, whereas strong EMG responses appear with longer latency. Further investigations have indicated that the primary afferents from leg and foot muscles are not likely to play a dominant role in mediating compensatory leg muscle EMG responses to translational perturbations (35,67).

It can be assumed that the compensatory polysynaptic responses in the leg muscles evoked by translational perturbations during gait are mainly mediated by muscle proprioceptive input from group II and even group III afferent fibers, although there is no direct and positive evidence for this assumption (37,68–70).

The polysynaptic spinal reflex mechanism belongs most probably to the spinal reflex pathways from the flexion reflex afferents (FRA), as there are several similarities with respect to the phasic modulation of the flexion reflexes during locomotion in humans (12,17,71–76). A major function of the FRA in motor control represents an interneuronal integration of reflex actions from muscle, joint, and cutaneous afferents, with influences and commands coming from supraspinal centers. In addition, these reflexes have alternative excitatory and inhibitory connections to both extensors and flexors (72–74). Reflexes from the FRA function, therefore, as a multisensory activating system, which also excite receptors (e.g., in the muscles).

Consequently the polysynaptic reflex system does not behave as a simple stretch reflex mechanism; rather, its function depends on multisensory afferent information and on supraspinal influences. The behavior of these reflexes during locomotion has to subserve the complex situation of a multivariable control that is designated to a certain goal dominant to numerous individual parameters (77–79). On the basis of the evidence that the covariation of muscle activity across several joints cannot simply be explained by differences in local muscles' stretch inputs, a close interaction between a central program and muscle proprioceptive input takes place to generate the appropriate pattern (35,55,63,77,80,81). The sensory information in the postural tasks might be used to identify the direction, velocity, and amplitude of the perturbation to restore the subject's center of mass to the equilibrium position over the base of support (i.e., the feet).

Further experiments have given an indication of other afferent information that might influence the polysynaptic spinal reflex system in addition to muscle stretch input. A different response pattern is obtained when subjects are tested in both bipedal and quadripedal stance postures; postural responses to the same perturbation change with initial stance posture and are biomechanically appropriate for restoring the center of mass (15). These observations indicate that during perturbations of gait, the body's center of mass is the essential parameter to be constrained within the base of support and, therefore, represents the "variable" to be controlled by the compensatory responses, with the purpose of preventing falling (82).

SIGNIFICANCE OF LOAD RECEPTOR INPUT

To study the relative contribution of a mechanism to motor control in human posture and gait, Nashner introduced the following experimental paradigm: Subjects stood on a movable platform that could be activated on command to slide horizontally forward or backward or tilt toes up or toes down (83). The EMG pattern induced by dorsiflexing rotation of the feet was basically different from that induced by backward platform translations, even though the triceps surae became stretched with a similar velocity in both conditions.

Following feet dorsiflexing *rotations* a small, short-latency response in the gastrocnemius is followed by a stronger activation of the tibialis anterior. The latter activity is required to compensate for the backward sway of the body induced by the rotation. Backward *translation* is followed only by strong, long-latency (about 80 ms) gastrocnemius activity. This EMG activity results in the restoration of a stable, vertical position over the displaced feet. It has been suggested by Nashner that the difference in the EMG pattern between the two conditions is owing to a *reflex adaptation* based on the assumption that postural stabilization is the product of diminishing muscular destabilization (83). It was assumed that this adaptation was achieved through a selection of appropriate postural reflexes (i.e., a successive "adaptation" of the reflex response, within two to four trials) if the signal is "inappropriate" to a functionally directed tibialis anterior (rotational) or gastrocnemius (translational) activation.

Subsequent experiments have clearly failed to support this concept of adaptation of the response pattern and have instead shown that an immediate change in pattern occurs within the first trial, after unexpectedly changing the type of perturbation (62,84). Therefore, the neuronal mechanisms are directed to the demands of equilibrium control (i.e., keeping the body's center of mass over the feet). Depending on the stance condition, muscle stretch does not necessarily result in a compensatory stretch reflex response but instead results in antagonistic muscle activation. It was suggested that the generation of an appropriate compensatory response pattern was achieved by the integration of multiple divergent sensory inputs on a spinal level (62,84).

How is the position of the body's center of mass relative to the feet signaled? This question has been neglected in most investigations of postural control, and we are just beginning to appreciate the influence that gravity has on sensory information and motor behavior (85,86). For an appropriate gain control of postural reflexes peripheral information is required that should signal the influence of "gravity" besides inputs from muscle stretch receptors and vestibular system (86).

The effect of reduced weight induced by water immersion, on those receptors involved in signaling changes in the position of the body's center of mass with respect to the support surface has been studied (87–89). The advantage of this particular technique compared with postural reactions during space flights is to leave vestibular function unaltered while still allowing manipulation of body mass (85). If a gravity-dependence of the compensatory EMG responses exists then manipulation of the force between the feet and the support platform should affect the responses to destabilize platform movements.

During immersion, postural reactions were qualitatively similar to those seen under normal conditions and also during space flights (85). There was a close relationship between actual body weight and the magnitude of the EMG responses after both backward and forward displacements (88). Out of water, however, no correlation existed between loading of the subjects and the EMG responses. This saturation of the response out of water might represent a natural limitation of muscle activation to prevent possible injury (e.g., rupture) of the musculoskeletal system.

In order to define both the type of the receptor and its properties that signals the projection of the center of body's mass vector to the feet, rotational and quasi "translational" dorsiflexing displacements were induced during horizontal body posture and also with different loads applied to the body (65). It was only during translational displacements that different torques were imposed by this loading. The rotational impulses were followed only by a small, short-latency gastrocnemius EMG response. The translational impulses were followed by a stronger gastrocnemius response of longer latency compared to the rotational response, although stretches of similar amplitude and velocity were applied. Application of a load to the body against the movable platform had a significant effect on the magnitude on the long-latency gastrocnemius response following translational perturbation, whereas no significant effect was seen on the short-latency gastrocnemius response following rotational and translational perturbations. A different distribution of pressure on the foot sole in the two conditions cannot account for the difference, as anesthetizing the foot did not alter the EMG pattern during upright stance. Increased loading of the body against the support area augments the torque only in the translational displacement condition. In the rotational condition, however, the torque remains unaffected. The magnitude of torque during translational impulses is directly proportional to the amount of the loading according to the formula:

$$T = L \times r$$

(T = torque, L = load; r = translation distance)

It was, therefore, assumed that load receptors in the leg extensors are mainly responsible for the different EMG patterns, which explains their antigravity function (65).

A potentially excitatory function of load receptors during locomotion and positive force feedback in the control of locomotor movement has already been described for the extensor muscles of the cat (90–95). Accordingly, the function of those reflexes known to be involved in the stabilization of human posture (e.g., muscle proprioceptive and vestibulospinal reflexes) might depend on the activity of receptors within the body that indicate deviations of the body's center of mass from a certain neutral position. Similar as in the cat experiments, also in humans, extensor load receptors input could provide such essential information. In the cat experiments it was suggested that these receptor signals arise from Golgi tendon organs and are mediated by Ib afferents to the spinal locomotor generator (96).

INTERACTION BETWEEN CENTRAL PROGRAMS AND AFFERENT INPUT

Central mechanisms and afferent input interact in such a way that the strength of a reflex in a synergistic group of muscles follows a program dependent on the actual task. The actual weighting of proprioceptive, vestibular, and visual inputs to the equilibrium control is context-dependent and can profoundly modify the actual program. An impaired interaction between central programs and afferent input again can lead to a movement disorder (82,97).

There is a general agreement that the control of gait is not based on local reflex responses but that a selection and integration of peripheral and supraspinal inputs occurs to generate an appropriate response pattern (22). This leads to the question of how such a great deal of information can be processed within a short time. Some interesting hypotheses concerning this problem have been put forward. All have a similar basis: error detection by comparison of the ongoing movement with a central reference pattern (i.e., by the incongruence between the anticipated and the actual stepping movements) (98). In 1950 von Holst and Mittelstaedt proposed the *Reafferenzprinzip* as the organizational principle of neuronal motor control (99). Held then expanded this idea (100). According to this theory, an "efference copy" in the central generator accompanies each efferent central command. The actual movement is signaled back as the reafference and compared with an efference copy. Deviations from this copy determine the compensatory reaction. Gurfinkel and coworkers put forward a similar organization for the adjustment of an ongoing movement to a central body representation (the "body scheme") for postural stabilization (101).

CONCLUSION

The control of gait selectively utilizes afferent information from a variety of sources, which then interacts with central programs to adjust a movement to actual requirements. Although a predominant working range exists for each receptor system, considerable overlap between systems is present. Thus, under normal conditions, stepping movements are little impaired in the absence of one of the main systems, namely visual information, proprioception, or labyrinth function. To separate contributions of each of these mechanisms remains necessarily artificial to some extent, because a close interaction among all these systems exists, in particular between central mechanisms and proprioceptive reflexes, to maintain the body's center of mass over the feet.

The selection of an appropriate program pattern underlying locomotion depends on a combination of afferent inputs and/or the instruction for a respective locomotor condition. This information determines the mode of organization of muscle synergies. Several reflex mechanisms interact with the programmed pattern. The short-latency stretch reflex in leg extensor muscles is profoundly modulated during locomotion, mainly by presynaptic inhibition of group Ia input. The functional implications of this modulation are not yet fully understood. However, polysynaptic spinal reflexes provide the main compensation for perturbations of gait. It is thought that these EMG responses are mediated by peripheral information from group II (and III) afferents. The function of proprioceptive reflexes involved in locomotion depends on the presence of contact forces opposing gravity. Extensor load receptors are thought to signal changes of the projection of body center of mass with respect to the feet. This afferent input probably arises from Golgi tendon organs and represents a newly discovered function of these receptors in the regulation of gait.

The *central mechanisms* involved in locomotion are reflected in a diphasic or triphasic pattern of leg muscle activation following displacement of the feet that is thought to be programmed in its basic structure. Close similarities with the triphasic EMG pattern described for ballistic voluntary movements suggest that there is an underlying analogous neuronal mechanism. The EMG pattern is assumed to be evoked by a multisensory afferent input and generated by spinal interneuronal circuits that are closely connected with spinal locomotor centers. The extent to which the timing of the pattern can be modified by afferent input is not yet fully explored. A basic requirement of bipedal locomotion is that both legs act in a cooperative manner; each limb affects the strength of muscle activation and the time-space behavior of the other. There is some evidence that spinal interneuronal circuits, which are themselves under supraspinal (e.g., cerebral and cerebellar) control, mediates interlimb coordination.

In regard to the *reflex mechanisms,* short latency stretch reflexes in leg extensor muscles are profoundly modulated during gait mainly by presynaptic inhibition group Ia input and less by fusimotor influences. During large translational perturbations a significant contribution of this reflex has not yet been demonstrated. However, short latency reflexes may be involved in compensation of small ground irregularities at distinct phases of gait. Polysynaptic spinal reflexes to a large extent provide compensation for foot displacement during gait. This includes an activation of synergistic muscle groups of both legs. It is thought that these EMG responses are mediated predominantly by peripheral information from group II afferents (converging with different peripheral and supraspinal inputs onto common spinal interneurons) on a spinal pathway. These reflexes modulate the basic motor pattern of spinal interneuronal circuits underlying the respective motor task. During recent years, increasing evidence has emerged for a crucial importance of load receptor input in the control of bipedal stance and gait. Yet we are just beginning to understand its interaction with other afferent inputs and control mechanisms.

ACKNOWLEDGMENT

This work was supported by grants of the Swiss National Science Foundation (No. 3153526.98).

REFERENCES

1. Herder JG. *Ideen zur Philosphie der Geschichte der Menschheit.* Leipzig: Hartknoch, 1785.
2. Marey EJ. *Le Mouvement.* Paris: Masson, 1894.
3. Bernstein NA. *Die Kymozyclographische Methode der Bewegungsuntersuchung.* In: Abderhalden E, ed. *Handbuch der Biologischen Arbeitsmethoden.* Wien: Urban Schwarzenberg, 1936:629–680.
4. Engberg I, Lundberg A. An electromyographic analysis of muscular activity in the hindlimb of the cat during unrestrained locomotion. *Acta Physiol Scand* 1969;75:614–630.
5. Grillner S. The role of muscle stiffness in meeting the changing postural and locomotor requirements for force development by ankle extensors. *Acta Physiol Scand* 1972;86:92–108.
6. Dietz V, Schmidtbleicher D, Noth J. Neuronal mechanisms of human locomotion. *J Neurophysiol* 1979;42:1212–1222.
7. Dietz V, Quintern J, Berger W. Stumbling reactions in man: release of a ballistic movement pattern. *Brain Res* 1986;362:355–357.
8. Hoffmann P. *Die Eigenreflexe (Sehnenreflexe) Menschlicher Muskeln.* Berlin: Springer, 1922.
9. Foerster O. Schlaffe und spastische Lähmung. In: Bethe A, Bergmann G, von Embden G, et al., eds. *Handbuch der Normalen und Patholgischen Physiologie.* Berlin: Springer, 1927:893–972.
10. Bickel A. *Über den Einfluss der sensiblen Nerven und der Labyrinthe auf die Bewegungen der Tiere. Pfluegers Arch Gesamte Physiol Menschen Tiere* 1897;67:299–344.
11. Hering HE. *Ueber Bewegungsstörungen nach centripetaler Lähmung. Arch Exp Pathol Pharmacol* 1897;38:266–283.
12. Lundberg A. Control of spinal mechanisms from the brain. In: Tower, ed. *The nervous system.* New York: Raven, 1975:253–265.
13. Grillner S. Control of locomotion in bipeds, tetrapods, and fish. In: Brookhart M, Mountcastle VB, eds. *Handbook of physiology.* Washington, DC: American Physiology Society, 1981:1179–1236.
14. Schomburg ED. Spinal sensorimotor systems and their supraspinal control. *Neurosci Res* 1990;7:265–340.
15. Macpherson JM, Hora FB, Dunbar DC, et al. Stance dependence of automatic postural adjustments in humans. *Exp Brain Res* 1989;78:557–566.
16. Nilsson J, Thorstensson A, Halbertsma J. Changes in leg movements and muscle activity with speed of locomotion and mode of progression in humans. *Acta Physiol Scand* 1985;123:457–475.
17. Duysens J, Pearson KG. The role of cutaneous afferents from the distal hindlimb in the regulation of the step cycle in thalamic cats. *Exp Brain Res* 1976;24:245–255.
18. Forssberg H, Grillner S, Rossignol S. Phasic gain control of reflexes from the dorsum of the paw during spinal locomotion. *Brain Res* 1977;132:121–139.
19. Grillner S. Interaction between sensory signals and the central networks controlling locomotion in lamprey, dogfish and cat. In: Grillner S, Stein PSG, Stuart DG, et al., eds. *Wenner-Gren International Symposium Series. Neurobiology of vertebrate locomotion.* London: Macmillan, 1986:505–512.
20. Jankowska E, Lundberg A. Interneurones in the spinal cord. *Trends Neurosci* 1981;4:230–233.
21. Amstrong DM. The supraspinal control of mammalian locomotion. *J Physiol (Lond)* 1988;405:1–37.
22. Baldissera F, Hultborn H, Illert M. Integration in spinal neuronal systems. In: Brookhart M, Mountcastle VB, eds. *Handbook of physiology.* Washington, DC: American Physiology Society, 1981:509–595.
23. Thorstensson A, Nilsson J, Carlson H, et al. Trunk movements in human locomotion. *Acta Physiol Scand* 1984;121:9–22.
24. Brooks VB. Motor programs revisited. In: Talbott RE, Humphrey DR, eds. *Posture and movement.* New York: Raven, 1979:13–49.
25. Keele SW. Movement control in skilled motor performance. *Psychol Bull* 1968;70:387–403.
26. Forssberg H. A developmental model of human locomotion. In: Grillner S, Stein PSG, Stuart DG, et al., eds. *Wenner-Gren International Symposium Series. Neurobiology of vertebrate locomotion.* London: Macmillan, 1986:485–501.

27. Prochazka A. Sensorimotor gain control: a basic strategy of motor systems? *Progr Neurobiol* 1989;33:281–307.
28. Hore JT, Vilis T. A cerebellar-dependent efference copy mechanism for generating appropriate muscle responses to limb perturbations. In: Bloedel JR, Dichgans J, Precht W, eds. *Proceedings in life sciences: cerebellar functions*. Heidelberg, Springer: 1985:1–23.
29. Schubert M, Curt A, Jensen L, et al. Corticospinal input in human gait: modulation of magnetically evoked motor response. *Exp Brain Res* 1997;115:234–246.
30. Schubert M, Curt A, Colombo G, et al. Voluntary control of human gait: conditioning of magnetically evoked responses in a precision stepping task. *Exp Brain Res* 1999;126:583–588.
31. Angel RW. Electromyography during voluntary movement: the two-burst pattern. *Electroencephalogr Clin Neurophysiol* 1974;36:493–498.
32. Dietz V, Quintern J, Boos G, et al. Obstruction of the swing phase during gait: phase-dependent bilateral leg muscle coordination. *Brain Res* 1986;384:166–169.
33. Nashner LM, McCollum G. The organization of human postural movements: a formal basis and experimental synthesis. *Behav Brain Sci* 1985;8:135–172.
34. Horak FB, Nashner LM, Diener HC. Postural strategies associated with somatosensory and vestibular loss. *Exp Brain Res* 1990;82:167–177.
35. Dietz V, Horstmann GA, Berger W. Interlimb coordination of leg muscle activation during perturbation of stance in humans. *J Neurophysiol* 1989;62:680–693.
36. Tax AAM, van Wezel BMH, Dietz V. Bipedal reflex coordination to tactile stimulation of the sural nerve during human running. *J Neurophysiol* 1995;73:1947–1964.
37. Berger W, Dietz V, Quintern J. Corrective reactions to stumbling in man: neuronal coordination of bilateral leg muscle activity during gait. *J Physiol (Lond)* 1984;357:109–125.
38. Dietz V, Berger W. Interlimb coordination of posture in patients with spastic paresis. Impaired function of spinal reflexes. *Brain* 1984;107:965–978.
39. Bonnet M, Gurfinkel S, Lipchits J, et al. Central programming of lower limb muscular activity in the standing man. *Agressologie* 1976;17:35–42.
40. Dietz V, Nakazawa K, Wirz M, et al. Level of spinal cord lesion determines locomotor activity in spinal man. *Exp Brain Res* 1999;128:405–409.
41. Sanes JN, Evarts EV. Motor psychophysics. *Hum Neurobiol* 1984;2:217–225.
42. Sanes J, Mauritz NKH, Dalakas MC, et al. Motor control in humans with large-fiber sensory neuropathy. *Hum Neurobiol* 1985;4:101–114.
43. Marsden CD. Neurophysiology. In: Stern G, ed. *Parkinson's disease*. London: Chapman and Hall Medical, 1990:57–98.
44. Lajoie Y, Teasdale N, Cole JD, et al. Gait of a deafferented subject without large myelinated sensory fibers below the neck. *Neurology* 1996;47:109–115.
45. Diener HC, Dichgans J, Guschlbauer B, et al. The significance of proprioception on postural stabilization as assessed by ischemia. *Brain Res* 1984;296:103–109.
46. Mauritz KH, Dietz V. Characteristics of postural instability induced by blocking of leg afferents by ischemia. *Exp Brain Res* 1980;38:117–119.
47. Sherrington CS. On the proprioceptive system, especially its reflex aspect. *Brain* 1906;29:476–482.
48. Gollhofer A, Schmidtbleicher D, Dietz V. Regulation of muscle stiffness in human locomotion. *Int J Sports Med* 1984;5:19–22.
49. Loeb GE, Hoffer JA. Activity of spindle afferents from cat anterior thigh muscles. II. Effects of fusimotor blockade. *J Neurophysiol* 1985;54:565–577.
50. Matthews PBC. *Mammalian muscle receptors and their central actions*. London: Arnold, 1972.
51. Stein PSG. Motor systems, with specific reference to the control of locomotion. *Ann Rev Neurosci* 1978;1:61–81.
52. Capaday C, Stein RB. Amplitude modulation of the soleus H-reflex in the human during walking and standing. *J Neurosci* 1986;6:1308–1313.
53. Capaday C, Stein RB. Difference in the amplitude of the human soleus H-reflex during walking and running. *J Physiol (Lond)* 1987;392:513–522.
54. Morin C, Katz R, Mazieres L, et al. Comparison of soleus H-reflex facilitation at the onset of soleus contractions produced voluntarily and during the stance phase of human gait. *Neurosci Lett* 1982;33:47–53.
55. Dietz V. Human neuronal control of automatic functional movements: interaction between central programs and afferent input. *Physiol Rev* 1992;72:33–69.
56. Crenna P, Frigo C. Excitability of the soleus H-reflex arc during walking and stepping in man. *Exp Brain Res* 1987;66:49–60.
57. Stein RB, Capaday C. The modulation of human reflexes during functional motor tasks. *Trends Neurosci* 1988;11:328–332.
58. Dietz V, Discher M, Faist M, et al. Amplitude modulation of the human quadriceps tendon jerk reflex during gait. *Exp Brain Res* 1999;82:211–213.
59. Dietz V, Faist M, Pierrot-Deseilligny E. Amplitude modulation of the quadriceps H–reflex in the human during the early stance phase of gait. *Exp Brain Res* 1990;79:221–224.
60. Llewellyn M, Prochazka A, Vincent S. Transmission of human tendon jerk reflexes during stance and gait. *J Physiol (Lond)* 1987;382:82P.
61. Sinkjaer T, Anderson JB, Larsen B. Soleus stretch reflex modulation during gait in humans. *J Neurophysiol* 1996;76:1112–1120.
62. Gollhofer A, Horstmann GA, Berger W, et al. Compensation of translational and rotational perturbations in human posture: stabilization of the center of gravity. *Neurosci Lett* 1989;105:73–78.
63. Dietz V. Interaction between central programs and afferent input in the control of posture and locomotion. *J Biomech* 1996;29:841–844.
64. Faist M, Dietz V, Pierrot-Deseilligny E. Modulation, probably presynaptic in origin, of monosynaptic Ia excitation during human gait. *Exp Brain Res* 1996;109:441–449.
65. Dietz V, Gollhofer A, Kleiber M, et al. Regulation of bipedal stance: dependence on "load" receptors. *Exp Brain Res* 1992;89:229–231.
66. Woollacott MH, Bonnet M, Yabe K. Preparatory process for anticipatory postural adjustments: modulation of leg muscles reflex pathways during preparation for arm movements in standing man. *Exp Brain Res* 1984;55:263–271.
67. Dietz V, Quintern J, Berger W, et al. Cerebral potentials and leg muscle e.m.g. responses associated with stance perturbation. *Exp Brain Res* 1985;57:348–354.
68. Lundberg A, Malmgren K, Schomburg ED. Reflex

pathway from group II muscle afferents. 3. Secondary spindle afferents and the FRA: a new hypothesis. *Exp Brain Res* 1987;65:294–306.
69. Nardone A, Grasso M, Giordano A, et al. Different effect of height on latency of leg and foot short- and medium-latency EMG responses to perturbation of stance in humans. *Neurosci Lett* 1996;206:89–92.
70. Matthews PBC. Evidence from the use of vibration that the human long–latency stretch reflex depends upon spindle secondary afferents. *J Physiol (Lond)* 1984;348:383–415.
71. Belanger M, Patla AE. Corrective responses to perturbation applied during walking in humans. *Neurosci Lett* 1984;49:291–295.
72. Duysens J, Trippel M, Horstmann GA, et al. Gating and reversal of reflexes in ankle muscles during human walking. *Exp Brain Res* 1990;82:351–358.
73. Duysens J, Tax AAM, Murrer L, et al. Backward and forward walking use different patterns of phase-dependent modulation of cutaneous reflexes in humans. *J Neurophysiol* 1996;76:301–310.
74. Duysens J, van Wezel BMH, Prokop T, et al. Medial gastrocnemius is more activated than lateral gastrocnemius in sural nerve induced reflexes during human gait. *Brain Res* 1996;727:230–232.
75. Kanda K, Sato H. Reflex responses of human thigh muscles to non-noxious sural stimulation during stepping. *Brain Res* 1983;288:378–380.
76. Yang JF, Stein RB. Phase-dependent reflex reversal in human leg muscles during walking. *J Neurophysiol* 1990;63:1109–1117.
77. Gurfinkel VS, Lipshits MI, Popov KE. On the origin of short-latency muscle responses to postural disturbances. *Agressologie* 1979;20:153–154.
78. Ito M. The CNS as a multivariable control system. *Behav Brain Sci* 1982;5:552–553.
79. Loeb GE, He J, Levine WS. Spinal cord circuits: are they mirrors of musculoskeletal mechanics? *J Motor Behav* 1989;21:473–491.
80. Gurfinkel VS, Latash ML. Segmental postural mechanisms and reversals of muscle reflexes. *Agressologie* 1979;20:145–146.
81. Matthews PBC. Proprioceptors and their contribution to somatosensory mapping: complex messages require complex processing. *Can J Physiol Pharmacol* 1988;66:430–438.
82. Dietz V Neurophysiology of gait disorders: present and future applications. *Electroenceph Clin Neurophysiol* 1997;103:333–355.
83. Nashner LM. Adapting reflexes controlling the human posture. *Exp Brain Res* 1976;26:59–72.
84. Hansen PD, Woollacott MH, Debu B. Postural responses to changing task conditions. *Exp Brain Res* 1988;73:627–636.
85. Clement G, Gurfinkel VS, Lestienne F, et al. Changes of posture during transient perturbations in microgravity. *Aviat Space Environ Med* 1985;56:666–671.
86. Mittelstaedt H. The formation of the visual and the postural vertical. In: Mergner T, Hlavacka F, eds. *Multisensory control of posture*. New York: Plenum, 1995:147–155.
87. Dietz V, Duysens J. Significance of load receptor input during locomotion. *Gait Posture* 2000;11:102–110.
88. Dietz V, Horstmann GA, Trippel M, et al. Human postural reflexes and gravity an under water simulation. *Neurosci Lett* 1989;106:350–355.
89. Dietz V, Colombo G. Effects of body immersion on postural adjustments to voluntary arm movements in humans: role of load receptor input. *J Physiol (Lond)* 1996;497:849–856.
90. Conway BA, Hultborn H, Kiehn O. Proprioceptive input resets central locomotor rhythm in the spinal cat. *Exp Brain Res* 1987;68:643–656.
91. Duysens J, Pearson KG. Inhibition of flexor burst generation by loading extensor muscles in walking cats. *Brain Res* 1980;187:321–332.
92. Pearson KG, Collins DF. Reversal of the influence of group Ib-afferents from plantaris on activity in medial gastrocnemius muscle during locomotor activity. *J Neurophysiol* 1993;70:1009–1017.
93. Gossard JP, Brownstone RM, Barajon I, et al. Transmission in a locomotor-related group Ib pathway from hindlimb extensor muscles in the cat. *Exp Brain Res* 1994;98:213–228.
94. Prochazka A, Gillard D, Bennett DJ. Positive force feedback control of muscles. *J Neurophysiol* 1997;77:3226–3236.
95. Prochazka A, Gillard D, Bennett DJ. Indication of positive feedback in the control of movement. *J Neurophysiol* 1997;77:3237–3251.
96. Pearson KG. Proprioceptive regulation. *Curr Opin Neurobiol* 1996;49:481–515.
97. Dietz V. Gait disorder in spasticity and Parkinson's disease. *Adv Neurol* 2000;87:143–154.
98. Nashner LM. Balance adjustments of humans perturbed while walking. *J Neurophysiol* 1980;44:650–664.
99. Von Holst E, Mittelstaedt H. *Das Reafferenzprinzip (Wechselwirkungen zwischen Zentralnervensystem und Peripherie). Naturwissenschaften* 1950;37:464–476.
100. Held R. Exposure history as a factor in maintaining stability of perception and coordination. *J Nerv Ment Dis* 1961;132:26–32.
101. Gurfinkel S, Levik YS, Popov KE, et al. Body scheme in the control of postural activity. In: Gurfinkel S, Joffe ME, Massion J, et al., eds. *Stance and motion facts and concepts*. New York: Plenum, 1988:185–193.

Gait Disorders. Advances in Neurology, Vol. 87,
edited by E. Růžička, M. Hallett, and J. Jankovic.
Lippincott Williams & Wilkins, Philadelphia © 2001.

6

Normal and Impaired Development of Gait

Wiltrud Berger

Department of Neurology, University of Freiburg, D-79106 Freiburg, Germany

This chapter presents an overview about the knowledge concerning gait development in humans. Data about impaired development in children with cerebral palsy supports the interpretation of physiological stages of development. Results from normal locomotion, corrective responses following perturbations, special demands for difficult postural and locomotory movements, and the maturation of afferent processing, is considered. A major difficulty with the study of developmental changes is to decide to which extent the observed changes during maturation are caused by physical or neurodevelopmental factors, or whether both factors are involved. Similar difficulties arise with early damage: Are the neurophysiological alterations directly owing to the lesion or to repair mechanisms, especially when normal motor function and an impaired central nervous system (CNS) develop in parallel?

LOCOMOTION

The evolution of bipedal gait has enabled humans to use their hands for cultural needs instead of locomotion. This fundamental aspect of upright stance requires a complex system for equilibrium control as a prerequisite. Some basic features of quadrupedal locomotion, however, seem to be preserved, and there is little doubt that a central pattern generator for automatic movements exists (1). Locomotorlike movements *in utero* can be observed at 10 weeks of gestation before central control exists (2). Also, the innate newborn stepping is a rhythmic, locomotorlike behavior that can be elicited directly after birth, when the baby is held under the arms and the feet touch the surface. The corresponding electromyographic (EMG) pattern, first described by Forssberg and Wallberg, consists of a coactivation of the antagonistic leg muscles (3). The disappearance of this pattern after 10 weeks of age may indicate a fundamental rearrangement with excitability changes in the spinal networks. The loss of the pattern might also result from inactivity because it can be trained by the environment (4). When the child is able to stand with little support and posture changes from quadrupedal to bipedal (7 to 10 months of age), the following pattern is seen with spontaneous locomotion or on a moving treadmill: (a) coactivation of antagonist leg muscles during the stance phase of gait, (b) low amplitude and tonically activated extensor EMG activity, (c) huge, biphasic potentials arising with a delay after a sharp decrease of the ankle angle in the beginning of the stance phase when making ground contact with the forefoot, compatible with a monosynaptic response (Fig. 6.1A) (5). The walking pattern at this stage of development is characterized by a digitigrade placing of the feet (Fig. 6.2). The coactivation pattern is gradually replaced by reciprocal activation after 2 to 3 years of age. The biphasic stretch reflexes are suppressed. A significant increase of leg extensor EMG takes place that is relevant for free and independent gait and the ability to react to ground irregularities (Fig. 6.1C).

Kinematic recordings illuminate these changes. During early development there is a digitigrade foot placement and a near vertical

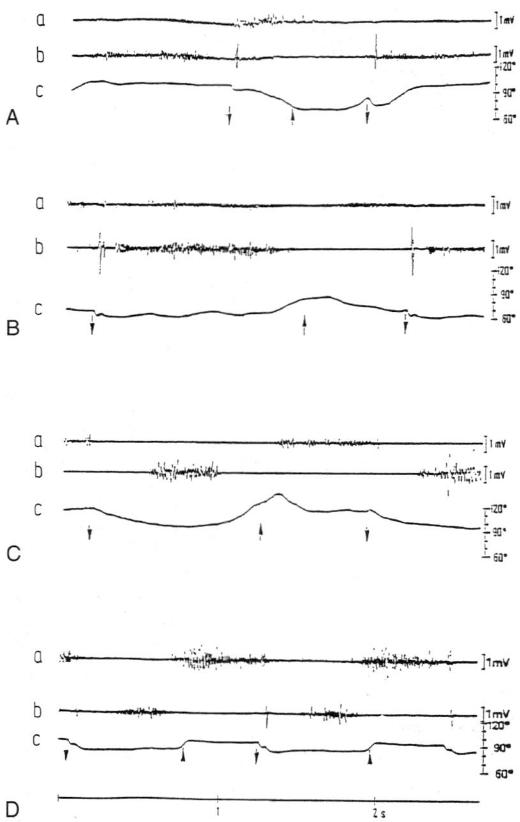

FIG. 6.1. Raw electromyographic (EMG) recordings from tibialis anterior (*a*) and gastrocnemius muscles (*b*) together with the goniometer trace of the ankle-joint angle (*c*) during normal gait on a treadmill. Arrows indicate onset (↑) and end (↓) of stance phase. **(A)** Normal child, 7 months. **(B)** Child with cerebral palsy, 13 years. **(C)** Normal child, 4 years. **(D)** Adult patient with spastic paresis. (From Berger W. Characteristics of locomotor control in children with cerebral palsy. *Neurosc Biobehav Rev* 1998;22:579–582, with permission.)

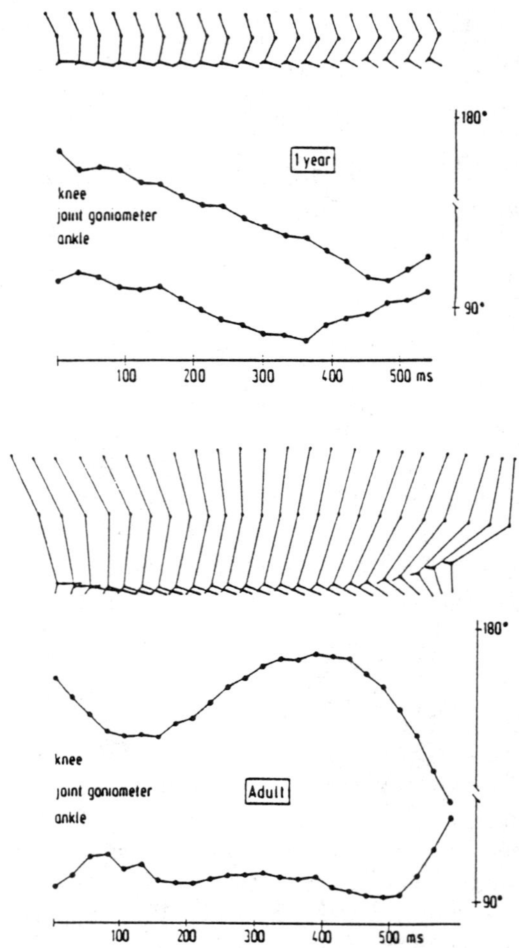

FIG. 6.2. Kinematic analysis together with knee- and ankle-joint angles of the stance phase during gait in a child and in a normal adult subject. (From Berger W. Characteristics of locomotor control in children with cerebral palsy. *Neurosc Biobehav Rev* 1998;22:579–582, with permission.)

position of the leg during the stance phase, supporting the body instead of propelling it forward. Forward propulsion is achieved by rotation of the hip of the unsupported leg. This is changed to plantigrade foot placement with heelstrike. The body rolls over the standing leg with a forward thrust at the end of stance from 4 years of age on and in adult stages (Fig. 6.2). This change implies an increase in the degrees of freedom of the articulations of the leg and requires a higher level of equilibrium control during bipedal locomotion. There is a similar change for head and trunk movements (6).

In conclusion, coactivation during the first stages of gait seems to be more related to holding the body in an upright position than propelling it forward because the crucial functions at the early stage are regulation and maintenance of body equilibrium. The increase of extensor EMG activity together with the suppression of the short latency reflexes seems to reflect the mutual influence of group I- and II-mediated reflexes on the background of the maturation of supraspinal control governing an autonomous spinal central pattern generator (CPG) network (5,7,8).

CORRECTIVE RESPONSES

The compensatory EMG responses following gait perturbations in children between 1 and 8 years of age confirm the findings during unperturbed gait (7). Single monosynaptic and oligosynaptic reflex potentials followed by a long-lasting polysynaptic extensor EMG response, along with coactivation of all antagonist muscles, were characteristic following a treadmill acceleration impulse in early infancy. From 4 years of age on, the short latency reflex potentials disappeared, the polysynaptic reflex responses became shorter, and a reciprocal mode of leg muscle activation occurred, with a consequent faster and more effective compensation for the perturbation. When the perturbation was triggered unilaterally during stance (on a split-belt), the displacements were followed by larger short latency reflexes in the younger children (present with a small amplitude also on the nondisplaced side), and the polysynaptic EMG responses were smaller on the displaced side and negligible on the nondisplaced side. Coactivation, again, was more expressed in the younger children (9).

In conclusion, maturation of corrective EMG responses is also expressed by reflex changes. Polysynaptic responses are effective with increasing age, whereas the oligosynaptic reflexes are suppressed. Decreasing coactivation with increasing age seems to represent the maturation of equilibrium control. Bilateral coordination following unilateral displacements shows similar changes with increasing age.

SPECIAL DEMANDS

To what extent are the observed changes during maturation caused by physical changes (e.g., body height and body weight)? Perturbations were unexpectedly applied to the back of subjects (children and adults) with different heights and weights. Electromyographic activity of the respective muscles and head, hip, and ankle joint movements were recorded. There was a close correlation between displacement amplitude at the ankle joints and the subjects' heights, with the largest displacements in small subjects. Perturbations of increasing strength resulted in a larger increment of both ankle joint displacements and extensor EMG responses in the smaller subjects. There is clear disadvantage of balance control in smaller subjects, irrespective of age. Not included in the study were children less than 5 years; therefore, one can speculate that children of 2 to 3 years of age, with still reduced extensor EMG activity (see the preceding), have both the difficulties of small body height and less established compensatory mechanisms (10). This is exactly what we observe in young children.

Further studies of enhanced body sway on a sinusoidally moving treadmill also reveal developmental changes. Damping of the oscillations from foot to head was greatest in adult subjects and smallest in the youngest children. The children showed an immature feed forward mechanism of body inclination (forward at the posterior turning point, and straight up at the anterior turning point). After the age of 10 years, posture is continually adjusted in such a way that the resulting torque acting on the body during the treadmill movement becomes minimized. Maturation of afferent control, especially gravity control by load receptors, might be relevant for this type of task (11,12).

Interlimb coordination during split-belt walking in children of 4 to 10 years, on the other hand, strongly suggests physical factors for most of the differences seen in the biomechanical measures, such as stride length and stride frequencies, compared to adults (13). Only a higher intersubject and intrasubject variability was found in the children, probably because of difficulties of postural control.

In conclusion, it depends on the age and the task whether physical "shortcomings" alone or in combination with a maturational delay contribute to the difficulties in demanding motor performances in younger children.

AFFERENT CONTROL

The role of sensorimotor integration or maturation seems to be relevant for motor control development, although it is not clear how

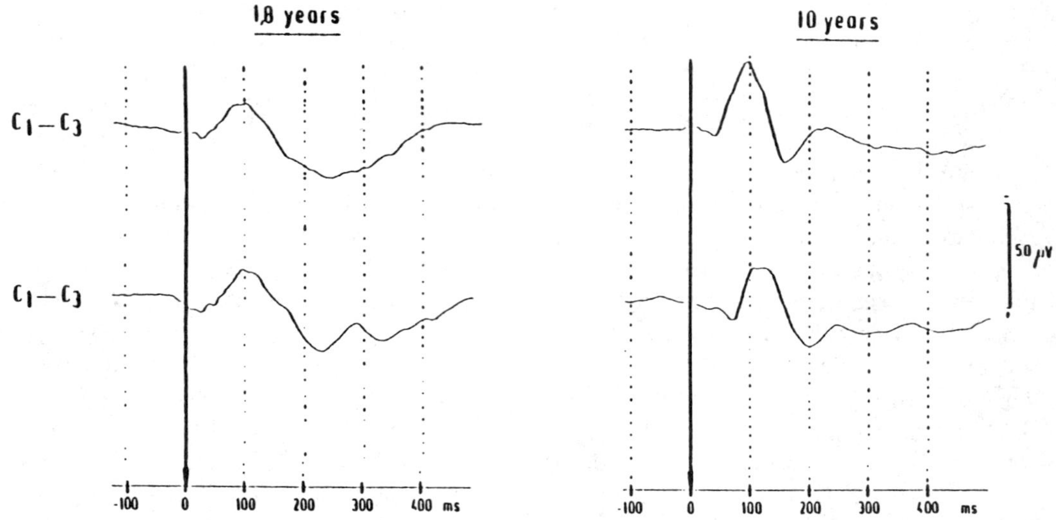

FIG. 6.3. Mechanically evoked cerebral potentials (backward displacement) during stance (**top**) and gait (**bottom**) in two children of different age. *Arrows* (0 ms) indicate decrease of ankle-joint angle. (From Berger W. Characteristics of locomotor control in children with cerebral palsy. *Neurosc Biobehav Rev* 1998;22:579–582, with permission.)

the environment may influence the developing nervous system. The development of automatic movements such as locomotion is based on innate information and less dependent on afferent control than finely tuned hand or finger movements, which develop through training. However, most of the results reported in the preceding can only be understood by understanding the parallel problem of maturation of afferent control. Babies at 20 to 28 weeks of age perform elbow extension movements with a high degree of coactivation of flexor and extensor muscles, which is not seen in adults. Active elbow extensions at a later stage (22 to 64 weeks of age) became increasingly smoother with their experience in predicting the magnitude and direction of external forces (14). Maturation is achieved by the ability to rely on and adapt to biomechanical demands by increasing afferent input processing and not only by an age-related increase of maximum muscle torque.

Our own studies of maturation of afferent control were performed using mechanically evoked cerebral potentials (9,15). Changes in the afferent control (in form of the cerebral potentials) and the efferent control (in form of EMG reflexes) during stance and gait perturbations in children between 1 and 10 years of age were compared with those of adults.

In the children of 1 to 2 years of age monosynaptic stretch reflex potentials appeared following perturbations during stance and gait, together with a reduced level of longer latency EMG responses. The cerebral potentials, too, had a profile that did not differ in the respective condition at this early stage (Fig. 6.3). The adult pattern was reached in children 6 to 10 years of age, with the suppression of monosynaptic stretch reflexes and the early part of the cerebral potentials during gait perturbation. This was interpreted as an inhibition of group I afferents at both segmental and supraspinal levels, involving both segmental stretch reflexes and group I signals to supraspinal centers. This control of afferent information has yet to be established in early infancy. We suggested that maturation of compensatory EMG responses during gait is achieved by the establishment of facilitation of polysynaptic spinal reflexes mediated via group II afferents. Immaturity of the afferent system processing could be the reason for reduced feed forward mechanisms during the sinusoidal treadmill movement.

Results with conflicting proprioceptive and visual stimuli are similar (16). An artificial optic flow during locomotion had a stronger modulatory effect in children than adults. Although this modulation was caused to stride length changes alone in adults, stride frequency and stride length were affected in children. The immaturity of the proprioceptive afferent control may be responsible for this stronger modulatory effect. The increase of central input on the spinal pattern generator in adults may be the reason for changes in the spatial parameter alone, whereas an immature supraspinal input leads to a restricted response pattern with affecting both parameters in children. This seems to be necessary for equilibrium control, which is crucial at this stage of development.

The literature about maturation as expressed by magnetically evoked motor potentials is mainly concerned with hand muscles, because monosynaptic transmission is expressed more in distal hand muscles than in proximal arm or lower leg muscles. The data suggest that the maturation of the corticospinal tract with consecutive changes of the central latency, as well as the changes of intracortical organization, interhemispherical inhibition, and the synaptical organization on a spinal level play an additional role (17–21).

In conclusion, some maturational changes of proprioceptive processing suggest that group I and group II central control play a major role for leg movements. The cortical influence is being studied only now for leg movements. The reason for this is that motor-evoked potentials are more difficult to elicit in the leg muscles because the fast corticospinal system may play a less important role in automatic movements such as locomotion.

IMPAIRED DEVELOPMENT

The diplegic child with cerebral palsy shows a locomotor pattern with coactivation of antagonist leg muscles during stance, a low and tonic activation of extensor EMG, and enhanced stretch reflex excitability quite similar to the gait pattern in the earliest stage of development (Fig. 6.1B) (22). This striking similarity in the children with cerebral palsy (8 to 16 years of age) with the immature locomotion pattern (1 to 2 years of age) led to the suggestion that an arrest of development takes place due to the early brain damage before a locomotor pattern has evolved (5,23). This pattern of children with cerebral palsy is different from that of spastic adult patients who show a preservation of reciprocal leg muscle activation (Fig. 6.1D) (24,25). For both spastic syndromes, however, there is a transformation of muscle fiber properties that is partly responsible for enhanced muscle tone (26).

Corrective responses following perturbations confirm the suggestion of maturation arrest, because ongoing enhanced short latency reflexes and suppressed polysynaptic reflexes persist. These polysynaptic reflexes perform the functionally meaningful part of EMG, and their reduction reflects the degree of paresis (27,28). It was shown in a preliminary study that transcallosal inhibition was absent in a group of adolescents with cerebral palsy during rest (29). Brouwer and Smits described abnormal cortical spinal projections to ankle muscles in individuals with cerebral palsy (30). Whether this reflects the early damage with defective maturation or the repair mechanisms of an early lesioned brain is still not clear. The different kinds of spasticity in adults, owing to a cerebral or paraspinal lesion, showed different modulatory effects during locomotion. The quadriceps tendon reflex during gait is depressed during the whole step cycle and profoundly modulated in healthy subjects. In paraparetic patients this depression was almost removed and was associated with weak or no modulation during the step cycle, whereas in hemiparetic patients reflex depression and modulation were only affected to a smaller degree. This is possibly owing to the unilateral preservation of fiber tracts in hemiparesis (31). Data from children with cerebral palsy are still lacking; therefore, spinal disorganization and reorganization following early brain damage remain to be discovered also in respect to physiotherapy.

ACKNOWLEDGMENTS

This work was supported over many years by the Deutsche Forschungsgemeinschaft

(DFG Be 936/4-1 and Be 936/5-1,2,3) and the Bundesministerium für Bildung und Forschung (BMBF 01 KL 9402).

REFERENCES

1. Grillner S, Zangger P. On the central generation of locomotion in the low spinal cat. *Exp Brain Res* 1979;34:241–261.
2. de Vries JIP, Visser GHA, Prechtl HFR. Fetal motility in the first half of pregnancy. In: Prechtl HFR, ed. *Continuity of neural functions from prenatal to postnatal life*. London: Spastics International Medical Publications, 1984:46–64.
3. Forssberg H, Wallberg H. Infant locomotion: a preliminary movement and electromyographic study. In: Berg K, Eriksson BD, eds. *Children and exercise*. Baltimore: University Park Press, 1980:32–49.
4. Zelazo PR. The development of walking: new findings and old assumptions. *J Mot Behav* 1983;15:99–137.
5. Berger W, Altenmüller E, Dietz V. Normal and impaired development of children's gait. *Hum Neurobiol* 1984;34:163–170.
6. Assaiante C, Amblard B. Head-trunk coordination and locomotor equilibrium in 3- to 8-year-old children. In: Berthoz A, Vidal P, Graf W, eds. *The head-neck sensory motor system*. Oxford University Press: New York, 1992:121–125.
7. Berger W, Quintern J, Dietz V. Stance and gait perturbations in children: developmental aspects of compensatory mechanisms *Electroenceph Clin Neurophysiol* 1985;61:385–395.
8. Myklebust BM, Gottlieb GL. Reciprocal excitation and reflex irradiation of short-latency reflexes in the healthy neonate. *Child Dev* 1993;64:1036–1045.
9. Berger W, Horstmann GA, Dietz V. Interlimb coordination of stance in children: divergent modulation of spinal reflex responses and cerebral evoked potentials in terms of age. *Neurosci Lett* 1990;116:118–122.
10. Berger W, Trippel M, Discher M, et al. Influence of subjects' height on the stabilization of posture. *Acta Otolaryng (Stockh)* 1992;112:22–30.
11. Berger W, Discher M, Trippel M, et al. Developmental aspects of stance regulation, compensation and adaptation. *Exp Brain Res* 1992;90:610–619.
12. Berger W, Trippel M, Assaiante C, et al. Developmental aspects of equilibrium control during stance: a kinematic and EMG study. *Gait Posture* 1995;3:149–155.
13. Zijlstra W, Prokop T, Berger W. Adaptability of leg movements during normal treadmill walking and split-belt walking in children. *Gait Posture* 1996;4:212–221.
14. Konczak J, Borutta M, Topka H, et al. The development of goal-directed reaching in infants: hand trajectory formation and joint torque control. *Exp Brain Res* 1995;106:156–168.
15. Berger W, Quintern J, Dietz V. Afferent and efferent control of stance and gait: developmental changes in children. *Electroenceph Clin Neurophysiol* 1987;66:244–252.
16. Berger W, Prokop T, Schubert M. Influence of optic flow on locomotion: differences between children, adults, elderly and pathophysiological states. *Gait Posture* 1999;9:17.
17. Eyre JA, Miller S, Ramesh V. Constancy of central conduction delays during development in man: investigation of motor and somatosensory pathways. *J Physiol (Lond)* 1991;434:441–452.
18. Müller K, Kass-Iliyya F, Reitz M. Ontogeny of ipsilateral corticospinal projections: a developmental study with transcranial magnetic stimulation. *Ann Neurol* 1997;42:705–711.
19. Gerloff C, Cohen LG, Floeter MK, et al. Inhibitory influence of the ipsilateral motor cortex on responses to stimulation of the human cortex and pyramidal tract. *J Physiol (Lond)* 1998;510:249–259.
20. Heinen F, Glocker FX, Fietzek UM, et al. The fast corticospinal system in school children: conduction proceeds skill. *Pediatr Neurol* 1998a;19:217–222.
21. Heinen F, Glocker FX, Fietzek UM, et al. Absence of transcallosal inhibition following focal magnetic stimulation in pre-school children. *Ann Neurol* 1998b;43:608–612.
22. Berger W, Quintern J, Dietz V. Pathophysiology of gait in children with cerebral palsy. *Electroenceph Clin Neurophysiol* 1982;53:538–548.
23. Berger W. Characteristics of locomotor control in children with cerebral palsy. *Neurosc Biobehav Rev* 1998;22:579–582.
24. Dietz V, Quintern J, Berger W. Electrophysiological studies of gait in spasticity and rigidity. Evidence that altered mechanical properties of muscle contribute to hypertonia. *Brain* 1981;104:431–449.
25. Forssberg H, Dietz V. Neurobiology of normal and impaired locomotor development. In: Conolly KJ, Forssberg H, eds. *Neurophysiology and neuropsychology of motor development*. London: MacKeith Press, 1997:78–100.
26. Dietz V, Berger W. Cerebral palsy and muscle transformation. *Dev Med Child Neurol* 1995;37:180–184.
27. Dietz V, Berger W. Interlimb coordination of posture in patients with spastic hemiparesis: impaired function of spinal reflexes. *Brain* 1984;107:965–978.
28. Berger W, Horstmann G, Dietz V. Spastic paresis: impaired spinal reflexes–intact motor programs. *J Neurol Neurosurg Psych* 1988;51:568–571.
29. Heinen F, Kirschner J, Fietzek UM, et al. Absence of transcallosal inhibition in adolescents with diplegic cerebral palsy. *Muscle Nerve* 1999;22:255–257.
30. Brouwer B, Smits E. Corticospinal input onto motor neurons projecting to ankle muscles in individuals with cerebral palsy. *Dev Med Child Neurol* 1996;38:787–796.
31. Faist M, Ertel M, Berger W, et al. Impaired modulation of quadriceps tendon jerk reflex during spastic gait: differences between spinal and cerebral lesions. *Brain* 1999;122:567–579.

Gait Disorders. Advances in Neurology, Vol. 87,
edited by E. Růžička, M. Hallett, and J. Jankovic.
Lippincott Williams & Wilkins, Philadelphia © 2001.

7

Use of Motion Analysis for Quantifying Movement Disorders

*Kenton R. Kaufman, †William J. Shaughnessy, and ‡John H. Noseworthy

**Biomechanics Laboratory, Department of Orthopedic Surgery; †Department of Orthopedics, Mayo Medical School, and Division of Pediatric Orthopedics, Department of Orthopedics, Mayo Clinic, and ‡Department of Neurology, Mayo Medical School and Mayo Clinic, Rochester, Minnesota 55905*

Every health professional treating patients with movement disorders must evaluate and treat the patient based on assumptions made about the relative functions of the central nervous system (CNS), selective motor control, weak or spastic muscles, joint contracture, and bony deformities. If methods to make objective measurements are not available or are not used, the usual methods of assessment include physical examination, manual muscle testing, and visual gait observation. A treatment plan is formed based on algorithms passed down by others and modified by experience gained from personal observations. However, many centers now have laboratories and skilled personnel to perform objective measurements rather than rely on intuition and assumptions. The role of a motion analysis laboratory is to provide quantitative information regarding the abnormal movement pattern as a basis for appropriate therapeutic intervention. Motion analysis should be used as part of the initial assessment to provide a basis for correct intervention and repeated to aid in the assessment of therapeutic outcome.

The purpose of this chapter is to describe how a motion analysis laboratory can be used to measure those aspects of a patient's neuromuscular performance that cannot be assessed quantitatively in a clinical setting.

HISTORICAL PERSPECTIVE

Motion analysis can be described as the objective, systematic analysis of movement. The concept of depicting and recording human motion began during the Renaissance Period. Giovanni Alphonso Borelli, a student of Galileo, was among the first scientists to analyze motion while developing his theory of muscle action based on mechanical principles (1). Duchenne conducted the first scientific systematic evaluation of muscle function. His findings were published in 1857 in the monumental work, *Physiologie des Mouvements,* 1857 (2). Eadweard Muybridge first performed photographic recording of human motion. Muybridge was asked to settle a bet by Governor Leeland Stanford of California regarding whether a trotting horse had all four feet off the ground at any instant in time. Muybridge placed cameras at regular intervals along a racetrack. Thin threads stretched across the track triggered the shutters. The horse's hooves triggered cameras in order, and a series of photographs clearly depicted the gait sequence. Muybridge subsequently compiled a detailed photographic exposé of human and animal locomotion, which was published in three volumes (3).

In Germany at the turn of the 20th century, Braune and Fischer became interested in measuring the motion of human body segments. They placed Geissler tubes, containing a rarified nitrogen gas, on various limb segments of a human subject dressed in black. Electrical circuits connected to the tubes created incandescence and the illuminated tubes were recorded by cameras as the subject walked. Experiments were carried out at night because there was no means to darken the room in which studies were performed. It took 10 to 12 hours to put this apparatus on the subject, whereas data collection was completed in minutes using four cameras. The images were digitized using a precision optical device. Geometry was used to extract three-dimensional coordinates. Equations needed to calculate resultant forces and moments at the joints of a 12-segment rigid body model were formulated. Although their quantitative results were published in 1895, their findings are still valid today (4).

Inman and colleagues combined rudimentary motion recordings with electromyography (EMG) in the mid-1900s. Their pioneering work in limb prosthetic research laid the foundation for modern gait analysis. Their book, *Human Walking,* was published in 1981 and represents the seminal text in the field (5).

Since this pioneering work was published, much effort has been put into developing the needed technology for human movement analysis. Automated movement tracking systems have replaced hand digitization. Advances in the aerospace industry have been utilized for the development of force plates for kinetic analysis. Computerized electromyography systems have replaced hand palpation. Currently, the technology and knowledge for gait analysis has advanced to a level that permits rapid evaluation.

EQUIPMENT AND METHODS

Observation

The simplest form of gait analysis is observational gait analysis. A systematic approach for observational gait analysis was developed at the Rancho Los Amigos Medical Center in Downey, California (6). An experienced observer can detect many gait deviations during both stance and swing phases. However, an obvious limitation of observation in gait analysis is the difficulty of observing multiple events and multiple body segments interacting concurrently. Further, it is not possible to visualize the location of force vectors in space or electromyographic activity of muscles. Events happening faster than 1/12 of a second (83 ms) cannot be perceived by the human eye (7). More consistent observations are obtained when motion videotapes are reviewed in slow motion (8). Saleh and Murdoch utilized experienced observers to study the gait of transtibial amputees (9). The prosthetic limbs of the amputees were intentionally misaligned in the sagittal plane. The agreement of experienced observers with a biomechanical model was 22%. Ford et al., in a 1995 study, asked prosthetic clinicians to rate videotape footage of transtibial amputees. The prosthetic limbs of the amputees were intentionally misaligned in the sagittal and coronal plane. The between rater reliability was quantified using the kappa statistic. The reliability was very low in the sagittal plane ($k = 0.08$) and only slightly better in the coronal plane ($k = 0.36$). Thus, it is easy to see that limitations in observational gait analysis can lead to misinterpretation of the patient's locomotion capabilities. Hence, it is important to utilize advances in gait analysis techniques to more precisely quantify the patient's functional status. Extensive instrumentation has been developed for recording of the various parameters during gait.

Movement Measurement

In the biomechanical analysis of motion, skeletal segments are studied as rigid links moving through space. These rigid links are assumed to be interconnected through a series of frictionless joints. Measurement systems that are aimed at capturing the spatial trajectories of body segments usually involve a camera system that tracks a series of body-fixed markers. Either passively reflective or actively illuminated markers are used with these systems. Using stereophotogrammetric principles, the planar projections of markers viewed by each camera are used to reconstruct the three-dimensional instantaneous

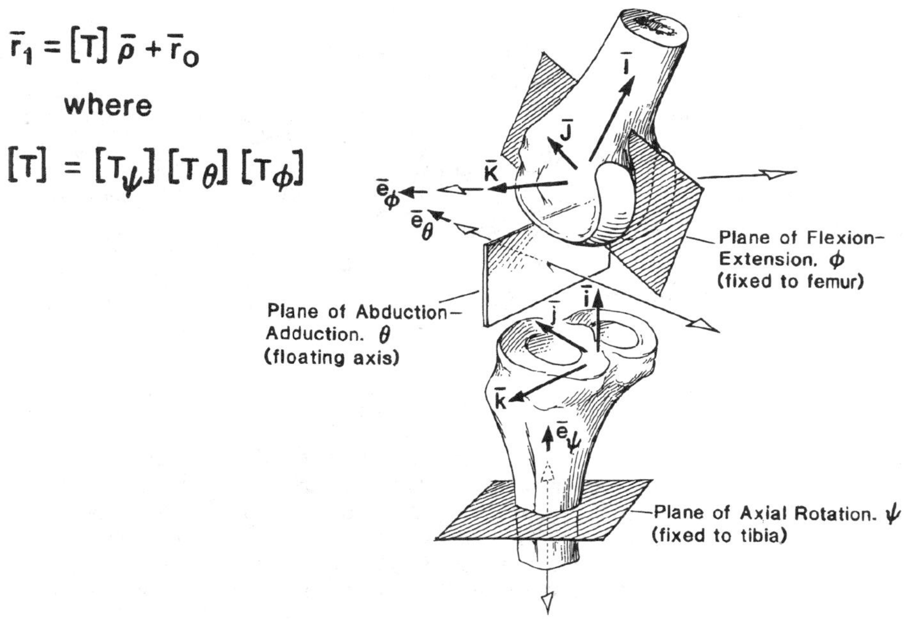

FIG. 7.1. Description of knee joint motion using an Eulerian angle system. An axis fixed to the distal femur defines flexion/extension motion, Φ. An axis fixed to proximal tibia along its anatomical axis defines internal-external rotation, Ψ. A floating axis is orthogonal to the other two axes and used to measure abduction–adduction, Θ. (From Chao EYS. Justification of triaxial goniometer for the measurement of joint rotation. *J Biomechan* 1980;13:989–1006.)

positions of the markers in a laboratory coordinate system. These markers are used to define anatomic coordinate systems for each limb segment. The marker system is coupled to a biomechanical model (10,11). If the positions of at least three noncolinear points fixed to the body segment are described (and the body segment is assumed to be rigid) then the position of the segment in space can be obtained. Once the position of adjacent limb segments has been determined, it is possible to determine the relative angle between adjacent limb segments in three dimensions. The Euler system is the most commonly used method clinically for describing three-dimensional motion (Fig. 7.1) (12,13).

Recently, advances have been made in the animation industry that will have future applications in the biomechanics field. Computerized motion analysis systems have been developed that provide marker trajectory data in real time. These systems are becoming available for applications in biomechanics. Once these applications are developed, it will be possible to obtain results of gait analysis studies much faster than is currently practical. This advance will make gait analysis much more clinically available.

Force Measurement

Gait analysis is also concerned with the forces that cause the observed movement and the assessment of their effect on locomotion (kinetic analysis). Forces acting on the human body can be divided into internal and external forces. The external forces represent all physical interactions between the body and the environment. These forces include gravitational, ground reaction forces, and inertial forces. The internal forces are those transmitted by body tissues that include muscular forces, ligament forces, and forces transmitted through joint contact.

Generally, only the ground reaction forces can be measured using a force plate. Current force plates typically use strain gauge or piezoelectric

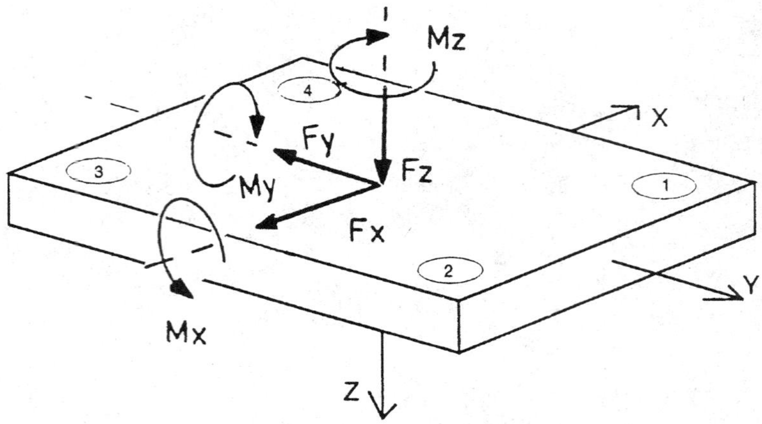

FIG. 7.2. A force plate is used to measure the location and magnitude of the ground reaction force. Transducers, numbered *1 through 4,* are located in the four corners of the plate. The ground reaction force is divided into three force (F_x, F_y, F_z) and three moment (M_x, M_y, M_z) components. F_x and F_y are shear forces. F_z is the vertical force. Some force plates only measure the moment around the vertical axis, that is M_z. This assumes that no tensile forces are imposed on the force plate, that is to say that the foot does not stick to the plate. Under this assumption, the other moments are zero.

transducers. Force platforms can be used to define the magnitude and direction of the resultant ground reaction force (GRF) applied to the foot by the ground (Fig. 7.2). The GRF vector is three-dimensional and consists of a vertical component plus two shear components acting along the force plate surface. The shear forces are applied parallel to the ground and require friction. These shear forces are usually resolved in the anterior-posterior and medial-lateral directions. An additional variable, the center of pressure, is needed to define the location of this GRF vector. The center of pressure is defined as the point about which the distributed force has zero moment when applied to the foot. It is found by determining the line of action of the forces measured by the platform and calculating where that line intersects the surface of the force platform.

These force data are combined with kinematic data using Newton's Second Law to calculate the forces causing motion. The process of proceeding from known kinematic data and external forces to obtain intersegmental joint forces and moments is called the inverse dynamics approach (Fig. 7.3) (14). The gravitational forces acting on each body segment can be determined from the

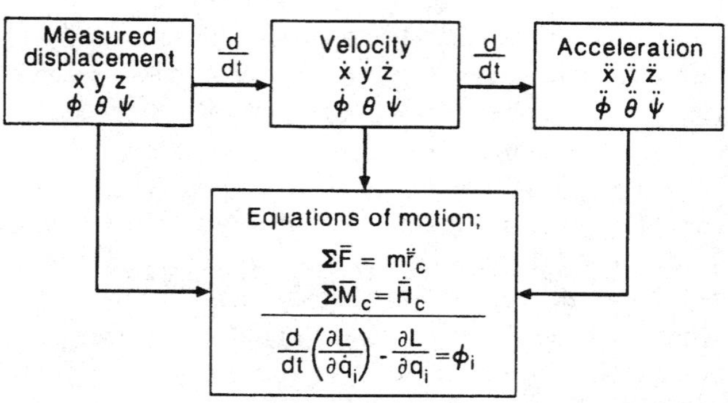

FIG. 7.3. Solution process for inverse dynamics problem. Displacement information must be differentiated twice to yield acceleration. Either Newtonian or Lagranian formulations can be used to formulate the equations of motion.

relevant mass and location of the center of mass for each segment. These quantities can be calculated together with the segmental mass moments of inertia using prediction techniques from anthropometric dimensions. The inertial forces can be obtained from calculations of angular and linear position, as well as velocity and acceleration of the body segments with respect to either a fixed laboratory coordinate system or referenced to another body segment using kinematic data. This information can be combined to solve the inverse dynamics problem. Joint power can also be calculated (15). These data provide understanding of the subtle musculoskeletal adaptations that are utilized by patients to maintain dynamic balance during gait. Kinetic data are available at the hip, knee, and ankle joint. When the position of this force line with respect to joint center has been established by combining force and movement data, the extrinsic joint moment, which is the product of lever arm and force, plus gravity and inertia, can be calculated. This moment is of great importance because it determines the requirements for intrinsic (muscle) force in the case of lower extremity muscles acting during load bearing. For example, when the force line falls behind the knee joint center, quadriceps muscle action is required to prevent knee collapse, and when the force line falls in front of the knee, extension muscle force is not needed.

At each joint, a state of equilibrium exists where the internal joint forces balance the external joint forces. The measurement of internal forces requires sophisticated invasive techniques. Analytical procedures have been developed for estimating internal joint forces. These analytical approaches use classical mechanics and mathematical optimization routines (16). These analytical approaches require the use of simplifying assumptions about the mechanical structure and knowledge of muscle physiology principles. Thus, the accuracy of the analytical predictions depends not only on the quality of the input data but also on the validity of the assumptions. In general, it is necessary to evaluate the estimated quantities by comparing them with experimental observations. Typically, electromyographic data are obtained to provide information regarding muscle activation patterns.

Electromyography

Neuromuscular coordination is required to adjust the varying muscular and ligamentous forces interacting with the abundant degrees of freedom in the joints and other parts of passive locomotive system to obtain dynamic balance during gait. Electromyographic data are useful to provide information about the timing of muscle activity and the relative intensity of muscle activity. Both surface and fine-wire electrodes have been used for gait kinesiologic EMG analysis. Each type of electrode has its advantages and disadvantages. Surface electrodes are convenient, easy to apply to the skin, and do not cause pain, irritation, or discomfort to the subject. However, they pick up signals from other active muscles in the general area of application. This feature makes surface electrodes the ideal choice for analysis of global activity in superficial muscle or muscle groups. However, surface electrodes are sensitive to movement of the skin under the electrodes and have poor specificity. They are influenced by significant muscle "cross-talk," in which the electrode signals of one muscle interfere with the signals from another (17). Thus, the activity of adjacent muscle groups can interfere and lead to false results. The major advantage of fine-wire electrodes is selectivity to measure the activity of specific muscles. The influence of electrical activity of nearby muscles is greatly reduced. Nonetheless, a number of disadvantages are associated with fine-wire electrodes. Pain on insertion, the difficulty of accurate placement, wire movement with muscle contraction, and the need for licensure to utilize wire electrodes are some of the drawbacks. Furthermore, subjects with indwelling electrodes walk more slowly after insertion of the electrodes (18). Because they are to be inserted transcutaneously with a needle, wire electrodes must be sterilized and sufficiently strong to resist breakage. Commonsense considerations, such as time, expense, pain experienced during a long study, the tolerance of the subject to multiple needle insertions, and the influence of indwelling electrodes on walking, necessitate a selection of the muscles most relevant to the specific movement abnormalities. Large muscles near the surface can be studied well with surface electrodes, whereas small muscles and those surrounded by other muscles require insertion of fine-wire electrodes. Electrical stimuli are usually given to confirm the accuracy of placement. A double differential technique has been shown to reduce cross-talk in surface EMGs (19). Electromyographic systems are available in either hardwired or telemetry versions. The hardwired versions now send multiple signals on a single cable. These systems are reliable and less expensive than telemetry. Telemetry systems do not encumber the subject with cables but are susceptible to electromagnetic interference.

Once the EMG data are acquired, they must be processed further to provide information about the timing of muscle activity and the relative intensity of the muscle activity. The EMG data are recorded throughout the gait cycle. The gait cycle is indicated either with synchronization of the kinematic data or with foot-switch information to indicate each foot strike and toe-off. Analysis of the EMG is performed by a phase-time plot of the activity of the muscle against events of the gait cycle. The raw EMG signal can be analyzed or processed further. The most common methods of EMG signal processing are full wave rectification, linear envelope, and integration of the rectified EMG. Low-pass filtering the full wave rectified signal creates the linear envelope. Integrated processing of the rectified signal is usually performed over a short duration (e.g., 2% gait cycle), and then the integration is reset and accumulated again. Normalization schemes may also be used to aid in analysis. Normalization may be based on the maximum manual muscle test or maximum EMG signal obtained during gait. The muscle is considered to be activated when at least 5% of the maximum electrical activity obtained during a manual muscle test is present for 5% of the gait cycle (20).

The electromyogram provides a means for studying muscle activity. The signals that result from action potentials and muscle fibers are stochastic and nonstationary adding to uncertainty in interpretation. Although the ultimate source of locomotor activity is muscle force, no study has established that electromyographic signals represent muscle force. The EMG signal is a measure of the bioelectric events that occur in conjunction with contraction of the muscle fibers. Thus, it is a phenomenon related to the initiation of muscle contraction rather than an effect of the muscle's mechanical action. There are many difficulties in correlating the EMG signal amplitude with muscle force magnitude. Both linear and nonlinear relationships between the force level of skeletal muscles and the EMG signal have been reported (17,21–28). Consequently, the EMG is commonly used in clinical gait analysis mainly to determine phasic patterns for individual muscles or muscle groups. It is possible to examine simple on/off patterns (29), or the EMG can be processed to find a graduation of signal level, after which EMG patterns are examined as defined by the level of activity over the gait cycle (30–32). In the latter process, it is common to normalize the signal as a percentage of voluntary maximum muscle contraction. The process of detecting when a muscle is "turned on or off" is usually one of testing whether the average level of the signal is above some predefined limit. This limit is often defined as a percentage of the maximum voluntary muscle contraction. Calculating the EMG level and then testing for occasions when the level exceeds some threshold value often determine on/off time. EMG on/off times are generally more variable from step to step than either kinematic or kinetic gait measurements.

Problems occur in dynamic situations when using electromyographic activity as a measure of muscle functional capability. A dynamic force produced by a muscle is not proportional to the degree of muscular activity. Other factors may affect the muscle force, such as a change of the muscle length, change of the contraction velocity, the rate and type of muscle contraction, joint position, and muscle fatigue. It is desirable to find an alternative measurable mechanical parameter related to muscle force. The electromyographic signal does not assess the tension produced by a muscle, because the tension reflects the sum of both the active contraction and the passive stretch. A technique that may provide information about muscle force is measurement of intramuscular pressure. Intramuscular pressure (IMP) is a mechanical variable that is proportional to muscle tension. It is possible to obtain IMP measurements during gait and relate these measurements to the timing and intensity of muscle contraction. IMP has been used to quantify

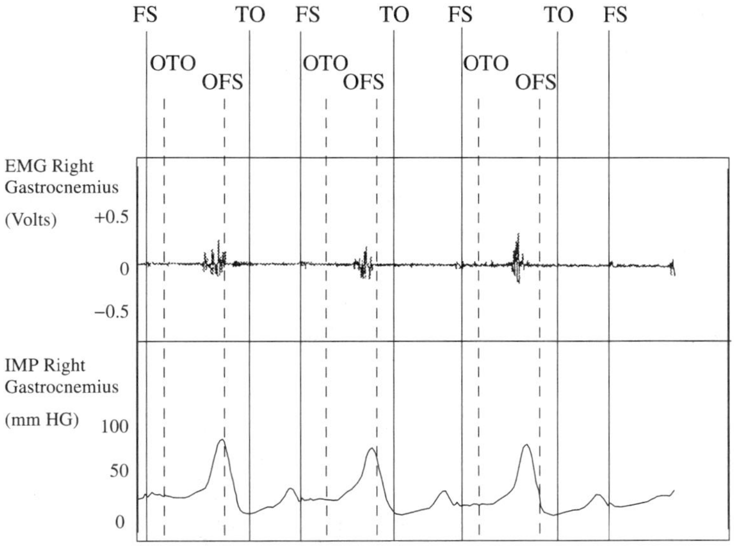

FIG. 7.4. Raw data for a single subject during gait. Both electromyographic (*EMG*) and intramuscular pressure (*IMP*) are being recorded from the gastrocnemius muscle. The stance phase of gait occurs from foot-strike to toe-off (*FS* to *TO*). The swing phase of gait occurs from TO to FS. Single limb stance occurs from opposite toe-off to opposite foot-strike (*OTO* to *OFS*). Peaks in intramuscular pressure during gait can be correlated with peaks of active contraction and passive stretch of the gastrocnemius. (From Kaufman KR, Sutherland DH. Dynamic intramuscular pressure measurements during gait. *Op Tech Sports Med* 1995;3:250–255.)

muscle function during dynamic activities (33). Intramuscular pressure measurements obtained during walking parallel the electromyographic activity, and also account for passive stretch of the muscle (Fig. 7.4) (33).

INTERPRETATION OF GAIT DATA

The most crucial step of interpreting the data remains to be performed once the data that describe the biomechanics of the patient's gait have been collected. The data must be synthesized and integrated in order to supply clinically relevant information based on the clinical examination and measurements performed. Human locomotion is very complex and multifaceted. The clinical interpretation of pathologic gait disorders includes holding in human memory a large number of graphs, numbers, and clinical tests from data presented on hard copy, charts, radiographs, video, and computer generated three-dimensional graphics from multiple trials of a subject walking. Further, comparisons must be made to data from a normal population in order to identify the potential movement problems for a given individual. The referring clinician, who may not be an expert in gait analysis, is overwhelmed by the magnitude of the number of measurements included in a typical gait report. The person interpreting the data obtained must integrate this information. Although data collection techniques for gait analysis have continually evolved over the last 50 years, the method of data presentation has not changed over this time. The data are still reported in two-dimensional charts with the abscissa usually defined as a percentage of the gait cycle and the ordinate displaying the gait parameter.

Recent developments in computer animation make it possible to apply advanced methods to visualize human movements. The large volume of variables currently found in a typical clinical report can be replaced with a few graphic images that succinctly provided the needed information. It is difficult to fully appreciate and understand the relationships between motion dynamics and biomechanical variables without scientific graphic visualization. Presently, computer software packages have advanced to the stage where it is possible to provide a gait analysis report using animation of fully three-dimensional, realistic graphical depictions of human locomotion. The format used for reporting test results is a matter of considerable importance. The results will be of little use to the clinician regardless of quality if they are not communicated in an effective format. The data must be presented in an accurate, clear, and concise format.

TREATMENT PLANNING AND ASSESSMENT

When treatment is being planned, the main objective is to differentiate the primary causes and compensations for the patient's functional problems. If the treatment is directed at compensation, the patient will lose the ability to compensate and movement problems will worsen. The patient will display adaptations in the gait pattern because of pain, injury, deformity, instability, and/or inappropriate muscle activation patterns. The ramifications of these problems cannot be fully assessed without an instrumented gait study. Patients can undergo dynamic adaptation related to the biomechanics of walking that must be factored into the treatment algorithm. For example, it has been shown that when planning corrective osteotomy knee surgery, patients with the same bony deformity will have differing knee loading because of dynamic adaptations (34). These dynamic adaptations will have a direct effect on surgical outcome. Those patients who dynamically compensated for their malalignment had a better long-term outcome (34,35). For patients with progressive disorders, these dynamic adaptations also change with time as the disease progresses. It is possible to use motion analysis studies to quantify these dynamic changes in locomotor patterns.

We are currently conducting a study to quantify gait changes in patients with progressive multiple sclerosis. These patients are studied at 6-month intervals over an 18-month period. Using gait analysis techniques, it is possible to show changes in joint motion that can be attributed to disease progression. An example of changes in knee motion is shown in Figure 7.5. The patient had an EDSS (Kurtzke) rating of 3.0 when first studied, and progressed to an Expanded Disability Status Scale (EDSS) score of 5.5 at the end of the 18-month study period, thus requiring a cane for ambulation. Comparing the data from the initial (0 week) and second visit (1 week), it can be seen that the data are very repeatable. The motion curves for theses two timepoints differed by less than 3 degrees on average throughout the entire gait cycle. The data also demonstrated that the patient lacked the normal knee flexion (shock absorption) wave during early stance. Further, the patient's knee went into hyperextension in mid-stance. These gait characteristics were consistent for all visits during the study period. The knee flexion during swing was

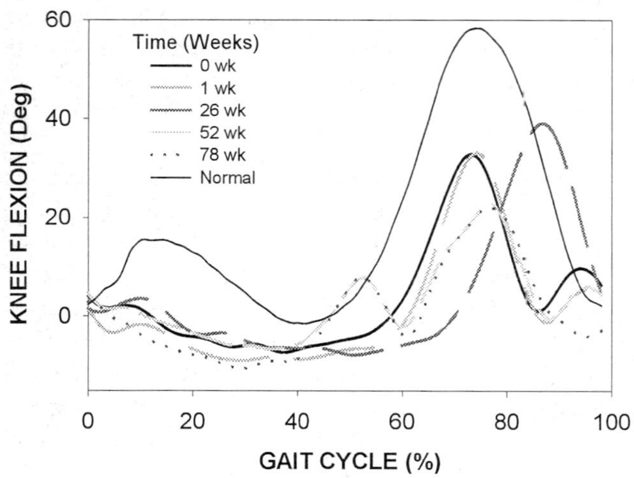

FIG. 7.5. Changes in knee motion over an 18-month period in a patient with primary progressive multiple sclerosis. A normal knee motion curve is given for comparison. The patient lacks knee flexion during early stance and goes into hyperextension during midstance. The knee flexion during swing is less than normal at the initial study and progressively declines over the 18-month study period. The results for the initial visit (0 weeks) and a second study done 1 week later demonstrate excellent measurement repeatability.

less than normal at the initial visit and declined further over the 18-month study period. This example clearly illustrates the objective nature of instrumented gait analysis and the ability to document subtle changes that may not be remembered over time if only clinical observation is used.

RATIONALE

The ability to document the need and effectiveness of a particular treatment will assume an increasingly important role in this era of government reimbursement for medical services. Managed care will require validation for many types of therapeutic interventions. Pretreatment and post-treatment measurement will become mandatory. Outcomes will have to be compared. Practitioners and facilities will be rated on their outcomes. Maximizing anticipated outcomes will be required to document that a treatment plan is worthwhile. Objective gait analysis is an essential tool to meet these demands. The technology is at a level where it is both feasible and affordable to provide an objective form of patient assessment.

A need exists for instrumentation and procedures to aid in a differential diagnosis and treatment of patients in all areas of medical care. Further, information is required to objectively document patient response to treatment. The ability to diagnose, prescribe treatment, and document results is common to all areas of medical care. However, the technology available in different medical specialties varies widely. This is particularly evident when the current medical technology for treating patients with cardiovascular conditions is compared to the technology for treating patients with neuromuscular conditions (Table 7.1). For both types of patients the technology can be divided into three levels: static examinations, dynamic examinations, and invasive procedures. Typically, the approach is to utilize the technology available at the lowest level that will meet the requirements for aiding in differential diagnosis and treatment planning. When a patient reports to a physician that they are experiencing chest pain and the risk factors for a myocardial infarction exist, the patient is monitored with an electrocardiogram. In some centers, an electron beam computed tomography (EBCT) scan is obtained to assess the amount of arteriosclerosis in the vessels of the heart muscle. These tests are obtained while the patient is either sitting or lying down; therefore, these constitute static exams. Other static modalities include magnetic resonance imaging (MRI), positron emission tomography (PET), ultrasound, and nuclear imaging. Dynamic tests may be undertaken if the physician has a high index of suspicion. These include a stress test or echocardiograph. Finally, angiography may be utilized as an invasive procedure to further examine the heart.

Conversely, for a patient with neuromuscular dysfunction, most of the modalities utilized are

TABLE 7.1. *Current medical technology*

		Treatment modality	
Level	Exam	Cardiovascular patients	Neuromuscular patients
I	Static	ECG EBCT MRI PET Ultrasound Nuclear Imaging	X-ray CT MRI Nuclear Imaging
II	Dynamic	Stress Test Echocardiography	Motion Analysis
III	Invasive	Angiography	Diagnostic EMG Kinesiological EMG

CT, computed tomography; EBCT, electron beam CT; ECG, electrocardiography; EMG, electromyography; MRI, magnetic resonance imaging; PET, positron emission tomography.

static modalities. Current modalities include radiography, computed tomography (CT), MRI, and nuclear imaging. It is also common to obtain diagnostic EMG to further elucidate a determination regarding the neuromuscular status of the patient. However, during all these examinations, the patient is static and non-weight bearing. Dynamic assessment of patients with neuromuscular dysfunction can only be obtained using motion analysis techniques along with acquisition of kinesiologic EMG.

Sometimes these studies are objected to as being too costly. However, this objection is unfounded. In terms of cost-benefit ratio, the most compelling consideration is the high cost of inappropriate treatment. It is important to remember that unsuccessful treatment will result in unfavorable changes in function and may require subsequent procedures to deal with the original problem. There is, of course, no assurance that gait studies performed prior to treatment planning will always ensure favorable outcome, but careful planning, based on objective data, will provide a solid foundation for decision making. Post-treatment studies will give the information required for objective evaluation of treatment results. The rate at which gait analysis technologies will become more common will depend on the market, manufacturers, and managed care requirements. Objective patient assessment using gait analysis techniques will facilitate the identification of optimal treatment regimens, and provide a solid foundation for clinical decision making.

CONCLUSION

Human function cannot be fully understood without studies of movement. The modern motion analysis laboratory that has evolved with technologic advances has the potential to open new opportunities for progress in the treatment of patients with movement disorders. Gait analysis systems have evolved to sophisticated automatic tracking systems, force platforms, and EMG activity. When coupled with a biomechanical model, this equipment is able to provide a complete, three-dimensional, dynamic description of the patient's kinematics and kinetics along with information on the timing and intensity of muscle activity during gait. The function of a motion analysis laboratory is to objectively measure the dynamic aspects of an individual patient's performance that cannot be quantitatively assessed in the clinical setting. Interpretation of these data make it possible to integrate morphology and functional adaptations in order to understand and treat the pathophysiology of movement disorders.

REFERENCES

1. Borelli GA. *De motor animalium.* Batavis: Lugduni, 1685.
2. Basmajian JV, De Luca CL. *Muscles alive: their functions revealed by electromyography,* 5th ed. Baltimore: Williams & Wilkins, 1985.
3. Muybridge E. *Human and animal locomotion.* New York: Dover, 1979 (original published in 1887).
4. Braune W, Fischer O. *Der Gang des Nenschen.* Leipzig: BG Teubner, 1895.
5. Inman VT, Ralston HJ, Todd F. *Human walking.* Baltimore: Williams & Wilkins, 1981.
6. Perry J. *Gait analysis: normal and pathological function.* Thorofare, NJ: Slack, 1992.
7. Gage JR, Onpuu S. Gait analysis in clinical practice. *Semin Orthop* 1989; 2:72–87.
8. Krebs DE, Edelstein JE, Fishman S. Reliability of observational kinematic gait analysis. *Phys Ther* 1985;65:1027–2033.
9. Saleh M, Murdoch G. In defense of gait analysis. *J Bone Joint Surg* 1985;67B:237–241.
10. Kadaba MP, Ramakrishnan WK, Wootten ME. Measurement of lower extremity kinematics during level walking. *J Orthop Res* 1990;8:383–392.
11. Kaufman KR, An KN, Chao EYS. A comparison of intersegmental joint dynamics to isokinetic dynamometer measurements. *J Biomechan* 1995;28:1243–1265.
12. Chao EYS. Justification of triaxial goniometer for the measurement of joint rotation. *J Biomechan* 1980;13:989–1006.
13. Grood ES, Suntay WJ. A joint coordinate system for the clinical disclusion of 3-dimensional motions: applications to the knee. *J Biomechan Eng* 1983;105:136–144.
14. Chao EYS. *Determination of applied forces in linking systems with known displacements: with special application to biomechanics.* Iowa City, Iowa: University of Iowa, 1971.
15. Winter DA. *Biomechanics and motor control of human movement,* 2nd ed. New York: Wiley & Sons, 1990.
16. Kaufman K, An K, Litchy W, et al. Physiological prediction of muscle forces. I. Theoretical formulation. *Neuroscience* 1991;40:781–792.
17. Zuniga EN, Simons DG. Nonlinear relationship between averaged electromyogram potential and muscle tension in normal subjects. *Arch Phys Med Rehab* 1969;50:613–620.
18. Young CC, Rose SE, Biden EN, et al. The effect of surface and internal electrodes on the gait of children

with cerebral palsy, spastic diplegia type. *J Orthop Res* 1989;7:732.
19. Koh TJ, Grabiner MD. Cross-talk in surface electromyograms of human hamstring muscles. *J Orthop Res* 1992;10:701–709.
20. Bogey RA, Barnes LA, Perry J. Computer algorithms to characterize individual subject EMG profiles during gait. *Arch Phys Med Rehab* 1992;73:835–841.
21. Woods JJ, Bigland-Ritchie B. Linear and nonlinear surface EMG/force relationships in human muscles. *Am Phys Med* 1983;62:287.
22. Matral M, Casser G. Relationship between force and integrated EMG activity during voluntary isometric and isotonic contraction. *Eur J Appl Physiol* 1977;46:185.
23. Bigland-Ritchie B, Kukulka CJ, Woods JJ. Surface EMG-force relationships in human muscles of different fibre composition. *J Physiol (Lond)* 1980;308:103P.
24. Maton B, Bouisset S. The distribution of activity among the muscles of a single group during isometric contraction. *Eur J Appl Physiol* 1972;37:101.
25. Komi PV, Buskirk ER. Effective eccentric and concentric muscle conditioning on tension and electrical activity of human muscle. *Ergonomics* 1972;15:417.
26. Moritani T, de Vries HA. Reexamination of the relationship between the surface integrated electromyogram (IEMG) and force of isometric contraction. *Am J Phys Med* 1978;57:263.
27. Lippold OCJ. The relation between integrated action potentials in a human muscle and its isometric tension. *J Physiol (Lond)* 1952;117:492.
28. Messier RH, Duffy J, Litchman HM, et al. The electromyogram as a measure of tension in the human biceps and triceps muscles. *Int J Mechan Sci* 1981;13:585.
29. Sutherland DH, Olshen RA, Biden EN, et al. *The development of mature walking*. Oxford, England: MacKeith Press, 1988.
30. Limbird TJ, Shiavi R, Frazer M, et al. EMG profiles of knee joint musculature during walking: changes induced by anterior cruciate ligament deficiency. *J Orthop Res* 1988;6:630.
31. Shiavi R, Green N. Ensemble averaging of locomotor electromyographic patterns using interpolation. *Med Biol Eng Comput* 1983;21:573.
32. Wooten ME, Kadaba MP, Cochran GUB. Dynamic electromyography. II. Normal patterns during gait. *J Orthop Res* 1990;8:259.
33. Kaufman KR, Sutherland DH. Dynamic intramuscular pressure measurement during gait. *Op Tech Sports Med* 1995;3:250–255.
34. Prodromos CC, Andriacchi TP, Galante JO. A relationship between gait and clinical changes following high tibial osteotomy. *J Bone Joint Surg* 1985;67A:1188–1194.
35. Wang JW, Kuo NN, Andriacchi TP, et al. The influence of walking mechanics and time on the results of proximal tibial osteotomy. *J Bone Joint Surg* 1990;6:905–909.

Gait Disorders. Advances in Neurology, Vol. 87,
edited by E. Růžička, M. Hallett, and J. Jankovic.
Lippincott Williams & Wilkins, Philadelphia © 2001.

8

Neuroimaging and Gait

Joseph C. Masdeu

Department of Neurology, University of Navarre, University Hospital of Navarre, Pamplona 31008, Spain

CLINICAL APPLICATIONS OF MAGNETIC RESONANCE IMAGING AND COMPUTED TOMOGRAPHY

Lumbosacral Spine

Magnetic resonance imaging (MRI) is not needed in most instances for the workup of spinal claudication. Computed tomography (CT) depicts a narrow canal with crowding of the lateral recesses because of facet hypertrophy. CT also shows the thickened ligamentum flavum and, possibly, calcification of the posterior longitudinal ligament. However, if CT is negative, MRI may be needed to rule out other lesions in the region of the cauda equina, such as a filum terminalis ependymoma or a neurilemoma.

Cervical Spine

Magnetic resonance imaging is the diagnostic tool of choice for the workup of patients with a clinical picture suggestive of cervical spondylosis (1,2). Spin-echo sequences should be obtained, including T2-weighted images depicting any possible edema or microcavitation in the cord itself. At first glance, the recently popularized FLAIR sequence (*Fl*uid *A*ttenuated *I*nversion *R*ecovery) appears ideal for the study of changes within the cord, because it combines the sensitivity for local water increase of a T2-weighted image with a background free of the bright signal of cerebrospinal fluid (CSF). Although the FLAIR sequence has not been studied in this process, its lack of sensitivity for other lesions of the spinal cord may be a harbinger of poor results here as well (3–5).

Cerebellar and Vestibular Disease

Cerebellar atrophy can be visualized with CT, but is depicted with greater accuracy with MRI. In patients symptomatic for disorders such as olivopontocerebellar degeneration, the changes are so prominent that they can be easily visualized with CT. On the other hand, ischemic lesions in the cerebellum or vestibular nuclei are reliably seen only with MRI. Even MRI may be negative in the first few hours or even days after the event. T2-weighted images are most sensitive for the intraparenchymal changes. The FLAIR sequence is more sensitive than spin echo T2 sequences for supratentorial, but not for infratentorial ischemic lesions (6). Because the location of an infarct often can be deduced from the clinical examination, MRI helps more by depicting the vascular changes than by showing the exact localization of the infarct. The most characteristic pattern in MRI of the posterior circulation is dissection of the vertebral artery. On T1-weighted images, a bright semilunar ring can be seen encircling the narrowed lumen of the vessel. Vessels occluded by local atheromatous changes or emboli can be seen, as well as perforator occlusion by atheromatous plaques in the wall of the basilar artery. Changes in the vessel wall are best visualized by MRI, but magnetic resonance (MR) angiography allows for the visualization in three dimensions of the lumen of large to mid-sized vessels.

MRI is also the procedure of choice to image other potentially treatable lesions of the posterior fossa causing gait impairment, such as tumors or arteriovenous malformations.

Lacunar Disease

Acutely, ischemic lacunar disease is poorly visualized by CT or MRI. MRI is eventually more sensitive than CT for the detection of lacunes. Because lacunes can cause unexplained gait and balance impairment in an older adult, MRI of the brain should be obtained a few days after an acute onset of balance or gait impairment. Depending on the location and extent of the lesion, it more likely will be related to small vessel disease (lipohyalinosis, arteriolosclerosis, CADASIL [*C*erebral *A*utosomal *D*ominant *A*rteriopathy with *S*ubcortical *I*nfarcts and *L*eukoencephalopathy]) or embolic. Giant lacunes are often embolic, but they seldom present with pure gait impairment, a frank hemiparesis being more common. The management of these lesions differs; therefore, a precise etiologic diagnosis is important. For ischemic lesions of the supratentorial compartment, FLAIR sequences are more sensitive than conventional spin-echo sequences (6,7).

White Matter Disease

White matter disease of aging can be visualized either with CT or MRI (8,9). Actually, MRI may be too sensitive for white matter disease. High intensity areas on T2 MR are often undetected on CT. On T2-MR images, it may be difficult to differentiate areas of increased water content because of dilation of perivascular spaces with normal aging or transependymal CSF absorption from areas of tissue damage because both have increased intensity values (10–12). For this reason it seems preferable to make the diagnosis of significant white matter changes only when the abnormalities are visible on T1-weighted images (13). Proton-density images are also helpful. High-intensity changes on this sequence seem to correlate with the presence of gliosis, a pathologic finding in some patients with white matter disease and gait disorder (14).

Hydrocephalus

Although hydrocephalus can be visualized with CT as well as with MRI, MRI shows CSF flow-related findings that may help separate hydrocephalus *ex vacuo* from communicating hydrocephalus. The flow void in the Sylvian aqueduct is prominent in patients with communicating hydrocephalus, and decreases after shunting (15,16). Bradley and coworkers studied CSF stroke volume and aqueductal CSF flow void score before and after shunting (17). All 12 patients with CSF stroke volumes greater than 42 μL responded favorably to CSF shunting. They and others failed to find a relationship between aqueductal CSF flow void score and responsiveness to shunting (18). Because older subjects often have atrophy, the sulci at the base may be dilated, sometimes markedly, in communicating hydrocephalus (19,20). Compression of the cortical sulci in the high convexity helps in some cases to define symptomatic hydrocephalus.

CLINICAL APPLICATIONS OF SINGLE PHOTON EMISSION COMPUTED TOMOGRAPHY AND POSITRON EMISSION TOMOGRAPHY

Single photon emission computed tomography (SPECT) can be used to evaluate cerebral perfusion in patients with brain disorders. Regional cerebral blood flow and metabolism can be obtained with positron emission tomography (PET). Both techniques also can be used to depict the regional density of a number of neurotransmitters. The role of these two procedures in the workup of patients with gait disorders is still in an investigational stage and is discussed in the next section, except that lower frontal to posterior perfusion ratio on SPECT was found to predict which patients with hydrocephalus will improve after shunting (21). Patients with decreased perfusion in the parieto-temporal association cortex are more likely to have Alzheimer's disease (AD) and enlarged ventricles because of atrophy. This information is important, because shunting is not without risk at any age, particularly in the elderly (22).

About one-fifth of them, or more, may be undiagnosed after completing the standard workup of patients with gait disorders (23,24). Because most of these patients have gait patterns suggestive of dysfunction of the control centers in the brain, it is logical to look for changes in these brain structures with techniques potentially more sensitive than MRI (25). For this reason, PET or SPECT may be used to image the medial frontal region, putamen, and lateral thalami of these patients, in order to assess hypoperfusion changes or decreased metabolism that still has not resulted in structural changes. There are multiple examples of the greater sensitivity of functional neuroimaging in degenerative disorders of the brain, including Huntington's chorea and AD (26). Nakamura and coworkers studied a group of 45 patients with AD at different clinical stages and 15 controls with *N*-isopropyl-*p*-[^{123}I]iodoamphetamine SPECT. At a moderate stage, reduced mean values of cortical perfusion, particularly in the frontal lobe, were associated with increased postural sway and stride length variability and with decreased stride length. At a severe stage, reduced perfusion in the basal ganglia and in the frontal lobe additionally were associated with increased postural sway, double support time, and stride length variability, and with decreased walking speed and stride length (27).

RESEARCH APPLICATIONS

For the study of normal gait and of idiopathic gait disorders, there are multiple applications of neuroimaging.

- Brain activation during standing and gait in normal subjects
- Measurement of regional and global atrophy of brain or spinal cord structures
- Localization and measurement of white matter abnormalities, shown to cause unsteadiness and a propensity to falling, particularly in the elderly
- Identification of brain regions that are abnormal in patients with gait disorders
- Biochemical characterization of areas that are abnormal in patients with gait disorders
- Brain activation by maneuvers that improve gait, such as the paradoxical gait of parkinsonian patients
- Identification of more homogeneous populations for the study of genetically transmitted disorders

Brain Activation Studies

Brain activation by standing posture has been studied with PET (28). Regional cerebral blood flow was determined with $H_2{}^{15}O$. The subjects were eight right-handed (right-footed) female volunteers, 31.8 ± 6.5 years of age. Eye movements were carefully monitored, to ensure a lack of eye movements during the task as much as possible. Recording could be performed with the subjects lying on the scanner (control condition) and with the patients standing in the various experimental conditions because the PET gantry could be tilted. Compared with the supine posture, standing with feet together activated the cerebellar anterior lobe and the right visual cortex (Brodmann area 18/19), and standing on one foot increased cerebral blood flow in the cerebellar anterior vermis and the posterior lobe lateral cortex ipsilateral to the weight-bearing side. Standing in tandem was accompanied by activation within the visual association cortex, the anterior and posterior vermis, and the midbrain. Standing with eyes closed activated the prefrontal cortex (Brodmann area 8/9).

Brain activation has been studied during walking with SPECT. Unlike PET, SPECT can record brain activity while the patient is not in the scanner, because the isotopes used for SPECT have a longer half-life than the isotopes used for PET. Brain perfusion is measured for a few minutes after the isotope is injected and can be recorded by scanning from about 15 minutes to several hours after injection. For this reason, SPECT lends itself to the study of gait. Fukuyama and coworkers studied gait in 14 subjects (25). The activation consisted of a 4-minute walk. Shortly after initiation of walking, 259 MBq of ^{99}Tc HMPAO were injected. At the end of the task, the patients were scanned with a three-head SPECT unit. The scanning procedure took 30 minutes. By injecting 777 MBq of ^{99}Tc HMPAO, the baseline perfusion study was then obtained, without repositioning the patient's head. The second scanning time was 15 minutes. Comparison between the baseline and activated conditions and among subjects was performed by conforming individual data to Talairach's atlas and using statistical parametric mapping. The supplementary motor area, medial primary sensorimotor area, striatum, cerebellar vermis, and visual cortex were activated.

Measurement of Regional and Global Atrophy of Brain or Spinal Cord Structures

Clues as to the cause of some gait disorders might be provided by regional patterns of atrophy in the brain, brainstem, or spinal cord. Automated procedures have been developed to measure the volume of the brain on MRI (29). Head MRI segmentation was used to separate the skull from the brain, the brain from the CSF and the gray from the white matter. The method is described in some detail. It combines histogram-based automatic thresholding with sequences of morphologic operations to separate the different head tissues. Four steps were involved: (a) A binary image is first obtained by automatic thresholding; discriminant analysis searches for the optical gray level that best separates these two classes by variance optimization; it is then assumed that each pixel belongs either to brain or background. (b) Morphological opening separates brain from skull. (c) Connected component analysis consists of three operations: (i) connection of components with nonzero pixels (CSF and tissues previously occupied by the skull and covering tissues), (ii) labeling and counting the connected components, and (iii) selecting the largest component as the brain. (d) The resultant binary image of the brain is masked to the original gray image and displayed separate from the covering tissues. The nonzero voxels are counted and multiplied by their size to measure size (29).

The diameter of the spinal cord could be decreased in some gait disorders. Transverse MRI sections can be used to measure the diameter of the cord at different levels and compare it to normative data (30).

Localization and Measurement of White Matter Abnormalities

White matter lesions have been shown to be more frequent in elderly with impaired balance and a tendency to fall (8,9,13,24,31–37). Most of the studies have used rater-determined scoring methods. Some have tried to measure the extent of white matter involvement using semiautomatic methods based on the operator defining the location of the lesion on MRI slices and computerized calculation of neighboring pixels with similar intensity (13). This procedure is helpful, but radiofrequency-pulse inhomogeneity can cause artefacts, particularly when mapping large areas or areas located away from the center of the radiofrequency coil (38). For this reason, most current software uses the comparison of multiple MRI pulses of the same slide (Multiparametric Segmentation Techniques) (39).

The direction of white matter tracts can be identified with diffusion-weighted MRI (40). Anisotropy maps of the brain can produce striking anatomic renditions of the white matter tracts of the brain (41). Lesion information combined with this kind of anatomic information could help make more precise the functional correlation of white matter lesions.

Identification of Brain Regions That Are Abnormal in Patients with Gait Disorders

In idiopathic gait disorders, where clinical imaging is unremarkable and measurements of brain atrophy are not specific, comparing brain activity between patients and controls might help uncover dysfunctional regions. Brain activity can be measured with metabolic markers by PET, with perfusion agents by SPECT, or by labels of neurotransmitter receptors or transporters using either technique. The study by Ito and coworkers exemplifies a commonly employed methodology (42). They used a dopamine marker, ^{18}F-dopa, to compare dopaminergic activity in controls and patients with early Parkinson's disease (PD). For each subject, PET data were superimposed to the subject's MRI, in order to sharpen anatomic definition. To allow for intersubject comparison, the composite images were fit within a standard coordinate space, such as the Talairach coordinates. Brain activity of patients and controls, expressed in mean Ki values, was then compared voxel by voxel. Statistically significant differences were determined by using statistical parametric mapping (SPM) software. With this procedure, it was determined that striatal and nigral dopaminergic activity was significantly decreased in the patient group. A similar technique could be applied to gait impaired patients who do not have PD or other identified cause of gait impairment. In addition to dopaminergic agents, other neurotransmitters could be labeled or regional metabolism compared.

Another strategy consists in labeling structures known to be involved in gait mechanisms and then compare the extent of neurotransmitter activity in patients and controls. Ichise has described a method to calculate the amount of dopaminergic activity of the striatum with the use of a presynaptic dopaminergic transporter ligand, [^{123}I]-β-CIT, and SPECT (43). The volume of the striatal dopamine labeled in this manner is smaller in patients with early PD, whereas the map of striatal receptors is increased, reflecting the upregulation of these receptors caused by decreased dopamine availability (44).

Biochemical Characterization of Areas That Are Abnormal in Patients with Gait Disorders

In addition to PET, SPECT, and functional MRI, other techniques are available for the biochemical characterization of brain areas that may be involved in the genesis of gait disorders. Brooks and coworkers used magnetic resonance spectroscopy (MRS) to study white matter lesions in three populations matched by age: normal elderly controls, aging individuals who had white matter lesions on T2 MRI but no gait impairment, and patients with white matter lesions and impaired gait (31). The last group was clinically diagnosed with subcortical arteriosclerotic encephalopathy and was the only group to have an abnormal MR spectrum. The ratios of *N*-acetyl-aspartate (NAA) to creatinine and NAA to choline were decreased, suggesting the loss of normal cells, whereas the ratio of choline to creatinine was increased. Thus, they were able to separate with MRS patient groups whose MRI findings, at least on T2-weighted images, were similar.

In parkinsonian patients, dopamine loss can be shown in the striatum with [^{123}I]-β-CIT, and SPECT, as mentioned in the preceding (43). In addition, upregulation of receptors, hungry for dopamine, can also be shown with SPECT, this time using a dopamine-receptor ligand, such as [^{123}I]-IBF (44). Similar results can be obtained with PET using a variety of radioligands (45,46).

PET and MRS have been used to follow tissue changes in monkeys rendered parkinsonian with the long-term administration of low doses of methyl-phenyl-tetrahydropyridine (MPTP) (47). This model of human parkinsonism was obtained by injecting low-dose MPTP to five cynomolgus monkeys over 18 months. Presynaptic dopamine uptake was monitored with ^{11}C-CFT PET over 24 months. The authors found that presynaptic dopaminergic terminals were progressively lost, even after MPTP was stopped. With MRS, they found that the NAA to Cr ratio became low and stayed that way, reflecting permanent neuronal loss. On the other hand, there was a transient rise in lactate levels, reflecting tissue injury. Interestingly, lactate levels continued to increase shortly after MPTP administration ceased but reversed 2 years after stopping MPTP administration. This study illustrates how neuroimaging can be used to study the pathogenetic mechanisms of chronic disease.

Brain Activation by Maneuvers That Improve Gait

It is conceivable that strategies could be devised to improve gait in a variety of clinical situations if the mechanisms underlying maneuvers that improve the quality of gait in some disorders could be better understood. Using ^{99}Tc-HMPAO SPECT, Hanakawa and coworkers showed activation of the frontal lateral premotor region during "paradoxical gait" in 10 patients with PD (48). In the control condition the patients walked on a treadmill with two white lines placed parallel to the direction of gait. In the study condition, there were transverse lines in the treadmill and the patients' gait improved ("paradoxical gait"). This finding may suggest that a "cortical strategy," with the patient walking more intent on his or her gait, may benefit gait in patients with lesions of the basal ganglia or its connections.

Identification of More Homogeneous Populations for the Study of Genetically Transmitted Disorders

The genetic study of diseases with a long incubation period is hindered by the delay in clinical symptomatology. Twin studies of PD have shown little concordance among identical twins. However, the question remained whether individuals who were normal at the time of the study might not go on to eventually develop PD. A recent PET study suggests that this may well be the case. Piccini and coworkers found that the concordance for subclinical striatal dopaminergic dysfunction was found to be significantly higher in 18 monozygotic than in 16 dizygotic twin pairs (55% versus 18%, respectively) (49). The asymptomatic monozygotic cotwins all showed progressive loss of dopaminergic function over 7 years and four developed clinical PD. None of the dizygotic twin pairs became clinically concordant. At follow-up, the combined concordance levels for subclinical dopaminergic dysfunction and clinical PD were 75% in the 12 monozygotic and 22% in the nine dizygotic twin pairs evaluated twice. This study exemplifies how the use of neuroimaging improved the classification of patients and controls, thereby suggesting a substantial genetic role in the genesis of PD.

REFERENCES

1. Statham PF, Hadley DM, Macpherson P, et al. MRI in the management of suspected cervical spondylotic myelopathy. *J Neurol Neurosurg Psychiatry* 1991;54:484–489.
2. Sadasivan KK, Reddy RP, Albright JA. The natural history of cervical spondylotic myelopathy. *Yale J Biol Med* 1993;66:235–242.
3. Keiper MD, Grossman RI, Brunson JC, et al. The low sensitivity of fluid-attenuated inversion-recovery MR in the detection of multiple sclerosis of the spinal cord. *AJNR Am J Neuroradiol* 1997;18:1035–1039.
4. Stevenson VL, Gawne-Cain ML, Barker GJ, et al. Imaging of the spinal cord and brain in multiple sclerosis: a comparative study between fast FLAIR and fast spin echo. *J Neurol* 1997;244:119–124.
5. Yousry TA, Filippi M, Becker C, et al. Comparison of MR pulse sequences in the detection of multiple sclerosis lesions. *AJNR Am J Neuroradiol* 1997;18:959–963.
6. Brant-Zawadzki M, Atkinson D, Detrick M, et al. Fluid-attenuated inversion recovery (FLAIR) for assessment of cerebral infarction. Initial clinical experience in 50 patients. *Stroke* 1996;27:1187–1191.
7. Noguchi K, Ogawa T, Inugami A, et al. MRI of acute cerebral infarction: a comparison of FLAIR and T2-weighted fast spin-echo imaging. *Neuroradiology* 1997;39:406–410.
8. Briley DP, Wasay M, Sergent S, et al. Cerebral white matter changes (leukoaraiosis), stroke, and gait disturbance. *J Am Geriatr Soc* 1997;45:1434–1438.
9. Baloh RW, Yue Q, Socotch TM, et al. White matter lesions and disequilibrium in older people. I. Case-control comparison. *Arch Neurol* 1995;52:970–974.
10. Awad I, Johnson P, Spetzler R, et al. Incidental subcortical lesions identified on magnetic resonance imaging in the elderly. II. Postmortem pathological correlations. *Stroke* 1986;17:1090–1097.
11. Kirkpatrick J, Hayman L. White-matter lesions on MR imaging of clinically healthy brains of elderly subjects: possible pathologic basis. *Radiology* 1987;162:509–511.
12. Zimmerman R, Fleming C, Lee B, et al. Periventricular hyperintensity as seen by magnetic resonance: prevalence and significance. *Am J Radiol* 1986;146:443–450.
13. Gass A, Oster M, Cohen S, et al. Assessment of T2- and T1-weighted MRI brain lesion load in patients with subcortical vascular encephalopathy. *Neuroradiology* 1998;40:503–506.
14. Baloh RW, Vinters HV. White matter lesions and disequilibrium in older people. II. Clinicopathologic correlation. *Arch Neurol* 1995;52:975–981.
15. Gideon P, Stahlberg F, Thomsen C, et al. Cerebrospinal fluid flow and production in patients with normal pressure hydrocephalus studied by MRI. *Neuroradiology* 1994;36:210–215.
16. Mascalchi M, Arnetoli G, Inzitari D, et al. Cine-MR imaging of aqueductal CSF flow in normal pressure hydrocephalus syndrome before and after CSF shunt. *Acta Radiol* 1993;34:586–592.
17. Bradley W Jr, Scalzo D, Queralt J, et al. Normal-pressure hydrocephalus: evaluation with cerebrospinal fluid flow measurements at MR imaging. *Radiology* 1996;198:523–529.
18. Krauss JK, Regel JP, Vach W, et al. Flow void of cerebrospinal fluid in idiopathic normal pressure hydrocephalus of the elderly: can it predict outcome after shunting? *Neurosurgery* 1997;40:67–73; discussion 73–64.
19. Holodny AI, George AE, de Leon MJ, et al. Focal dilation and paradoxical collapse of cortical fissures and sulci in patients with normal-pressure hydrocephalus. *J Neurosurg* 1998;89:742–747.
20. Kitagaki H, Mori E, Ishii K, et al. CSF spaces in idiopathic normal pressure hydrocephalus: morphology and volumetry. *AJNR Am J Neuroradiol* 1998;19:1277–1284.
21. Graff-Radford N, Godersky J, Jones M. Variables predicting outcome in symptomatic hydrocephalus in the elderly. *Neurology* 1989;39:1601–1604.
22. Weiner HL, Constantini S, Cohen H, et al. Current treatment of normal-pressure hydrocephalus: comparison of flow-regulated and differential-pressure shunt valves. *Neurosurgery* 1995;37:877–884.
23. Sudarsky L. Clinical approach to gait disorders of aging:

an overview. In: Masdeu J, Sudarsky L, Wolfson L, eds. *Gait disorders of aging. Falls and therapeutic strategies.* Philadelphia: Lippincott-Raven, 1997:147–157.
24. Atchison PR, Thompson PD, Frackowiak RS, et al. The syndrome of gait ignition failure: a report of six cases. *Mov Disord* 1993;8:285–292.
25. Fukuyama H, Ouchi Y, Matsuzaki S, et al. Brain functional activity during gait in normal subjects: a SPECT study. *Neurosci Lett* 1997;228:183–186.
26. Leblhuber F, Brucker B, Reisecker F, et al. Single photon emission computed tomography in subjects at risk for Huntington's chorea. *J Neurol* 1990;237:496–498.
27. Nakamura T, Meguro K, Yamazaki H, et al. Postural and gait disturbance correlated with decreased frontal cerebral blood flow in Alzheimer disease. *Alzheimer Dis Assoc Disord* 1997;11:132–139.
28. Ouchi Y, Okada H, Yoshikawa E, et al. Brain activation during maintenance of standing postures in humans. *Brain* 1999;122:329–338.
29. Losseff NA, Wang L, Lai HM, et al. Progressive cerebral atrophy in multiple sclerosis. A serial MRI study. *Brain* 1996;119:2009–2019.
30. Hedera P, DiMauro S, Bonilla E, et al. Phenotypic analysis of autosomal dominant hereditary spastic paraplegia linked to chromosome 8q. *Neurology* 1999;53: 44–50.
31. Brooks WM, Wesley MH, Kodituwakku PW, et al. 1H-MRS differentiates white matter hyperintensities in subcortical arteriosclerotic encephalopathy from those in normal elderly. *Stroke* 1997;28:1940–1943.
32. Camicioli R, Moore MM, Sexton G, et al. Age-related brain changes associated with motor function in healthy older people. *J Am Geriatr Soc* 1999;47:330–334.
33. Kerber KA, Enrietto JA, Jacobson KM, et al. Disequilibrium in older people: a prospective study. *Neurology* 1998;51:574–580.
34. Masdeu J, Wolfson L, Lantos G, et al. White matter disease in the elderly prone to falling. *Arch Neurol* 1989;46:1292–1296.
35. Tell GS, Lefkowitz DS, Diehr P, et al. Relationship between balance and abnormalities in cerebral magnetic resonance imaging in older adults. *Arch Neurol* 1998;55:73–79.
36. Trenkwalder C, Paulus W, Krafczyk S, et al. Postural stability differentiates "lower body" from idiopathic parkinsonism. *Acta Neurol Scand* 1995;91:444–452.
37. van Zagten M, Lodder J, Kessels F. Gait disorder and parkinsonian signs in patients with stroke related to small deep infarcts and white matter lesions. *Mov Disord* 1998;13:89–95.
38. Tofts PS. Standardisation and optimisation of magnetic resonance techniques for multicentre studies. *J Neurol Neurosurg Psychiatry* 1998;64:S37–43.
39. Filippi M, Horsfield MA, Hajnal JV, et al. Quantitative assessment of magnetic resonance imaging lesion load in multiple sclerosis. *J Neurol Neurosurg Psychiatry* 1998;64:S88–93.
40. Horsfield MA, Larsson HB, Jones DK, et al. Diffusion magnetic resonance imaging in multiple sclerosis. *J Neurol Neurosurg Psychiatry* 1998;64:S80–84.
41. Makris N, Worth AJ, Sorensen AG, et al. Morphometry of in vivo human white matter association pathways with diffusion-weighted magnetic resonance imaging. *Ann Neurol* 1997;42:951–962.
42. Ito K, Morrish PK, Rakshi JS, et al. Statistical parametric mapping with ^{18}F-dopa PET shows bilaterally reduced striatal and nigral dopaminergic function in early Parkinson's disease. *J Neurol Neurosurg Psychiatry* 1999;66:754–758.
43. Ichise M, Kim YJ, Erami SS, et al. Functional morphometry of the striatum in Parkinson's disease on three-dimensional surface display of ^{123}I-beta-CIT SPECT data. *J Nucl Med* 1999;40:530–538.
44. Ichise M, Kim YJ, Ballinger JR, et al. SPECT imaging of pre- and postsynaptic dopaminergic alterations in L-dopa-untreated PD. *Neurology* 1999;52:1206–1214.
45. Eidelberg D, Moeller JR, Kazumata K, et al. Metabolic correlates of pallidal neuronal activity in Parkinson's disease. *Brain* 1997;120:1315–1324.
46. Kazumata K, Dhawan V, Chaly T, et al. Dopamine transporter imaging with fluorine-18-FPCIT and PET. *J Nucl Med* 1998;39:1521–1530.
47. Brownell AL, Jenkins BG, Elmaleh DR, et al. Combined PET/MRS brain studies show dynamic and long-term physiological changes in a primate model of Parkinson disease. *Nat Med* 1998;4:1308–1312.
48. Hanakawa T, Fukuyama H, Katsumi Y, et al. Enhanced lateral premotor activity during paradoxical gait in Parkinson's disease. *Ann Neurol* 1999;45:329–336.
49. Piccini P, Burn DJ, Ceravolo R, et al. The role of inheritance in sporadic Parkinson's disease: evidence from a longitudinal study of dopaminergic function in twins. *Ann Neurol* 1999;45:577–582.

Gait Disorders. Advances in Neurology, Vol. 87,
edited by E. Růžička, M. Hallett, and J. Jankovic.
Lippincott Williams & Wilkins, Philadelphia © 2001.

9

The Posturo-Locomotion-Manual Test

A Simple Method for the Characterization of Neurological Movement Disturbances

[*†]Bo Johnels, [*]Páll E. Ingvarsson, [*]Göran Steg, and [‡]Torsten Olsson

[*]*Department of Neurology, Göteborg University and* [†]*Sahlgrenska University Hospital, SE-41345 Göteborg, Sweden;* [‡]*Department of Signals and Systems, Chalmers University of Technology, SE-41296 Göteborg, Sweden*

The Posturo-Locomotion-Manual (PLM) test was developed from the need of a linear and simple clinical neurological procedure to test in an objective way the movement capacity of freely moving individuals performing acts of relevance for activities of daily life. The test movement should be familiar to the subject and demand little or no training. This procedure should give an overall estimate of the movement capacity because each patient has a specific profile of motor deficits regarding activities such as walking, equilibrium control, and manual dexterity; but also, as far as possible, reflect the condition in different parts of the motor system. It was important for us that the procedure utilize current neurophysiologic knowledge of motor control.

The basic hypothesis used was one considering the basal ganglia as coordinative centers for posture and volitional movement. The supportive area under the body is small in the upright position. Therefore, it is important that there is preparatory control of posture and equilibrium counterbalancing any force on the body that depends on loads, accelerations, and postural changes during the movement. In a simplified scheme of nervous function the cerebral cortex is thought to generate a plan for the volitional movement (movement plan) that recruits lower central nervous centers as soon as the requirements for (dynamic) equilibrium control are met. The movements generate forces (and loads) that have to be met by changes of muscle tone in an anticipatory way. An example is the erector spinae, which is activated in advance of the arm before lifting an object (1). The importance of the basal ganglia for coordination is illustrated in patients with Parkinson's disease (PD) by the loss of the capacity to vary posture according to the needs of a movement and to turn around in a single movement when standing. These patients must instead turn around with repeated small adjustments of the feet in order to maintain balance. The cortex–basal ganglia circuitry utilizes brainstem centers for various innate or learned generators or motor programs. Locomotion is dependent on the spinal pattern generator for gait (2). The correction of posture relies on brainstem centers for the balance between flexor and extensor antigravity muscles, and different spinal pathways relay the different phases of a manual transport movement such as reaching and grip hand functions (Fig. 9.1) (3–5). The picture of a distributed system emerges. The cerebral cortex is important for the planning of a movement, but the executive details are formed by pattern generators at different levels in the central nervous system (CNS), such as

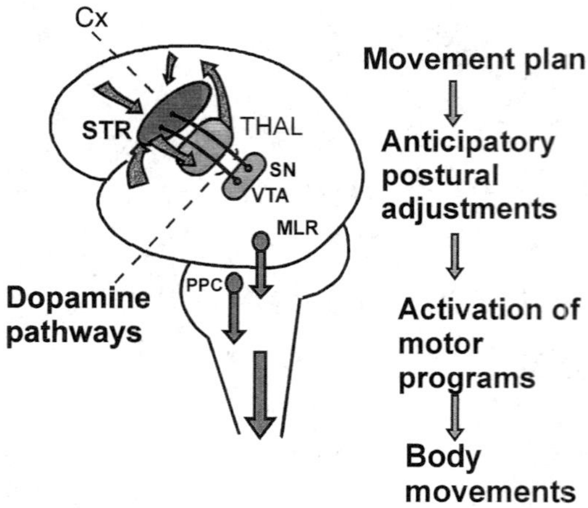

FIG. 9.1. Hypothetical levels of organization in the motor system. Abbreviations: *Cx*, cortex; *STR*, striatum and pallidum; *THAL*, thalamus; *SN*, substantia nigra; *VTA*, ventral tegmental area; *MLR*, mesencephalic locomotor region; *PPC*, pontine postural centers.

the brainstem and spinal cord. The basal ganglia (and cerebellum) play an important role in coordination, at least of volitional movement in postural control. On the basis of this, we decided to use a test movement to put strain on postural and equilibrium control, locomotion, and goal-directed manual transport, especially because these functions are known to be disturbed in each patient with unmedicated PD to a different degree (6).

METHOD

The PLM test is a simple procedure that normally can be handled by one laboratory assistant. The procedure is patient-friendly: It can be performed by all who can walk, the single measurements are quick, and the patient can rest between recordings. Markers covered with infrared light-reflective tape are placed on the head, shoulder, arm, hip, and both legs of the subject and also on a small (500-g) handle placed on a circular support (Fig. 9.2). The entire procedure usually takes less than 5 minutes. The markers are viewed by a video camera system that has an infrared flashlight around its lens and a microprocessor that calculates the position in space of these points of the body with high precision (MacReflex, Qualisys AB, Partille, Sweden). The Cartesian coordinates of the markers are delivered to a personal computer system with a repetition rate of 50 Hz.

The patient is instructed to stand at the starting position with the object placed on the floor beside him or her. At the start command, the patient bends down to take the object, transports

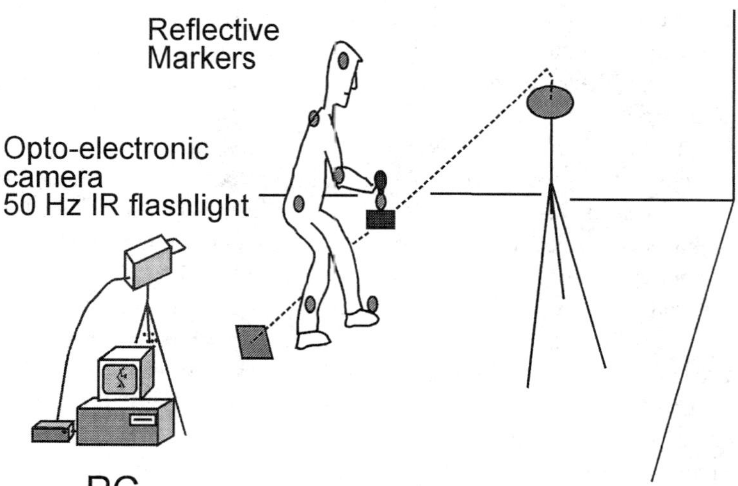

FIG. 9.2. Recording equipment and the Posturo-Locomotion-Manual Test. *IR*, infrared; *PC*, personal computer.

it 150 cm forward, and places it on a stand at the height of the chin. Without loosening his or her grip of the object, the patient transports it back to the starting position and repeats the movement as quickly as possible two or three times. This usually takes 10 to 40 seconds, but may take more time if the patient is very bradykinetic or has gait initiation difficulties. Gentle psychological support or a hand on the shoulder during recording can act as a security measure for patients with a history of frequent falls, such as those where progressive supranuclear palsy or multiple system atrophy is suspected.

The computer software (PLM program, distributed by Qualisys AB) works by inspecting the velocity profiles of the markers placed on the patient and object (7). The following measures of the test movement are identified and determined:

- The movement time (MT) spent for the forward transport of the object from the starting position on the floor to the stand
- The time spent to raise the body from the moment the object is gripped until the body is fully straightened out (P-phase)
- The time for locomotion determined from inspection of the movements of the legs (L-phase)
- The time used for the forward aiming and placing movement of the arm (M-phase)

The Simultaneity Index (SI) is calculated from the following formula to assess the degree of coordination of the PLM phases to a smooth movement.

$$SI = (P + L + M)/MT$$

This index is increased when gait and arm movements are initiated at an earlier moment during the test. Figure 9.3 shows that an increased SI gives a shorter movement time, even though PLM-phase duration has not changed. Thus, in this case the higher speed is accomplished without increase of muscle force. However, this will probably increase the "computational" demands on the CNS for keeping the body balanced. The result of the PLM program is a table with MT and PLM phase data and SI for each recorded moment. A simple spreadsheet script is used as report generator.

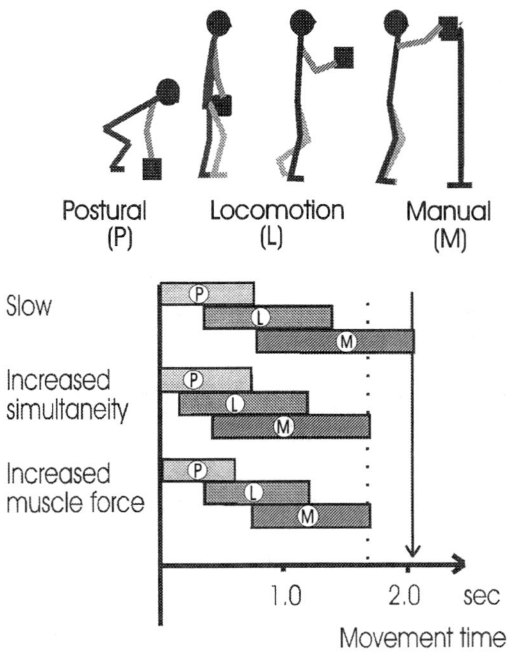

FIG. 9.3. Simultaneity of the postural (*P*), locomotion (*L*), and manual (*M*) phases of body movement. Increased speed can be accomplished by an increase in simultaneity or muscle force, leading to a shortening of the phase duration.

RESULTS

Normal Subjects

Sixty healthy individuals between the ages of 20 and 85 were recorded. As expected, there was a large variation in MT among individuals in the same age group. However, as estimated with linear regression, the mean MT increased from 0.8 to 1.6 seconds for subjects between 20 and 85 years. Although age dependence is not fully linear, for practical clinical purposes we utilize the mean values calculated from the linear regression equation as reference values and express the movement time and phase duration in percent of this value for each person to compensate for the age effect. The regression line equations are given in Table 9.1, from which normal

TABLE 9.1. *Linear regression coefficients*

MT	y = 0.012x + 0.598	R = 0.80
P	y = 0.002x + 0.565	R = 0.52
L	y = 0.0078x + 0.463	R = 0.69
M	y = 0.0082x + 0.360	R = 0.76

L, locomotion phase; M, manual phase; MT, movement time; P, postural phase; x, age in years

reference data were calculated. The MT (in percent of normal performance) gives an approximate value for the degree of bradykinesia. The L- and M-phase duration also increased, but the P-phase showed much less augmentation with age (Fig. 9.4). Thus, it is unlikely that the increase of MT with age was caused by changes in muscle force, joint function, or other mechanical factors. It is more probable that the slowdown with age is caused by changes in CNS function. Inspection of the SI showed this to decrease somewhat with age, especially after age 70 (8). In contrast to the findings of others, no difference was found between the sexes (Fig. 9.5) (9). It is assumed that the slowdown with age is at least partly a result of loss of simultaneity in the performance of complex movements.

Parkinson's Disease

Patients with PD in Hoehn and Yahr stage 2 to 4 have participated in measurements with PLM during different drug tests. At the same time they were assessed with the United Parkinson's Disease Rating Scale (UPDRS) before and at the estimated time of maximal effect of treatment with different dopaminergic drugs. A drug test comparing normal and water-soluble tablets of L-Dopa showed the latter to have a much quicker onset of action, but otherwise quantitatively and qualitatively identical effects in PD. Significant differences among the groups were obtained with only eight patients in a crossover design (10).

Posturo-Locomotion-Manual Movement Time

Patients with PD showed an increased MT, up to more than 10 times the reference values for that age, calculated from the linear regression data of normal subjects. The variability between subsequent measurements was typically much greater before than after treatment with L-Dopa (11).

Phase Profiles

Each patient showed a specific pattern of prolongation of the P-, L-, and M-phase duration, which roughly corresponded with the clinical symptoms and the UPDRS (6,12). Thus, if a patient had difficulties with gait, the L-phase was

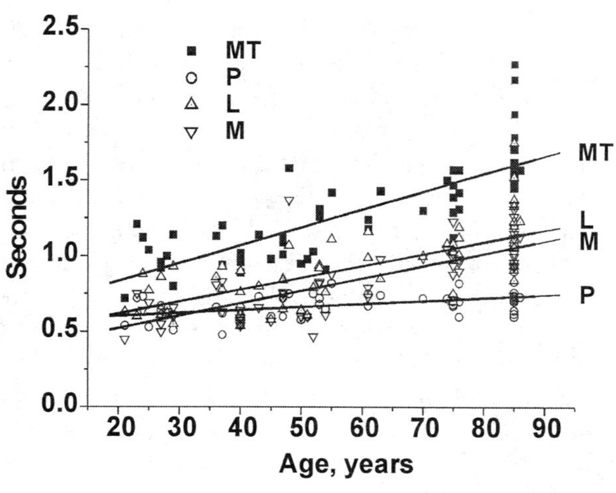

FIG. 9.4. Posturo-Locomotion-Manual (PLM) Test, normal subjects. Note the considerable normal variation of peak performance. Regression lines are used for comparison and age correction when measuring patients with movement disorders. *MT*, movement time.

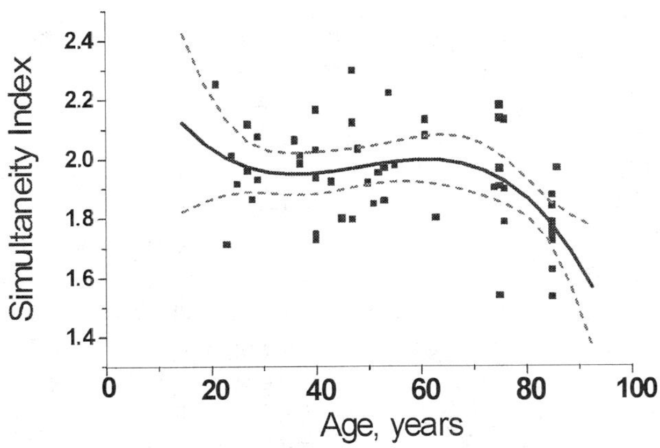

FIG. 9.5. Dependence of age for the simultaneity index (SI), normal subjects. The capacity for simultaneous performance of different movements decreases after approximately 60 years of age.

prolonged, whereas similar prolongation for the P- and M-phase were found when there were postural problems or decreased manual dexterity. There was also good correlation ($P < 0.0001$, $R = 0.8$, Spearman Rank Correlation) between PLM-MT and UPDRS (part 3, motor function) in the off-condition (no antiparkinson medication for >12 hours) and for the maximal effect of a test dose of 200 mg L-Dopa + benserazide (Madopar).

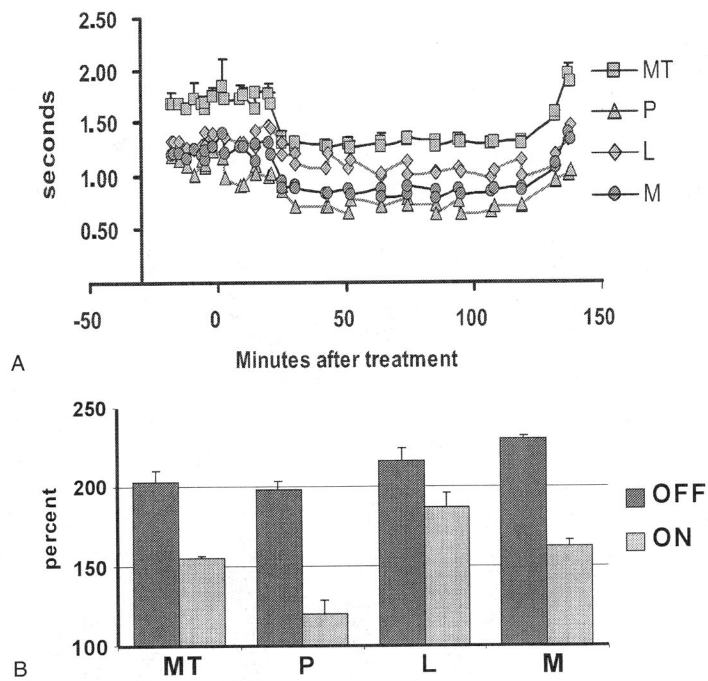

FIG. 9.6. L-Dopa test in a patient with Parkinson's disease. **A:** Movement time (*MT*), postural (*P*), locomotion (*L*) and manual (*M*) phase duration. **B:** Graphic representation of the mean value and standard error for the three consecutive phases before and after treatment with 200 mg L-Dopa that produce the shortest mean duration. Age adjusted and expressed in percent of linear regression data from normal subjects. *OFF* indicates before medication; *ON* indicates after medication.

L-Dopa Test

The L-Dopa test has been used as a routine clinical examination for diagnostic and therapeutic purposes for several years. The patient arrived at the laboratory after 12 hours without antiparkinson medication. Before treatment, 10 repeated PLM recordings were performed to account for the effect of training and act as baseline measurements. The three consecutive measurements with the lowest mean value were automatically selected as the off-value (Fig 9.6). Thereafter, the patient was given 200 mg of a soluble L-Dopa preparation plus benserazide (Madopark Quick, Roche) and was followed with new recordings at 5- to 10-minute intervals until the effect of the medication was seen to appear and disappear again, usually for 2 to 3 hours. There is seldom any need for premedication against nausea even in *de novo* patients who have not previously taken L-Dopa. Approximately every thirtieth patient developed significant nausea and/or vomiting, necessitating a few hours rest. The onset of effect was often abrupt in advanced PD, whereas there was a slower onset in *de novo* patients. As a rule the variation between individual movements during a recording was low in the patients with early PD; the standard error of the mean was typically 1% to 5% in three consecutive forward movements and among subsequent data files (Fig. 9.6A). The three consecutive measurements before L-Dopa that produced the lowest mean value were used as off-value and the three lowest after treatment were selected as the on-value. The degree of bradykinesia (MT) and the PLM-symptom profile could be determined by expressing the off/on

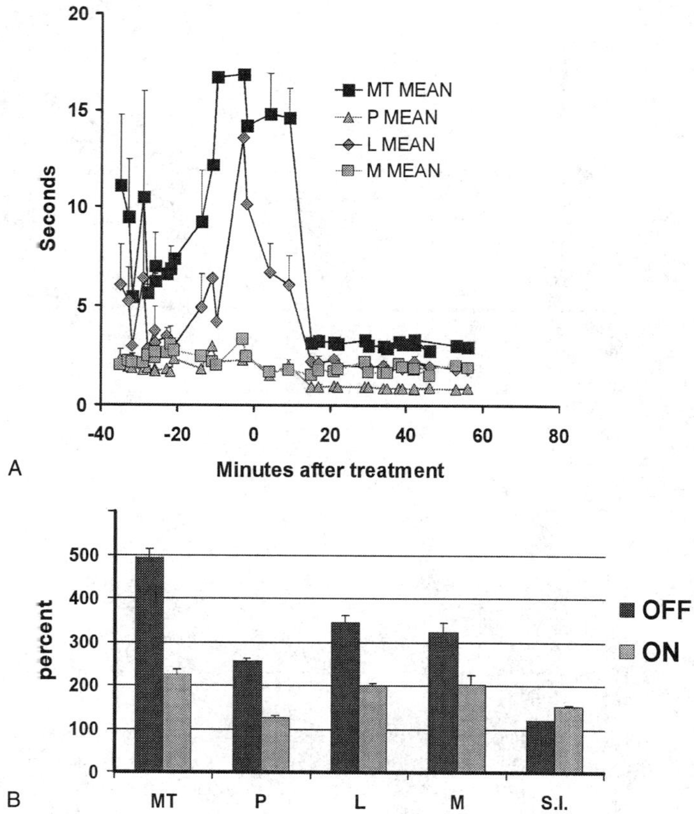

FIG. 9.7. Apomorph ne test in a patient with Parkinson's disease. (For an explanation, see Figure 9.6.) Abbreviation: *S.I.*, simultaneity index.

measurements in percent of normal values for age (Fig. 9.6B). The symptom profile seems to be very stable during several years of PD both in the beginning and more advanced disease.

The PLM-symptom profile changed after treatment (Fig. 9.6B, *light gray bars*). There was almost full normalization in early disease, that is, the duration of the P-, L-, and M-phases approached 100% of normal; however, there was often an uneven effect on the PLM-phases and an incomplete reduction of MT in more advanced disease.

L-Dopa and apomorphine tests can be used to diagnose as well as assess the degree of improvement an individual can expect from increased dopaminergic treatment. Like L-Dopa, apomorphine is a dopamine D1 + D2 receptor agonist and similar clinical effects can be expected (Fig. 9.7). There is a large variation of MT before treatment, mainly owing to blocking of gait (prolonged L-phase). After treatment this patient appears clinically to move normally, but still has substantial bradykinesia (MT = 220%). There is little variation in motor performance when gait and postural control are improved.

Drug Profiles

Dopamine agonists show some selectivity on motor function. The single-dose effect of a

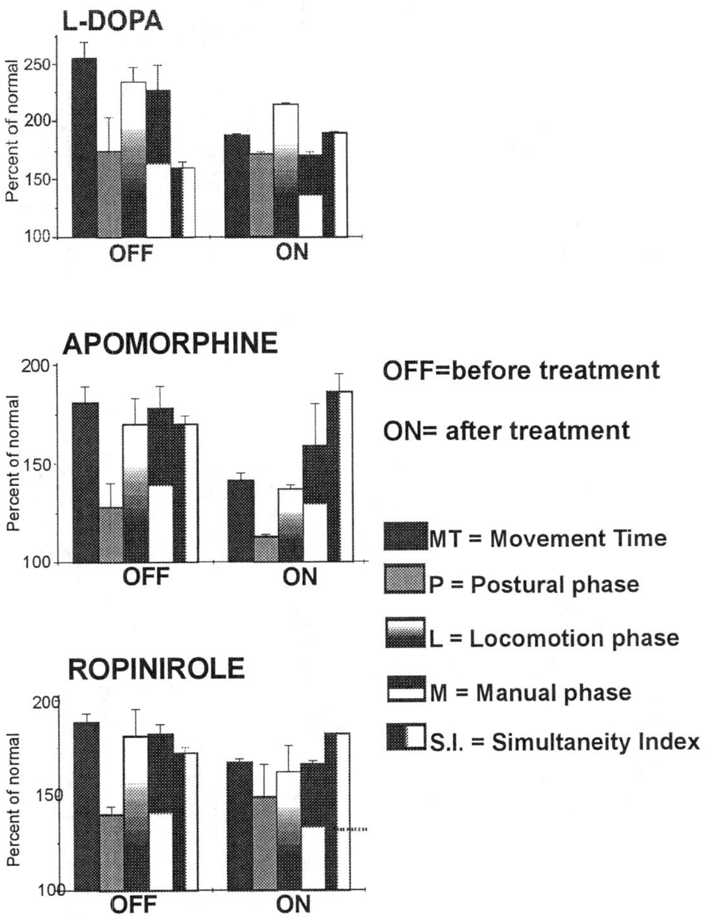

FIG. 9.8. PLM test data from subsequent single-dose testing in a patient with Parkinson's disease of L-Dopa (300 mg per os), apomorphine (3 mg subcutaneously), and ropinirole (3 mg intramuscularly). There is a 1-week interval between doses.

specific drug on the PLM-profile is very stable in repeated measurements in individuals with PD. A comparison between the single dose effect of three different dopamine agonists performed at 1-week intervals in a patient with PD showed that the PLM-profile in the off-state was stable but the effect in the on-state on different movement phases changed with the drug given. An example is shown in Figure 9.8. This patient had a dominant prolongation (deterioration) of the L- and M-phases. In this case apomorphine had a more pronounced effect on postural and locomotor function than L-Dopa. This illustrates that it may be useful to try different dopaminergic drugs against specific motor symptoms, "profiled" drug treatment. In patients with PD, SI showed a significant increase in 85% of the L-Dopa tests performed.

Differential Diagnosis

In a comparative study between patients with PD and Normal (Adult) Pressure Hydrocephalus (NPH), the SI increased in all PD patients after L-Dopa treatment. In contrast, patients with NPH reduced movement time (MT) in the test after shunt operation, but there was no change in SI. This might indicate that dopaminergic tone in the basal ganglia is important for simultaneous execution of the different phases in the PLM test movement (13).

In recent studies using the PLM–L-Dopa test for differential diagnosis in various parkinsonian syndromes, the test predicted the clinical diagnoses of PD or non-PD in 85% of the cases and in 90% (77 of 85) after additional determination of CSF-neurofilament levels (14,15).

DISCUSSION

The PLM test is based on a physiological hypothesis of motor function in freely moving individuals and was originally constructed as a pathophysiological tool. It has been used successfully as a standard test for clinical evaluation. This test is truly quantitative and objective because the software (PLM program) automatically calculates the result and is independent of the observer. It has linear properties and is more sensitive to changes than scoring systems

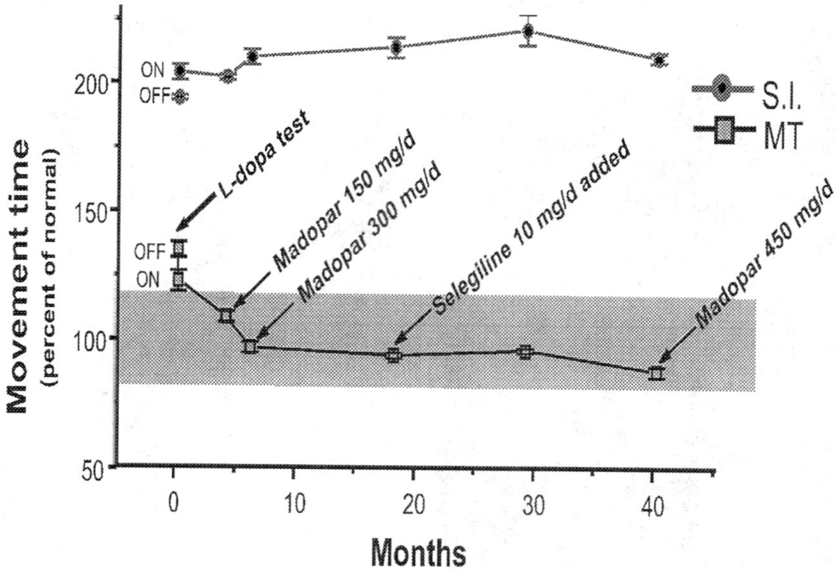

FIG. 9.9. Follow-up treatment with antiparkinsonian drugs in a patient with Parkinson's disease. *MT*, movement time; *S.I.*, simultaneity index.

that use a scale with a only few steps. Short time stability or reproducibility of the test is very good, as demonstrated in several drug tests. The PLM test is also a practical tool for the long-term follow-up of the effect of changes in medication, as illustrated in Figure 9.9. This figure shows iterated recordings from a *de novo* patient with PD. It can be seen that this patient had little bradykinesia at the time of admission (MT = 140% of normal performance). After a test dose of 200 mg L-Dopa (Madopar), MT dropped to 123%. The difference was significant ($P < 0.001$). The performance was further improved after 4 months treatment with 150 mg L-Dopa (plus benserazide) and the patient performed within normal limits (shadowed area in the graph). Addition of selegiline or increase of the L-Dopa dose did not speed up the test. There was also a substantial improvement of the simultaneity of the PLM-phases, that is, a smoother movement pattern.

The PLM profile gives a rough estimation of the degree of postural, locomotor, and manual deficits and the degree to which these are improved by different treatments.

Ingvarsson investigated the SI (unpublished data). He varied the complexity of the movement task and concluded that the most impressive increase of simultaneity was found in more compound rather than simple movements. Dopaminergic treatment as well as electrical stimulation of the subthalamic nucleus in PD improves the SI, indicating that the basal ganglia are important for coordination of different motor programs to natural movements.

It is important that new objective procedures are developed for the future. The PLM test does not measure tremor or hyperkinesias, but these functions could be integrated into the present procedure. The optoelectronic cameras of today are inexpensive and uncomplicated to use. Software is commercially available to combine them with measurement of EMG, forces, and other sensors. We hope that other laboratories will develop and refine these measurement principles, in order to develop a better international standard for the measurement of movement capacity. This would considerably decrease the cost of clinical treatment trials because they would be more precise, measurements from different clinics in the world would be easily comparable, and the number of patients participating in the studies would be reduced. The PLM test, together with electrical or chemical stimulation in the brain, can be used as a pathophysiological tool.

REFERENCES

1. Cordo PJ, Nashner LM. Properties of postural adjustments associated with rapid arm movements. *J Neurophysiol* 1982;47:287–302.
2. Grillner S, Parker D, el Manira A. Vertebrate locomotion—a lamprey perspective. *Ann NY Acad Sci* 1998;860:1–18.
3. Mori S. Integration of posture and locomotion in acute decerebrate cats and in awake freely moving cats. *Progr Neurobiol* 1987;28:161–195.
4. Pettersson LG, Lundberg A, Alstermark B, et al. Effect of spinal cord lesions on forelimb target-reaching and on visually guided switching of target-reaching in the cat. *Neurosci Res* 1997;29:241–526.
5. Alstermark B, Isa T, Tantisira B. Integration in descending motor pathways controlling the forelimb in the cat. 18. Morphology, axonal projection and termination of collaterals from C3-C4 propriospinal neurones in the segment of origin. *Exp Brain Res* 1991;84:561–568.
6. Johnels B, Ingvarsson PE, Thorselius M, et al. Disability profiles and quantitative assessment in Parkinson's disease. *Acta Neurol Scand* 1989;79:227–238.
7. Thorselius M, Johnels B, Ingvarsson PE, et al. Computer-aided analysis of a composite human movement. On peak representation of biological waveforms and an application to human movement analysis. *Technical report no. 77L.* Göteborg, Sweden: Chalmers University of Technology, 1989.
8. Valls M, Ingvarsson P, Johnels B, et al. Age-related slowing and fragmentation of a complex movement quantified by optoelectronic kinesiology. *Clin Rehabil* 1990;4:111–122.
9. Samson MM, Crowe A, Duursma SA, et al. Spatial-temporal analysis of mobility over the adult age range using the Postural-Locomotor-Manual Test. *J Gerontol A Biol Sci Med Sci* 1998;53:M242–247.
10. Jansson Y, Eriksson B, Johnels B. Dispersible levodopa has a fast and more reproducible onset of action than the conventional preparation in Parkinson's disease. *Parkinsonism Rel Disord* 1999;4:201–205.
11. Johnels B, Ingvarsson PE, Holmberg B, et al. Single-dose l-dopa response in early Parkinson's disease. Measurements with optoelectronic recording technique. *Mov Disord* 1993;8:56–62.
12. Ingvarsson PE, Johnels B, Steg G, et al. Objective assessment in Parkinson's disease: optoelectronic movement and force analysis in clinical routine and research. *Adv Neurol* 1999;80:447–458.

13. Matousek M, Wikkelsö C, Blomsterwall E, et al. Motor performance in Normal Pressure Hydrocephalus assessed with an optoelectronic measurement technique. *Acta Neurol Scand* 1995;91:500–505.
14. Holmberg B, Rosengren L, Karlsson JE, et al. Increased cerebrospinal fluid levels of neurofilament protein in progressive supranuclear palsy and multiple system atrophy compared to Parkinson's disease. *Mov Disord* 1998;13:70–77.
15. Holmberg B, Johnels B, Ingvarsson PE, et al. CSF neurofilament and Levodopa tests as diagnostic tools in Parkinsonian syndromes. *Parkinsonism and Related Disorders*, in press.

Gait Disorders. Advances in Neurology, Vol. 87,
edited by E. Růžička, M. Hallett, and J. Jankovic.
Lippincott Williams & Wilkins, Philadelphia © 2001.

10

Simple Assessments of Mobility

Methodology and Clinical Application of Kinetic Gait Analysis

*Georg Ebersbach and †Werner Poewe

**Movement Disorders Clinic, Movement Disorders and Parkinson's Disease Clinic, 14547 Beelitz-Heilstätten, Germany; †Department of Neurology, University of Innsbruck, A-6020 Innsbruck, Austria*

A variety of technical approaches have been introduced for the analysis of human gait. According to the specific aims of the respective investigation, attention has been focused on kinetic, kinematic, and/or electrophysiological aspects of gait control. Gait analysis is mainly performed in order to quantify motor performance in different defined disorders of walking and has yielded valuable information about the effect of therapeutic interventions or specific characteristics of gait disorders. In contrast, attempts to enhance differential diagnosis of gait disturbances by quantitative gait analysis have not yet led to conclusive results. A possible reason for the major diagnostic precision of subjective observational gait analysis is that clinical diagnosis of gait syndromes, such as ataxic or spastic gait, relies on "gestalt" features that are hardly accessible by technical measurements. Clinical observation thus still remains the "gold standard" for the differential diagnosis of gait disorders.

The choice of a particular approach to gait analysis depends on the information needed for study purposes but also on the availability of resources. Although three-dimensional kinematic studies usually require expensive and sophisticated equipment, kinetic data can be obtained considerably faster and cheaper using stopwatch and ruler, video, footswitches, conductive pathways, and/or "fishing lines."

According to Patla, the major requirements for successful walking are equilibrium (i.e., the ability to maintain balance under dynamic conditions), locomotion (i.e., the ability to regulate rhythmic stepping), and the adaptation of these movements corresponding to intrinsic and environmental demands (1). Following a model proposed by Gabell and Nayak, assessment of gait kinetics allows analysis of many of these aspects (2). It was suggested in a gait study in a highly selected sample of 64 healthy subjects that gait patterning is expressed by stride length and stride duration, whereas double-support time and step width were assumed to reflect control of equilibrium. Parameters of gait patterning were further differentiated into force-related (stride length) and rhythm-related (stride duration) measures. Increases or decreases of the parameters were interpreted as an adaptation of balance and gait rhythm to environmental or intrinsic demands, whereas increases of step-to-step variability of the measures were considered to indicate disturbed gait patterning and disequilibrium, respectively. This concept is not universally accepted, although it is widely used. This chapter reviews technical requirements, methodology, data processing, interpretation, and clinical applications of kinetic gait analysis.

TECHNICAL EQUIPMENT

The easiest approach to assessment of gait kinetics requires no more than a *stopwatch* and a defined walking distance. A timed walking test is part of the CAPSIT protocol (*C*ore *A*ssessment *P*rogram for *S*urgical *I*ntervention *T*herapies in *P*arkinson's disease) for measurement of mobility of patients with Parkinson's disease (PD) and requires subjects to walk as fast as possible 7 meters back and forth, including turns (3). This test, although imprecise, is sensitive for treatment effects. Counting the number of steps while measuring the time required to walk a defined distance allows calculation of mean stride-duration and stride-length. The objectivity of this procedure depends on the ability to operate the stopwatch precisely and to correct for the distance between the limit of the walkway and the location of final foot placement. A further shortcoming of this "no-budget" approach is the impossibility of elimination of the effect of deceleration and acceleration on mean values of gait parameters.

Footswitches, which can be attached to the soles of shoes, allow for a precise recording of stride, stance, swing, and double support duration. Furthermore, step-to-step variability of these temporal measures can be obtained. Data acquisition may be performed with portable or stationary devices. Setups, including application of more than one trigger to each foot, enable the investigator to analyze additional features of gait, such as the temporal relation between ground contact of heel and forefoot. Footswitches do not allow for a precise recording of spatial gait parameters, however.

Spatial gait measures can be recorded with some types of *conductive pathways* and—less expensively—with devices based on *"fishing lines"* (4). Bessou et al. developed a so-called locometer, which has been used frequently for gait analysis (5). In this simple device, locomotor displacements are transmitted to the recording apparatus by means of threads attached to each foot at the level of the head of the second metatarsal. The traction of the threads during gait leads to rotation of a pulley system monitored by an optical recording device. Signal output is transmitted to a desktop computer with appropriate software, which allows calculation of all longitudinal temporal and spatial parameters for each foot separately. The length of the threads allows for a walking distance of 10 meters without gait being restrained by relevant resistance because the energy absorption exerted by backward-traction of the pulley only corresponds to 3% of the kinetic energy of the mass center of a lower limb (5). The measures that can be obtained with simple devices for gait analysis are shown in Table 10.1.

METHODOLOGY

Subjects should be given the opportunity to familiarize themselves with the laboratory environment in order to obtain representative data by gait analysis. Several passes off-record have to be permitted in order to eliminate alterations of gait owing to the artificial condition of walking in a laboratory. For assessment of steady-state walking the first three and the last two steps of each pass need to be eliminated from the data set to avoid bias owing to acceleration and deceleration. Surface of the pathway, visual environment, and illumination should be standardized.

TABLE 10.1. *Information given by different approaches to gait analysis*

	Velocity	Stride duration	Stride length	Step-width	Segments of stride, e.g., double support	Variability (temporal)	Variability (spatial)	Accelerations
Stopwatch, ruler	(+)	(+)	(+)	–	–	–	–	–
Foot-switches	(+)	+	(+)	–	+	+	–	–
Conductive pathway	+	+	+	+	+	+	+	–
Fishing line	+	+	+	–	+	+	+	+

An increasing number of studies have used additional strategies to enhance the sensitivity of gait analysis for subtle changes. The simplest approach in this respect is to record walking at different freely chosen gait velocities. Instructing subjects to walk in correspondence to externally imposed rhythms or velocities is more artificial but easier to standardize (6). Susceptibility of gait to different constraints can be assessed by paradigms that include interfering sensory conditions such as stripes being attached to the pathway in irregular patterns or stroboscopic illumination (7,8). Interference of concomitant motor or cognitive behavior can be assessed using dual task designs requiring subjects to perform different activities simultaneously while walking. With gait being used as a primary task, and assuming that gait performance remains constant, performance of the secondary tasks was thought to reflect the amount of attention required by walking devices or changing postural requirements during the step cycle (9,10). Using gait as the secondary task, Bardy and Laurent (11) demonstrated the influence of an auditory reaction time task on braking strategy, and Ebersbach and coworkers (12) found double support time influenced by a fine motor task and digit retention performed simultaneously during gait.

DATA PROCESSING

Gait parameters are not independent measures but related to each other. For example time spent in double support increases with a longer stride duration. In addition, it is generally accepted that gait patterning is influenced by further variables, such as age, gender, and stature. Various strategies to correct for such interdependencies have been proposed, including expression of temporal variables as a percentage of stride duration or relation of stride length to body height or length of the legs. Gabell and Nayak suggested conversion of the standard deviation of measures recorded for every single step to a percentage of the mean value in order to correct measures of step-to-step variability for different gait patterns (2). They suggested using the coefficient of variability (CoVar), which is expressed by the equation

$$\text{CoVar} = \text{standard deviation} \times 100/\text{mean}$$

It was shown using this approach that gait patterning parameters have a very low variability, with a CoVar of less than 7% for stride duration and stride length physiologically. In contrast, a higher variability was found for balance-related parameters with a CoVar of 27% for double support time and 17% for step width, respectively (2).

INTERPRETATION

The mutual dependency of gait measures requires careful interpretation of raw values. The idea that perceived disequilibrium leads to a gait pattern with increased time spent with both feet on the ground has inspired many authors to assess double support time in neurological gait disturbances. Increased time spent in double support has been reported in PD and hydrocephalus (13–17). However, the validity of double support time as an indicator for dynamic equilibrium is restricted by the observation that not only the absolute but also the relative timing of different phases of stride vary with walking velocity (18,19). The proportion of time spent in stance and double support increases with slower gait (15).

Similarly, the clinical interpretation of stride length does not depend on the absolute measure (even when corrected for stature), but rather on the relation between stride length and velocity. Various studies in healthy subjects have shown that the relationship between velocity and stride is linear with small differences between sex and age groups (20,21). This finding allows expression of the relationship between these gait parameters as an equation of linear regression. Transformations of regressions among any of these measures are possible because cadence, stride length, and velocity are related (velocity = cadence × stride length/2). In the following all data are referred to using the regression between stride length and velocity in order to facilitate comparisons. The y-axis represents velocity and the x-axis represents stride length ($y = ax + b$).

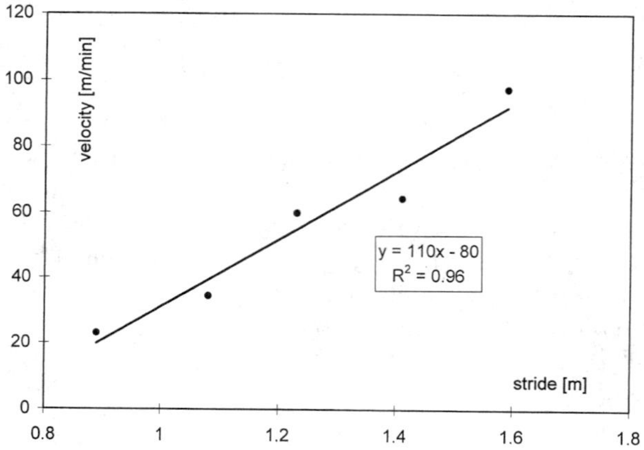

FIG. 10.1. Linear regression of stride vs. velocity in a healthy subject walking with different freely chosen walking velocities.

Flattening of the regression line (indicated by a low coefficient a) means a relatively stronger contribution of stride length to velocity. Differences of intercepts (b) are more difficult to interpret because low intercepts can be owing to flat slopes or a parallel rightward shift of the regression lines with lower stride length for any velocity. Thus, only when bias caused by different slopes is controlled for can intercepts be compared. Figure 10.1 depicts an exemplary plot established in a healthy subject walking with five freely chosen different gait velocities (very slow, slow, normal, fast, very fast). It can be inferred that the inclination of the slope reflects the individual mode of temporo-spatial regulation of locomotion. Intercepts are determined by the slope and (if slope is constant) by the gain of stride. In "normal gait" high intra-individual consistency of linear regression is contrasted by a wide range of normal values for slope and intercept in inter-individual comparisons (22).

Linear relationship of stride length to velocity is only consistent for the medium velocity range with a flattening or even a breakpoint occurring when the upper individual limits of velocity are approached (18,23).

Linear regression analysis cannot only be applied to the relationships between stride, velocity, and cadence. Morris et al. used regression analysis for gait data recorded at different walking velocities and found inverse linear relations for proportion of time spent in double support versus gait velocity (24). This finding is in line with a previous study by Elble et al. in 20 young and 20 elderly healthy subjects using computerized stroboscopic photometry during normal and fast gait (25). In this study, higher double support time in elderly subjects was found to be entirely attributable to reduced stride length when multiple regression (analysis of covariance) was performed. In our laboratory stride and double support were assessed at different walking velocities in 48 healthy subjects and 24 patients with cerebellar ataxia. Linear regression analysis disclosed almost identical relationships between these measures in both groups (Fig. 10.2).

CLINICAL STUDIES ON GAIT KINETICS

Variability of Gait Parameters

Various authors applied Gabell and Nayak's concept (2) in order to relate alterations of gait parameters to clinical disturbances of walking. In patients with idiopathic PD, Blin et al. and Vieregge et al. reported increase of stride length variability without disturbance of rhythmic timing and related this feature to deficient production of internal cues in the basal ganglia (26,27). Gait control in 22 healthy subjects and 22 patients with early PD was challenged in a recent study by Ebersbach et al. by means of a paradigm requiring subjects to decrease their step rate (cadence) by 20% in response to a metronome signal (rhythmic constraint) (28). Gait kinetics were recorded by means of a mechanical device (locometer) in 16 patients and 16 healthy controls. Whereas

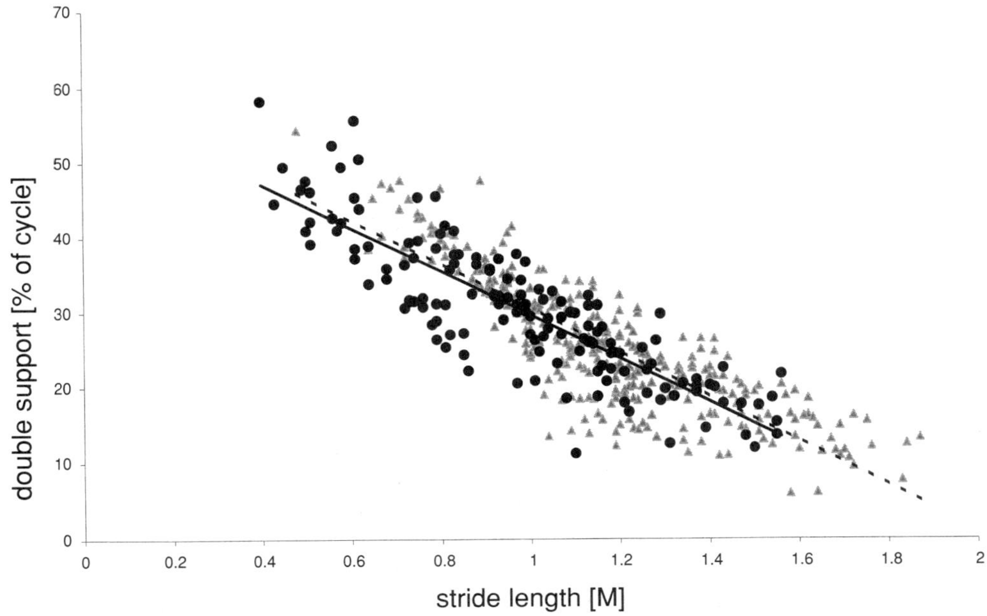

FIG. 10.2. Linear regression of stride [M] and double support [% of stride time] in 48 healthy subjects (*grey pyramids*) and patients with cerebellar ataxia (*black dots*) walking with different velocities. Regression lines for controls and patients (*dotted*) are almost identical suggesting that double support is determined by stride but not by disequilibrium.

regulation of step length became irregular during rhythmic constraint in both patients and controls, irregular timing of steps was only observed in patients, which suggests disturbance of periodic locomotor activity generation (Fig. 10.3; Fig. 10.4).

Increased step-to-step variability of stride duration and length was assumed to reflect two basic components of locomotor pattern generation. These components—possibly subserved by different neural elements—comprise an effector system controlling proper phase relations between muscles within a cycle and a timekeeper system that is thought to produce a periodic signal that determines cycle-to-cycle timing (29). Irregular intracycle motor execution as indicated by increased variability of stride length can be attributed to disturbance of motor circuits regulating force generation during gait. This decrease of subcortical servo control of stride amplitude can occur physiologically in contextual settings requiring modification of stereotyped locomotor routine or in pathological conditions such as PD.

A disturbance of the timekeeper system, that is, an abnormal increase of variability of stride duration was found during rhythmic constraint in patients with PD in contrast to healthy controls (28). Variability of cycle-to-cycle intervals in rhythmic movements increases when oscillations of a physiological system depart from the preferred frequency band, according to Turvey and coworkers (29). The results of the study suggest that the range of stepping frequencies allowing for rhythmic locomotion is narrowed in PD. Recently, Hausdorff et al. confirmed disturbance of gait rhythmicity in PD (30). In this study, temporal gait parameters were measured in 15 patients with PD, 20 patients with Huntington's disease (HD), and 16 healthy controls using insole footswitches connected to a portable storage device. Variability of stride duration in both patient groups was two to three times that observed in control subjects. It has been hypothesized that a disturbance characterized by irregular timing of steps might be caused by dysfunction of neural systems

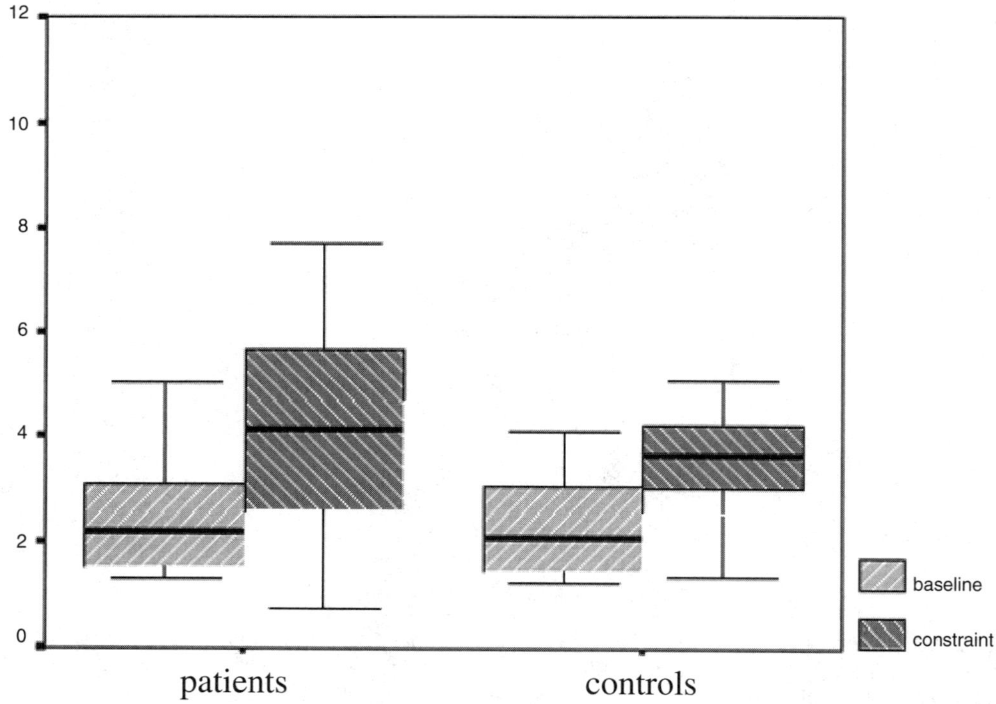

FIG. 10.3. Variability of step length in patients with Parkinson's disease (n = 16) and healthy controls (n = 16) under normal conditions and when subjected to an externally imposed slowing of cadence. Box-plots are showing the distribution of the coefficient of variability (CoVar = standard deviation × 100/mean). (From Ebersbach G, Heijmenberg M, Kindermann L, et al. Interference of rhythmic constraint on gait in healthy subjects and patients with early Parkinson's disease: evidence for impaired locomotor pattern generation in early Parkinson's disease. *Mov Disord* 1999;14:619–625, with permission.)

connecting basal ganglia and the mesencephalic locomotor region (28).

In contrast to PD, quantitative studies of gait kinetics have only rarely been performed in ataxia and gait disturbance in subcortical arteriosclerotic encephalopathy (SAE) (31–33). Step-to-step variability of stride duration and length was considerably higher in patients with ataxia and SAE compared to healthy controls and patients with PD in a study by Ebersbach et al. on gait parameters in ataxia, PD, and SAE (22). Whereas irregular amplitudes and movement times are consistent with clinical observations in ataxia, these features have not been reported in SAE (31,34). These results suggest that irregular step length is not a distinct feature for PD but can be found even more pronounced in ataxia and gait disturbance owing to SAE.

Linear Regression Analysis

Whereas irregularity of stride-to-stride performance in clinical gait disturbances can be analyzed assessing only the individually preferred gait pattern, this approach does not allow for conclusive interpretation of absolute measures. The finding of reduced step length during preferred walking velocity in PD, for example, could be interpreted as pathological scaling of amplitude. Yet, because reduced stride occurs physiologically with low walking velocity, small stepped gait could also just be caused by nonspecific slowing of gait, reflecting a strategy to minimize

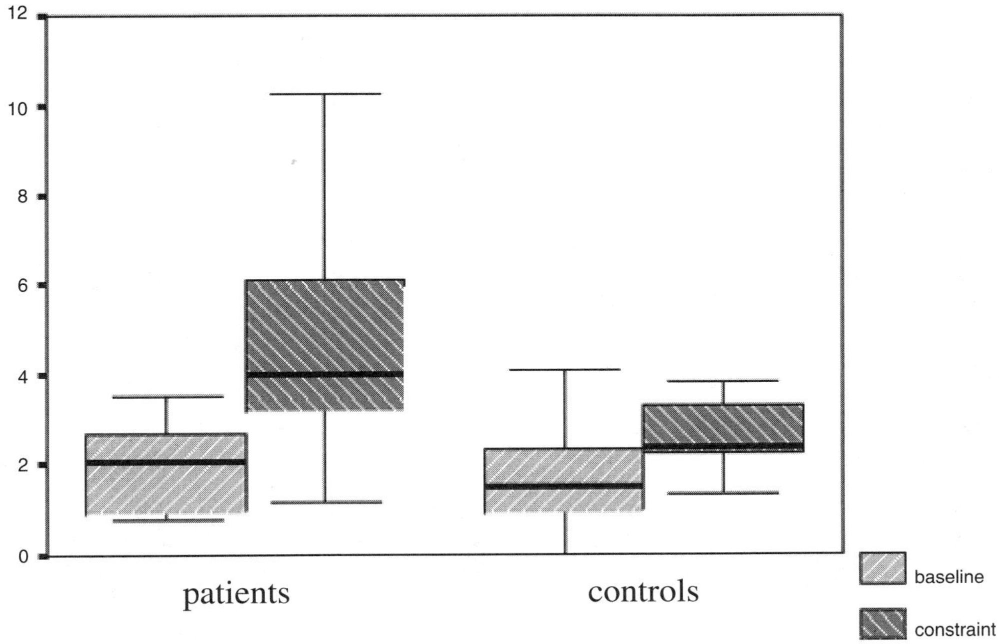

FIG. 10.4. Variability of stride duration in patients with Parkinson's disease (n = 16) and healthy controls (n = 16) under normal conditions and when subjected to an externally imposed slowing of cadence. Box-plots are showing the distribution of the coefficient of variability (CoVar = standard deviation × 100/mean). (From Ebersbach G, Heijmenberg M, Kindermann L, et al. Interference of rhythmic constraint on gait in healthy subjects and patients with early Parkinson's disease: evidence for impaired locomotor pattern generation in early Parkinson's disease. *Mov Disord* 1999;14:619–625, with permission.)

energy expenditure (35). Linear regression analysis of gait parameters obtained during walks at different velocities is helpful to clarify whether strides are short or *too* short for a given velocity. Morris et al. measured gait parameters in controls and patients with PD while walking with different velocities (24). Reduced stride length and higher cadence for any given velocity was reported in PD, whereas the rate at which cadence and stride length were increased to achieve higher velocities was similar in patients and controls. This scaling down of stride amplitude was attributed to a disorder in motor set. In a more recent study by Morris et al., subjects were instructed to adapt cadence to a metronome signal set at rates ranging from 40 to 180 steps/min (6). Linear regression of stride length versus velocity in healthy controls and 20 patients with PD showed that slopes did not differ significantly among groups, whereas higher mean intercepts were found in patients. Administration of L-Dopa led to lower intercepts with slope remaining unchanged.

Linear regression of stride versus velocity was also assessed in a study by Ebersbach et al. that included patients suffering from cerebellar ataxia or gait disturbance owing to SAE in addition to patients with PD (22). In this study, close linear relation, as reflected by high R^2 values, was demonstrated for all patient groups. In keeping with the findings of Morris et al., patients with PD showed normal slopes but higher intercepts than controls, indicating reduced amplitude of stride at any given velocity (24). In contrast to PD, patients with ataxia showed a disproportionate decrease of step length occurring during slow gait and disproportionate increase occurring during fast walking (Fig. 10.5).

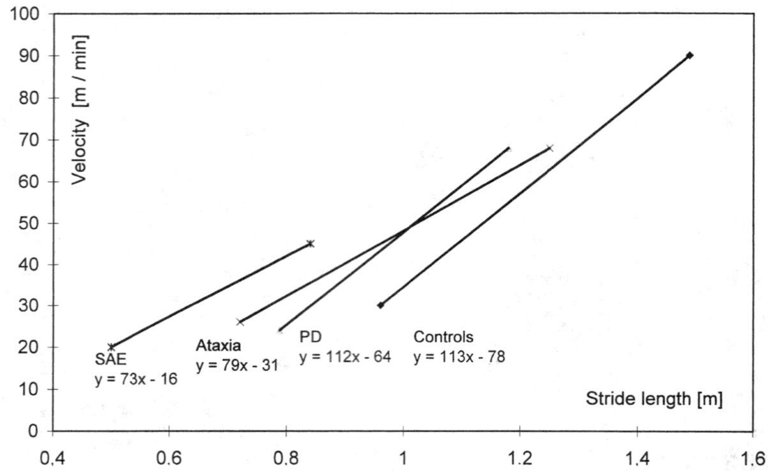

FIG. 10.5. Linear regressions of stride vs. velocity in healthy subjects (n = 30) and patients with Parkinson's disease (*PD*, n = 30), subcortical arteriosclerotic encephalopathy (*SAE*, n = 20) and ataxia (n = 20). (From Ebersbach G, Sojer M, Valldeoriola F, et al. Comparative analysis of gait in Parkinson's disease, cerebellar ataxia and subcortical arteriosclerotic encephalopathy. *Brain* 1999;122:1349–1355, with permission.)

Remarkably, regression equations in patients with SAE resembled more those established in cerebellar disease than those found in PD. With slope of stride versus velocity being altered regardless of the etiology of gait disturbance, the disproportionate contribution of stride length to the increase of velocity in patients with SAE and ataxia was attributed to a nonspecific feature of disequilibrium possibly reflecting a compensatory response to omnidirectional instability, analogous to the broadening of base. During slow gait, equilibrium is challenged by lateral sway vectors forcing the affected subject to reduce periods of single leg support disproportionately in order to keep lateral instability minimal. The sagittal vector becomes predominant with increasing velocity and large steps are needed to prevent the subject from falling forward.

Increased time spent in double support has been reported in gait disorders including PD and is related to disequilibrium according to the concept of Gabell and Nayak (2). Yet, when differences in walking velocity were considered using linear regression analysis for velocity versus double support time no difference could be found for slope and intercept between healthy controls and patients with PD (24). These results are in line with the findings of Elble and coworkers who found increased double support in senile gait to be attributable to decreased stride length. The data recorded in healthy subjects and patients with ataxia in our own laboratory (see Figure 10.2) suggest that double support time is not an independent variable associated with balance mechanisms as suggested by Gabell and Nayak (2) but a non-specific measure determined by stride amplitude.

Dual Task Studies

Recently, a number of studies addressed the relationship between gait performance and the execution of simultaneous tasks. Lundin-Olsson et al. found increased propensity to falls in subjects who stopped walking while talking (36). Ebersbach et al. showed that double-support time increases when gait is performed in dual-task conditions (simultaneous digit-retention) (12). Walking speed in subjects with Alzheimer's disease (AD) was shown to decrease when a verbal task was executed simultaneously during gait, whereas in a study by Camicioli et al. no such slowing was found with increasing age in healthy subjects (37). Reduction of gait velocity while approaching a target occurred earlier when a dual-task paradigm (auditory reaction time) was applied in the study of Bardy and Laurent (38). The ability of patients with PD to generate steps of normal length after attentional and sensory training was lost in a study by Morris et al. when a secondary task (reciting a sentence) was interspersed during gait (39).

Sensory Interference

Both helpful and confounding manipulations have been employed in the use of sensory stimuli to influence gait performance. Morris et al. showed that walking over floor stripes produced almost normal stride length, velocity, and cadence in patients with PD (24). Using acoustic facilitation, Thaut et al. and McIntosh et al. produced increased velocity with nearly equal percentage increases in cadence and stride length, whereas Morris et al. found that, in contrast to visual cues, increase of gait velocity induced by metronome walking is rather owing to a disproportionate increase of cadence compared to stride length (24,40,41). The use of such sensory cues has been incorporated in therapeutic training programs for PD, although carryover seems to be doubtful in the absence of constant vigilance (39–41). Using confounding visual stimuli, that is, artificially altered optical flow pattern while walking on treadmill or stroboscopic illumination of the walkway, gait parameters in patients with PD were shown to be pathologically susceptible to sensory interference (42).

CONCLUSION

Information obtained by assessment of gait kinetics is less abundant than three-dimensional kinematic gait analysis. Yet, depending on the individual aims of gait analysis, this limitation is recompensed by greater simplicity, easier setups, faster assessment procedures, and cheaper costs. Footswitches, conductive pathways, or "fishing-line" devices permit the acquisition of a variety of kinetic measures, and some basic parameters can even be recorded without special equipment. The interpretation of kinetic gait data needs to be performed with caution because most measures are not independent. Linear regression can be helpful to accommodate discrepant values recorded at different walking velocities and should be included in protocols dealing with rehabilitation assessments, drug monitoring, or follow-up observations of gait disturbances. Study designs, including dual task assessments or sensory stimuli, allow challenging walking performance and thus enhance sensitivity of gait analysis.

REFERENCES

1. Patla AE. Neurobiomechanical bases for the control of human locomotion. In: Bronstein AM, Brandt T, Woollacott M, eds. *Clinical disorders of balance posture and gait.* London: Arnold, 1996:19–41.
2. Gabell A, Nayak US. The effect of age on variability in gait. *J Gerontol* 1984;39:662–666.
3. Defer GL, Widner H, Mariè RM, et al. Core assessment program for surgical international therapies in Parkinson's disease (CAPSIT-PD). *Mov Disord* 1999; 14:572–584.
4. Nayak USL, Gabell A, Simons MA, et al. Measurement of gait and balance in the elderly. *J Am Geriat Soc* 1982;30:516–520.
5. Bessou P, Dupui P, Montoya R, et al. Simultaneous recording of longitudinal displacements of both feet during human walking. *J Physiol Paris* 1988;83:102–110.
6. Morris M, Iansek R, Matyas T, et al. Abnormalities in stride length-cadence relation in parkinson gait. *Mov Disord* 1998;13:61–69.
7. Ebersbach G, Kindermann L, Hösl M, et al. Influence of sensory and rhythmic interference on gait in Parkinson's disease. *J Neurol* 1995;242:136.
8. Azulay JP, Mesure S, Amblard B, et al. Visual control of locomotion in Parkinson's disease. *Brain* 1999;122:111–120.
9. Wright DL, Kemp TL. The dual-task methodology and assessing the attentional demands of ambulation with walking devices. *Phys Ther* 1992;72:306–315.
10. Lajoie Y, Teasdale N, Bard C, et al. Attentional demands for static and dynamic equilibrium. *Exp Brain Res* 1993;97:139–144.
11. Bardy BG. Visual cues and attention demand in locomotor positioning. *Percept Mot Skills* 1991;72:915–926.
12. Ebersbach G, Dimitrijevic MR, Poewe W. Influence of concurrent tasks on gait: a dual-task approach. *Percept Mot Skills* 1995;81:107–113.
13. Murray MP, Sepic SB, Gardner GM, et al. Walking patterns of men with parkinsonism. *Am J Phys Med* 1978;57:278–294.
14. Knutsson E. An analysis of parkinsonian gait. *Brain* 1972;95:475–486.
15. Stern GM, Franklyn SE, Imms FJ, et al. Quantitative assessments of gait and mobility in Parkinson's disease. *J Neural Transm* 1983;19:201–214.
16. Blin O, Ferrandez AM, Pailhous J, et al. Dopa-sensitive and dopa-resistant gait parameters in Parkinson's disease. *J Neurol Sci* 1991;103:51–54.
17. Sorensen P, Jansen EC, Gjerris F. Motor disturbances in normal-pressure hydrocephalus. Special reference to stance and gait. *Arch Neurol* 1986;43:34–38.

18. Larsson LE, Odenrick P, Sandlund B, et al. The phases of the stride and their interaction in human gait. *Scand J Rehab Med* 1992;12:107–112.
19. Nilsson J, Thorstensson A. Adaptability in frequency and amplitude of leg movements during human locomotion at different speeds. *Acta Physiol Scand* 1987;129:107–114.
20. Grieve DW. Gait patterns and the speed of walking. *Bio-Med Eng* 1968;119–122.
21. Hirokawa S. Normal gait characteristics under temporal and distance constraints. *J Biomed Eng* 1989;11:449–456.
22. Ebersbach G, Sojer M, Valldeoriola F, et al. Comparative analysis of gait in Parkinson's disease, cerebellar ataxia and subcortical arteriosclerotic encephalopathy. *Brain* 1999;122:1349–1355.
23. Bowes SG, Charlett A, Dobbs RJ, et al. Gait in relation to ageing and idiopathic parkinsonism. *Scand J Rehabil Med* 1992;24:181–186.
24. Morris ME, Iansek R, Matyas TA, et al. The pathogenesis of gait hypokinesia in Parkinson's disease. *Brain* 1994;117:1169–1181.
25. Elble RJ, Thomas SS, Higgins C, et al. Stride-dependent changes in gait of older people. *J Neurol* 1991;238:1–5.
26. Blin O, Ferrandez AM, Serratrice G. Quantitative analysis of gait in Parkinson patients: increased variability of stride length. *J Neurol Sci* 1990;98:91–97.
27. Vieregge P, Stolze H, Klein C, et al. Gait quantitation in parkinson's disease-locomotor disability and correlation to clinical rating scales. *J Neural Transm* 1997;104:237–248.
28. Ebersbach G, Heijmenberg M, Kindermann L, et al. Interference of rhythmic constraint on gait in healthy subjects and patients with early Parkinson's disease: evidence for impaired locomotor pattern generation in early Parkinson's disease. *Mov Disord* 1999;14:619–625.
29. Turvey MT, Schmidt RC, Rosenblum LD. "Clock" and "motor" components in absolute coordination of rhythmic movements. *Neuroscience* 1989;33:1–10.
30. Hausdorff JM, Cudkowicz ME, Firtion R, et al. Gait variability and basal ganglia disorders: stride-to-stride variations of gait cycle timing in Parkinson's disease and Huntington's disease. *Mov Disord* 1998;13:428–437.
31. Palliyath S, Hallett M, Thomas SL, et al. Gait in patients with cerebellar ataxia. *Mov Disord* 1998;13:958–964.
32. Zijlmans JCM, Poels PJE, Duysens J, et al. Quantitative gait analysis in patients with vascular parkinsonism. *Mov Disord* 1996;11:501–508.
33. Hennerici MG, Oster M, Cohen S. Are gait disturbances and white matter degeneration early indicators of vascular dementia? *Dementia* 1994;5:197–202.
34. Hallett M, Massaquoi SG. Physiologic studies of dysmetria in patients with cerebellar deficits. *Can J Neurol Sci* 1993;20:S83–92.
35. Brooks VB. *The neural basis of motor control*. New York: Oxford University Press, 1986.
36. Lundin-Olsson L, Nyberg L, Gustafson Y. "Stops walking when talking" as a predictor of falls in elderly people. *Lancet* 1997;349:617.
37. Camicioli R, Howieson D, Lehman S, et al. Talking while walking: the effect of a dual task in aging and Alzheimer's disease. *Neurology* 1997;48:955–958.
38. Bardy BG, Laurent M. Visual cues and attention demand in locomotor positioning. *Percept Mot Skills* 1991;72:915–926.
39. Morris ME, Iansek R, Matyas TA, et al. Stride length regulation in Parkinson's disease. Normalization strategies and underlying mechanisms. *Brain* 1996;119:551–568.
40. Thaut MH, McIntosh GC, Rice RR, et al. Rhythmic auditory stimulation in gait training for Parkinson's disease patients. *Mov Disord* 1996;11:193–200.
41. McIntosh GC, Brown SH, Rice RR, et al. Rhythmic auditory-motor facilitation of gait patterns in patients with Parkinson's disease. *J Neurol Neurosurg Psychiatry* 1997;62:22–26.
42. Prokop T, Berger W. Influence of optic flow on locomotion in normal subjects and patients with Parkinson's disease. *Electroenceph Clin Neurophysiol* 1996;99:402.

Gait Disorders. Advances in Neurology, Vol. 87,
edited by E. Růžička, M. Hallett, and J. Jankovic.
Lippincott Williams & Wilkins, Philadelphia © 2001.

11

Gait Disorders: Prevalence, Morbidity, and Etiology

Lewis Sudarsky

Department of Neurology, Havard Medical School; and Department of Neurology, Brigham and Women's Hospital, Boston, Massachusetts 02115

Gait disorders are a common and frequent presentation of neurologic disease, particularly during development and in old age. Reliable estimates of prevalence are difficult to obtain, as there is no standard definition or criteria to apply to this heterogenous group of disorders. An abnormality of gait was noted in 15% of subjects in a study in Durham, North Carolina in which a group of volunteers over 60 were examined by a neurologist (1). A study of functional status of a cohort of 79 year olds in Göteborg, Sweden found that one in four used mechanical aids to help with walking (2). The most current data come from the East Boston Neighborhood Health Study, in which care was taken to examine a representative subset of seniors from the community. An abnormal gait, defined by shuffling or a degree of difficulty with turns, was observed in 15% of the population aged 67 to 74, 29% of those 75 to 84, and 49% of the population 85 and older (3).

Of course, these numbers apply to elderly people living in the community. The prevalence of gait disorders is substantially higher in an acute care hospital or geriatric unit. In a review of 100 admissions to a geriatric unit by Prakash and Stern, 70 were freely independent in ambulation, 22 had gait disorders, and eight were bed-bound (4). Estimates suggest that up to half of people in a nursing home or chronic care facility are nonambulatory (5).

CHANGES IN GAIT WITH NORMAL AGING

Changes in gait occur as a product of normal aging and disease. It is sometimes difficult to sort out the difference. In his studies on the neurology of old age, Critchley called attention to characteristic changes in the gait of older people he encountered (6). He described a shortening of stride, a slightly widened base of support, a loss of elasticity, and a degree of disequilibrium. He also described flexed posture, small steps, and a subjective sense of propulsion; features often characterized as *marche a petit pas* (6). He coined the term *senile gait,* which persists in the literature. This term is vague and pejorative, and it begs the question by assuming that gait degenerates with age.

We approach the problem today by examining fit older people, who are examples of "successful aging." Murray and coworkers noted a shorter, broader stride in the gait of healthy male subjects over 65 (7). Subsequent studies have confirmed a reduction in velocity and stride of 10% to 20%, comparing healthy people in their seventies with subjects in their twenties (8,9). There is a slight increase in stance width and double support time, and less vigorous force development at the moment of push off. Changes in velocity and stride that are substantially larger most likely represent the effects of disease, particularly if stability or ergonomic efficiency is compromised.

MORBIDITY OF GAIT DISORDERS

Gait disorders are important because they compromise independence and contribute to the risk of falls and injury. Falls are a common event in the elderly, and not all falls result in injury. Studies suggest that 30% of people over 65 fall each year. Ten percent to 15% of these falls result in injury, and 5% to 10% result in a fracture. There are more than 200,000 hip fractures annually in the United States, and a comparable number of wrist fractures related to falling (10). Falls are thus a major source of morbidity and mortality. Accidental injury is the sixth leading cause of death in the elderly, and falls are the major cause after age 70 (11). The death rate for injuries in which falls are a contributing factor exceeds 100 per 100,000 population after age 85 (12).

Studies clearly establish a relationship between gait disorders and falls. Early studies looked at fall events, and tried to establish cause after the fact. In a widely quoted study from 1960, J.H. Sheldon looked at 500 falls in 202 individuals. A large number of slipping and tripping falls were attributed to environmental hazards and accidents (13). Some people had recurrent falls over a period of months, suggesting an underlying disturbance of postural mechanisms. In a meta-analysis of 3,628 falls from 12 published studies, Rubenstein noted that 31% were accidental or environment related. Seventeen percent were attributed to balance or gait disorders, or to leg weakness (14).

A more contemporary approach to the problem of falls is the controlled study in which risk factors are examined for correlation with fall events in a population over a period of time. Tinetti and coworkers did a prospective study of falls in the community of New Haven, Connecticut (15). Her group looked at seven items in a simple clinical gait and balance assessment. Patients who were scored abnormal in six or seven items had a 2.5-time increased risk of falls over the period of follow-up (15). Weakness and frailty, sedative medications, and cognitive impairment were other important risk factors in the analysis. Subsequent studies have confirmed that both balance disturbance and gait disorder increase the risk of falls threefold (14). The same correlation holds when these risk factors are examined with regard to injurious falls (16).

Since 1995, a number of biomechanics laboratories have examined the gait of older people who fall in more detail. The investigators have tried to understand what aspects of abnormal gait performance pose a particular risk for falls. This strategy assumes that falls are heterogeneous, but that relevant features will nonetheless stand out. Hausdorf et al. looked at 18 people over 70 with a history of falls, for comparison with 17 older people who had no falls in the prior 5 years (17). They used a device implanted in the shoe to record footfall, and measured stride-to-stride variability in duration of stride over a 6-minute walk. They found significantly larger variation in stride time and percent stance time in the falls group (17). They noted that gait variability itself might predispose to falls, or might be a marker for a deeper structural disorder of gait and balance.

Lee and Kerrigan studied 15 subjects (mean age 77) with repeated falls in the gait lab, for comparison with age-matched controls (18). Cadence and stride length were somewhat reduced in the falls group. Kinetic data showed increases in peak torque for hip flexion, knee extension, ankle inversion, and dorsiflexion in the falls group. Ankle plantar–flexion torque was decreased in the falls group, and power absorption was greater at the ankle in these patients. They speculate that the increases in peak torque across more proximal joints might reflect stiffness or cocontraction, and might represent a compensatory strategy (18). Vieregge has suggested that reductions in foot–floor clearance during the swing phase might predispose to stumbling and tripping falls (19).

The other major problem for patients with gait disorders is loss of independence. This may occur as a direct effect of the physical disability and loss of function. Patients are increasingly dependent on help when they can no longer walk to the store and walk freely around their community. Those patients who are no longer able to ambulate around the house may need to have live-in help or seek nursing home care. The limitation may also occur indirectly, as a result of anxiety and fear of falling. Many people voluntarily restrict their activity because of fear of falling (20). In one study, fear of falling was rated above fear of robbery and concern about financial difficulty among older people living in a community (21). A heightened anxiety and fear often occur following a fall, in which patients dramatically limit their physical activity. This "post-fall syndrome" may be associated with an increased morbidity and mortality (22).

ETIOLOGY OF GAIT DISORDERS

Gait is a complex performance and there are many possibilities for failure. Consequently, the gait disorders encountered in the clinic are enormously heterogeneous. Gait is sensitive to minor degrees of orthopedic deformity, and many patients with neurologic disorders of gait have comorbidity from arthritis. Separation of neurologic disorders from those that are primarily musculoskeletal is sometimes not easy or straightforward (23).

The spectrum of illness also varies depending on the population under consideration. Any study conducted in a chronic care facility will encounter a large number of poorly ambulatory and nonambulatory patients in whom it is difficult to identify the root cause of the problem. Restricting consideration to patients with gait disorders living in the community may help focus the search for etiologic cause.

Sudarsky and Ronthal in 1983 looked at the problem from the perspective of neurology office practice. Fifty patients over 65 were examined who were referred for an undiagnosed disorder of gait. Patients with hemiparesis, known Parkinson's disease, patients on neuroleptics, and those with an orthopedic deformity or limited joint mobility were excluded. Most of the patients in the study had imaging. A principal diagnosis was assigned (24). Table 11.1 expands the series to 120 patients, with the addition of another 70 patients examined between 1990 and 1993 with the aid of magnetic resonance imaging (MRI). Several general observations can be made from the data. In 28% of the study patients, the gait disorder was clearly multifactorial. In 10% to 20% of cases, patients were seen several times with laboratory testing, neurophysiology, and imaging and there was no clear diagnosis.

Myelopathy

Myelopathy from cervical spondylosis is one of the most common causes of gait disorder in the elderly. Spinal diseases account for 17% of the patients in our series (Fig. 11.1), and 22% of the neurologic admissions for gait disorder at the Veterans Hospital in Taiwan (25). Degenerative changes about the disc space and posterior ligamentous hypertrophy narrow the canal, causing mechanical compression and vascular compromise of the cervical spinal cord. A spastic

TABLE 11.1. *Classification of gait disorder in 120 patients, according to etiologic cause*

	1980–2	1990–4	Total	Percent
Myelopathy	8	12	20	16.7
Parkinsonism	5	9	14	11.7
Hydrocephalus	2	6	8	6.7
Multiple infarcts	8	10	18	15.0
Cerebellar degeneration	4	4	8	6.7
Sensory deficits	9	13	22	18.3
Toxic/metabolic	3	0	3	2.5
Psychogenic	1	3	4	3.3
Other	3	3	6	5.0
Unknown cause	7	10	17	14.2
Total	50	70	120	100

Initial fifty patients are from Sudarsky L, Ronthal M. Gait disorders among elderly patients: a survey study of 50 patients. *Arch Neurol* 1983;40:740–743, with permission.

Seventy additional patients are from Sudarsky L. Clinical approach to gait disorders of aging: an overview. In: Masdeu JC, Sudarsky L, Wolfson L, eds. *Gait disorders of aging: falls and therapeutic strategies.* Philadelphia: Lippincott–Raven Publishers, 1997:147–158, from which table is reproduced with permission.

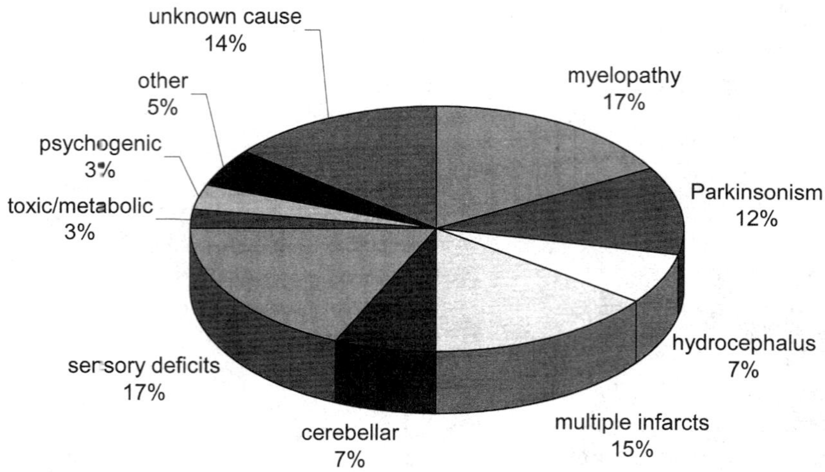

FIG. 11.1. Pie chart shows distribution of cases in combined series of Sudarsky and Ronthal.

or spastic–ataxic gait is typically observed, with stiffness and "bounce" in the legs, and a tendency to circumduct and scuff the feet. An occasional patient will experience a discrete exacerbation in relation to an injury or fall. The natural history is quite variable, and there is no consensus on the role of spondylosis surgery in older patients (26). Vitamin B_{12} deficiency is an occasional cause of myelopathy and gait impairment in the elderly.

Parkinsonism

Parkinson's disease (PD) is common, affecting 1.5% of the population over 65. In addition, some older people exhibit a flexed posture, a degree of postural instability and a shuffling gait, aspects of parkinsonism. An axial parkinsonian syndrome was observed in 6% to 9% of the oldest groups in the Rotterdam study, 30% in the 75- to 84-year-old age group in the East Boston community (27,28). Some of the features recognized in the East Boston study are extrapyramidal signs that have been associated with aging (29). We recognized PD or a related disorder in 12% of our gait disorder series, but note that obvious cases of PD and patients on neuroleptics were excluded from the study.

Drug-induced parkinsonism is increasingly prevalent as chronic psychiatric patients are discharged into the community. In one study from the United Kingdom, drug-induced parkinsonism was recognized in patients on a geriatric unit, many of whom had received neuroleptic medications for sedation or dizziness (30). Neuroleptic drugs that block D_2 receptors often produce an extrapyramidal syndrome. They are known to impair postural responses and increase the risk of falls. Drug-induced parkinsonism is reversible, but the disorder often takes 2 to 3 months to resolve after the medication has been discontinued.

Hydrocephalus

Adams, Froher, and Hakim, described the syndrome of normal pressure hydrocephalus 35 years ago, but controversy persists about its prevalence and indications for shunting (31). Gait disorder can be the salient or presenting feature, and is the aspect of the syndrome most responsive to treatment. Although hydrocephalus is rare as a cause of reversible dementia, we have encountered a number of cases presenting with a shuffling, hesitant, and unsteady gait. The feet often appear to be "stuck to the floor."

A method is needed to confirm the presence of a dynamic disorder and to distinguish true from *ex vacuo* hydrocephalus because there are many older patients with a gait disorder and enlarged ventricles. Responses to a large volume lumbar puncture and various cerebrospinal fluid (CSF) infusion tests have been used to predict response to shunting (32). Magnetic resonance imaging-based studies of CSF flow through the aqueduct may help in the evaluation of these patients (33).

Multiple Infarcts and Small Vessel Disease

The most common cause of frontal gait disorder is cerebrovascular disease. Patients with multiple cerebral infarcts and/or hypertensive small vessel disease account for 15% of our series. The consequences of multiple infarcts on postural control and locomotion are often substantial, because the system is sometimes unable to compensate for multiple lesions. Patients with hypertensive small vessel disease (Binswanger's disease) often have a gait disorder of the type described in the preceding, sometimes characterized as "lower body parkinsonism" (34). Correlation with imaging studies suggests that critical lesions are in the periventricular white matter and frontal centrum semiovale (35). A common mechanism has been proposed for this gait disorder and the gait disorder of hydrocephalus: a disconnection of frontal cortex and subcortical locomotor centers.

Cerebellar Degeneration

In our study, 6.7% of the patients had cerebellar gait disorders. Among these were patients with alcoholic cerebellar degeneration, the cerebellar presentation of multiple system atrophy, and patients with sporadic ataxia of late onset. Some of the hereditary ataxias can also present with late onset, particularly SCA-3 and SCA-5. The diagnostic evaluation of patients with progressive ataxia and a negative family history is reviewed in a number of standard texts (36).

Cerebellar gait is both a locomotor disorder and a balance disorder. Palliyath et al. described the characteristics of cerebellar gait (37). The gait is slow and halting, stepping is irregular, and there is a lurching quality as body segments struggle to maintain alignment. Patients may stumble or veer off to the side, particularly when they turn or change direction. There is decompensation on attempting to walk tandem heel to toe. The cerebellar gait is difficult to treat pharmacologically; a number of rehabilitation strategies have been explored.

Sensory Deficits

A large number of patients present with an unsteady gait owing to deficits in sensory afferent systems. Patients with sensory deficits account for 18% of our series and comprise the largest group. Balance during locomotion depends on high-quality information from the visual system, the vestibular system, and proprioceptive information from the lower limbs. Muscle spindle afferents may also play a role in postural control. There is a healthy redundancy of sensory information, but major disturbances in these systems produce a sense of disequilibrium and patients may exhibit a sensory ataxia of gait.

Fife and Baloh described a group of 26 patients over 75 presenting with disequilibrium of unknown cause, and found bilateral vestibular deficits in seven (38). Somatosensory deficits may be sufficient to compromise ambulation, particularly in older patients with poor vision. Locomotor ataxia was described in patients with tabetic neurosyphilis in the 19th century. There is erratic foot placement and a tendency to misstep. Some patients are visually dependent in their walking, and do poorly in the dark. Causes of a predominantly ataxic neuropathy in clinical practice include vincristine and cisplatin chemotherapy, paraproteinemia, and subacute sensory neuropathy, which may be paraneoplastic. Drachman and Hart in 1972 called attention to a group of older patients with multiple sensory deficits and imbalance (39). Some of these patients decompensate following cataract surgery.

Other Causes

Patients with metabolic encephalopathy often display an insecure gait. Antidepressant and sedative drugs may adversely affect postural control and increase the risk for falls (40,41). Toxic and metabolic disorders were observed in 2.5% of patients in our current series. We also observed an occasional patient with a mass lesion, including a man with a sphenoid meningioma and a patient with bilateral subdural hematomas (always a risk in patients who fall).

Gait is unconscious and automatic, but walking is nonetheless influenced by psychological state. Psychogenic disorders of gait are well described in the neurology literature from the 19th century to the present. We occasionally observe these disorders among older patients. Depression can be associated with characteristic changes in gait (42). Psychogenic gait disorder is important to recognize, because it is generally treatable.

Treatable Disorders

A clinical approach can be derived based on this experience with gait disorder in older patients. We can expect to make a diagnosis in 80% to 90% of outpatients with this presentation following examination and standard neurodiagnostic procedures (43). Treatable disorders are relatively common: A therapeutic intervention was available for 25% of the patients in our 1983 study (24). This compares quite favorably with our yield in evaluation of dementia in the elderly. In many patients with chronic disorders of gait and balance that are not specifically treatable, there are rehabilitation strategies to reduce the risk of falls and injury. Appropriate footwear and assistive devices are recommended. A home safety evaluation is sometimes productive to reduce environmental hazards.

REFERENCES

1. Newman G, Dovermuehle RH, Busse EW. Alterations in neurologic status with age. *J Am Geriatr Soc* 1960;8:915–917.
2. Wundgren-Linquist B, Aniansson A, Rundgren A. Functional studies in 79-year-olds III. Walking performance and climbing capacity. *Scand J Rehabil Med* 1983;15:121–131.
3. Odenheimer G, Funkenstein HH, Beckett L, et al. Comparison of neurologic changes in successfully aging persons vs the total aging population. *Arch Neurol* 1994;51:573–580.
4. Prakash C, Stern G. Neurologic signs in the elderly. *Age Aging* 1973;2:24–67.
5. Sudarsky L. Geriatrics: gait disorders in the elderly. *N Engl J Med* 1990 322:1441–1446.
6. Critchely M. The neurology of old age. *Lancet* 1931;1:1221–1230.
7. Murray MP, Kory RC, Clarkson BH. Walking patterns of healty old men. *J Gerontol* 1969;24:169–178.
8. Winter DA, Patla AE, Frank JS, et al. Biomechanical walking pattern changes in the fit and healthy elderly. *Phys Ther* 1990;70:340–347.
9. Elble RJ, Thomas SS, Higgins C, et al. Stride-dependent changes in gait of older people. *J Neurol* 1991;238:1–5.
10. Nevitt MC, Cummings SR. Type of fall and risk of hip and wrist fractures. *J Am Geriatr Soc* 1993;41:1226–1234.
11. Sattin RW. Falls among older persons: a public health perspective. *Ann Rev Public Health* 1992;13:489–508.
12. Nevitt MC. Falls in the elderly: risk factors and prevention. In: Masdeu J, Sudarsky L, Wolfson L, eds. *Gait disorders of aging: falls and therapeutic strategies*. Philadelphia: Lippincott–Raven, 1997:13–36.
13. Sheldon JH. On the natural history of falls in old age. *Br Med J* 1960;2:1685–1690.
14. Rubenstein L, Josephson KR. Interventions to reduce the multifactorial risks for falling. In: Masdeu J, Sudarsky L, Wolfson L, eds. *Gait disorders of aging: falls and therapeutic strategies*. Philadelphia: Lippincott–Raven, 1997:309–328.
15. Tinetti ME, Speechley M, Ginter SF. Risk factors for falls among elderly persons living in the community. *N Engl J Med* 1988;319:1701–1707.
16. O'Laughlin JL, Robiraille Y, Boivin J, et al. Incidence of and risk factors for falls and injurious falls among the community-dwelling elderly. *Am J Epidemiol* 1993;137:342–354.
17. Hausdorff JM, Edelberg HK, Mitchell SL, et al. Increased gait unsteadiness in community-dwelling elderly fallers. *Arch Phys Med Rehabil* 1997;78:278–283.
18. Lee LW, Kerrigan DC. Identification of kinetic differences between fallers and nonfallers in the elderly. *Am J Phys Med Rehabil* 1999;78:242–246.
19. Vieregge P. Gait disorders and falls from the neurologic viewpoint 2: clinical aspects. *Z Gerontol Geriatr* 1997;30:263–266.
20. Maki BE, Holliday PJ, Topper AK. Fear of falling and postural performance in the elderly. *J Gerontol* 1991;46:M123–131.
21. Walker JE, Howland J. Falls and fear of falling among elderly persons living in the community. *Am J Occup Ther* 1991;45:119–122.
22. Murphy J, Isaacs B. The post-fall syndrome: a study of 36 elderly patients. *Gerontology* 1982;28:265–270.
23. Rasker JJ, Jansen ENH, Haan J, et al. Normal-pressure hydrocephalus in rheumatic patients: a diagnostic pitfall. *N Engl J Med* 198;312:1239–1241.
24. Sudarsky L, Ronthal M. Gait disorders among elderly patients: a survey study of 50 patients. *Arch Neurol* 1983;40:740–743.
25. Fuh JL, Lin KN, Wang SJ, et al. Neurologic disease presenting with gait impairment in the elderly. In: Woollacott M, Horak F, eds. *Posture and gait: control mechanisms, vol. II*. Eugene, OR: University of Oregon Books, 1992:71–74.
26. Roland LP. Surgical treatment of cervical spondylotic myelopathy. *Neurology* 1992;42:5–13.
27. deRijk MC, Breteler MB, Graveland GA, et al. Prevalence of Parkinson's disease in the elderly. *Neurology* 1995;45:2143–2146.
28. Bennett DA, Beckett LA, Murray AM, et al. Prevalence of Parkinsonian signs and associated mortality in a community population of older people. *N Engl J Med* 1996;334:71–76.

29. Barbeau A. Aging and the extrapyramidal system. *J Am Geriatr Soc* 1973;21:145–149.
30. Stephen PJ, Williamson J. Drug-induced parkinsonism in the elderly. *Lancet* 1984;2:1082–1083.
31. Vanneste JA. Three decades of normal pressure hydrocephalus: are we wiser now? *J Neurol Neurosurg Psychol* 1994;57:1021–1025.
32. Wikkelso C, Anderson H, Blomstrand C, et al. The clinical effect of lumbar puncture in normal-pressure hydrocephalus. *J Neurol Neurosurg Psychol* 1982;45: 64–69.
33. Bradley WG, Whittemore AR, Kortman DE, et al. Marked cerebrospinal flow void: indicator of successful shunt in patients with suspected normal-pressure hydrocephalus. *Radiology* 1991;178:459–466.
34. Fitzgerald PM, Jankovic J. Lower body parkinsonism: evidence for a vascular etiology. *Mov Disord* 1989;4:249–260.
35. Sudarsky L. Frontal gait disorder: clinical correlation with MRI. In: Woollacott M, Horak F, eds. *Posture and gait: control mechanisms, vol. II.* Eugene, OR: University of Oregon Books, 1992:156–159.
36. Harding AE. Ataxic disorders. In: Bradley WG, Daroff RB, Fenichel GM, et al, eds. *Neurology in clinical practice.* Boston: Butterworth Heinemann, 1996:289–296.
37. Palliyath S, Hallett M, Thomas SL, et al. Gait in patients with cerebellar ataxia. *Mov Disord* 1998;13:958–964.
38. Fife TD, Baloh RW. Disequilibrium of unknown cause in older people. *Ann Neurol* 1993;34:694–702.
39. Drachman DA, Hart CW. An approach to the dizzy patient. *Neurology* 1972;22:323–334.
40. Ray WA, Griffin MR, Schaffner W, et al. Psychotropic drug use and the risk of hip fracture. *N Engl J Med* 1987;316:363–369.
41. Thapa PB, Gideon P, Cost TW, et al. Antidepressants and the risk of falls among nursing home residents. *N Engl J Med* 1998;339:875–882.
42. Sloman L, Berridge M, Homatidis MA, et al. Gait patterns of depressed patients and normal subjects. *Am J Psychiatry* 1982;139:94–97.
43. Sudarsky L. Clinical approach to gait disorders of aging: an overveiw. In: Masdeu JC, Sudarsky L, Wolfson L, eds. *Gait disorders of aging: falls and therapeutic strategies.* Philadelphia: Lippincott–Raven, 1997:147–158.

Gait Disorders. Advances in Neurology, Vol. 87,
edited by E. Růžička, M. Hallett, and J. Jankovic.
Lippincott Williams & Wilkins, Philadelphia © 2001.

12

Classification, Diagnosis, and Etiology of Gait Disorders

*†Joseph Jankovic, ‡John G. Nutt, and §¶Lewis Sudarsky

**Parkinson's Disease Center and Movement Disorders Clinic; †Department of Neurology, Baylor College of Medicine, Houston, Texas 77030; ‡Department of Neurology, Oregon Health Sciences University, Portland, Oregon 97201; §Department of Neurology, Harvard Medical School, Boston, Massachusetts; and ¶Department of Neurology, Brigham and Women's Hospital, Boston, Massachusetts 02115*

Gait is a complex motor skill that, when properly executed, requires the integration of mechanisms of locomotion with those of balance, motor control, and musculoskeletal function (1). Locomotion, a generation of sequence of command signals to advance, load, and unload the limbs, is not a consciously learned motor act but rather a repetitive motor pattern generated by spinal mechanisms and turned on and modified by brainstem structures (1a–6) (also, see chapter 2). Once learned, gait can be performed automatically and without conscious effort. In contrast to fourlegged animals whose walking is dependent on spinal pattern generators, automatic walking can be elicited in primates by electrical stimulation of the midbrain tegmentum (midbrain locomotor center), laterodorsal pontomesencephalic junction, including the pedunculopontine nucleus (PPN), and the posterior subthalamus (6–8). The PPN, a collection of cholinergic neurons located in the caudal mesencephalic tegmentum, receives direct bilateral descending projections from the subthalamic nucleus (STN), the dorsal and ventral striatum, the pallidum, and the substantia nigra reticulata (SNr). Descending projections from the pallidum and the SNr are mediated by the inhibitory neurotransmitter GABA; the PPN in turn provides excitatory ascending projections to the striatal output nuclei via acetylcholine and glutamate. Although the functional role of these PPN projections is not well known, PPN appears to mediate the influence of the basal ganglia on motor mechanisms of the brainstem and spinal cord, including gait, posture, and balance and as such it constitutes a major component of the mesencephalic locomotor center (8a). Studies have shown that stimulation of the PPN in the cat produces stepping and other rhythmic events, whereas an inhibition of the PPN leads to a reduction of locomotor activity (8). Elements of spinal stepping have been described in humans with paraplegia (9,10). Besides the spinal cord, dorsal midbrain corresponding to the brainstem locomotor region in experimental animals was found to be active during bipedal gait, as determined by regional cerebral blood flow measured by single photon emission tomography (SPECT) during gait on a treadmill (11). Although the basal ganglia, brainstem, and spinal cord play an important role in the control of posture and movement, the posterior parietal cortex also has been postulated to be involved in the perception of body stance and sway and may contribute to normal gait and balance (12).

Bipedal gait, along with language and speech, are the abilities that differentiate humans from their ancestors. Fossil evidence indicates that humans have used the bipedal form of locomotion for more than a million years (13). Over the centuries, gait disorders often have been associated with drunkenness and senility, but with the introduction of localization as the basis of neurologic diagnosis, attempts have been made to develop a clinical-anatomical etiologic classification of gait disorders (14,15). Bruns introduced the term frontal ataxia to describe severe disequilibrium owing to mass lesions in the frontal lobe (16). Petrén reported patients with start hesitation, freezing, and turning pauses and termed the condition *trepidant abasia* (17). Von Malaise described the gait pattern *marché à petit pas* in patients with frontal lobe disorders (18). These and other classic reports have contributed to the current understanding of nosology and classification of gaits.

Gait pattern changes with age: body sway increases, whereas dynamic balance declines (19–21). In addition, lower extremity strength, particularly ankle extension, declines. Furthermore, velocity of gait, length of stride, and pushoff power decrease, and double-limb support interval increases with a more flatfooted landing (22–25). These changes indicate adaptation by older adults toward a safer, more stable gait pattern owing to deterioration in strength and motor responses for an efficient control of balance during walking. Because of reduced reserves to support balance and gait, older adults are more prone to gait disturbances and falls. In addition, as many as half of elderly individuals living in the community voluntarily restrict their activity because they are fearful of falling (20,26).

Normal gait is critical to an individual's quality of life, and disorders of gait are a source of considerable handicap and distress. In one population-based study, 15% of the subjects over 60 years of age had some abnormality of gait that was the leading cause of significant neurologic impairment (27). The prevalence of gait disturbance may be considerably higher among very old persons (28,29). Forty percent to 50% of people in nursing homes have difficulty with walking, and they frequently fall (30). In one study, the most common causes of gait disorders in 120 patients in a neurologic referral practice were sensory deficits (17%), myelopathy (17%), multiple infarcts (15%), parkinsonism (12%), hydrocephalus (7%), cerebellar disorders (7%), and a variety of other causes. Falls in older adults, caused by loss of balance rather than tripping, are often associated with deep white matter abnormalities (31–35). The rate of fall-induced injuries and deaths in older adults appear to be increasing (36). There are many reasons why elderly people are more prone to falls, not least of which are various environmental hazards common in the homes of older persons (37). One neurophysiologic mechanism contributing to the falls may be owing to a delay in electromyographic (EMG) activity noted in older adults during a free fall startle in response to an auditory stimulus (38).

The purpose of this chapter is to provide a framework for assessment and clinical-anatomical etiologic classification of gait disorders.

DIAGNOSIS

Patients with gait or walking problems may attribute their difficulties to weakness, unsteadiness, slowness, stiffness, pain, and other impairments. Whatever the primary cause may be, gait and balance difficulties are often complicated by additional motor, musculoskeletal, and psychological factors, such as a fear of falling (39). Because the pathogenesis of gait disorders is often multifactorial, a systematic and comprehensive approach to the diagnosis is critical. This approach should be designed to assess the two essential components of gait: (a) locomotion (generation of alternating, repetitive sequence), and (b) maintenance of dynamic balance. Gait has been classically studied in the forms of the walking cycle (40). The cycle begins when the heel of one foot touches the floor. Stance is the entire period during which the foot is on the ground. Swing applies to the time the foot is in the air for limb advancement. Stride is the actions of one limb during a walking cycle. The average normal time distribution of a cycle is 60% for stance and 40% for swing. The duration of the gait cycle varies with a person's walking speed. Both stance and swing phases are shortened as walking speed increases. Also, walking faster proportionally lengthens single-limb support and shortens the double-limb support intervals. During running both feet are airborne some of the time, but during walking at least one foot is in contact with the ground at all times and 20% to 25% of the time both are on the ground (double-limb support) (28). The stride-to-stride variability is highest in young children, diminishes with normal aging, but increases again in disease states, such as Parkinson's disease (PD) and Huntington's disease (HD) (41,42). The process of locomotion, the capacity to initiate and maintain rhythmic stepping, is highly dependent on equilibrium, the capacity to assume and maintain upright posture and balance, musculoskeletal system, muscle strength, normal motor-sensory integration, normal execution of central motor programs, righting, anticipatory, and reactive postural reflexes, and supporting, rescue, and protective reactions (34,43–45). Impairment in any single component of gait, particularly stance and equilibrium, initiation and maintenance of rhythmic pattern of leg contraction, and postural reflexes, results in abnormal locomotion (46,47).

In addition to understanding the mechanisms of gait abnormalities, it is also important to assess the gait disorder in terms of severity and functional impairment. Although there are many techniques and instruments designed to quantitatively measure gait, most require a special gait laboratory and computerized video-EMG analysis. Because such equipment is expensive and cumbersome, it is usually reserved for research purposes and very few centers routinely utilize such quantitative assessments. There is, therefore, a need to develop a user-friendly gait rating scale, similar to the Unified Parkinson Disease Rating Scale (UPDRS) and other scales such as the functional reach, performance-oriented mobility assessment, timed walking tests, and other quantitative assessments of gait and balance (48–54). Such a Gait And Balance Scale (GABS) is currently being developed and validated.

CLASSIFICATION

The different gait disorders can be characterized phenomenologically by typical manifestations and physical signs into the following categories: hemiparetic, paraparetic, sensory, steppage, petits pas, apraxic, propulsive or retropulsive, ataxic, waddling, dystonic, choreic, antalgic, vertiginous, and hysteric (psychogenic) (Table 12.1). Although there are limitations to this categorization and some features of the various gait disorders overlap, this classification is useful to facilitate communication among clinicians. Also, this classification may be helpful in localizing the responsible lesion or lesions and in finding the most likely pathogenesis or etiology of the gait disorder. Because many of the abnormal gait patterns represent syndromes rather than a distinct entity, the etiology for each pattern may vary.

The classification of abnormal gaits is challenging because the various gait patterns often overlap and one pattern can evolve into another in the same individual as a consequence of the natural progression of the underlying disease process. The gait disorder observed clinically is the product of an abnormal physiology and a compensatory response. Furthermore, complex gait patterns can occur in mixed movement disorders. For example, patients with cerebral palsy may manifest a combination of athetosis, spasticity, dystonia, and ataxia. Similarly, patients with parkinsonism may have slow and shuffling gait and at the same time their gait may be impaired by L-Dopa–induced dyskinesias, most notably stereotypy and dystonia, superimposed on parkinsonism. Nearly all gait disorders are associated with other neurologic disturbances that may be contributing to the impaired locomotion.

The proposed classification is organized into two major categories: clinical gait patterns and anatomic–clinical classifications (Table 12.1; Table 12.2). An attempt is made to define a set of clinical criteria that will predict with a certain degree of certainty the anatomic–pathological findings. Only detailed pathological studies, however, will be able to determine whether such clinical–anatomic–pathological correlations are valid.

Anatomically, the primary gait disorders may be categorized as: (a) frontal gait disorders, (b) corticobasal gait disorders, and (c) subcortical gait disorders (Table 12.2). Although there is some overlap among these three types of primary gait disorders, they can be differentiated relatively easily in early stages.

Frontal gait disorders, combination of locomotor disorder and disequilibrium, have been described by a variety of terms, including *Bruns'*

TABLE 12.1. *Gait patterns*

Physical signs	Description	Associated signs
Hemiparetic gait	Extension and circumduction of one leg	Weakness on the affected side; hyperreflexia; extensor plantar response; flexed arm
Paraparetic gait	Stiffness, extension, adduction, and scissoring of both legs	Bilateral leg weakness, hyperreflexia, spasticity, and extensor plantar responses
Sensory gait	Unsteadiness of walking when visual input is withdrawn	Positive Romberg sign; decreased position sense
Steppage gait	Weakness of foot dorsiflexors; foot drop; excessive flexion of hips and knees when walking; short strides; unilateral or bilateral	Atrophy of distal leg muscles; decreased ankle reflex; possible sensory loss
Cautious gait[a]	Wide-based, careful, slow	Associated often with anxiety, fear of open spaces and fear of falling
Freezing gait[a]	Difficulty initiating a step; freezing; feet almost stuck to floor; turn hesitation; shuffling gait	Hypokinesia; muscular rigidity; grasp reflexes; possible resting tremor, dementia, or urinary incontinence
Propulsive or retropulsive gait[a]	Body's center of gravity appears to be either in front or behind the patient, who is struggling to keep his or her feet up to center of gravity; festination	Hypokinesia; muscular rigidity; postural instability
Ataxic gait	Wide-based gait; incoordination; staggering; decomposition of movements	Dysmetria; dysdiadochokinesia; tremor; postural instability
Astasia	Primary balance disorder	Postural instability
Waddling gait	Wide-based gait; swaying; toe-walk; lumbar lordosis; symmetrical	Proximal muscle weakness of lower extremities
Dystonic gait[a]	Sustained abnormal posture of the foot or leg; distorted gait; hyperflexion of hips	Action-related gait disturbance; atypical presentations
Choreic gait[a]	Irregular, dancelike gait; slow and wide-based; spontaneous knee flexion and leg raising	Athetotic and choreic movements of the upper extremities
Antalgic gait	Limping; avoidance of bearing full weight on the affected leg; limitation of range of movement	Pain in lower extremity aggravated by leg, hip, thigh movement and weight bearing
Vertiginous gait	Unsteady gait; falling to one side; postural imbalance	Vertigo; nausea; nystagmus
Psychogenic (hysteric) gait	Bizarre and nonphysiologic gait; different varieties; rare fall or injury	Give-way weakness; Hoover's sign; other signs of conversion

[a] These gaits may be seen in patients with Parkinson's disease.

ataxia, marché à petits pas, arteriosclerotic parkinsonism, lower body parkinsonism, vascular parkinsonism, and *gait apraxia* (16,56–65). In addition to inability to appropriately execute the act of walking, patients with gait apraxia may also have apraxia of rising or sitting (66,67). These patients appear perplexed with the task of rising or sitting and make bizarre, inappropriate attempts to accomplish changes in position.

The frontal gait disorders are commonly caused by anterior cerebral artery stroke, multi-infarct state, subcortical arteriosclerotic encephalopathy (Binswanger's disease), normal pressure hydrocephalus, Alzheimer's disease (AD), and corticobasal degeneration, and other bilateral frontal lobe disorders (68–73). In one study of 55 patients with AD, 22 (40%) had a higher level of gait disorder compared to 10 (18%) age-matched controls ($P < 0.01$) (74). The pattern of gait disturbance in patients with AD varied according to the stage of the disease. Cautious gait was the most common gait disorder in AD patients with mild dementia, whereas frontal gait disorder was the most common disturbance in patients with severe dementia. The prevalence of frontal release signs (gegenhalten or any primitive reflex) was highest among patients with frontal gait disorder. The finding of

(*Text continued on page 125*)

TABLE 12.2. *Anatomic-clinical-etiologic classification of gait disorders*

Anatomic classification [previous terminology]	Clinical features	Pathology/pathogenesis
Frontal gait disorders [frontal disequilibrium, gait apraxia, frontal apraxia, frontal (Bruns') ataxia, parkinsonian ataxia, astasia–abasia, marché à petits pas, magnetic gait, senile gait, senile paraplegia, magnetic gait, slipping clutch gait, arteriosclerotic parkinsonism, lower body parkinsonism]	A. Pure 1. Short stride 2. Abnormal stance (wide > narrow base, variable, crossing of legs) 3. Freezing (motor blocks) 4. Loss of balance (disequilibrium in response to perturbation, unable to stand or sit unsupported) 5. Inappropriate postural adjustments when arising from chair (extending instead of flexing trunk and legs) or turn in bed 6. Stiff trunk/legs (military gait) 7. Leg apraxia (difficulty with stepping or bicycling movements) 8. Minimal or no improvement with cues. B. Associated findings 1. Pseudobulbar palsy 2. Cognitive impairment 3. Pyramidal signs 4. Urinary disturbance 5. Foot grasp 6. Frontal release signs.	Bilateral frontal lobe white matter lesions, anterior cerebral artery infarction, periventricular multiinfarct state, Binswanger's disease, Pick's disease, frontal mass, normal pressure hydrocephalus. Disconnection between motor, premotor and supplementary motor cortex and subcortical motor areas such as the basal ganglia, brainstem, and cerebellum.
Subcortical hyperkinetic gait disorders	I. Choreic (random brief movements, wide-based stance, variable stride and timing, disequilibrium in later stages) II. Dystonic (inversion of foot or other foot/leg deformities, bizarre gait pattern, improved by walking backwards, "dystonic paraparesis" in dopa-responsive dystonia) III. Athetotic (slow, often associated with dystonia and spasticity) IV. Stereotypic (bizarre, but patterned gait) V. Myoclonic (wide-based, bouncing stance, drop attacks) VI. Tremulous (orthostatic tremor present while standing but disappears while walking) VII. Other	Huntington's disease, primary and secondary dystonia, tardive dyskinesia, cerebral palsy, other hyperkinetic movement disorders
Subcortical astasia (thalamic astasia, thalamic ataxia, subcortical disequilibrium)	1. Marked disequilibrium (unable to stand or even sit, falls "like a falling log") 2. Normal strength and sensation.	Thalamotomy, thalamic strokes, thalamic arteriovenous malformation, putaminal or pallidal strokes
Pyramidal gait (hemiparetic, hemiplegic, spastic gait)	1. Shoulder adducted 2. Elbow flexed 3. Forearm pronated and wrist flexed	Cerebral hemisphere (internal capsule) stroke, demyelination, tumor, or other lesions

Continued

TABLE 12.2. *Continued*

Anatomic classification [previous terminology]	Clinical features	Pathology/pathogenesis
	4. Hip slightly flexed and knee extended 5. Slow circumduction of affected leg with toe dragging 6. Wide stance 7. Spasticity on the affected side.	
Cerebellar gait (ataxic gait)	1. Wide-based stance 2. Marked disequilibrium particularly rapid postural adjustments 3. Dyssenergia of leg movements (irregular and variable) 4. Dysmetria (erratic foot placement) 5. Titubation 6. "Bouncing" gait when combined with spasticity (spastic ataxia).	Strokes, demyelination, cerebellar degenerations, other cerebellar disorders.
Subcortical hypokinetic gait disorders (parkinsonian gait)	A. Pure 1. Short stride 2. Slow 3. Shuffling 4. Narrow base 5. Festination 6. Freezing (motor blocks) 7. Start hesitation 8. Turns en bloc 9. Abnormal postural responses (retropulsion > propulsion) and falling 10. Motor blocks improve with cues. B. Associated findings I. Parkinson's disease a. Rest tremor b. Body bradykinesia c. Hypomimia d. Dysarthria e. Flexed posture and knees f. Other parkinsonian features. II. Parkinsonism plus a. Parkinsonism-plus gait (stiff, knees extended, wide base, freezing, unsteady, frequent falls, crossing of feet and pivoting on turning, toe walking) b. Ocular palsy (vertical > horizontal) c. Neck extension/flexion d. Pseudobulbar palsy e. Dysautonomia.	Vascular (or other) lesions in the thalamus, basal ganglia, brainstem (pedunculo-pontine nucleus), Parkinson's disease, progressive supranuclear palsy, multiple system atrophy.
Cortical-subcortical gait disorders (isolated gait ignition failure, primary progressive freezing gait, motor blocks, lower body parkinsonism, pure akinesia, trepidant abasia, Petren's gait)	A. Pure 1. Freezing (motor blocks) 2. Start hesitation 3. Turn hesitation 4. Blocking in narrow spaces 5. Shuffling 6. Stride normal or lengthens with walking (no festination)	Nonspecific cortical and subcortical white matter lesions, frontal cortical hypometabolism, early stages of progressive supranuclear palsy and other parkinsonian disorders. Cortical-brainstem disconnection.

Continued

TABLE 12.2. *Continued*

Anatomic classification [previous terminology]	Clinical features	Pathology/pathogenesis
	7. Normal stepping or bicycling movements (in sitting or supine position)	
	8. Normal postural responses	
	9. Normal arm swing	
	10. Improvement with cues.	
	B. Associated findings	
	1. Cognitive impairment	
	2. Dysarthria	
	3. Loss of manual dexterity	
	4. Loss of balance and postural responses	
	5. Bradykinesia	
	6. Rigidity	
	7. Loss of associated movements.	

altered spatio-temporal gait strategy in order to compensate for postural instability in patients with subcortical arteriosclerotic encephalopathy and in those with cerebellar ataxia suggested common mechanisms in both gait disorders (70).

Cortical–subcortical gait disorders have been also termed *trepidant abasia, gait ignition failure, primary progressive freezing gait, motor blocks,* and *pure akinesia* (14,17,75–79) (also see chapter 19). The characteristic feature of freezing gait is inability to initiate and maintain locomotion. Patients often describe the phenomenon as if the foot is "glued" to the ground. When attempting to start walking, patients cannot get the foot to advance, so-called start hesitation. In mild cases, start hesitation is characterized by a pause before beginning to walk and a series of short steps before the normal stride length is reached. In some cases, the patient does not appear to make any weight shifts that would allow one foot to leave the ground; the patient appears truly frozen to the spot. Other times, the lateral and forward weight shifts are inadequate to permit a full step but may allow the foot to advance an inch or so to produce a slow, shuffling progression. In other cases, there may be exaggerated swaying of the body in an attempt to free one foot and even so, the toe may seem to stick to the floor while the heel is lifted. Frequently, once underway, the stride lengthens and speeds up, giving the appearance of a slipping clutch engaging (slipped clutch phenomenon). Locomotion may be interrupted by turning (turn hesitation) or passage through constricted areas such as doorways and may be quite disabling and embarrassing when getting out of the elevator. Minor obstacles on the floor, asking the patient a question, an unexpected touch or sound, or any other distraction will cause the patient to slow down or arrest the locomotion (80). Conversely, the patient can resume normal locomotion when he or she deliberately concentrates on walking. In addition to start hesitation, festination, and freezing, many patients with pure akinesia develop severe disequilibrium and frequent falling, as well as dysarthria and micrographia, but no rigidity, tremor, or dementia. Although some patients develop square-wave jerks and slow saccades, it is not clear how many actually evolve into progressive supranuclear palsy (PSP) (79). Although a minority of patients have been reported to improve with L-threo-3, 4-dihydroxyphenylserine (DOPS) or tricyclic antidepressants, suggesting underlying noradrenergic deficiency, the vast majority of such patients do not improve with any pharmacologic therapy.

Surprisingly, patients may overcome the freezing with a variety of visual, auditory, and tactile cues, and they may ascend and descend stairs better than they walk on the level. This phenomenon is referred to as *kinésie paradoxale* or paradoxical gait. Other tricks used by patients to initiate gait include stepping on targets on the floor, stepping over stripes on the floor, stepping over the handle of an upturned walking cane, trying to kick the cane, stepping to marching music or command, and stepping sideways (81–85). Each patient tends to discover tricks that will help with initiation of gait but the tricks are only effective sometimes. It appears that the tricks must be somewhat novel to be effective. Walking in the patient with freezing is influenced by the same factors that aid or hinder a novice dancer learning the footwork of a new dance. Although normal walking is a learned motor skill carried out without conscious effort, when this normal gait pattern is impaired, walking becomes less automatic and requires more conscious control.

The mechanism of tricks seems to involve helping the patient to focus on moving one leg to or over a target rather than simply thinking of walking. Thus, the actions that interrupt locomotion and aid initiation appear to be those that hinder or promote attention necessary for motor acts carried out under conscious cortical control. This is consistent with the finding of enhanced lateral premotor activity, as demonstrated by increased regional cerebral blood flow, during paradoxical gait observed in some patients with PD (86).

Freezing (motor blocks) cannot be explained by any specific neurologic abnormality (weakness, incoordination, or sensory loss), and, therefore, it is often considered a form of an apraxia (61–65). However, the freezing gait pattern is usually seen in patients without other signs of apraxia and patients with bilateral apraxia may have normal gait (14,75,77). No stimulus is adequate to cue performance in these patients. It thus seems that freezing is best envisioned as loss of access to diencephalic and brainstem locomotor centers rather than loss of a learned skill. Viewed as a basic defect in internal rhythm formation, freezing of gait has been found to correlate well with manual motor blocks as measured by a finger-tapping task (87). Freezing has been attributed to frontal cortical dysfunction and a similarity has been noted between freezing and grasp. In this regard, it is of interest that a supplementary motor area has been implicated in the mechanism of grasp and may be also involved in patients who freeze (88).

Anatomically, freezing is associated with disturbances of the basal ganglia, frontal lobe and their interconnections, hence the designation corticobasal gait disorders (Table 12.1). Frontal and basal ganglia lesions cause difficulties with attention, switching between tasks and simultaneous execution of tasks, and these functions may relate to the phenomenon of freezing (89). Freezing is typically seen in parkinsonian disorders (PD, PSP, multiple system atrophy, corticobasal ganglionic degeneration, and vascular parkinsonism), hydrocephalus, and frontal lobe lesions (59,68,78). These disorders may present as gait ignition failure, lower-half or lower-body parkinsonism (56,57,69,75,79). This disorder is characterized by difficulties with gait initiation, shuffling and hesitant gait, but well-preserved arm swing. The base may be normal but more frequently the base is widened, possibly owing to associated atrophy of the cerebellar vermis (68). Likewise, balance may be perfectly normal but more often is disturbed. Lower body parkinsonism is frequently associated with white matter ischemic changes. In multiinfarct state, freezing may be associated with bizarre features, such as exaggerated arm swing and excessive truncal sway from side to side to alternately unweigh the feet and initiate or maintain stepping. The base may be extremely wide; therefore, they are often termed ataxic (68). In these patients, the efforts at walking appear to be a caricature of normal gait. The possible contribution of chronic ischemia to disequilibrium seen in older, even normotensive people, has been suggested by the finding of increased sclerotic index and subcortical leukoencephalopathy (along with frontal atrophy, ventriculomegaly, and reactive astrocytes) on neuropathological examination when compared to control subjects (90).

Normal pressure hydrocephalus can also cause a freezing gait pattern (71,91). Frontal lobe infarcts, tumors, and degenerative processes may also produce freezing, although disequilibrium is often more prominent than freezing. Finally, there are some patients in whom the freezing gait pattern is a progressive disorder without other neurologic signs or MRI abnormalities. Imaging is important in sorting out these various etiologies of freezing.

Freezing (motor blocks) in parkinsonism is assumed to be related to dopamine deficiency, yet the response to L-Dopa is unpredictable. In some patients, L-Dopa and dopamine agonists relieve freezing; in others freezing is worsened, but in most cases dopaminergic therapy has no effect (92,93). In many patients, dopaminergic drugs have no effect on freezing. Similarly, the effect of pallidotomy on freezing is unpredictable. Some patients clearly experience improvement in contralateral freezing after pallidotomy, but this may not necessarily result in a meaningful improvement in walking because the ipsilateral freezing may impair balance during gait propulsion (94). This apparent discrepancy may be resolved by the findings that posterior ventral globes pallidus internus (GPi) stimulation worsened gait and more dorsal GPi stimulation improved gait (95).

Subcortical hypokinetic gait disorders are also known as *akinetic-rigid gait or parkinsonian gait,* and are typically seen in patients with parkinsonism. Patients with PD, PSP, and multiple system atrophy typically exhibit this abnormality in which the normal postural-locomotor synergies are impaired, the stance is narrow based, posture and knees are flexed, the step height is low resulting in shuffling and in turning *en bloc* (49,79,96–99). In addition, festination and postural instability are common. Although these gaits are classified as *subcortical,* referring to primary abnormality in the basal ganglia and their connections, there is evidence that lateral premotor cortex and the cerebellum may be also contributing to the gait abnormality seen in patients with PD and related disorders (86). The involvement of the cortex in parkinsonian gait is suggested by the observation that the gait abnormality is markedly exacerbated when mental concentration is impaired and patients attempt to execute a second task (e.g., talking) while walking. Indeed, an impairment of gait by a simultaneous performance of multiple tasks is a sensitive predictor of postural instability and falling (100).

The gait speed in PD is markedly reduced and the stride-to-stride variability of gait cycle timing is two to three times greater than in normal controls (41). It is important to note, however, that the gait parameters are dependent on the speed of gait and setting various temporal constraints when testing gait allows identification of abnormalities that may not be revealed when only the preferred velocity of walking is studied (85,97,101). When patients with PD are instructed to voluntarily increase their speed of walking, the step rate is disproportionally increased as compared to controls, whereas the increase in stride length is lower (97,102). Patients with PD, therefore, have a higher cadence rate than control subjects for any given velocity, possibly as a compensatory mechanism for reduced step size. The gait hypokinesia, exhibited by patients with PD, has been attributed to an inability to internally generate sufficiently large steps and defective scaling of stride length has been considered to be the main gait disturbance in PD (97,98,103). Furthermore, impairment in force load control may also contribute to the gait and balance problems associated with PD (104). In a study of 15 patients with PD complicated by motor complications, O'Sullivan et al. found improvements in stride length and gait velocity after L-Dopa, but there was no improvement in cadence (49). Likewise, surgical treatments have been shown to improve velocity, stride length, and other parameters of gait and balance, but they usually do not correct the abnormalities in stride length–cadence relationship (see chapters 28 and 30).

The earliest and most disabling symptom of PSP usually relates to gait and balance impairment, as a result of which patients frequently fall and sustain injuries. The marked instability is presumably a result of visual–vestibular impairment, axial rigidity, and bradykinesia (105). In contrast to short and shuffling steps, stooped posture, narrow base, and flexed knees, typically seen in patients with PD, patients with PSP have a stiff and broad-based gait, with a tendency to have their knees (and trunk) extended and arms slightly abducted. Instead of turning en bloc they tend to pivot, which further compromises their balance. Although the gait disorder of PSP appears ataxic, the patients usually do not exhibit prominent cerebellar findings. Postural control in patients with PSP often resembles a toy soldier who stands motionless when unperturbed, but falls like a log when pushed (96). The uncompensated loss of postural reflexes and motor blocks (freezing) especially on turning, coupled with a peculiar lack of insight into the difficulties with equilibrium (possibly secondary to frontal lobe dysfunction), lead to frequent falling. This is often present even in the early stages of the disease and helps to differentiate PSP from PD (106).

Subcortical hyperkinetic gait disorders include dystonic gait, choreic gait, and gait and stance disorders associated with other hyperkinetic movement disorders such as orthostatic tremor and myoclonus (Table 12.2) (107). Dystonic gaits may vary from simple limping, high-stepping, or leg dragging owing to dystonic foot inversion or eversion or other abnormal postures owing to low limb dystonia to a complex gait (108). As a result of trunk and leg dystonia, many patients have bizarre gaits phenomenologically linked to gaits of various animals; hence, the terms *dromedary, monkey,* and *ducklike gait*. Various sensory tricks, such as placing the hands in the pockets, behind the neck or back, or on the hip, might enable the patients to walk relatively normally. Also, running, walking backward, or dancing might improve the quality of the gait.

Chorea, typically present in patients with HD, may produce a very irregular gait pattern often described as a stuttering or dancing gait (41,109). The contact of the foot with the support surface is unpredictable because of the superimposed involuntary movements of trunk and legs. The steps are of variable length and deviate from the direction of travel. The heel, toe, or side of the foot may make initial contact with the ground repetitive, giving the stuttering appearance. Despite the gait appearing extremely precarious, the patients often do not fall until the gait is grossly abnormal and the balance becomes compromised. Similar to patients with PD, patients with HD have a slower velocity of gait that can be modulated during selfpaced and rhythmic metronome cuing, but in contrast to PD, there is no synchronization between step cadence and rhythmic stimulus (110).

Some patients with tardive dyskinesia or L-Dopa–induced dyskinesia develop a stereotyped gait such as goose stepping, sometimes wrongly attributed to psychogenic causes. Although patients with essential tremor usually do not complain of gait difficulties, some do develop unsteady gait and on examination have difficulties walking in tandem (111,112). In one study of 33 patients with essential tremor, the sharpened Romberg and walk on floor tests with eyes open and closed were significantly impaired as compared to normal controls (112). The mean scores of the ET group were worse than those of the control group for each test, but significant differences were found only with the most challenging motor control tasks. The ET group performed significantly worse than the control subjects with the eyes open SR ($P = 0.0167$, Mann–Whitney U) and WOF ($P = 0.021$, Mann–Whitney U) tests. Orthostatic tremor is a fast (14 to 16 Hz) tremor, involving mainly legs and trunk, which appears on standing after a latency of several seconds or minutes (113,114). It is associated with a feeling of unsteadiness and calf cramps, relieved by sitting or supine position, and with clonazepam. Positron emission tomography (PET) indicates bilateral cerebellar (and contralateral lentiform and thalamic) dysfunction (115).

Myoclonic gait is interrupted by a jerklike movement (positive myoclonus) or by sudden give in muscle tone (negative myoclonus), often resulting in a buckling of the knees, collapse, and a fall. This is most typically seen in patients with generalized myoclonus as a result of a hypoxic/ischemic event (116). One form of spinal myoclonus is the propriospinal myoclonus that produces axial jerks, usually beginning in the abdominal muscles (117).

Subcortical disequilibrium previously referred to as thalamic astasia, thalamic ataxia, or subcortical disequilibrium, is usually associated with thalamic or basal ganglia lesions (118–120). Subcortical disequilibrium is usually produced by unilateral lesions of dorsolateral thalamus (primarily the ventrolateral or posterior nucleus involving the dentatoorubrothalamic pathway) or the lenticular nucleus. Infarcts or hemorrhages in these areas often result in tendency to fall backward or contralateral to the lesion when standing or even sitting. Although patients are generally aware of their instability, they appear to neglect or ignore it and they are often unable to correct the drift or to prevent falls. Some patients exhibit motor neglect, failing to use the limbs contralateral to the lesion for spontaneous activities or in tasks requiring bilateral limb involvement although they can carry out command tasks with the limb. Not all patients with subcortical (thalamic) abasia exhibit sensory impairment. Some patients exhibit unilateral asterixis, a recognized sign of thalamic lesions. Subcortical disequilibrium (thalamic astasia) improves over days to months following acute unilateral lesions, possibly because the vestibulocerebellar pathway that projects to the medial ventrolateral nucleus of the thalamus and may be responsible for thalamic abasia, is bilateral (118).

Pyramidal gait disorders present in a hemiparetic and spastic pattern (Table 12.2). Spastic gaits are frequently associated with stroke, demyelination, mass, or trauma to the motor cortex or the corticospinal tracts (121,122) (also see chapter 14). Although spasticity clearly contributes to overall disability of patients after stroke, it may not significantly contribute to the stroke-related impairment in walking (123). Focal epilepsy may cause a paroxysmal gait disorder (124). *Cerebellar gait disorders* are characterized by ataxia and can be produced by any insult to the cerebellum (125,126) (also see chapter 15). In contrast to normal subjects, patients with cerebellar degeneration have been found to have reduced step and stride length, delayed heel-off time, toe-off time, and time of peak flexion of the knee in swing (126). In addition, the patients exhibited multijoint incoordination and increased variability in all gait measures. *Brainstem gait disorders* and *myelopathic gait disorders* are characterized by spastic or stiff (scissoring) gait (53,127). In addition, a lesion in the pontomesencephalic junction (involving the PPN) can produce severe disequilibrium and gait failure characterized by difficulty initiating gait and by steps of irregular amplitude and direction (127). The involvement of central vestibular pathways also contributes to this balance and gait abnormality (128).

Cautious gait disorders have been labeled variously as *senile gait, pseudoagoraphobia, post-fall syndrome, space phobia, adaptive gait,* and *astasobasophobia* (14,23,26,129–132). It is characterized by a slow, slightly wide-based, and short steps as if walking on ice, probably representing a compensatory strategy for instability. This abnormal gait pattern is most frequently seen in older adults, but cautious gait can occur at any age; therefore, the term is preferable to senile gait. Although there is some overlap between cautious gait and senile gait, kinematics in older, healthy adults typically shows slower speed, shorter stride, reduced arm swing, flexed knees, and reduced toe clearance (23,24). In contrast to parkinsonian gait, patients with senile gait do not manifest other features of PD, such as tremor, hypomimia, dysarthria, and other parkinsonian features. In many cases, cautious gait first appears after a fall, even if the fall is not associated with any injury. As a result of the fall, some patients, particularly older adults, lose confidence in their ability to walk and maintain normal balance. They then suddenly or gradually adopt the wide-based, careful gait with a need to hold to the wall, objects, or an attendant. They may be unable to walk in open spaces (pseudoagoraphobia) but are able to walk inside their house. In some cases, however, the patient becomes completely disabled because of severe fear of falling that is not proportionate to motor and sensory deficit. Patients with such overcautious gait often become incapacitated, although some respond to intensive gait training and anxiolytic medications.

In addition to gait disorders of central origin, there are many different gait disorders caused by damage to or dysfunction of the peripheral nervous system. Waddling is the characteristic feature of *myopathic gait disorders,* resulting from proximal muscle weakness. Etiologies include muscular dystrophies, myopathies, and other neuromuscular diseases. Patients with *neuropathic gait disorders* have distal muscle weakness that may be unilateral or bilateral. In order to compensate for a foot drop patients develop a steppage gait. If sensory alterations accompany weakness, the diagnosis of peripheral neuropathy is more assured. Sensory deprivation gait disorders are commonly produced by the loss of proprioceptive input from the legs. Lesions that interrupt large-diameter sensory afferent fibers, such as peripheral neuropathies and posterior root, ganglion, or column damage, can cause this unsteady gait pattern. In addition, vestibular dysfunction, such as acute vestibulopathy, or deprivations of auditory and visual inputs can also evoke such conditions (133). The veering during a walk in patients with this *vestibular gait and balance disorder* actually improves with running (134). *Orthopedic gait disorders* are associated with arthritis or other joint and skeletal abnormalities (135). They are characterized by a slow, stiff, and painful (antalgic) pattern.

Psychogenic gait disorders are also termed hysterical gaits or acrobatic gaits (136–138). Their presentations are often bizarre and inconsistent. In addition to the dramatic, lurching quality to the gait patients often exhibit a tendency to collapse with knee buckling, but without self-injury and without any weakness or evidence of an organic cause (139). The gait is incongruous with any organic gait described in the preceding. When asked to tandem walk they may balance on one foot while waving the other foot in the air before placing it on the floor, or they cross their feet (astasia–abasia). When distracted, elements of normal gait may become apparent, although transiently. When asked to perform the Romberg test, there may be increasing sway with improvement by distraction.

It is important to note that apparent inconsistencies are present in some organic gaits. For example, patients with generalized dystonia may not be able to walk forward without severe abnormal posturing, but may be able to walk backward without much difficulty. This feature of dystonia, a form of a sensory trick, often leads to the wrong diagnosis of a psychogenic gait. Some patients with cautious gaits (e.g., pseudoagoraphobia) may not be able to walk unless they lightly touch a wall or accompanying person, but this should not be misinterpreted as a psychogenic gait, because the light touch may provide an important proprioceptive clue or even a form of psychological support that legitimately improves gait. Another characteristic of a psychogenic gait is its fluctuation from minute to minute and hour to hour. This should not be difficult to differentiate from organic intermittent or paroxysmal gait disorders, such as seen in patients with periodic paralyses, episodic ataxias, and paroxysmal dystonias.

The diagnosis of psychogenic gait disorder should be a positive diagnosis rather than merely a diagnosis of exclusion (137,138). It is usually supported by other features indicative of a psychogenic disorder, such as false weakness, false sensory symptoms, multiple somatizations, bizarre movements or pseudoseizures, seeming indifferent to the disability, relief with psychotherapy, powerful suggestion, placebo, or physiotherapy, and evidence of psychological conflicts or previous psychiatric history.

REFERENCES

1. Dinkinson MH, Farley CT, Full RJ, et al. How animals move: an integrative view. *Science* 2000;288:100–106.
1a. Orlovsky GN, Shik ML. Control of locomotion: a neurophysiological analysis of the cat locomotor system. *Int Rev Physiol* 1976;10:281–317.
2. Garcia-Rill E. The basal ganglia and the locomotor regions. *Brain Res Rev* 1986;11:47–63.
3. Mori S. Integration of posture and locomotion in acute decerebrate cats and in awake, freely moving cats. *Prog Neurobiol* 1987;28:161–195.
4. Armstrong DM. Supraspinal control of locomotion. *J Physiol* 1988;405:1–37.
5. Grillner S, Deliagina T, Ekeberg O, et al. Neural networks that co-ordinate locomotion and body orientation in lamprey. *TINS* 1995;18:270–279.
6. Grillner S. Ion channels and locomotion. *Science* 1997; 278:1087–1088.
7. Eidelberg E, Walden JG, Nguyen LH. Locomotor control in Macaque monkeys. *Brain* 1981;104:647–663.
8. Garcia-Rill E. The pedunculopontine nucleus. *Prog Neurobiol* 1991;36:363–389.
8a. Pahapill PA, Lozano AM. The pedunculopontine nucleus and Parkinson's disease. *Brain* 2000;123:1767–1783.
9. Calancie B, Needham-Shropshire B, Jacobs P, et al. Involuntary stepping after chronic spinal cord injury: evidence for a central rhythm generator for locomotion in man. *Brain* 1994;117:1143–1159.
10. Dietz V, Colombo G, Jensen L. Locomotor activity in spinal man. *Lancet* 1994;344:1260–1263.
11. Hanakawa T, Katsumi Y, Fukuyama H, et al. Mechanisms underlying gait disturbance in Parkinson's disease. A single photon emission computed tomography study. *Brain* 1999;122:1271–1282.
12. Schieppati M, Tacchini E, Nardone A, et al. Subjective perception of body sway. *J Neurol Neurosurg Psychiatry* 1999;66:313–322.
13. Napier J. The antiquity of human walking. *Sci Am* 1967; 216:56–66.
14. Nutt JG, Marsden CD, Thompson PD. Human walking and higher-level gait disorders, particularly in the elderly. *Neurology* 1993;43:268–279.
15. Schiller F. Staggering gait in medical history. *Ann Neurol* 1995;37:127–135.
16. Bruns L. *Uber storungen des gleichgewichtes bei stirnhirntumoren. Dtsch Med Wochenschr* 1892;18:138–140.
17. Petrén K. *Über den Zusammenhang swischen anatomisch bedingter und functioneller Gangstörung (besonders in der Form von trepid ander Abasie) im*

Griesenalter. Arch Psych Nerven 1901;33:818–871; 34:444–489.
18. Von Malaise E. *Studien uber wese grundlagen senile getstoringen. Arch Psychiat* 1910;46:902–1009.
19. Murray MP, Kory RC, Clarkson BH. Walking patterns in healthy old men. *J Gerontol* 1969;24:169–178.
20. Imms FJ, Edholm OG. Studies of gait and mobility in the elderly. *Age Aging* 1981;10:147–156.
21. Larish DD, Martin PE, Mungiole M. Characteristic patterns of gait in the healthy old. *Ann NY Acad Sci* 1988;515:18–31.
22. Winter DA, Patla AE, Frank JS, et al. Biomechanical walking pattern changes in the fit and healthy elderly. *Phys Ther* 1990;70:340–347.
23. Elble RJ, Higgins C, Hughes L. The syndrome of senile gait. *J Neurol* 1991;239:71–75.
24. Elble RJ, Sienko-Thomas S, Higgins C, et al. Stride-dependent changes in gait of older people. *J Neurol* 1991;238:1–5.
25. Wolfson L, Whipple R, Derby CA, et al. A dynamic posturography study of balance in healthy elderly. *Neurology* 1992;42:2069–2075.
26. Overstall RW, Exton-Smith AN, Imms FJ, et al. Falls in the elderly related to postural imbalance. *Br Med J* 1977;1:261–264.
27. Newman G, Dovermuehle RH, Busse EW. Alterations in neurologic status with age. *J Am Geriatr Soc* 1960;8:915–917.
28. Sudarsky L. Geriatrics: gait disorders in the elderly. *N Engl J Med* 1990:322:1441–1446.
29. Alexander NB. Gait disorders in older adults. *J Am Geriatr Soc* 1996;44:434–451.
30. Tinetti ME, Baker DI, McAvay G, et al. A multifactorial intervention to reduce the risk of falling among elderly people living in the community. *N Engl J Med* 1994;331:821–827.
31. Masdeu JC, Wolfson L, Lantos G. Brain white–matter changes in the elderly prone to falling. *Arch Neurol* 1989;46:1292–1296.
32. Rubestein LZ, Robbins AS, Josephson KR, et al. The value of assessing falls in an elderly population. A randomized clinical trial. *Ann Int Med* 1990;113:308–316.
33. Baloh RW, Yue Q, Socotch TM, et al. White matter lesions and disequilibrium in older people: I. Case-control comparison. *Arch Neurol* 1995;52:970–974.
34. Rudge P, Bronstein AM. Investigations of disorders of balance. *J Neurol Neurosurg Psychiatry* 1995;59:568–578.
35. Tell GS, Lefkowitz DS, Diehr P, et al. Relationship between balance and abnormalities in cerebral magnetic resonance imaging in older adults. *Arch Neurol* 1998;55:73–79.
36. Kannus P, Parkkari J, Koskinen S, et al. Fall-induced injuries and deaths among older adults. *JAMA* 1999;281:1895–1899.
37. Gill TM, Williams CS, Robison JT, et al. A population-based study of environmental hazards in the homes of older persons. *Am J Public Health* 1999;89:553–556.
38. Bisdorff AR, Bronstein AM, Wolsley C, et al. EMG responses to free fall in the elderly subjects and akinetic rigid patients. *J Neurol Neurosurg Psychiatry* 1999;66:447–455.
39. Nutt J. Gait and balance disorders: a syndrome approach. In: Jankovic J, Tolosa E, eds. *Parkinson's disease and movement disorders,* 3rd ed. Baltimore: Williams & Wilkins, 1998:687–700.
40. Dietz V, Zijlstra W, Prokop T, et al. Leg muscle activation during gait in Parkinson's disease: adaptation and interlimb coordination. *Electroenceph Clin Neurophysiol* 1996;97:408–415.
41. Hausdorff JM, Cudkowicz ME, Firtion R, et al. Gait variability and basal ganglia disorders: stride-to-stride variations of gait cycle timing in Parkinson's disease and Huntington's disease. *Mov Disord* 1998;13:428–437.
42. Hausdorff JM, Zemany L, Peng C, et al. Maturation of gait dynamics: stride-to-stride variability and its temporal organization in children. *J Appl Physiol* 1999;86:1040–1047.
43. Melvill-Jones G, Watt DGD. Observations on the control of stepping and hopping movements in man. *J Physiol* 1971;219:709–727.
44. Nasher LM. Fixed patterns of rapid postural responses among leg muscles during stance. *Exp Brain Res* 1977; 30:13–24.
45. Marsden CD, Merton PM, Morton HB. Human postural responses. *Brain* 1981;104:513–534.
46. Elble RJ, Moody C, Leffer K, et al. The initiation of normal walking. *Mov Disord* 1994;9:139–146.
47. Dietz V. Neurophysiology of gait disorders: present and future applications. *Electroencephalogr Clin Neurophysiol* 1997;103:333–355.
48. Fahn S, Elton RI, Members of the UPDRS Development Committee. Unified Parkinson's Disease Rating Scale. In: Fahn S, Marsden CD, Calne DB, eds. *Recent developments in Parkinson's disease,* vol 2. Florham Park, NJ: Macmillan Health Care Information, 1987:153–164.
49. O'Sullivan JD, Said CM, Dillon LC, et al. Gait analysis in patients with Parkinson's disease and motor fluctuations: influence of levodopa and comparison with other measures of motor function. *Mov Disord* 1998;13:900–906.
50. Duncan PW, Studenski S, Chandler J, et al. Functional reach: Predictive validity in a sample of elderly male veterans. *J Gerontol Med Sci* 1992;47:M93–98.
51. Weiner DK, Bongiorni DR, Studenski SA, et al. Does functional reach improve with rehabilitation? *Arch Phys Med Rehabil* 1993;74:796–800.
52. Tinetti ME. Performance-oriented assessment of mobility problems in elderly patients. *J Am Geriatr Soc* 1986;34:119–126.
53. Singh A, Crockard HA. Quantitative assessment of cervical spondylotic myelopathy by a simple walking test. *Lancet* 1999;354:370–373.
54. Berg K, Maki B, Williams JI, et al. A comparison of clinical and laboratory measures of postural balance in an elderly population. *Arch Phys Med Rehabil* 1992;73: 1073–1083.
55. Critchley M. Arteriosclerotic parkinsonism. *Brain* 1929;52:23–83.
56. FitzGerald PM, Jankovic J. Lower body parkinsonism: evidence for vascular etiology. *Mov Disord* 1989;4:249–260.
57. Elble RJ, Cousins R, Leffler K, et al. Gait initiation by patients with lower-half parkinsonism. *Brain* 1996; 119:1705–1716.
58. Zijlmans JCM, Poels PJE, Duysens J, et al. Quantitative gait analysis in patients with vascular parkinsonism. *Mov Disord* 1996;11:501–508.

59. Winikates J, Jankovic J. Clinical correlates of vascular parkinsonism. *Arch Neurol* 1999;56:98–102.
60. Meyer JS, Barron D. Apraxia of gait: a clinicopathological study. *Brain* 1960;83:261–284.
61. Geschwind N. The apraxias: neural mechanisms of disorders of learned movement. *Am Sci* 1975;63:188–195.
62. Nadeau SE, Roeltgen DP, Sevush S, et al. Apraxia due to a pathologically documented thalamic infarction. *Neurology* 1994;44:2133–2137.
63. Freund H-J. The apraxias. In: Kennard C, ed. *Recent advances in clinical neurology,* vol. 8. London: Churchill Livingstone, 1995:29–49.
64. Poizner H, Clark MA, Merians AS, et al. Joint coordination deficits in limb apraxia. *Brain* 1995;118:227–242.
65. Heilman KM, Maher LM, Greenwald ML, et al. Conceptual apraxia from lateralized lesions. *Neurology* 1997;49:457–464.
66. Kremer M. Sitting, standing and walking. *Br Med J* 1958;2:63–68.
67. Dick JPR, Snowden J, Northen B, et al. Slowly progressive apraxia. *Behav Neurol* 1989;2:101–114.
68. Thajeb P. Gait disorders of multi-infarct dementia. CT and clinical correlation. *Acta Neurol Scand* 1993;87:239–242.
69. Thompson PD, Marsden CD. Gait disorder of subcortical arteriosclerotic encephalopathy: Biswanger's disease. *Mov Disord* 1987;2:1–8.
70. Ebersbach G, Sojer M, Valldeoriola F, et al. Comparative analysis of gait in Parkinson's disease, cerebellar ataxia and subcortical arteriosclerotic encephalopathy. *Brain* 1999;122:1349–1355.
71. Adams RD, Fisher CM, Hakim S, et al. Symptomatic occult hydrocephalus with "normal" cerebrospinal fluid pressure: a treatable syndrome. *N Engl J Med* 1965;273:117–126.
72. Fisher CM. Hydrocephalus as a cause of disturbances of gait in the elderly. *Neurology* 1982;32:1358–1363.
73. Rossor MN, Tyrrell PJ, Warrington EK, et al. Progressive frontal gait disturbance with atypical Alzheimer's disease and corticobasal degeneration. *J Neurol Neurosurg Psychiatry* 1999;67:345–352.
74. O'Keeffe ST, Kazeem H, Philpott RM, et al. Gait disturbance in Alzheimer's disease: a clinical study. *Age Aging* 1996;25:313–316.
75. Atchison PR, Thompson PD, Frackowiak SJ, et al. The syndrome of gait ignition failure: a report of six cases. *Mov Disord* 1993;8:285–292.
76. Vidaihet M, Atchison PR, Stocchi F, et al. The Bereitschafts potential preceding stepping in patients with isolated gait ignition failure. *Mov Disord* 1995;10: 18–21.
77. Achiron A, Ziv I, Goren M, et al. Primary progressive freezing gait. *Mov Disord* 1993;8:293–297.
78. Giladi N, McMahon D, Przedborski S, et al. Motor blocks in Parkinson's disease. *Neurology* 1992;42:333–339.
79. Riley DE, Fogt N, Leigh RJ. The syndrome of "pure akinesia" and its relationship to progressive supranuclear palsy. *Neurology* 1994;44:1025–1029.
80. Mestre D, Blin O, Serratrice G. Contrast sensitivity is increased in a case of nonparkinsonian freezing gait. *Neurology* 1992;42:189–194.
81. Stern GM, Lander CM, Lees AJ. Akinetic freezing and trick movements in Parkinson's disease. *J Neural Transm* 1980;16:137–141.
82. Dietz MA, Goetz CG, Stebbins GT. Evaluation of a modified inverted walking stick as treatment for parkinsonian freezing episodes. *Mov Disord* 1990;5:243–247.
83. Thaut MH, McIntosh GC, Rice RR, et al. Rhythmic auditory stimulation in gait training for Parkinson's disease patients. *Mov Disord* 1996;11:193–200.
84. Dunne JW, Hankey GJ, Edis RH. Parkinsonism: upturned walking stick as an aid to locomotion. *Arch Phys Med Rehabil* 1987;68:380–381.
85. McIntosh GC, Brown SH, Rice RR, et al. Rhythmic auditory-motor facilitation of gait patterns in patients with Parkinson's disease. *J Neurol Neurosurg Psychiatry* 1997;62:22–26.
86. Hanakawa T, Fukuyama H, Katsumi Y, et al. Enhanced lateral premotor activity during paradoxical gait in Parkinson's disease. *Ann Neurol* 1999;45:329–336.
87. Ziv I, Avraham M, Dabby R, et al. Early-occurrence of manual motor blocks in Parkinson's disease: a quantitative assessment. *Acta Neurol Scand* 1999;99:106–111.
88. Hashimoto R, Tanaka Y. Contribution of the supplementary motor area and anterior cingulate gyrus to pathological grasping phenomenon. *Eur Neurol* 1998; 40:151–158.
89. Yanagisawa N, Ueno E, Takami M. Frozen gait of Parkinson's disease and vascular parkinsonism: a study with floor reaction forces and EMG. In: Shimamura M, Grillner S, Edgerton VR, eds. *Neurobiological basis of human locomotion.* Tokoyo: Japan Scientific Societies Press, 1991:291–304.
90. Whitman GT, DiPatre PL, Lopez IA, et al. Neuropathology in older people with disequilibrium of unknown cause. *Neurology* 1999;53:375–382.
91. Estanol BV. Gait apraxia in communicating hydrocephalus. *J Neurol Neurosurg Psychiatry* 1981;44:305–308.
92. Ambani LM, Van Woert MH. Start hesitation: a side effect of long-term levodopa therapy. *N Engl J Med* 1973;288:1113–1115.
93. Ahlskog JE, Muenter MD, Bailey PA, et al. Dopamine agonist treatment of fluctuating parkinsonism: D-2 (controlled-release MK-458) vs combined d-1 and d-2 (pergolide). *Arch Neurol* 1992;49:560–568.
94. Robert-Warrior D, Overby A, Jankovic J, et al. Postural control and functional changes in patients with Parkinson's disease after posteroventral pallidotomy. *Brain* 2000;123:2141–2149.
95. Bejjani B, Damier P, Arnulf I, et al. Pallidal stimulation for Parkinson's disease: two targets? *Neurology* 1997;49:1564–1569.
96. Horak FB, Nutt JG, Nashner LM. Postural inflexibility in parkinsonian subjects. *J Neurol Sci* 1992;111:46–52.
97. Morris ME, Iansek R, Matyas TA, Summers JJ. Ability to modulate walking cadence remains intact in Parkinson's disease. *J Neurol Neurosurg Psychiatry* 1994;57:1532–1534.
98. Morris ME, Iansek R, Matyas TA, et al. Stride length regulation in Parkinson's disease: normalization strategies and underlying mechanisms. *Brain* 1996;119: 551–568.
99. Litvan I, Goetz C, Jankovic J, et al. What is the accuracy of the clinical diagnosis of multiple system atrophy? A clinicopathological study. *Arch Neurol* 1997;54:937–944.

100. Lundin-Olsson L, Nyberg L, Gustafson Y. "Stops walking when talking" as a predictor of falls in elderly people. *Lancet* 1997;34:617.
101. Ebersbach G, Heijmenberg M, Kindermann L, et al. Interference of rhythmic constraint on gait in healthy subjects and patients with early Parkinson's disease: evidence for impaired locomotor pattern generation in early Parkinson's disease. *Mov Disord* 1999;14:619–625.
102. Ferrandez A-M, Blin O. A comparison between the effect of intentional modulations and the actions of L-dopa on gait in Parkinson's disease. *Behav Brain Res* 1991;45:177–183.
103. Morris M, Iansek R, Mayas T, et al. Abnormalities in the stride length–cadence relation in parkinsonian gait. *Mov Disord* 1998;13:61–69.
104. Dietz V, Colombo G. Influence of body load on the gait pattern in Parkinson's disease. *Mov Disord* 1998;13:255–261.
105. Jankovic J, Friedman DI, Pirozzolo FJ, et al. Progressive supranuclear palsy: motor, neurobehavioral, and neuro-ophthalmic findings. *Adv Neurol* 1990;53:293–304.
106. Litvan I. Progressive supranuclear palsy revisited. *Acta Neurol Scand* 1998;98:73–84.
107. Bussel B, Roby-Brami A, Azouvi P, et al. Myoclonus in a patient with spinal cord transection: possible involvement of spinal stepping generator. *Brain* 1988;111:1235–1245.
108. Jankovic J, Fahn S. Dystonic disorders. In: Jankovic J, Tolosa E, eds. *Parkinson's disease and movement disorders,* 3rd ed. Baltimore: Williams & Wilkins, 1998: 513–551.
109. Koller WC, Trimble J. The gait abnormality of Huntington's disease. *Neurology* 1985;35:1450–1454.
110. Thaut MH, Miltner R, Lange HW, et al. Velocity modulation and rhythmic synchronization of gait in Huntington's disease. *Mov Disord* 1999;14:808–819.
111. Singer C, Sanchez-Ramos J, Weiner WJ. Gait abnormality in essential tremor. *Mov Disord* 1994;9:193–196.
112. Henderson E, Overby A, Jankovic J. Postural control in essential tremor. *Neurology* 1996;46:A273.
113. FitzGerald PM, Jankovic J. Orthostatic tremor: an association with essential tremor. *Mov Disord* 1991; 6:60–64.
114. Sander HW, Masdeu J, Tavoulareas G, et al. Orthostatic tremor: an electrophysiological analysis. *Mov Disord* 1998;13:735–748.
115. Wills AJ, Thompson PD, Findley LJ, et al. A positron emission tomography study of primary orthostatic tremor. *Neurology* 1996;46:747–752.
116. Werhahn KJ, Brown P, Thompson PD, et al. The clinical features and prognosis of chronic posthypoxic myoclonus. *Mov Disord* 1997;12:216–220.
117. Brown P, Rothwell JC, Thompson PD, et al. Propriospinal myoclonus: evidence for spinal "pattern" generators in humans. *Mov Disord* 1994;9:571–576.
118. Masdeu JC, Gorelick PB. Thalamic astasia: inability to stand after unilateral thalamic lesions. *Ann Neurol* 1988;23:596–603.
119. Labadie EL, Awerbuch GI, Hamilton RH, et al. Falling and postural deficits due to acute unilateral basal ganglia lesions. *Arch Neurol* 1989;45:492–496.
120. Solomon DH, Barohn RJ, Bazan C, et al. The thalamic ataxia syndrome. *Neurology* 1994;44:810–814.
121. Sudarsky L, Ronthal M. Gait disorders among elderly patients: a survey study of 50 patients. *Arch Neurol* 1983;40:740–743.
122. Friedman PJ. Gait recovery after hemiplegic stroke. *Int Disabil Stud* 1990;12:119–222.
123. Ada L, Vattanasilp W, O'Dwyer J, et al. Does spasticity contribute to walking dysfunction after stroke. *J Neurol Neurosurg Psychiatry* 1998;64:628–635.
124. Neville BG, Boyd SG. Selective epileptic gait disorder. *J Neurol Neurosurg Psychiatry* 1995;58:371–373.
125. Subramony SH. Degenerative ataxias. *Curr Op Neurol* 1994;7:316–322.
126. Palliyath S, Hallett M, Thomas SL, et al. Gait in patients with cerebellar ataxia. *Mov Disord* 1998;13:958–964.
127. Masdeu JC, Alampur U, Cavaliere R, et al. Astasia and gait failure with damage of the pontomesencephalic locomotor region. *Ann Neurol* 1994;35:619–621.
128. Felice KJ, Keilson GR, Schwartz WJ. 'Rubral' gait ataxia. *Neurology* 1990;40:1004–1005.
129. Marks I. Space "phobia," a pseudo-agoraphobic syndrome. *J Neurol Neurosurg Psychiatry* 1981;44:387–391.
130. Koller WC, Glatt SL, Fox JH. Senile gait. A distinct neurologic entity. *Clin Geriatr Med* 1985;1:661–669.
131. Murphy J, Isaacs B. The post-fall syndrome: a study of 36 elderly patients. *Gerontology* 1982;82:265–270.
132. Sattin RW. Falls among older persons: a public health perspective. *Ann Rev Public Health* 1992;85:489–508.
133. Baloh RW. Dizziness in older people. *J Am Geriatr Soc* 1992;40:713–721.
134. Brandt T, Strupp M, Benson J. You are better off running than walking with acute vestibulopathy. *Lancet* 1999;354:746.
135. Messier SP. Osteoarthritis of the knee and associated factors of age and obesity: effects on gait. *Med Sci Sports Exerc* 1994;26:1446–1452.
136. Hayes MW, Graham S, Heldorf P, et al. A video review of the diagnosis of psychogenic gait: appendix and commentary. *Mov Disord* 1999;14:914–921.
137. Keane JR. Hysterical gait disorders, 60 cases. *Neurology* 1989;39:586–589.
138. Lempert T, Brandt T, Dieterich M, et al. How to identify psychogenic disorders of stance and gait. *J Neurol* 1991;238:140–146.
139. Williams DT, Ford B, Fahn S. Phenomenology and psychopathology related to psychogenic movement disorders. *Adv Neurol* 1995;65:231–257.

Gait Disorders. Advances in Neurology, Vol. 87,
edited by E. Růžička, M. Hallett, and J. Jankovic.
Lippincott Williams & Wilkins, Philadelphia © 2001.

13

Classification of Gait and Balance Disorders

John G. Nutt

Department of Neurology, Oregon Health Sciences University, Portland, Oregon 97201

Classification is "the systematic arrangement of items into groups or categories according to a definite plan expressive of natural relationships" *(Webster's Third International Dictionary).* Classifications are important in medicine. They represent our understanding of pathophysiological mechanisms and the relationships among different diseases and syndromes. Classifications aid in the diagnostic evaluation of patients. Currently, the classifications for gait and balance disorders are rudimentary and problematic for several reasons.

First, the term *gait,* defined by Webster as the "manner of walking" or "sequence of foot movements," does not recognize the importance of balance or equilibrium to walking. The clinical arena also does not explicitly acknowledge balance as a key and perhaps critical element in safe ambulation. The name of this meeting, International Symposium on Gait Disorders, is yet another example of the neglect of balance. Many so-called gait disorders are in reality balance disorders, not disorders in the sequence of foot movements. For example, Bruns' *frontal ataxia* and van Bogart and Martins' *apraxia of gait* are descriptions of patients who could not even stand independently (1,2). Although gait or locomotion can sometimes be separated from balance or postural equilibrium, locomotion and balance are more often inextricably intertwined; consequently, classifications need to include disorders of gait and balance (3).

Second, existing gait classifications in neurology texts are lists of abnormal gaits that are named by anatomic substrates (e.g., frontal gaits), clinical features (e.g., festinating gait), and diseases or syndromes (e.g., gait of normal pressure hydrocephalus). Table 13.1 lists the gaits described in a widely used neurology text, the fifth edition of Adams and Victor (4). It is typical of most texts that even cover the topic of gait disorders separately rather than considering abnormal gaits as simply physical signs of various neurological diseases. Lists of gait abnormalities are not classifications; they do not recognize relations among various gait disorders.

Third, many terms used in gait classifications are not explicitly defined. Common problematic terms are gait apraxia and senile gait. Nor are synonyms acknowledged or terminology reconciled. For example, to what extent are *freezing, festination, slipping clutch, parkinsonian gait, marché a petits pas, lower body parkinsonism,* and *gait apraxia* identical, related, or dissimilar gait patterns?

Finally, many gait and balance abnormalities encountered in the clinic do not fit into current descriptive classifications.

CLASSIFICATION BY GAIT AND BALANCE SYNDROMES

There can be more than one method to classify clinical entities that would serve different purposes. I will propose two: a syndrome classification of patterns of gait and balance dysfunction and a pathophysiological or systems classification.

The syndrome classification is based on the assumption that there are gait and balance features

TABLE 13.1. *Typical gait classificatons*

Anatomical
Cerebellar
Frontal lobe
Signs/Syndromes
Sensory ataxia
Hemiplegic and paraplegic
Festinating
Choreoathetotic and dystonic
Steppage
Waddling
Drunken or staggering
Toppling
Disorders/Diagnoses
Hysterical gait
Normal pressure hydrocephalus
Senile
Mentally retarded

Adapted from Adams RD, Victor M. *Principles of Neurology*, Fifth edition. New York: McGraw–Hill, 1993.

that allow a meaningful division of abnormalities of ambulation that assist the clinician in evaluating patients. It is complicated by the fact that part of what is observed may not be a direct consequence of pathology but instead be compensatory changes in ambulation to compensate for loss of balance, strength, or confidence. The syndrome classification is based on the history and observation of gait and postural responses. History is particularly important for patients with falls, because they are generally not directly observed. Gait and balance features are observed with the patient rising from sitting, walking, turning, and responding to the "pull test." These features describe gait and balance syndromes. Each syndrome has a differential. Other clinical features, imaging, and laboratory testing help differentiate between causes of a syndrome but are not used to define the syndrome. The proposed syndrome classification has three categories: fall, disequilibrium, and gait syndromes.

Fall syndromes are based on history (Table 13.2). Collapsing falls are caused by loss of muscle tone. "Collapsing in a heap" is a common description. Akinetic seizures, negative myoclonus, syncope, and orthostatic hypotension cause collapsing falls. Toppling falls are falls where muscle tone is present so that the patient "topples like a falling tree." They may occur when the subject is just standing, as seen in progressive supranuclear palsy (PSP) or thalamic astasia or when the subject is changing position, as is characteristic of parkinsonism. Tripping falls occur because the feet do not clear the support surface adequately. The falls are generally forward. Foot drop, spasticity, and parkinsonism are common causes of tripping falls. Freezing falls occur when the feet do not move quickly enough to stay under the center of balance. The patient typically falls forward onto the knees and outstretched arms. Finally, nonpatterned falls, falls that do not seem to fit a consistent pattern, may represent failure of attention and insight producing carelessness as can occur in dementia.

TABLE 13.2. *Fall syndromes*

1. Collapsing
a. akinetic seizures
b. syncope
c. orthostatic hypotension
2. Toppling
a. while standing
b. while changing position/posture
3. Tripping
4. Freezing
5. Non-patterned

Disequilibrium syndromes are identified by inspection of arising, standing, response to perturbation, and turning (Table 13.3). Dysmetric, often hypermetric, postural responses are characteristic of cerebellar disorders, the prototype for dysmetric disequilibrium. The postural responses are appropriately organized but improperly scaled (5).

Bradykinetic postural responses are frequent in parkinsonism. Despite responses that clinically appear delayed, weak, or even absent, the latency of postural responses is not prolonged but the development of force is slow; therefore, the execution is slow (6,7).

Sensory deprivation or disorganization is characteristic of vestibular disorders and sometimes

TABLE 13.3. *Disequilibrium syndromes*

1. Dysmetric
2. Bradykinetic
3. Sensory deprivation or disorganization
4. Apraxic

TABLE 13.4. *Gait features on which to base syndromes*

1. Proximal or distal weakness
2. Base (standing and walking)
3. Stride length
4. Cadence (regularity of stride and base while walking)
5. Deviation from direction of travel
6. Rigidity/fluidity
7. Initiation and maintenance of walking
8. Adaptability

TABLE 13.5. *Gait syndromes features*

1. Dysmetric: dysmetric leg movements and irregular progression
2. Stiff/rigid: loss of fluidity, stiffness of legs and trunk
3. Weakness: waddling and foot drop
4. Veering: deviation of gait or falls to one side
5. Freezing: start and turn hesitation
6. Marche à petits pas: very short steps with widened base
7. Cautious: slowing, short steps and enbloc turns—is compensation for imbalance
8. Psychogenic: bizarre, inconsistent, destractible

peripheral neuropathies. Disequilibrium occurs because there is inadequate sensory information to trigger and modify postural responses (7–9). Conceivably, PSP or thalamic lesions may disrupt sensory processing and thereby affect balance.

Apraxic disequilibrium is the disorganization of arising and standing because the organization of limb and truncal movements is inappropriate. Examples are patients who try to arise from sitting without bringing the feet under the chair or who push backward while standing. These types of disequilibrium disorders are common with frontal lobe dysfunction and perhaps advanced parkinsonism (10).

Gait syndromes are based on abnormalities that are apparent while the patient is walking (Table 13.4). Proximal or distal weakness may be deduced by gait pattern. The distance between the feet (base) may be widened or, less commonly, narrowed while standing or walking. Stride length is frequently shortened with any gait disorder. The cadence or regularity of steps, both length and base, may vary during walking. Deviation or veering from intended direction of travel may be observed. Stiffness or rigidity of the legs or trunk may be apparent by the loss of the normal fluidity of gait. Difficulty initiating or maintaining gait (freezing) is one of the most obvious abnormalities of gait. Adaptability is a more nebulous feature. It may be estimated by the patient's ability to modify walking to avoid obstacles, perform precision walking, or perhaps just turning about.

Seven gait syndromes are proposed (Table 13.5; Table 13.6). Dysmetric leg movements and irregular progression (locomotion) characterize dysmetric gaits. Typically, these abnormalities are associated with a widened base and somewhat shorter stride. Cadence is obviously abnormal. Examples are cerebellar ataxia, sensory ataxia, and chorea.

Stiff or rigid gaits are gaits in which the usual fluidity of walking is lost. Rotation of trunk is reduced or absent. The range of motion at the knees and hips may be reduced. Base may be abnormally narrow or wide; stride is shortened. Examples are spasticity, parkinsonism, dystonia, and musculoskeletal diseases. The stiffness may be unilateral, as in spastic hemiparesis or hemidystonia

Gaits disturbed by proximal or distal weakness are well recognized. Proximal weakness prevents fixation of the pelvis during single support portions of gait. Myopathies and dystrophies that typically affect proximal muscles more than distal produce waddling gaits. Distal weakness generally affects dorsiflexors of the ankle, requiring the leg to be lifted more for the toe to clear the ground. Peripheral neuropathies are the common cause of this problem.

Veering gaits are those in which the patient tends to lean, fall, or deviate in one direction

TABLE 13.6. *Gait syndromes disease examples*

1. Dysmetric (cerebellar ataxia, chorea, sensory ataxia)
2. Stiff/rigid (spasticity, parkinsonism, dystonia, musculoskeletal)
3. Weakness (myopathy, peripheral neuropathy)
4. Veering (vestibular disorders, thalamic astasia)
5. Freezing (multiinfarct, parkinsonism)
6. Marche à petits pas (multiinfarct)
7. Cautious (nonspecific, multifactorial)
8. Psychogenic

while walking. Vestibular disorders are the common cause but other brainstem and thalamic lesions (thalamic astasia) may cause the same problems without obvious interruption of central vestibular pathways.

Freezing gaits are those characterized by difficulty initiating (start hesitation and "slipping clutch" phenomena) and maintaining locomotion (turn hesitation). Patients exhibiting freezing generally will also have a stiff or rigid gait, but not necessarily so. Freezing is associated with parkinsonism and frontal lobe and diffuse deep white matter lesions. It may also be idiopathic with no associated neurologic or imaging abnormalities.

Cautious gait is marked by mild to moderate slowing, shortening of stride, and en bloc turns with only mild widening of base and no freezing. It is termed cautious because it is the gait pattern assumed by a normal person when concerned about balance, such as when walking on a slippery surface. Cautious gait is an appropriate response to perceived threats to postural balance. As such, cautious gait is nonspecific and may be associated with a variety of problems that impact a person's ability to walk safely. Cautious gait may also be of multifactorial etiology.

A final category is psychogenic gait disorders. Although balance may be disturbed in patients with psychogenic origin for the problem, most can ambulate as well and therefore are considered gait disorders. A variety of bizarre patterns that fit none of the preceding descriptions are possible. Distractibility, inconsistencies and other nonphysiological signs are common tipoffs to the diagnosis. An "overcautious" pattern sometimes termed space phobia or fear of falling occurs in some older women, generally in response to a fall or some other event arousing their anxiety about falling. Gait is often wide-based, staggering, and the person must hold on to another person, furniture, or the wall.

The proposed gait syndromes are not exclusive; patients may show elements of more than one syndrome. Also, gait patterns are not fixed but may change or progress across time in conjunction with the evolution of the neurologic problems. Many gait syndromes will begin as a cautious gait and evolve into other syndromes.

It should be emphasized that this is a proposed syndrome classification. It needs to be tested in the clinic to determine if it adequately covers the balance and gait patterns observed and if the distinctions among the various syndromes are clinically obvious and useful.

CLASSIFICATION BY NEURAL SYSTEMS

A classification of gait disorders by the systems underlying gait and balance is necessarily tentative because much of the integration of sensory and context information and selection and modification of motor strategies to produce an appropriate or optimal postural and locomotor response is not understood at the current time. A hierarchical system, modeled after Hughlings Jackson's approach, considers three levels of systems or neural function, the lower, middle, and higher levels (Table 13.7).

The lower level has three components. The first component consists of the intrinsic locomotor synergies in the spinal gray matter (central pattern generators that produce the patterned limb movements of locomotion) and the intrinsic postural responses in brainstem. These locomotor and postural responses are the building blocks of successful balance and locomotion. The spinal locomotor synergies can be

TABLE 13.7. *Systems classification*

I. Lower level
   1. Spinal locomotor and brainstem postural synergies
   2. Primary afferent input (vestibular, visual, proprioception)
   3. Force production (muscle and nerve—strength)

II. Middle level
   4. Perception/orientation (organization of primary sensation into spatial maps of body in gravitational field)
   5. Force scaling (modulation of force by basal ganglia, cerebellum and corticospinal system for optimization of motor patterns)

III. Higher level
   6. Synergy selection (spinal cord for locomotor and brainstem for balance synergies) and adaptation to immediate circumstances (unconscious functions)
   7. Cognitive [attention, insight for adaptation to person's goals (conscious functions)]

demonstrated in lumbar spinal cord that is entirely separated from the remainder of the central nervous system (CNS) by a mid-thoracic spinal transection in cats and by spinal cord injuries in humans (11–13). Brainstem postural responses are evident in the cat with decerebrate posture induced by transection of the upper brainstem (3). Focal stimulation in the pons can induce postural adjustments in the intact cat (3). In humans, brain damage from a variety of causes can apparently release brainstem postural responses such as decerebrate or decorticate posturing and tonic neck responses.

The second component of the lowest level is the primary sensory modalities with which the person locates the self in the gravitational field and the relation of the limbs and trunk to each other. The information required for spatial orientation largely comes from the visual, vestibular, and proprioceptive sensory systems. Under most conditions, the information is redundant so that accurate spatial sense is possible with input from just one or two of the sensory systems. Conflicting information from sensory systems or under conditions when insufficient information is available for orientation of the body in space leads to impaired or improper balance and locomotor strategies. The disequilibrium of acute and chronic vestibular dysfunction and the sensory ataxia related to proprioceptive dysfunction are examples of gait and balance disorders associated with disordered sensory input.

The third component of the lowest system is the musculoskeletal system and peripheral motor nerves connecting it to the CNS. These organs are responsible of generating forces to preserve balance and move in space. Damage or disease affecting these structures, the effectors of postural and locomotor strategies, obviously alter the execution of the strategies. Skeletal deformities, arthritis, muscle disease, and peripheral motor neuropathies affect gait and postural responses. For the neurologist, the waddling gait of muscular dystrophies and polymyositis and the steppage gait of peripheral neuropathies such as Charcot Marie Tooth disease are prime examples of this type of dysfunction.

At the middle level of this classification, there are two components. The first is the integration of sensory information into spatial maps. This function probably takes place in many areas of the brain. Spatial maps concerned with motor function have been identified in putamen and premotor cortex. Maps concerned with visual function exist in frontal eye fields and the superior colliculus. Surprisingly, the parietal lobes appear to be more important in creating the spatial maps, which may actually reside elsewhere in the brain (14). The idea of disorders that affect spatial orientation is currently a theoretical construct; no diseases that affect this function have been definitively identified. Candidates are syndromes such as PSP, thalamic and putaminal astasia, and some parietal lesions. It is difficult to know if these syndromes are attributable to lack of synthesizing information into maps (an agnosia for location in space?), sensory and motor neglect, or other types of dysfunction because patients with these clinical syndromes have not been studied carefully.

The second component of the middle level is the modulation of force for optimal locomotor and postural responses. The central motor system has this role. Basal ganglia, cerebellum, and corticospinal tracts sharpen locomotor and postural responses but do not create the synergies. The clinical manifestations of dysfunction at this level are parkinsonism (bradykinetic postural and locomotor synergies), chorea/dystonia (synergies with superimposed involuntary movements), ataxia (dysmetric synergies), and spasticity (slowed, imprecise synergies). These clinical syndromes are a distortion, not a loss, of appropriate postural and locomotor synergies caused by the imprecise execution of appropriate synergies.

At the highest level of the classification, two components are hypothesized. The first largely operates at an unconscious level. It is responsible for accessing the appropriate brainstem and spinal synergies for balance and walking. The selection of synergies is based on the information about the body, its location in space and the goals of the individual. Sensitivity to context is an important component of this function. For example, balance and locomotor synergies should be different walking on the edge of a cliff, walking on a slick surface, and walking in a wide-open level space. Another example is the unconscious awareness of other objects in the immediate vicinity of the person, such as walls, that may offer postural support if equilibrium is perturbed. Clinical examples of problems at this level may include freezing where there appears to be loss of access to locomotor synergies and impaired anticipatory postural responses or inappropriate and bizarre postural responses associated with frontal lobe lesions (10,15–17).

A second component of the highest system operates more at a conscious level to modify locomotor synergies. It is responsible for precision stepping such as on stepping-stones or performing unfamiliar dance steps. The corticospinal tract mediates some of these effects (18). If there are lower and middle level postural and locomotor difficulties, this higher level compensates as best it can to allow ambulation within the constraints imposed by the lower level dysfunction. Under these circumstances, walking and balance are elevated from operation at the largely unconscious level to operation at a conscious level. Attention and insight then become important because of their role in voluntary motor actions. Falls occur in older patients who do not direct sufficient attention to walking and balance or who do not have the insight to avoid posturally challenging situations. This may be the reason that dementia and centrally active drug use in the elderly emerge in epidemiological studies as predisposing factors to falls. Psychogenic gait disorders would also be seen as representative of dysfunction at this level.

CONCLUSIONS

This chapter has attempted to point out the problems with current classifications of gait disorders and propose two new classifications that would serve different purposes. The syndrome classification, intended to help the clinician consider the diagnostic possibilities for falls, abnormal postural responses, and abnormal gait patterns, is untested. The more systems-oriented balance and gait disorders classification is intended to provide a logical hierarchy and interrelations of gait disorders. It is hypothetical because higher-level disorders have received little attention in clinic or laboratory investigations and the proposed higher level functions of the classification are unproved. Both clinicians and laboratory investigators are more comfortable dealing with lower level dysfunction, which is complicated enough because of the redundancy in the locomotor and postural systems.

What is needed to advance our understanding of gait and balance disorders? First, and most pressing, an agreement on terminology for the clinical phenomena needs to be developed. Currently the field is bedeviled by the various terms that are used. One possibility is for a group of experts to meet and bring video examples of the various disordered gait and balance patterns that they recognize and to work out a standard terminology accompanied by video examples of the patterns.

Second, the accuracy and utility of the syndrome scheme needs testing in the clinic. Does it divide balance and gait disorder patterns into a scheme that is diagnostically helpful?

Finally, clinicians and clinical investigators need to examine patients with enigmatic postural and locomotor dysfunction, particularly those associated with cortical lesions, using physiological and neuroimaging techniques. Animal studies need to explore the contribution from higher structures to execution of postural and locomotor responses.

Safe, efficient ambulation is a wonderful attribute of health. Understanding the many ways in which it may be disturbed by neurological disease should lead to better methods to treat or cope with dysfunction.

REFERENCES

1. Bruns L. *Uber storugen des gleichgewichtes bei stirnhirntumoren. Dtsch Med Wochensch* 1892;18:138–140.
2. van Bogart L, Martin P. *Sur deux signes du syndrome de desequilibration frontale: l'apraxie de la marché et l'antonie statique. Encephale* 1929;24:11–18.
3. Mori S. Integration of posture and locomotion in acute decerebrate cats and in awake freely moving cats. *Prog Neurobiol* 1987;28:161–195.
4. Adams RD, Victor M. *Principles of Neurology*, Fifth edition. New York: McGraw–Hill, 1993.
5. Horak FC, Diener HC. Cerebellar control of postural scaling and central set in stance. *J Neurophysiol* 1994;72:479–493.

6. Horak FB, Nutt JG, Nashner LM. Postural inflexibility in parkinsonian subjects. *J Neurol Sci* 1992;111: 46–58.
7. Horak FB, Nashner LM, Diener HC. Postural strategies associated with somatosensory and vestibular loss. *Exp Brain Res* 1990;82:167–177.
8. Inglis JT, Horak FB, Shupert CL, et al. The importance of somatosensory information in triggering and scaling automatic postural responses in humans. *Exp Brain Res* 1994;101:159–164.
9. Horak FB, Shupert CL, Dietz V, et al. Vestibular and somatosensory contributions to responses to head and body displacements. *Exp Brain Res* 1994;100:93–106.
10. Nutt JG, Marsden CD, Thompson PD. Human walking and higher level gait disorders, particularly in the elderly. *Neurology* 1993;43:268–279.
11. Grillner S, Wallen P. Central pattern generators for locomotion with special reference to vertebrates. *Annu Rev Neurosci* 1985;8:233–261.
12. Calancie B, Needham-Shropshire B, Jacobs P, et al. Involuntary stepping after chronic spinal cord injury: evidence for a central rhythm generator for locomotion in man. *Brain* 1994;117:1143–1159.
13. Dietz V, Colombo G, Jensen L. Locomotor activity in spinal man. *Lancet* 1994;344:1260–1263.
14. Gross CG, Graziano MSA. Multiple representations of space in the brain. *Neuroscientist* 1995;1:43–50.
15. Gurfinkel VS, El'ner AM. Contribution of the frontal lobe secondary motor area to organization of postural components in human voluntary movement. *Neirofiziologiya* 1988;20:7–15.
16. Massion J. Movement, posture, and equilibrium: interaction and coordination. *Prog Neurobiol* 1992;38:35–56.
17. Palmer E, Downes L, Ashby P. Associated postural adjustments are impaired by a lesion of the cortex. *Neurology* 1996;46:471–475.
18. Armstrong DM. Supraspinal control of locomotion. *J Physiol* 1988;405:1–37.

Gait Disorders. Advances in Neurology, Vol. 87,
edited by E. Růžička, M. Hallett, and J. Jankovic.
Lippincott Williams & Wilkins, Philadelphia © 2001.

14

Gait Disorder in Spasticity and Parkinson's Disease

Volker Dietz

Department of Paraplegiology, University of Zurich; and Swiss Paraplegic Centre, University Hospital Balgrist, CH-8008 Zurich, Switzerland

Movement disorders are prominent features of an impaired function of the motor system and are frequently best reflected during gait. The movement disorder usually represents the first symptom of a lesion within the central motor system in a patient. The neurological examination notes changes in reflex excitability and muscle tone and leads to the appropriate diagnosis underlying the gait disorder. The physical signs obtained during the clinical examination, however, can give little information about the pathophysiology underlying the movement disorder: Stretch reflex excitability and muscle tone are basically different in the *passive* (clinical examination) compared to the *active* motor condition (movement). In addition, several reflex systems are involved in the execution and control of a movement such as gait. Therefore, we have to know about the function of reflexes and supraspinal motor centers involved in the respective motor task for the adequate treatment of a movement disorder. A movement such as locomotion is determined by the strength of electromyographic (EMG) activation of antagonistic leg muscles as well as intrinsic and passive muscle properties. The EMG activity recorded from the leg muscles reflects the action and interaction between central programs and afferent inputs from various sources, which can only be separated to a limited degree. Therefore, we have to record the EMG activity from several antagonistic leg muscles and the resulting biomechanical parameters such as joint movements and, eventually, of muscle tension in order to assess the neuronal control of locomotor movements. Thus it is possible to evaluate the behavior of neuronal and biomechanical parameters during the gait disorder. Any changes in the neuronal or biomechanical systems may lead to the pathophysiologic basis of movement disorder. One must be aware, however, that such deviations may already be secondary and compensatory to the primary dysfunction of the motor systems involved in the respective movement.

GAIT DISORDER IN PARKINSON'S DISEASE

Evidence is accumulating that the different regions of the basal ganglia have direct descending output connections to different parts of brainstem motor-regulating centers: to the locomotor drive centers in the subthalamic area and mesencephalon, and to the centers involved in posture regulation in the pontine reticular formation (1,2). The mesencephalic locomotor system exerts its descending control via bulbopontine and reticulospinal pathways. Tests of activity in reticulospinal pathways indicate an inadequate function in these systems in Parkinson's disease (PD) (3).

Pathophysiologically, an impaired neuronal control of gait associated with rigid and poorly modulated motor performance represents a major deficit of PD (4). These abnormalities are thought to result from varying combinations of hypokinesia, rigidity, and deficits of posture and equilibrium (5,6). Furthermore, distinct differences can be evaluated by quantitative gait analysis between the gait pattern of patients with vascular parkinsonism and idiopathic PD (7) and of those with normal pressure hydrocephalus and PD (7a). Little is known, however, about the extent to which such postural instability reflects deficits in the programmed adjustments or reflex mechanisms of compensation.

Central Mechanisms

Several studies on gait indicate impaired programming in patients with PD (8). The electrophysiological gait analysis of patients with PD, in addition to showing slow and reduced movements reveals a characteristic pattern of leg muscle activation with reduced amplitude and little modulated EMG activity in the leg extensor muscles during the stance phase and increased tibialis anterior activity during swing. Furthermore, the characteristic coordination of normal plantigrade gait is lost (9). The close similarity of gait between parkinsonian patients before medication and children who had not yet developed a plantigrade gait has led to the suggestion that an immature pattern may reappear in PD as a result of deficits in the neuronal circuits controlling plantigrade locomotion (9).

The leg muscle EMG pattern induced by feet displacement also indicates an impairment of programmed muscle activation (10,11). During stance perturbations, the compensatory gastrocnemius response is followed by a tibialis anterior activation. The latter activity is significantly stronger in parkinsonian patients than in age-matched healthy subjects. This late activation of the tibialis anterior muscle is thought to be part of a programmed pattern; therefore, the enhanced late tibialis anterior activity may reflect an impaired central generation of the EMG pattern. The enhanced tibialis anterior activation corresponds to the so-called shortening reaction first described by Westphal (12–14). In addition, parkinsonian patients are inflexible in adapting and modifying their postural responses to changing support conditions (15). The idea of an impaired central regulation is in agreement with the concept of an overcompensated and faulty predictive feedback system suggested elsewhere (16).

In a recent study, leg muscle activity adaptation and coordination between lower limbs were studied during walking on a treadmill with split-belts at different speeds in parkinsonian patients and age-matched healthy subjects (17). Two main differences were observed in the EMG patterns: (a) Leg muscle EMG activity was less modulated and gastrocnemius EMG amplitude was small during normal and split-belt walking. However, there was no significant difference between the two groups in respect to the reorganization of the EMG pattern required for the various split-belt walking conditions. (b) The amount of coactivation of antagonistic leg muscles during the support phase of the stride cycle was greater in the patients compared to the healthy subjects during normal and split-belt walking. It was suggested that reduced EMG modulation and recruitment in the leg extensors might contribute to impaired walking. This in turn may be a result of an impaired proprioceptive feedback from extensor load receptors. This defective control was partially compensated for in parkinsonian patients by a greater amount of leg flexor activation that leads to a higher degree of coactivation. Visual input plays a role in the control of this increased activation (18,19).

Proprioceptive Reflexes and Muscle Tone

Impaired function of proprioceptive reflexes in patients with PD contributes to gait instability. This may be a major reason why these patients rely more on visual information for the regulation of gait (20). The dysfunction of proprioceptive reflexes differs, however, from that described for spasticity. Monosynaptic reflex activity in the gastrocnemius muscle of patients with PD is negligible, as in healthy subjects. The polysynaptic compensatory gastrocnemius EMG responses are present but significantly smaller than those obtained in age-matched healthy subjects because of reduced reflex sensitivity (10). The impaired function of polysynaptic reflexes confirms earlier suggestions of alterations in central responsiveness and defective utilization of sensory input in these patients (21,22). Reduced sensitivity of polysynaptic reflexes in the leg extensor muscles appears to be a direct consequence of the dopamine deficiency in parkinsonian patients, because it is also observed (without other changes) in young normal subjects following intake of a single dose of haloperidol (23). When applying various dopamine receptor antagonists, it becomes evident that this effect is owing to an impaired function of central dopamine D_2 receptors (23). Conversely, only some gait parameters (kinematic) are L-Dopa–sensitive, whereas others (temporal) are L-Dopa–resistant (24).

Changes in the behavior of central mechanisms and reflexes described for patients with PD do not require the introduction of a qualitatively new pattern. These changes also characterize differences between elderly and young normal subjects, although they are significantly more pronounced in parkinsonian patients (10).

Evidence for associated changes of inherent muscle stiffness in PD was first established on the basis of gait studies (10). In line with these observations, perturbation experiments revealed a slower ankle joint displacement trajectory in patients with PD than in age-matched healthy subjects (10). This effect has to be attributed to altered mechanical properties of gastrocnemius muscle in PD and contributes to rigid muscle tone. These changes of muscle fiber properties are, however, less pronounced in PD than in long-lasting spasticity. Such changes in muscle stiffness may be advantageous insofar as a higher resistance to stretch helps to compensate for a perturbation. Changes of inherent mechanical properties of muscle in PD also have been reported in upper limb muscles (25,26).

The observations made in parkinsonian patients as established in the preceding are remarkable in that such profound differences can be observed in reflex function and inherent muscle stiffness, dependent on which muscle is under study and on the conditions of the investigation: (a) The reflex function and inherent muscle stiffness are normal in the tibialis anterior in contrast to the leg extensors (10). The differential behavior of the antagonist leg muscles can best be explained by differences in neuronal control owing to the different function fulfilled by these muscles in the regulation of gait. (b) A great number of electrophysiological studies in PD are concerned with the function of peripheral feedback mechanisms during limb displacement in a *sitting* position. In contrast to the compensatory responses described for perturbations of stance or gait, most of these investigations show an *increase* in the amplitude and duration of the long-latency EMG response in lower limbs (21,27). An increase of reflex gain at a central site has been postulated because muscle spindle recordings show normal $\alpha\gamma$-coactivation in these patients (28). Controversy arose, however, as to whether this finding results from an increase of a cortical (16) or spinal reflex loop (21), or rather from the absence of an inhibitory mechanism (29). The discrepant finding of a reduced stretch sensitivity of proprioceptive postural reflexes may arise primarily from the difference in motor tasks investigated. Perturbation of gait represents a functional condition, with a convergence of several afferent inputs (e.g., from extensor load receptors) and interaction with central mechanisms.

Load Receptor Function

The regulation of body equilibrium in patients with PD and age-matched healthy subjects was studied (11). Postural reactions were investigated with subjects standing on a sinusoidally moving treadmill. The body oscillations of the patients induced in this condition were compensated more by activation of leg flexor muscles in compensation for reduced leg extensor activation. Reduced activation of the leg extensor muscles was assumed to result from impaired proprioceptive feedback input from extensor load receptors (11). This defective control may be partially compensated for in parkinsonian patients by a greater amount of leg flexor activation, which leads to a higher degree of coactivation. Several studies on motor control in patients with PD are in line with the assumption of a defective load control in these patients (30,31).

The influence of body unloading on leg muscle activation during treadmill locomotion was investigated (19,32). Load sensitivity in both groups of subjects was seen only in leg extensor muscles. The absolute level of leg extensor

EMG amplitude during the stance phase was, however, smaller in the patients with PD than in the age-matched healthy subjects for all unloading conditions. However, the slope of decrease in EMG amplitude with successive unloading (up to 75% of body weight) was about the same in both groups. This suggests that the threshold of load receptor reflex loop is maladjusted or biased in PD, but not the slope or gain of this reflex mechanism. This leads to a changed magnitude of this reflex response, which is essential for the maintenance of body equilibrium. In comparison with cerebellar gait disorders, the defective control involves a similar mechanism acting in the opposite direction however.

SPASTIC GAIT DISORDER

Spasticity produces numerous physical signs, such as exaggerated reflexes, clonus, and muscle hypertonia. Clinically spastic hypertonia has been defined as a resistance of passive muscle to stretch in a velocity-dependent manner following activation of tonic stretch reflexes (33).

The physical signs of spasticity, however, bear little relationship to the patient's movement-disorder–related disability. The widely accepted conclusion that exaggerated reflexes are responsible for muscle hypertonia, and therefore movement disorder, was drawn from clinical observations on the pathophysiology and treatment of spasticity. The function of these reflexes during natural movements and the relationship between exaggerated reflexes and movement disorder is not often considered. Patients with spinal cord lesions exhibit characteristic gait impairment. This can be evaluated by the recording of electrophysiological and biomechanical parameters. Of course, there is some difference between spasticity of cerebral and spinal origin, but the main features are quite similar, such as leg muscle activation during locomotion and pathophysiology of spastic muscle tone (34).

Reflexes and Muscle Tone

It has been suggested that neuronal reorganization occurs following central lesions in both cat (35) and humans (36). Novel connections (e.g., sprouting, functional strengthening of existing connections, removed depression of previously inactive connections) may cause changes in the strength of inhibition. In addition, supersensitivity caused by denervation may occur (35). Although recent observations have indicated that spinal cord lesions do not cause sprouting of primary afferents in either cat (37) or humans (38), changes in the reduction of presynaptic inhibition of group Ia fibers does occur, which correlates with enhanced excitability of tendon tap reflexes (39). In addition, reduction of presynaptic inhibition is stronger in patients with paraplegia than in those with hemiplegia (40). However, no correlation is seen between decreased presynaptic inhibition of Ia terminals and the degree of spasticity measured by Ashworth's scale (40).

The treatment of spasticity is usually directed toward reducing stretch reflex activity, because it is thought that exaggerated reflexes are responsible for increased muscle tone and therefore spastic movement disorders. Studies on muscle tone and reflex activity usually have been performed under *passive* motor conditions (41,42). In such a condition, increased elbow torque following displacement was associated with an increased EMG activity in the flexor muscles of the spastic side compared to the unaffected side in patients with spastic hemiparesis (43). Nevertheless, in patients with spastic hemiparesis following stroke, muscle hypertonia was found to be closely associated with muscle fiber contracture but not reflex hyperexcitability (44).

Extensive investigations on *functional* movements of leg and arm muscles have not revealed any causal relationship between exaggerated reflexes and movement disorder (45–49). The reciprocal mode of leg muscle activation during gait was preserved in spasticity in adult patients with cerebral or spinal lesions. Exaggerated stretch reflexes in spasticity were associated with an absence or reduction of functionally essential polysynaptic (long-latency) reflexes. Both cutaneous and stretch reflex modulation was shown to be impaired during walking in patients with spinal cord lesions (50,51). In the latter experiments, ankle joint rotations were induced in any phase of the step cycle. It was proposed that impaired modulation of the stretch reflex along with increased ankle joint stiffness contribute to impaired walking ability of these patients.

In spastic patients the EMG activity in the calf muscles during gait is smaller in amplitude and less well modulated compared to healthy subjects. This observation is most probably owing to the impaired function of polysynaptic reflexes. Fast regulation of motoneuron discharge, which characterizes the normal muscle, is absent in spasticity (52,53). This corresponds to a loss of EMG modulation during gait. In patients with spastic hemiparesis caused by cerebral lesion, the strength of EMG activity in the affected leg is reduced compared to the unaffected leg. This corresponds to the degree of paresis observed during both gait and elbow movements (45,48). Thus, it becomes clear that inhibition and facilitation of spinal reflexes depends on supraspinal control, which is impaired in spasticity.

A fundamentally different development of tension of the triceps surae takes place during the stance phase of the stride cycle in spastic paresis (acquired at an early or later stage) (45,46). In the unaffected leg, the tension development correlates with the modulation of EMG activity (the same is true in healthy subjects), whereas in the spastic leg tension development is connected to the stretching period of the tonically activated muscle (with small EMG amplitude). There is no visible influence of monosynaptic reflex potentials on the tension developed by the triceps surae during gait. A similar discrepancy between the resistance to stretch and the level of EMG activity has been described for flexor muscles of the upper limb in spastic patients (54,55). Muscle hypertonia in hemiparetic patients was found to be primarily associated with muscle contracture but not with exaggerated reflexes (44).

Muscle tone during functional movements in patients with spastic paresis cannot be explained by an increased activity of motoneurons assessed by EMG recordings. Instead, a transformation of motor units such that a higher tension to EMG activity relationship occurs during the stretching phase of the triceps surae. This has the consequence that regulation of muscle tension takes place at a lower level of neuronal organization. Therefore, the changed regulation of spastic gait should be considered as optimal for the given state of the motor system (56).

Motor Unit Transformation

There are several findings that support the suggestion that changes in mechanical muscle fiber properties occur in spasticity. Contraction times are prolonged in hand as well as gastrocnemius muscles in patients with spastic hemiparesis (57,58). Torque motor experiments applied to upper and lower limb muscles indicate a major, nonreflex contribution to the spastic muscle tone in the antigravity muscles, that is, in the leg extensors and elbow flexors (59,60). Histochemistry and morphometry studies of spastic muscle have revealed neurogenic changes of the muscle fibers (52,61). These include (a) increased levels of muscle fiber atrophy (especially of type II fibers), (b) a predominance of type I fibers in the gastrocnemius during later stages, when spasticity of cerebral origin has been established, and (c) structural changes, such as the appearance of target fibers, mainly in type I fibers. A significant part of changes of mechanical muscle fiber properties may also be attributed to a shortening of muscle length as a result of a decrease in the number of sarcomeres in series along the myofibrils accompanied by an increase in resistance to stretch (62). Such muscle contracture can be produced in experimental animals by plaster cast immobilization of muscles in shortened positions.

The alteration to a simpler regulation of muscle tension following paresis owing to spinal or supraspinal lesions is basically advantageous for the patient as it enables him to support the body during gait and, consequently, to achieve mobility (47). However, rapid movements are no longer possible owing to the absence of modulation of muscle activity. Following a severe spinal or supraspinal lesion, these transformative processes can have unwelcome consequences (e.g., painful spasms and involuntary movements).

The latter patients are usually much less able to perform stepping movements because spinal locomotor centers do not provide sufficient basic activation of leg muscles. In the last year it has been shown that specific locomotor training could enhance locomotor activity and thereby improve mobility (see "Locomotion in Paraplegic Patients" section).

Specific Aspects of Gait Disorder in Children with Cerebral Palsy

Studies in children with cerebral palsy (CP), as in spastic adults, are frequently restricted to the physical signs of spasticity (63–65). This may also be owing to the fact that about half of the children with CP could not yet walk at 6 years of age (66).

Leg–muscle activity during *functional movements,* such as locomotion, of children with congenital CP has characteristic signs of impaired maturation of the normal gait pattern (67). The pattern recorded in children with CP of around 10 years of age mainly consists of a coactivation of antagonistic leg muscles during the stance phase of a gait cycle and a general reduction in EMG amplitude. In contrast, when the cerebral lesion is acquired at a later stage and the reciprocal mode of leg muscle activity is already established (i.e., at around 4 years), reciprocal activation of antagonistic leg muscles is preserved during spastic gait.

Although neurophysiological studies indicate that muscle tone in children with CP represents an inhomogeneous condition (63), there are typical features, such as the coactivation of all antagonistic leg muscles during the stance phase of gait, associated with a reduced and tonic mode of leg extensor muscle activation (starting before ground contact), and the appearance of isolated EMG potentials after ground contact (68). These potentials are probably monosynaptic stretch reflex potentials mediated by group I afferents, because they appear with short latency after the onset of gastrocnemius stretch. This pattern closely resembles the pattern of stepping in newborn infants (71–73). Myotatic reflex irradiation, usually observed in children with CP, is present in nondisabled infants under 2 years of age (71–73). Both abnormal corticospinal input and a deficient modulation of spinal interneuronal circuits with impairment of reciprocal inhibition may contribute to the coactivation pattern (74,75).

Monosynaptic reflex potentials disappear, the polysynaptic reflex response becomes stronger and more phasic, and a reciprocal mode of leg muscle activation becomes established from 4 years of age onward only in healthy children. These changes represent a shift from a predominance of rigid and functionally ineffective monosynaptic stretch reflexes to that of polysynaptic spinal reflexes. According to kinematographic analysis, this shift is reflected in a sticklike usage of the legs in the early stage of stepping, whereas the body is rolled off over the standing leg in older children.

Little is known about the natural evolution of CP. There are few controlled studies documenting the positive effect of a specific treatment or training program (76–78). It appears that children with CP have a delayed development of infant stepping and supported locomotion, and fail to develop the plantigrade gait.

Summary

The central programming, timing, and reciprocal mode of leg muscle activation during gait are basically intact in patients with spastic paresis. Exaggerated monosynaptic reflexes are associated with a loss of the functionally essential polysynaptic reflex mechanisms, both being dependent on supraspinal control. When this control is either not yet matured (small children) or impaired (spastic paresis), inhibition of monosynaptic stretch reflexes is missing in combination with a reduced facilitation of polysynaptic reflexes.

A spinal or cerebral lesion associated with paresis is followed by a transformation of motor units (and most probably shortening of muscle fibers leading to muscle contracture), such that tension development in the muscle occurs in a simpler fashion. Calf muscle tension during gait is normally determined by modulated gastrocnemius or soleus EMG activity. In the spastic leg, calf muscle tension is associated with the stretching of the tonically activated muscle. This regulation of muscle tension at a lower level is efficient insofar as it enables the patient to support body weight during gait.

Consequently, physiotherapeutic approaches should be applied primarily and antispastic drug therapy secondarily in mobile patients; whereas antispastic drugs may relieve muscle spasms and improve nursing care in immobilized patients.

LOCOMOTION IN PATIENTS WITH PARAPLEGIA

Neuronal Capacity of the Spinal Cord

For more than 30 years functional electrical stimulation of paralyzed limb muscles was the only technique used to improve mobility in patients with paraplegia (79). Despite technical developments, this method is still experimental for locomotion, and no pioneering breakthrough has occurred that allows for more extensive application of the technique (80). Basic problems include rapid development of muscle fatigue and adverse interactions with spinal reflexes, which obviously cannot be overcome by technical means. However, a new approach has been developed in the last few years that improves the mobility of patients with incomplete paraplegia. This is achieved by external activation and training of spinal locomotor centers.

Recovery of locomotor function following spinal cord transection in the *cat* was believed for several years to be restricted to immature animals (81). It was later shown that the recovery of locomotor patterns could be improved using regular training even in adult animals (82). When spontaneous stepping was not stimulated, the cat lost the ability to step spontaneously. During locomotor training the animal was supported and thus only bore a part of its body weight. A treadmill induced locomotor movements of the hindlimbs, whereas the forelimbs stood on a platform. Body support was decreased in proportion to the animals' improving locomotor abilities with ongoing training. After some weeks of training the cat was able to completely take over body weight and perform well-coordinated stepping movements (83). The locomotor pattern at this stage closely resembled the pattern of the normal adult cat. In other experiments, the effect of hindlimb exercise on the modulation of reflex activity was studied in adult rats after spinal cord transection (84). It could be shown that exercise helps to normalize the excitability of specific spinal reflexes. Thus, the training represents an important factor in the recovery of locomotor function. Stepping movements were even demonstrated in a monkey after transection of the spinal cord, which suggests that the isolated primate spinal cord is also capable of generating hindlimb stepping movements (85).

Steplike movements in *humans* are present at birth and can be initiated spontaneously or by peripheral stimuli. The EMG activity underlying this newborn stepping is centrally programmed and, as in anencephalic children, it is likely that spinal mechanisms generate the EMG activity (86). The apparent loss of locomotor movements in accidentally spinal-lesioned humans has been suggested to result from a greater predominance of supraspinal over spinal neuronal mechanisms (87). Nevertheless, there are indications that spinal interneuronal circuits in humans exist that are involved in the generation of locomotor EMG activity in leg muscles similar to those described for the cat (83,88). Furthermore, involuntary steplike leg movements recently described in a patient with an incomplete injury to the spinal cord as well as the behavior of a propriospinal clonus released after cervical trauma indicate a spinal pattern generator in humans (89–92).

Effect of Locomotor Training in Patients with Paraplegia

In recent studies, researchers have tried to determine the degree to which locomotor EMG activity and movements can be both elicited and trained in leg muscles of patients with either complete or incomplete paraplegia (93,94).

The induction of complex bilateral leg muscle activation combined with coordinated stepping movements in patients with incomplete and complete paraplegia was achieved by partially unloading (up to 60%) patients who were on a moving treadmill. The leg movements had to be assisted externally, especially during transitions from stance to swing, during the first phases of the training (usually 2 to 6 weeks, depending on the severity of paresis) in patients with incomplete paraplegia, and during the whole training period (3 to 5 months) in patients with complete paraplegia. Patients with paraplegia displayed a less dynamic mode of muscle activation (less well modulated in amplitude) compared to healthy subjects. This may result from the impaired function of polysynaptic spinal reflexes in patients with spinal lesions (67). The pattern of leg muscle EMG activity was similar to that seen in healthy subjects in other respects, such as timing. Different amplitude levels of leg extensor (the main antigravity muscle during gait) EMG activity occurred in the different subject groups that largely exceeded the interindividual variability. The amplitude level of EMG activity was considerably smaller in patients with complete paraplegia compared to patients with incomplete paraplegia, although both patient groups had smaller EMG levels compared to healthy subjects. Spastic symptoms (e.g., increased muscle tone, exaggerated reflexes) were present in both patient groups despite the reduced level of EMG activity. This supports earlier suggestions claiming that alterations of mechanical muscle fiber properties of the tonically active muscle are mainly responsible for the clinical signs of spasticity (see "Spastic Gait Disorder" section).

The EMG pattern observed during locomotor training in patients with complete paraplegia may result from rhythmic stretches of the leg muscles (95). The integrated EMG of tibialis anterior and gastrocnemius muscles was collected every 50 ms over the whole step cycle and was related to the lengthening or shortening (determined by ankle and knee joint movements) of the respective muscle in order to analyze the EMG activity that may be evoked by stretch reflexes. It became evident that leg muscle EMG activity during locomotion (muscle lengthening and shortening) is approximately equally distributed in both healthy subjects and patients. This indicates that stretch reflexes are unlikely to play a major role in the generation of leg muscle EMG patterns in these patients, but instead that the locomotor pattern is programmed at a spinal level.

The amplitude of gastrocnemius EMG activity increased significantly throughout the stance phase during the course of a daily locomotor training program, whereas an inappropriate tibialis anterior activation decreased. These training effects were seen in both patients with incomplete paraplegia and those with complete paraplegia. This was related to a greater weight-bearing function of the extensors (i.e., body unloading during treadmill locomotion could be reduced). The slope of the increase of gastrocnemius EMG was similar in patients with both incomplete and complete paraplegia. This indicates that the isolated human spinal cord contains the capacity not only to generate a locomotor pattern, but also to learn. Only patients with incomplete paraplegia benefited from the training program insofar as they learned to perform unsupported stepping movements on solid ground (93,94). Patients with complete paraplegia experienced positive effects on the cardiovascular and musculoskeletal systems, that is, they suffered less from spastic symptoms. In comparison to leg extensor EMG, only a small effect of training on leg flexor EMG amplitude was seen, which may result from different neuronal control of leg flexor and extensor muscles during locomotion (96). Successive body reloading during training may serve as a stimulus for extensor load receptors, which are essential for leg extensor activation during locomotion in both cats and humans (88,97,98). The lower gain of extensor EMG (i.e., generally smaller EMG amplitude), in patients with complete paraplegia may be owing to a loss of input from descending noradrenergic pathways to spinal locomotor centers (83).

OUTLOOK

The advantage of gait analysis represents the quantitative assessment of a functional movement with its underlying neuronal mechanisms and biomechanical consequences. In the future, this approach may be developed further to extract the factors responsible for a movement disorder. Gait analysis may help to select the most effective pharmacologic and physiotherapeutic approach to future *rehabilitation*. This may not only benefit the patient but also might lead to reduced health care costs, because most physiotherapeutic approaches are not based on controlled studies or convincingly demonstrated effectiveness. For future application in *clinical* diagnosis, gait analysis may help to achieve an early diagnosis, detection, and appropriate training of movement disorder subtypes.

With the recordings of electrophysiologic and biomechanical parameters during gait of patients with *PD,* the best therapeutic approach for improved gait performance can be selected. In addition we can follow the effect of any treatment on the locomotor pattern. Analysis of neuromuscular changes following *cerebral* or *spinal motor lesions* has revealed that the development of spastic muscle tone can be advantageous in providing body support during stepping movements. Consequently, neuromuscular changes can be treated adequately and should become incorporated into the physiotherapeutic approach to the patient.

The strength of leg muscle activation is insufficient to build up enough muscle tone or control limb movements for locomotion in severely affected paretic patients. One approach to enhance spinal locomotor activity in patients with incomplete and complete paraplegia represents the search for substances that influence the gain of leg extensor EMG activity. Although substances that have been investigated to date have not been convincing in their action, stronger substances might be explored in the future. The most promising approach for the future may be to induce partial regeneration of the lesioned spinal cord tract fibers. Recent experiments in the rat indicated that after inhibition of neurite growth inhibitors, partial regeneration could occur (99,100). This approach may improve functional mobility even in patients with almost complete paraplegia when used in conjunction with appropriate locomotor training. Currently, electrophysiologic and biomechanical recordings during locomotion in rats after spinal cord lesions should provide information about how far this model can be applied to humans with spinal cord injury. This research should also help to answer questions such as how many spinal tract fibers have to be preserved or regenerated after a spinal cord injury for the performance of stepping movements.

CONCLUSION

This chapter deals with the neuronal mechanisms underlying impaired gait as a paradigm of movement disorder, assessed by electrophysiologic means with the aim of first, a better understanding of the underlying pathophysiology and second, the selection of an adequate treatment. For the patient usually one of the first symptoms of a lesion within the central motor system represents the *movement disorder,* which is most characteristic during locomotion in patients with spasticity or PD. The *clinical* examination reveals typical changes in tendon tap reflexes and muscle tone typical for one of the movement disorders. However, today we know that there exists only a weak relationship between the physical signs obtained during the clinical examination in a passive motor condition and the impaired neuronal mechanisms in operation during an active movement. By recording and analyzing electrophysiologic and biomechanical parameters during a functional movement (e.g., locomotion), one can reliably assess the significance of impaired reflex behavior or pathophysiology of muscle tone and its contribution to the movement disorder. Consequently, adequate treatment should be based on the pathophysiology and significance of the mechanisms underlying the patient's functional movement disorder in addition to including cosmetic therapy and correction of an isolated clinical parameter.

ACKNOWLEDGMENTS

This work was supported by grants from the Swiss National Science Foundation (grant no. 31-53526.98). The author is grateful to Dr. I. Gibson for correcting the English text.

REFERENCES

1. Marsden CD. Neurophysiology. In: Stern G, ed. *Parkinson's disease*. London: Chapman and Hall, 1990:57–98.
2. Murray MP, Clarkson BH. The vertical pathways of the foot during level walking. II. Clinical examples of distorted pathways. *J Am Phys Ther Ass* 1996;46:590–599.
3. Delwaide PJ, Pepin JL, Maertens de Noordhout A. The audiospinal reaction in parkinsonian patients reflects functional changes in reticular nuclei. *Ann Neurol* 1999;33:63–69.
4. Martin JP. *The basal ganglia and posture*. London: Pitman, 1967.
5. Knutsson E. An analysis of parkinsonian gait. *Brain* 1972;95:475–486.
6. Murray MP. Gait as a total pattern of movement. *Am J Phys Med* 1967;46:290–332.
7. Zijlmans JCM, Poels PJE, Duysens J, et al. Quantitative gait analysis in patients with vascular parkinsonism. *Mov Disord* 1996;11:501–508.

7a. Stolze H, Kühtz-Büschbeck JP, Drücke H, et al. Comparative analysis of the gait disorder of normal pressure of hydrocephalus and Parkinson's disease. *J Neurol Neurosurg Psychiatry* 2001 (in press).
8. Dietz V. Human neuronal control of automatic functional movements: interaction between central programs and afferent input. *Physiol Rev* 1992;72:33–69.
9. Forssberg H, Johnels B, Steg G. Is Parkinsonian gait caused by a regression to an immature walking pattern? In: Hassler RG, Christ JF, eds. *Advances in Neurology*, Vol 40. New York: Raven Press, 1984:375–379.
10. Dietz V, Berger W, Horstmann GA. Posture in Parkinson's disease: impairment of reflexes and programming. *Ann Neurol* 1988;24:660–669.
11. Dietz V, Zijlstra W, Assaiante C, et al. Balance control in Parkinson's disease. *Gait Posture* 1993;1:77–84.
12. Westphal E. *Unterschenkelphänomen und Nervendehnung. Arch Psychiat Nervenkr* 1987;7:666–670.
13. Angel RW. Muscular contractions elicited by passive shortening. In: Desmedt JE, ed. *Advances in Neurology*, Vol 39. New York: Raven Press, 1983:555–563.
14. Berardelli A, Hallett M. Shortening reaction of human tibialis anterior. *Neurology* 1984;34:242–246.
15. Schieppati M, Nardone A. Free and support stance in Parkinson's disease: the effect of posture and "postural set" on leg muscle responses to perturbation, and its relation to the severity of the disease. *Brain* 1991;114:1227–1244.
16. Tatton WG, Bedingham V, Verrier MC, et al. Characteristic alterations in response to imposed wrist displacement in parkinsonian rigidity and dystonia musculorum deformans. *Can J Neurol Sci* 1984;11:281–287.
17. Dietz V, Zijlstra W, Prokop T, et al. Leg muscle activation during gait in Parkinson's disease: adaptation and interlimb coordination. *Electroenceph Clin Neurophysiol* 1996;97:408–415.
18. Brouwer B, Ashby P. Corticospinal projections to lower limb motoneurons in man. *Exp Brain Res* 1992;89:649–654.
19. Dietz V, Leenders KL, Colombo G. Leg muscle activation during gait in Parkinson's disease: influence of body unloading. *Electroenceph Clin Neurophysiol* 1997;105:400–405.
20. Bronstein AM, Hood JD, Gresty MA, et al. Visual control of balance in cerebellar and parkinsonian syndromes. *Brain* 1990;113:767–779.
21. Berardelli A, Sabra AF, Hallett M. Physiological mechanisms of rigidity in Parkinson's disease. *J Neurol Neurosurg Psychiatry* 1983;46:45–53.
22. Tatton WG, Eastman MJ, Bedingham W, et al. Defective utilization of sensory input as the basis for bradykinesia, rigidity, and decreased movement repertoire in Parkinson's disease: a hypothesis. *Can J Neurol Sci* 1984;11:136–143.
23. Dietz V, Feuerstein TJ, Berger W. Significance of dopamine receptor antagonists in human postural control. *Neurosci Lett* 1990;117:81–86.
24. Blin O, Ferrandez AM, Pailhouse J, et al. Dopa-sensitive and Dopa-resistant gait parameters in Parkinson's disease. *J Neurol Sci* 1991;103:51–54.
25. Berardelli A, Dick JPR, Rothwell JC, et al. Scaling of the size of the first agonist EMG burst during rapid wrist movements in patients with Parkinson's disease. *J Neurol Neurosurg Psychiatry* 1986;49:1273–1279.
26. Watts RL, Wiegner AW, Young RR. Elastic properties of muscles measured at the elbow in man. II. Patients with parkinsonian rigidity. *J Neurol Neurosurg Psychiatry* 198;49:1177–1181.
27. Chan CWY, Kearney RE, Melvill-Jones G. Tibialis anterior response to sudden ankle displacements in normal and parkinsonian subjects. *Brain Res* 1979;173:303–314.
28. Burke D, Hagbarth KE, Wallin G. Reflex mechanisms in parkinsonian rigidity. *Scand J Rehabil Med* 1977;9:15–23.
29. Cody FWJ, MacDermott N, Matthews PBC, et al. Observations on the genesis of the stretch reflex in Parkinson's disease. *Brain* 1986;109:229–249.
30. Stelmach GE. Basal ganglia impairment and force control. In: Requin J, Stelmach GE, eds. *Tutorials in motor neuroscience*. Dordrecht: Kluwer, 1991:137–148.
31. Burne JA, Lippold OCJ. Loss of tendon organ inhibition in Parkinson's disease. *Brain* 1996;119:1115–1121.
32. Dietz V, Colombo G. Influence of body load and gait pattern in Parkinson's disease. *Mov Disord* 1998;13:255–261.
33. Lance JW. Symposium synopsis. In: Feldman RG, Young RR, Koella WP, eds. *Spasticity: disordered motor control*. Chicago: Year Book, 1980:485–495.
34. Dietz V. Spasticity: exaggerated reflexes or movement disorder? In: Forssberg H, Hirschfeld H, eds. *Movement disorders in children*. Basel: Karger, 1992:225–233.
35. Mendell LM. Modifiability of spinal synapses. *Physiol Rev* 1984;64:260–324.
36. Carr LJ, Harrison LM, Evans AL, et al. Patterns of central motor reorganization in hemiplegic cerebral palsy. *Brain* 1993;116:1223–1247.
37. Nacimiento W, Mautes A, Töpper R, et al. B-50 (GAP-42) in the spinal cord caudal to hemisection: indication for lack of intraspinal sprouting in dorsal root axons. *J Neurosci Res* 1993;35:603–617.
38. Ashby P. Discussion I. In: Emre M, Benecke R, eds. *Spasticity. The current status of research and treatment*. Carnforth: Parthenon, 1989:68–69.
39. Burke D, Ashby P. Are spinal "presynaptic" inhibitory mechanisms suppressed in spasticity? *J Neurol Sci* 1972;15:321–326.
40. Faist M, Mazevet D, Dietz V, et al. A quantitative assessment of presynaptic inhibition of Ia afferents in spastics: differences in hemiplegics and paraplegics. *Brain* 1994;117:1449–1455.
41. Thilmann AF, Fellows SJ, Garms E. Pathological stretch reflexes on the "good" side of hemiparetic patients. *J Neurol Neurosurg Psychiatry* 1990;53:208–214.
42. Ihilmann AF, Fellows SJ, Garms E. The mechanism of spastic muscle hypertonus: variation in reflex gain over the time course of spasticity. *Brain* 1991;114:233–244.
43. Ibrahim IK, Berger W, Trippel M, et al. Stretch-induced electromyographic activity and torque in spastic elbow muscles. *Brain* 1993;116:971–989.
44. O'Dwyer NJ, Ada L, Neilson PD. Spasticity and muscle contracture following stroke. *Brain* 1996;114:1737–1749.
45. Berger W, Quintern J, Dietz V. Tension development and muscle activation in the leg during gait in spastic hemiparesis: the independence of muscle hypertonia and exaggerated stretch reflexes. *J Neurol Neurosurg Psychiatry* 1984;47:1029–1033.
46. Dietz V, Berger W. Normal and impaired regulation of

muscle stiffness in gait: a new hypothesis about muscle hypertonia. *Exp Neurol* 1983;79:680–687.
47. Dietz V, Quintern J, Berger W. Electrophysiological studies of gait in spasticity and rigidity. Evidence that altered mechanical properties of muscle contribute to hypertonia. *Brain* 1981;104:431–449.
48. Dietz V, Trippel M, Berger W. Reflex activity and muscle tone during elbow movements of patients with spastic paresis. *Ann Neurol* 1991;30:767–784.
49. Power RK, Campbell DL, Rymer WZ. Stretch reflex dynamics in spastic elbow flexor muscles. *Ann Neurol* 1989;25:32–42.
50. Jones CA, Yang JF. Reflex behavior during walking in incomplete spinal-cord-injured subjects. *Exp Neurol* 1994;128:239–248.
51. Sinkjaer T, Andersen JB, Nielsen JF. Impaired stretch reflex and joint torque modulation during spastic gait in multiple sclerosis patients. *J Neurol* 1996;243:566–574.
52. Dietz V, Ketelsen UP, Berger W, et al. Motor unit involvement in spastic paresis: relationship between leg muscle activation and histochemistry. *J Neurol Sci* 1986;75:89–103.
53. Rosenfalck A, Adreassen S. Impaired regulation of force and firing pattern of single motor units in patients with spasticity. *J Neurol Neurosurg Psychiatry* 1980;43:907–916.
54. Powers RK, Marder-Meyer J, Rymer WZ. Quantitative relations between hypertonia and stretch reflex threshold in spastic hemiparesis. *Ann Neurol* 1988;23:115–124.
55. Lee WA, Boughton A, Rymer WZ. Absence of stretch reflex gain enhancement in voluntarily activated spastic muscle. *Exp Neurol* 1987;98:317–335.
56. Latash ML, Anson JG. What are "normal movements" in atypical populations. *Behav Brain Sci* 1996;19:55–106.
57. Young JL, Mayer RF. Physiological alterations of motor units in hemiplegia. *J Neurol Sci* 1982;54:401–412.
58. Dietz V, Berger W. Interlimb coordination of posture in patients with spastic paresis. Impaired function of spinal reflexes. *Brain* 1984;107:965–978.
59. Hufschmidt A, Mauritz KH. Chronic transformation of muscle in spasticity: a peripheral contribution to increased tone. *J Neurol Neurosurg Psychiatry* 1985;48:676–685.
60. Sinkjaer T, Toft E, Larsen K, et al. Non-reflex and reflex mediated ankle joint stiffness in multiple sclerosis patients with spasticity. *Muscle Nerve* 1993;16:69–76.
61. Edström L. Selective changes in the sizes of red and white muscle fibres in upper motor lesions and Parkinsonism. *J Neurol Sci* 1970;11:537–550.
62. O'Dwyer NJ, Ada L. Reflex hyperexcitability and muscle contracture in relation to spastic hypertonia. *Curr Opin Neurol* 1996;9:451–455.
63. Brown JK, Rodda J, Walsh EG, et al. Neurophysiology of lower-limb function in hemiplegic children. *Dev Med Child Neurol* 1991;33:1037–1047.
64. Brouwer B, Wheeldon RK, Stradiotto-Parker N, et al. Reflex excitability and isometric force production in cerebral palsy: the effect of serial casting. *Dev Med Child Neurol* 1998;40:168–175.
65. Lin JP, Brown JK, Brotherstone R. Assessment of spasticity in hemiplegic cerebral palsy. II: distal lower-limb reflex excitability and function. *Dev Med Child Neurol* 1994;36:290–303.
66. Trahan J, Marcoux S. Factors associated with the inability of children with cerebral palsy to walk at six years: a retrospective study. *Dev Med Child Neurol* 1995;36:787–795.
67. Berger W, Quintern J, Dietz V. Pathophysiological aspects of gait in children with cerebral palsy. *Electroenceph Clin Neurophysiol* 1982;53:538–548.
68. Dietz V, Berger W. Cerebral palsy and muscle transformation. *Dev Med Child Neurol* 1995;37:180–184.
69. Forssberg H, Wallberg H. Infant locomotion: a preliminary movement and electromyographic study. In: Berg K, Eriksson BD, eds. *Children and exercise*. Baltimore: University Park Press, 1980:32–49.
70. Leonard CT, Hirschfeld H, Forssberg H. The development of independent walking in children with cerebral palsy. *Dev Med Child Neurol* 1991;33:567–577.
71. Leonard CT, Hirschfeld H. Myotatic reflex responses of non-disabled children and children with spastic cerebral palsy. *Dev Med Child Neurol* 1995;37:783–799.
72. Mykleburst BM, Gottlieb GL, Agarwal GC. Stretch reflexes of the normal infant. *Dev Med Child Neurol* 1986;28:440–449.
73. O'Dwyer NJ, Neilson P, Nash J. Reduction of spasticity in cerebral palsy using feedback of the tonic stretch reflex: a controlled study. *Dev Med Child Neurol* 1994;36:770–786.
74. Brouwer B, Smits E. Corticospinal input onto motor neurons projecting to ankle muscles in individuals with cerebral palsy. *Dev Med Child Neurol* 1996;38:787–796.
75. Leonard CT, Moritani T, Hirschfeld H, et al. Deficits in reciprocal inhibition of children with cerebral palsy as revealed by H-reflex testing. *Dev Med Child Neurol* 1990;32:974–984.
76. Tardieu C, Lespargot A, Tabary C, et al. For how long must the soleus muscle be stretched each day to prevent contracture? *Dev Med Child Neurol* 1988;30:3–10.
77. Forssberg H. Preface. In: Forssberg H, Hirschfeld H, eds. *Movement disorders in children*. Basel: Karger, 1992:7–8.
78. McLaughlin JF, Astley SJ, Bjornson KF, et al. Selective dorsal rhizotomy: efficacy and safety in an investigator masked randomized clinical trial. *Dev Med Child Neurol* 1998;40:220–232.
79. Kantrowitz A. Electronic physiologic aids. Brooklyn, NY: *Report of the Maimonides Hospital* 1960:4–5.
80. Quintern J, Minwegen P, Mauritz KH. Control mechanisms for restoring posture and movements in paraplegics. In: Allum JHJ, Hulliger M, eds. *Afferent control of posture and locomotion*. Amsterdam: Elsevier, 1989:489–502.
81. Forssberg H, Grillner S, Halbertsma J. The locomotion of the low spinal cat. I. Coordination within a hind-limb. *Acta Physiol Scand* 1980;108:269–281.
82. Barbeau H, Rossignol S. Recovery of locomotion after chronic spinalization in the adult cat. *Brain Res* 1987;412:84–95.
83. Barbeau H. Rossignol S. Enhancement of locomotor recovery following spinal cord injury. *Curr Opin Neurol* 1994;7:517–524.
84. Skinner RD, Houle JD, Reese NB, et al. Effects of exercise and fetal spinal cord implants on the H-reflex in chronically spinalized adult rats. *Brain Res* 1996; 729:127–131.

85. Vilensky JA, O'Connor BL. Stepping in humans with complete spinal cord transection: a phylogenetic evaluation. *Motor Control* 1997;1: 284–292.
86. Forssberg H. A developmental model of human locomotion. In: Grillner S, Stein PSG, Stuart DG, eds. *Neurobiology of vertebrate locomotion*. London: Macmillan, 1986:485–501.
87. Kuhn RA. Functional capacity of the isolated human spinal cord. *Brain* 1950;73:1–51.
88. Dietz V, Gollhofer A, Kleiber M, et al. Regulation of bipedal stance: dependence on "load" receptors. *Exp Brain Res* 1992;89:229–231.
89. Calancie B, Needham-Shropshire B, Jacobs P, et al. Involuntary stepping after chronic spinal cord injury: evidence for a central rhythm generator for locomotion in man. *Brain* 1994;117:1143–1159.
90. Nicol DJ, Granat M, Baxendale RH, et al. Evidence for a human spinal stepping generator. *Brain Res* 1995;9: 451–455.
91. Harkema SJ, Requejo PS, Hurley SL, et al. Human lumbosacral spinal cord interprets loading during stepping. *J Neurophysiol* 1997;77:797–811.
92. Brown P, Rothwell JC, Thompson PD, et al. Propriospinal myoclonus: evidence for spinal "pattern" generators in humans. *Mov Disord* 1994;9:571–576.
93. Dietz V, Colombo G, Jensen L. Locomotor activity in spinal man. *Lancet* 1994;344:1260–1263.
94. Dietz V, Colombo G, Jensen L, et al. Locomotor capacity of spinal cord in paraplegic patients. *Ann Neurol* 1995;37:574–582.
95. Dietz V. Locomotor training in paraplegic patients. *Ann Neurol* 1995;38:965.
96. Dietz V, Horstmann GA, Berger W. Interlimb coordination of leg muscle activation during perturbation of stance in humans. *J Neurophysiol* 1989;62:680–693.
97. Pearson KG, Collins DF. Reversal of the influence of group Ib-afferents from plantaris on activity in medial gastrocnemius muscle during locomotor activity. *J Neurophysiol* 1993;70:1009–1017.
98. Dietz V, Colombo G. Effects of body immersion on postural adjustments to voluntary arm movements in humans: role of load receptor input. *J Physiol (Lond)* 1996;497:849–856.
99. Schwab ME. Regeneration of lesioned CNS axons by neutralisation of neurite growth inhibitors: a short review. *Paraplegia* 1991;29:294–298.
100. Schwab ME, Bartholdi D. Degeneration and regeneration of axons in the lesioned spinal cord. *Physiol Rev* 1996;76:319–370.

Gait Disorders. Advances in Neurology, Vol. 87,
edited by E. Růžička, M. Hallett, and J. Jankovic.
Lippincott Williams & Wilkins, Philadelphia © 2001.

15
Cerebellar Ataxic Gait

Mark Hallett

Human Motor Control Section, National Institute of Neurological Disorders and Stroke, National Institutes of Health, Bethesda, Maryland 20892-1428

Difficulty with gait is often a major problem in patients with cerebellar dysfunction. From a clinical point of view, the principal features are irregularity of stepping, both in direction and distance. This may lead to veering to one side or lurching in different directions. Stability of upright stance is poor and patients may fall. Just as with standing balance, the base, or distance between the feet, is said to be broad. Despite numerous clinical descriptions, there has been no quantitative assessment until our recent detailed analysis using standard gait laboratory methodology (1). That study will be reviewed and put into the context of what is known about the pathophysiology of ataxic movement.

KINEMATICS OF CEREBELLAR GAIT

Method

We studied six men with hereditary cerebellar cortical atrophy (CCA) and three men and one woman with olivopontocerebellar atrophy (OPCA) ranging in age from 21 to 64 years. All patients exhibited clinically pure ataxia without significant other neurologic signs. Ten neurologically normal volunteers served as age- and sex-matched controls.

Kinematic data were sampled within a laboratory coordinate system defined by a vertically oriented z-axis and a y-axis parallel to the path of progression. Two strain gauge force plates were positioned along the y-axis to measure consecutive contralateral stance phase kinetics. Gait events, such as heel-strike and toe-off, were determined visually from the kinetic and kinematic data. A five-camera video-based kinematic data acquisition system (VICON, Oxford Metrics, Tampa, Florida) synchronously collected the unprocessed kinematic and force plate data at 50 Hz. Spherical retroreflective targets were bilaterally attached to the skin surface at the following sites: anterior to the tragus of the ear, greater tubercle of the humerus, lateral epicondyle of the humerus, posterior surface of the forearm between the styloid processes of the radius and ulna, greater trochanter of the femur, lateral femoral condyle, lateral malleolus, and fifth metatarsal-phalangeal joint.

The subjects, dressed in shorts, walked with bare feet at a self-determined pace. Six to 10 gait cycles were analyzed for each subject. Standard gait descriptors were determined (Table 15.1).

Results

Whereas all the trials from the control subjects could be analyzed, many of the trials from the patients could not. If the patients veered out of the view of the cameras or stumbled, the data could not be properly assessed. Hence, the patient trials analyzed are the best performances.

Examples of angular motion at ankle, knee, and hip from a patient compared with the matched control subject are shown in Figures 15.1 and 15.2. In these figures, ankle, knee, and hip angles are displayed versus time and versus each other (angle/angle diagrams). In the angle versus times plots, the dashed line

TABLE 15.1. *Definitions of gait descriptors*

Cadence:	The number of steps per minute.
Step length:	The Y-axis displacement between the lateral malleolus target positions of the two feet between heel strike and the subsequent contralateral heel strike.
Stride length:	The sum of two consecutive step lengths measured as the Y displacement of the lateral malleolus of one foot from heel strike to subsequent heel strike of the same foot.
Step width:	The X-axis displacement between the lateral malleolus target positions of the two feet between heel strike and the subsequent contralateral heel strike.
Step length symmetry:	The step length on the right divided by the step length on the left, figured in percent.
Stride length summetry:	The stride length measured from the right foot devided by the stride length measured from the left foot, figured in percent.
Step width symmetry:	The step width on the right divided by the step width on the left, figured in percent.
Foot height:	Maximum distance of the fifth metatarsal-phalangeal joint from the floor during swing.
Stance time:	The time that the foot is on the floor, measured as the time between heel strike and toe or heel off, whichever is last.
Swing time:	The time that the foot is in the air, measured as the time between toe off and heel strike.
Step time:	The time between heel strike of one foot to the subsequent heel strike of the contralateral foot.
Gait cycle or stride time:	The time between two consecutive heel strikes of the same foot.
Average gait velocity:	The stride length divided by the stride time.
Heel off time:	Moment in stance when the heel leaves the floor, measured in percent of gait cycle when the ankle angle begins to plantar flex.
Toe off time:	End of stance phase when the toe leaves the floor, measured in percent of gait cycle when the ankle angle shows maximum of plantar flexion and begins to dorsiflex.

Stride length, step length, and step width were normalized by the subject's height.

Variability of the measurements was determined using the coefficient of variation, which is defined as the standard deviation of a measurement for each subject divided by the corresponding mean value and expressed as a percentage.

indicates the normal tolerance band of mean plus or minus two standard deviations. The normal events are clear in the plots of the control subject. The ankle shows a brief plantar flexion at heel-strike, followed by a gentle dorsiflexion in stance as the body moves over the foot. The ankle then shows a brisk plantar flexion producing push-off lasting from heel-off to toe-off. During swing there is a dorsiflexion of the ankle to avoid hitting the toe on the ground and to prepare for heel-strike. The knee shows a slight flexion during stance and a more pronounced flexion during swing. The hip extends in stance and flexes during swing.

The angle/angle diagrams can best be interpreted in terms of the normal gait cycle. In the ankle/knee diagram, heel strike is at the upper right. Early stance phase is C-shaped ending at the lower right resulting from the dorsiflexion of the ankle and brief flexion of the knee. Later stance moves up and to the left with knee flexion and ankle plantarflexion. Swing phase completes the counterclockwise oval with the major movement down and to the right coming from dorsiflexion of the ankle with simultaneous knee extension. In the knee/hip diagram, heel strike is at the upper left, and the gait cycle progresses around the plot clockwise. Stance phase is located at the top of the oval and going slightly beyond, with the early dip owing to knee flexion and the general motion to the right owing to hip extension. Swing phase shows a return of the graph to the left owing to hip flexion, whereas the graph goes down and up owing to flexion and extension of the knee.

The patient graphs show marked variability compared to the control graphs. The general pattern of angular motion has the main normal characteristics, but some systematic abnormalities can be appreciated. Some events appear late, such as the push-off of the ankle and time of peak knee flexion. The knee flexion in stance is deficient. The angle/angle diagrams appear more deviant. The ankle/knee diagram is flattened out

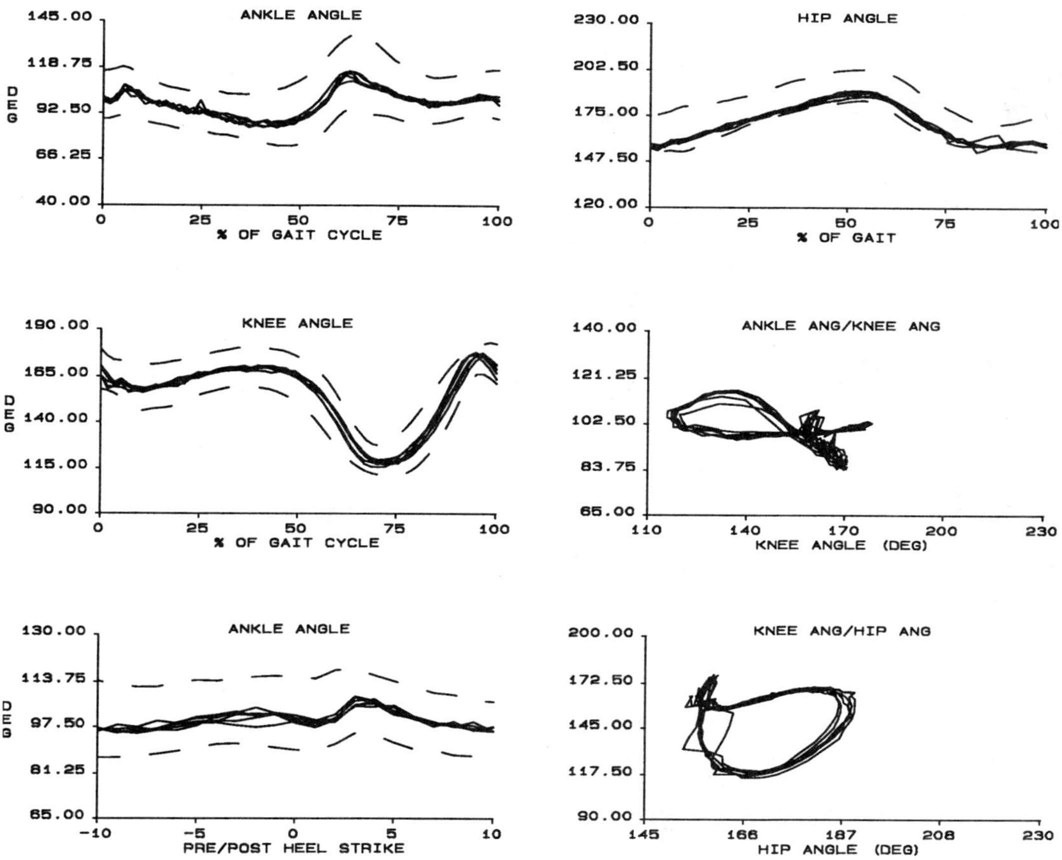

FIG. 15.1. The right-sided angular motions of a normal control subject. For joint angles versus time, single trials (*solid lines*) are superimposed with the normal confidence limits (*dashed lines*) plus or minus two standard deviations. Ankle plantarflexion (physiological extension), knee extension, and hip extension are plotted upward. For the angle/angle diagrams, single trials are superimposed. For the ankle/knee plot, increasing values are for ankle plantarflexion and knee extension. For the knee/hip plot, increasing values are for knee and hip extension. See the text for a detailed description.

because of reduced range of rotation of the ankle. Additionally, the upward movement of the graph at the onset of swing is delayed because of relatively more delay of the ankle than of the knee. The knee/hip diagram is compressed in the hip angle direction suggesting reduced hip angle range of rotation. The lower right-hand part of the oval is not as round, indicating relatively tardy knee flexion compared with hip flexion.

In quantitative terms, the first observation is that the patients are slower than the controls. Step and stride length are significantly reduced and there is a trend to reduced cadence. These factors together lead to a significant diminution of gait velocity. Events significantly delayed are heel-off time, toe-off time, and time of peak flexion of the knee in swing. All these late events could be owing to prolonged stance time in the patients for which there was a trend that just missed significance. Ankle range of rotation, knee range of rotation, knee range of rotation during stance and hip range of rotation all were reduced in the patients, but only ankle range of rotation reached significance. Despite clinical impression, there was no significant difference in step width or height that the toe was lifted from the floor in swing phase.

Patients differed significantly from controls in terms of variability of performance for virtually all measures, including step and stride length,

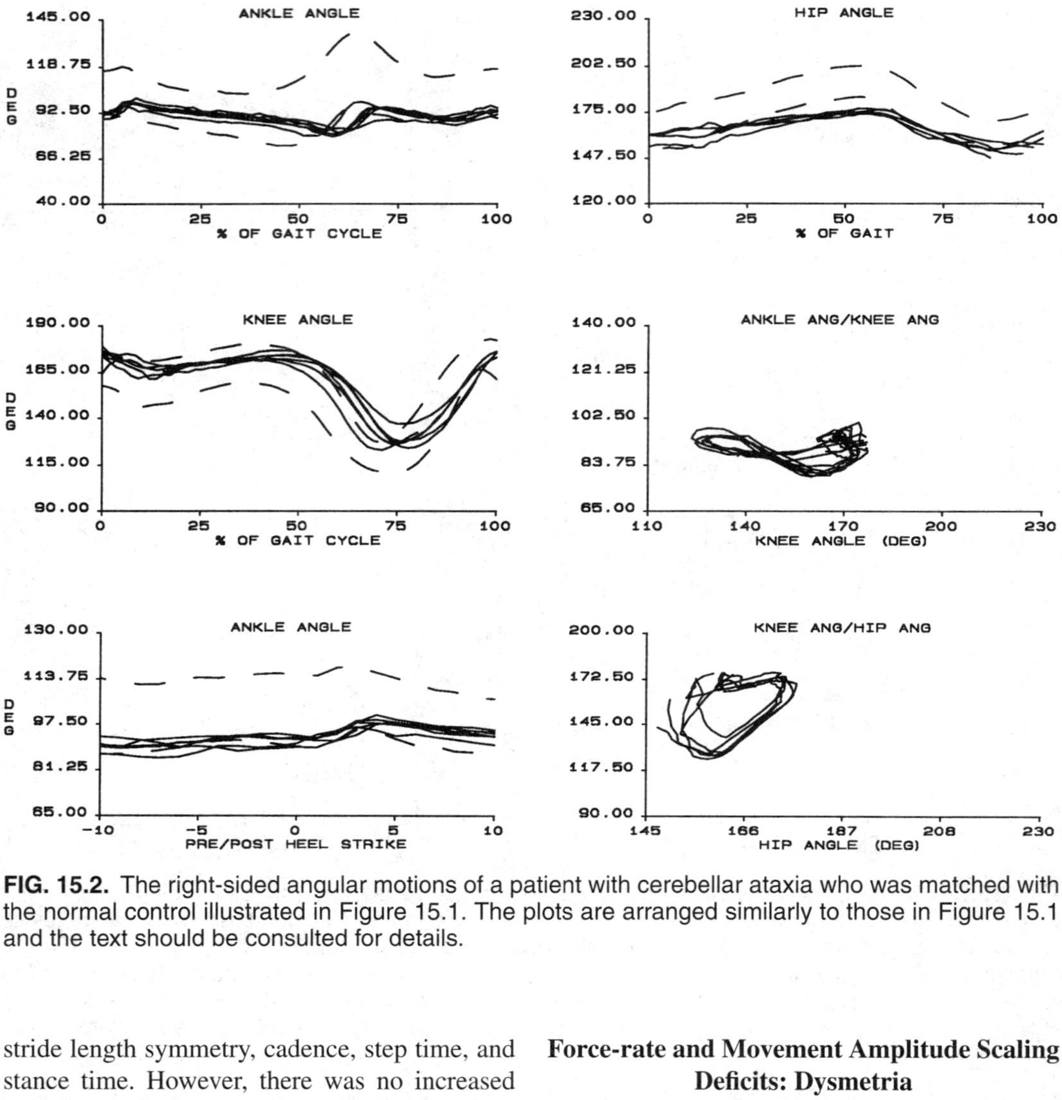

FIG. 15.2. The right-sided angular motions of a patient with cerebellar ataxia who was matched with the normal control illustrated in Figure 15.1. The plots are arranged similarly to those in Figure 15.1 and the text should be consulted for details.

stride length symmetry, cadence, step time, and stance time. However, there was no increased variability with either step width or step width symmetry. There was increased variability of ankle range of rotation, the ankle angle at heel strike and distance of the foot from the floor in swing. The knee showed increased variability with range of rotation during stance and for the time of peak flexion during swing.

MOTOR ABNORMALITIES IN CEREBELLAR DYSFUNCTION

This section is abridged and modified from Massaquoi and Hallett, where more details may be found (2).

Force-rate and Movement Amplitude Scaling Deficits: Dysmetria

Classical descriptions of cerebellar ataxia include various clinical signs such as *dysmetria, dyssynergia (asynergia, decomposition of movement), dysdiadochokinesia, dysrhythmia,* and *kinetic (intention)* and *postural tremors* (3,4). Characteristically, ataxic individuals have particular difficulty in properly generating, guiding, and terminating high-speed movements. Movements accelerate somewhat slowly and are relatively late in onset if executed in reaction to a cue. Movements may then either partially arrest prior to reaching their targets, or gradually accelerate to excessive speed and overshoot their targets to an abnormal degree. These two types of errors are examples of dysmetria, hypometria, and hypermetria, respectively. Two distinct motor control abnormalities appear to underlie dysmetria: force-rate inadequacy and step amplitude misscaling. The former causes brief, more consistent velocity-sensitive inaccuracies and the latter, more variable protracted errors.

At a fundamental level, the patient with cerebellar ataxia has difficulty changing voluntary force levels abruptly (5). Both acceleration and braking are impaired. In point-to-point movements, for example, this voluntary force-rate deficit is generally corroborated by slowness in the build-up of agonist electromyography (EMG) and a prolonged agonist action with delayed onset of antagonist EMG (6,7). In patients attempting rapid, single-joint movement, the first agonist burst is frequently prolonged regardless of the distance and speed of the movement, and the most striking kinematic abnormality is prolonged acceleration time. The pattern of acceleration time exceeding deceleration time is common in patients but uncommon in normal subjects. Duration of the first agonist burst correlates with, and is largely responsible for, acceleration time. Altered production of appropriate acceleration for rapid voluntary movements therefore may be the primary abnormality in cerebellar dysfunction for attempted rapid voluntary movements. Hypermetria would be the expected resultant movement error unless there is compensation. Hypometria has been attributed to overcompensation, asthenia in the acute setting, tremor, or failure of timely relaxation of the antagonist during movement initiation (8). Any of these mechanisms may be contributory in a given movement, and the topography of the lesion might correlate with the type of deficit (8).

For point-to-point movements of any given duration, ataxic movements exhibit greater overshoot than normal. In their study of rapid point-to-point elbow flexions, Hore and Diener noted in normal subjects a transient overshoot of about 5% to 10% of the movement distance (9). Ataxic patients overshot the target by more than 20% and as much as 35% of the movement distance. On the other hand, whenever there is no observable overshoot, the movements of ataxic individuals are usually abnormally slow or are hypometric. From the point of view of Fitts' speed-accuracy tradeoff, ataxic patients display decreased motor control bandwidth. Generally, therefore, in the assessment of ataxia it is important to note both the degree of overshoot and the movement time. Appropriate abnormality of either may be consistent with ataxia. Because, however, there may be alternative explanations for increased movement time, slowness is a much less specific finding than overshoot. Owing to the inherent tradeoff between speed and accuracy, patients often slow down intentionally in order to maintain error levels that are acceptable to them. Therefore, if it is important to observe maximal speed in a motor task, the examiner must explain that large errors are acceptable and may, in fact, be unavoidable. Even with this encouragement, the examiner is sometimes uncertain that the maximum achievable speed has been elicited.

Patients with cerebellar deficits also have abnormalities in termination of movement. This problem has been explicitly studied in a task where subjects were asked to make a rapid elbow flexion on the background of tonic elbow extension needed to hold a position against a background force (10). In this circumstance, the tonic triceps activity typically stops before the phasic biceps activity occurs (the "Hufschmidt phenomenon"). Patients with cerebellar dysfunction have a delay in terminating the triceps activity so that it overlaps the beginning of the biceps activity. This delay in stopping leads to overlap of the end of one movement with the beginning of the next.

Abnormal Control of Simple Multijoint Movements: Dyssynergia

In ataxic simple multijoint movements, such as intended straight point-to-point hand movements, there is a breakdown in the normal coordination of joint rotations. This has been termed *dyssynergia* or *asynergia* and is described as a type of *movement decomposition*. This typically causes abnormal movement path deviations. As the movements of normal subjects usually display some natural deviation from perfect linearity, abnormality in path is a matter of degree of curvature and specific pattern. Evidence is now accumulating that ataxic multijoint movements exhibit characteristic trajectory abnormalities (11). Thach et al. have attributed the pronounced ataxia seen in multijoint movements to a hypothetically preferential role for the cerebellum in the coordination of multijoint movement (12). Although the neuroanatomic organization of the cerebellum makes it particularly well-suited for coordinating muscle actions of different body parts, cerebellar function in both single and multijoint control may be fundamentally similar.

Analysis of simple, horizontal planar two-joint arm movements suggests that the deficits in acceleration and braking observed at single joints may account, at least in part, for the dyssynergia observed (6,11). It appears that the force-rate deficit may be accentuated at the joint having the greatest torque rate demand, which causes an imbalance in the joint accelerations leading to hand movement curvature. This suspected mechanism is consistent with the marked worsening of dyssynergia with increases in intended acceleration.

As noted by Holmes, ataxia may be especially apparent in multijoint movements because the control problem is more demanding. In addition to the need for forces to launch and stop, there is a requirement for rapid compensation for the disturbing effects of multiple interaction torques between body segments, as well as the need to coordinate more muscles having different individual actions. Because of the additional degrees of force and motion freedom available, failure to compensate for muscular forces and body interaction torques may lead to multidirectional path errors in addition to overall dysmetria. Indeed, several groups have specifically related multijoint trajectory errors in cerebellar ataxia to deficits in interaction torque compensation (13,14).

Several investigators have suggested other mechanisms for asynergia. Multijoint movements sometimes may be decomposed into multistep single joint movement components as a voluntary strategy to simplify programming by minimizing interaction torques between the joints (14). Dyssynergy may be owing to the general difficulties cerebellar patients have with timing tasks (15). These might yield problems with coordinating the actions of the different joints or muscles within the synergy as suggested by Thach et al. (16). From this perspective, dysmetria and dyssynergy within simple (single intended velocity peak) single and multijoint movements may have a mechanism similar to that which underlies *dysdiadochokinesia*, a disruption of compound movements involving more than one intended velocity peak (see the following).

Abnormalities in Timing and Coupling Movements and Other Processes

Ataxia also includes disruption of the normally smooth concatenation and coordination of compound movement subcomponents. This gives rise to a particular degradation of the rhythm of repetitively alternating single movements (*dysrhythmia*), and of the synchronization of single-joint movement components within repetitively alternating multijoint movements yielding *dysdiadochokinesia,* a second type of movement decomposition. Although clinical testing for dysrhythmia and dysdiadochokinesia typically employs rapidly alternating oppositely directed movements that maximize the sensitivity for detecting errors in the timing of movement onsets and offsets, timing difficulties may be noted in a variety of tasks that involve sequential movements. Bedside testing for dysrhrythmia can be performed by asking the patient to tap out a rhythm with a single-joint movement. Tests for dysdiadochokinesia include alternately slapping the palmar and dorsal surfaces of the hand on the thigh, or making rapid pincer movements of the index finger tip to the opposing midthumb crease. Accurate slapping or tapping requires precise synchronization of rotations of more than one joint (the elbow and radioulnar joints in the first case, the interphalangeal and metacarpophalangeal joints in the latter). In these two tasks, ataxic patients display both an irregular underlying rhythm and inaccurately placed contacts owing to failed multijoint coordination; therefore, dysdiadochokinesia can be seen as a combination of dysrhythmia and dyssynergia.

Thus, in multicomponent movements, considering that each subcomponent movement is subject to imprecise execution owing to simple movement control deficits discussed in the preceding, it is clear that at least some timing derangement is associated with, if not owing to, abnormal acceleration, braking, or scaling. That is, it results from serial dysmetria, as well as serial dyssynergia in the multijoint case. If a patient is asked to perform even multicomponent movements very slowly, both temporal and spatial accuracy tend to improve substantially.

In addition to timing aberrations that are associated with and in fact may result from clumsy movement execution, there appears to be a separate timing abnormality owing to failure of a cerebellum-dependent "central clock" (15). Theoretically, this clock assists in the timely launching of movements with respect to preceding movements (17,18). The same system may generally help to launch movements with respect to other events, both external and internal. In all types of reaction tasks, not only does agonist EMG build up more slowly in cerebellar patients, but also the EMG onset itself is significantly delayed with respect to the time of the stimulus, as if a triggering system were defective (18).

Increased Movement Variability

Ataxic motor performance is frequently described as being more variable than normal (1,6). However, aside from the presence of involuntary movements, ataxic variability may arise more as a consequence of enhanced susceptibility to perturbation and the sequential compounding of errors than of an inherent noise, as might result from the presence of an unstable autonomous generator.

Increased Postural Sway and Titubation

Ataxic patients exhibit increased irregular sway when standing and sometimes a more regular tremor (titubation). The increase in sway is exaggerated by loss or alteration of sensory input, and excessive sway leads to falls (19). The characteristics of sway vary according to the site of the cerebellar system lesion. Diener and Dichgans performed extensive studies of postural balance in patients with cerebellar system disease (20,21). Common to all ataxic patients except those with lesions restricted to the hemispheres is the tendency to have abnormally large amplitude sway when the eyes are closed. Patients with anterior lobe atrophy owing to chronic alcohol intake and malnutrition, and patients with Friedreich's ataxia have a high "Romberg quotient," meaning that they sway considerably more with eyes closed. In general, the eyes-closed instability is greater in Friedreich's patients, who typically have significant proprioceptive loss and may fall without vision. By contrast, anterior lobe lesion patients tend to oscillate markedly without falling when their eyes are closed. Patients with anterior lobe damage also tend to move much more in an anteroposterior direction, whereas those with Friedreich's ataxia have an abnormal degree of lateral sway.

Patients with vestibulocerebellar lesions display increased, omnidirectional, low frequency (approximately 1 Hz) sway and may fall with eyes both open and closed, and therefore have a normal Romberg quotient. Patients that have hemispheric lesions may exhibit slightly increased sway relative to normal subjects, but balance instability is not prominent. Those with diffuse cerebellar damage exhibit a mixture of characteristics. They may be differentiated from normal subjects, but not from each other on the basis of posturography.

In addition to low frequency (approximately 1 Hz) sway, a characteristic 2- to 3-Hz body tremor is seen exclusively in patients with anterior lobe dysfunction when the eyes are closed. Unlike the irregular head and trunk titubation that may be seen with various other cerebellar lesions, the anterior lobe tremor consists of regular anteroposterior oscillation at the head, hip, and ankle. The hip is 180 degrees out of phase with the head so that the center of gravity moves little and balance is maintained despite marked titubation. This tremor has been attributed to increased duration and amplitude of long-latency stretch responses. These long-latency responses are likely to be the scalable, secondary responses observed by Horak and Diener following exaggerated postural responses (22). Although abnormally large, these responses eventually stabilize the body after a few decaying oscillations at about 2- to 3-Hz when the eyes are open. Presumably, persistent titubation occurs especially with eyes closed because the gain of these scalable responses is increased in an effort to compensate for the loss of visual input. This is consistent with the view of titubation as a postural tremor.

INTERPRETATION OF GAIT RESULTS

The gait of patients with cerebellar dysfunction is characterized by stumbling, scraping the toe, lurching to one side, and falls. Because such performance cannot be captured and quantified easily, the data we have analyzed represent the best performance of the patients and not their average performance. The patients walked slower than the matched controls, usually as a result of reduced step length, but there was also a trend toward a slower cadence. Slowness characterizes limb movement in patients with cerebellar dysfunction and certainly some is because of prolongation of EMG burst patterns required for movement, but the majority of the slowness is probably because of compensation (6,7). Balance is poor in these patients, and the movements while walking and the need to periodically balance on one foot stress the system (19,20). Slowing down should make the balance problem less severe. Compensatory slowness of walking is seen in most neurological conditions affecting the motor system.

Some of the "abnormalities" observed here are simple consequences of slowness of walking. Slowing down will increase the percent of the gait cycle devoted to stance (23). This is certainly the main explanation of the delayed rotations of the ankle and knee. Other abnormalities, including reduced flexion of the knee in stance and decreased range of rotation at the ankle, are less likely to be ascribed to slowness of walking. Reduced knee flexion in stance and decreased ankle range of rotation might reflect a regression to earlier stages of ontogeny of locomotion as described by Forssberg and colleagues (24).

We were unable to demonstrate a wide base while walking despite the clinical impression of this and the fact that these patients prefer to stand with a widened base of support. A wide base is likely of less value when walking than when standing still.

An analysis of interjoint coordination, illustrated with the angle/angle diagrams, reveals problems that are not immediately apparent by looking at one joint at a time. For example, the diagrams showed that there was relative delay of plantar flexion of the ankle compared with knee flexion at the end of stance and relative delay of knee flexion to hip flexion at the onset of swing. This is likely because of the difficulty patients with cerebellar dysfunction have in coordinating multijoint movement (11,14).

The variability of even the best performances of the patients is a principal abnormality. Although increased variability may characterize all movement disorders, it is particularly marked in cerebellar dysfunction. This variability is clearly the source of problems in gait. For example, even though the foot on average clears the floor with a good distance, the variability is such that the foot will hit the floor on some occasions.

REFERENCES

1. Palliyath S, Hallett M, Thomas SL, et al. Gait in patients with cerebellar ataxia. *Mov Disord* 1998;13:958–964.
2. Massaquoi SG, Hallett M. Ataxia and other cerebellar syndromes. In: Jankovic J, Tolosa E, eds. *Parkinson's disease and movement disorders*, 3rd ed. Baltimore: Williams & Wilkins, 1998:623–686.
3. Holmes G. The cerebellum of man. *Brain* 1939;62:1–30.
4. Gilman S, Bloedel JR, Lechtenberg R. *Disorders of the cerebellum*. Philadelphia: FA Davis, 1981.
5. Mai N, Bolsinger P, Avarello M, et al. Control of isometric finger force in patients with cerebellar disease. *Brain* 1988;111:973–998.
6. Hallett M, Massaquoi S. Physiologic studies of dysmetria in patients with cerebellar deficits. *Can J Neurol Sci* 1993;20:S83–S89.
7. Hallett M, Berardelli A, Matheson J, et al. Physiological analysis of simple rapid movements in patients with cerebellar deficits. *J Neurol Neurosurg Psychiatry* 1991;53:124–133.
8. Manto MU, Setta F, Jacquy J, et al. Different types of cerebellar hypometria associated with a distinct topography of the lesion in cerebellum. *J Neurol Sci* 1998;158:88–95.
9. Hore J, Wild B, Diener HC. Cerebellar dysmetria at the elbow, wrist, and fingers. *J Neurophysiol* 1991;65:563–571.
10. Hallett M, Shahani BT, Young RR. EMG analysis of patients with cerebellar deficits. *J Neurol Neurosurg Psychiatry* 1975;38:1163–1169.
11. Massaquoi S, Hallett M. Kinematics of initiating a

two–joint arm movement in patients with cerebellar ataxia. *Can J Neurol Sci* 1996;23:3–14.
12. Thach WT, Perry JG, Kane SA, et al. Cerebellar nuclei: rapid alternating movement, motor somatotopy, and a mechanism for the control of muscle synergy. *Rev Neurol (Paris)* 1993;149:607–628.
13. Topka H, Konczak J, Schneider K, et al. Multijoint arm movements in cerebellar ataxia: abnormal control of movement dynamics. *Exp Brain Res* 1998;119:493–503.
14. Bastian AJ, Martin TA, Keating JG, et al. Cerebellar ataxia. Abnormal control of interaction torques across multiple joints. *J Neurophysiol* 1996;76:492–509.
15. Keele SW, Ivry R. Does the cerebellum provide a common computation for diverse tasks? A timing hypothesis. *Ann NY Acad Sci* 1990;608:179–207.
16. Thach WT, Goodkin HP, Keating JG. The cerebellum and the adaptive coordination of movement. *Annu Rev Neurosci* 1992;15:403–442.
17. Diener HC, Hore J, Ivry R, et al. Cerebellar dysfunction of movement and perception. *Can J Neurol Sci* 1993;20:S62–S69.
18. Grill SE, Hallett M, McShane LM. Timing of onset of afferent responses and of use of kinesthetic information for control of movement in normal and cerebellar-impaired subjects. *Exp Brain Res* 1997;113:33–47.
19. Gatev P, Thomas S, Lou J-S, et al. Effects of diminished and conflicting sensory information on balance in patients with cerebellar deficits. *Mov Disord* 1996;11:654–664.
20. Diener HC, Dichgans J, Bacher M, et al. Quantification of postural sway in normals and patients with cerebellar diseases. *Electroencephalogr Clin Neurophysiol* 1984;57:134–142.
21. Diener HC, Dichgans J. Pathophysiology of cerebellar ataxia. *Mov Disord* 1992;7:95–109.
22. Horak FB, Diener HC. Cerebellar control of postural scaling and central set in stance. *J Neurophysiol* 1994;72:479–493.
23. Winter DA. *The biomechanics and motor control of human gait: normal, elderly and pathological*, 2nd ed. Waterloo: University of Waterloo Press, 1991.
24. Forssberg H, Hirschfeld H, Stokes VP. Development of human locomotor mechanisms. In: Shimamura M, Grillner S, Edgerton VR, eds. *Neurobiological basis of human locomotion*. Tokyo: Japan Scientific Societies Press, 1991:259–273.

Gait Disorders. Advances in Neurology, Vol. 87,
edited by E. Růžička, M. Hallett, and J. Jankovic.
Lippincott Williams & Wilkins, Philadelphia © 2001.

16

Vestibulopathic Gait

Walking and Running

Thomas Brandt, Michael Strupp, Judy Benson, and Marianne Dieterich

Department of Neurology, Ludwig-Maximilians University, Grosshadern Clinic, 81377 Munich, Germany

The first part of this chapter deals with typical peripheral or central vestibular syndromes and their impact on balance control during static posture and gait. In the second part, we report our preliminary and hypothetical reflections on the seemingly paradoxical observation that running is safer than slow walking in cases of acute vestibulopathy.

Vestibular dysfunction is a significant differential diagnosis in patients who present with falls or weaving, veering, and toppling gaits that occur without concurrent unconsciousness, paresis, sensory loss, or cerebellar deficit. Clinically, peripheral or central vestibular syndromes are commonly characterized by a combination of vertigo, nystagmus, postural imbalance, and nausea. These four manifestations correlate with different aspects of vestibular function. The vertigo itself results from a disturbance of cortical spatial orientation. Nystagmus is secondary to a direction-specific imbalance in the vestibulo-ocular reflex, which activates brainstem neuronal circuitry. Postural imbalance is caused by inappropriate or abnormal activation of monosynaptic or polysynaptic vestibulospinal pathways. Finally, the unpleasant vegetative effects of nausea and vomiting are caused by activation of the medullary vomiting center.

Basically there are three types of vestibular dysfunction. Each has typical key signs and symptoms that help to establish the correct diagnosis of patients with vestibulopathic gaits.

BILATERAL VESTIBULAR LOSS

Key symptoms of bilateral vestibular loss (congenital or acquired bilateral vestibular failure) are oscillopsia associated with head movements (owing to the defective vestibulo-ocular reflex) and unsteadiness of gait, particularly in the dark or on unlevel ground (when visual and somatosensory input cannot substitute for the missing vestibulospinal control). These patients typically have no complaints when standing still and not moving the head. Diagnosis is made by a bedside test for defective vestibulo-ocular reflex and by the absence of nystagmic reaction to both caloric and rotatory pendular testing.

VESTIBULAR TONE IMBALANCE

Key symptoms of vestibular tone imbalance (acute unilateral lesions of the labyrinth, vestibular nerve, or central vestibular pathways) are rotatory vertigo or perceived body tilt with spontaneous nystagmus, ocular torsion, or skew deviation associated with a direction-specific deviation of gait and body falls (because of the lesion-induced vestibular tone imbalance). A lesion-induced vestibular tone imbalance typically manifests as an acute syndrome that slowly and gradually resolves within days to weeks either by central compensation or healing of the lesion. Diagnosis is made on the basis of a combination of perceptual, ocular motor, and postural signs and symptoms. The direction of nystagmus or deviation of posture and gait indicates that the particular tone imbalance occurs in one of the three major planes of action of the vestibular system (yaw, pitch, or roll).

Vestibular neuritis is a clinical prototype of acute unilateral vestibulopathy, which causes a vestibular tone imbalance. In vestibular neuritis the fast phase of the spontaneous rotational nystagmus and the initial perception of apparent body motion are directed away from the side of the lesion, and the postural reactions initiated by vestibulospinal reflexes are usually in a direction opposite to that of vertigo. These reactions result in both the Romberg fall and past pointing toward the side of the lesion. Patients with this type of vertigo often make confusing and contradictory statements about the direction of their symptoms. There are, in fact, two sensations that are opposite in direction, and the patient may be describing either one (Fig. 16.1). The first is the purely subjective sense of self-motion in the direction of the nystagmus fast phases, which is not associated with any measurable body sway. The second is the "compensatory" vestibulospinal reaction, which results in objective, measurable postural destabilization, deviation of gait, and a possible Romberg fall in the direction opposite to the fast phases.

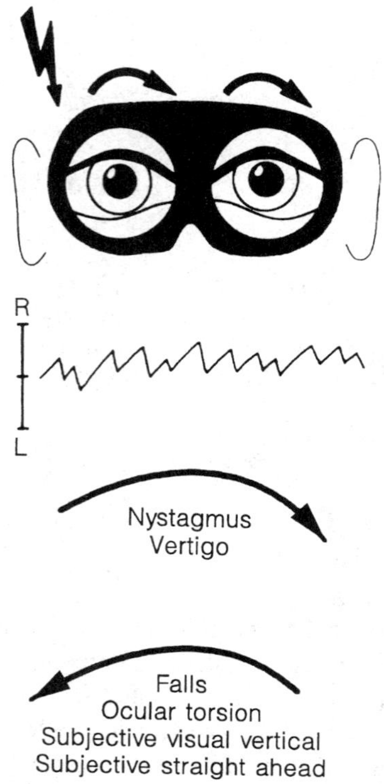

FIG. 16.1. Ocular signs, perception, and postural deviation in the acute stage of right-sided vestibular neuritis. Spontaneous vestibular nystagmus is always horizontal-rotatory away from the side of the lesion (best observed with Frenzel's glasses). The initial perception of apparent body motion (vertigo) is also directed away from the side of the lesion, whereas measurable destabilization (Romberg fall) is always toward the side of the lesion. The latter is the compensatory vestibulospinal reaction to the apparent tilt. The same is true for adjustments of perceived visual vertical and subjective straight ahead.

VESTIBULAR ATTACK

Key symptoms of vestibular attack (paroxysmal stimulation of the vestibular system) include attacks of vertigo, ocular motor dysfunction, and postural imbalance. These symptoms may occur spontaneously (basilar migraine, paroxysmal vertigo of childhood, episodic ataxia type I or II, epilepsy) or be elicited by changes in head position (benign paroxysmal positioning vertigo, vestibular paroxysmia). Carefully taking the patient's history, clinical examination, and testing of the vestibular function may determine the different etiologies of these attacks. The direction-specific perceptual, ocular motor, and postural signs and symptoms during the attack indicate the particular vestibular structure involved. The neuro-ophthalmological findings during the attack-free interval and the possible triggers such as changes in head position help to identify the mechanism and etiology. These three basic vestibular dysfunctions—bilateral vestibular loss, vestibular tone imbalance, vestibular attacks—clearly differ from each other. In bilateral vestibular failure, unsteadiness is only obvious in darkness and on unlevel ground; in acute unilateral lesions, the vestibular tone imbalance slowly improves over time; and in paroxysmal vestibular stimulation, vestibulopathic gait occurs as acute attacks rather than continuously.

TABLE 16.1. *Peripheral vestibular falls*

Disorder	Direction	Mechanism
Vestibular neuritis	Lateral Ipsiversive	Vestibular tone imbalance (yaw, roll) due to horizontal and anterior canal (and utricle) paresis
Benign paroxysmal positioning vertigo (BPPV)	Forward Ipsiversive	Ampullofugal stimulation of posterior canal by canalolithiasis and a heavy clot-induced endolymph flow
Menière's drop attacks (Tumarkin's otolithic crisis)	Vertical (Down)	Loss of postural tone due to abnormal otolith stimulation in sudden endolymphatic fluid pressure changes
Otolith Tullio phenomenon	Backward Contraversive (Diagonal)	Sound-induced mechanical stimulation of utricle by luxated stapes footplate
Vestibular paroxysmia	Forward Contraversive Multidirectional	Neurovascular cross-compression causing ephaptic stimulation of vestibular nerve
Bilateral vestibulopathy	Multidirectional Fore-aft	Impaired (vestibulospinal) postural reflexes particularly in darkness

DIFFERENTIATION OF PERIPHERAL AND CENTRAL VESTIBULAR DISORDERS

Peripheral and central vestibular pathways run from the labyrinths via vestibular and ocular motor nuclei to the thalamus and vestibular cortex. Thus, both peripheral and central vestibular disorders cause postural instability, which results in falls in characteristic directions (Tables 16.1 and 16.2). Some of these characteristic directions can be attributed either to the particular plane of the affected semicircular canal or to a central pathway that mediates the three-dimensional vestibulo-ocular reflex in yaw, pitch, and roll (1–2). Ipsiversive lateral falls occur in vestibular neuritis or in Wallenberg's syndrome, where they are known as lateropulsion (3). Contraversive falls are typical for the otolith Tullio phenomenon, vestibular epilepsy,

TABLE 16.2. *Central vestibular falls*

Disorder	Direction	Mechanism
Vestibular epilepsy	Contraversive	Simple or complex partial seizures due to epileptic discharges of vestibular cortex
Thalamic astasia	Contraversive or ipsiversive	Vestibular tone imbalance (yaw, roll) in posterolateral vestibular thalamic lesions
Ocular tilt reaction	Contraversive in pontomesencephalic lesions Ipsiversive in pontomedullary lesions	Tone imbalance of VOR[a] in roll due to lesions of otolith and vertical canal pathways
Paroxysmal ocular tilt reaction	Ipsiversive with pontomesencephalic stimulation Contraversive with peripheral vestibular stimulation	Pathological excitation of otolith and vertical canal pathways mediating VOR[a] in roll
Lateropulsion (Wallenberg's syndrome)	Ipsiversive Diagonal	Lesion-induced tone imbalance of VOR[a] in roll and yaw with concurrent deviation of subjective vertical
Downbeat nystagmus/vertigo	Backward	Lesional vestibular tone imbalance of the VOR[a] in pitch

[a] VOR, vestibulo-ocular reflex

TABLE 16.3. *Typical signs and symptoms suggesting vestibular unsteadiness or falls in disorders of the peripheral or central vestibular system*

Signs/symptoms	Lesion sites (disorder)
Peripheral vestibular system	
Unsteadiness of gait, particularly in the dark or on unlevel ground, and oscillopsia associated with head movements or when walking	Both labyrinths or vestibular nerves (bilateral vestibular failure)
Ipsiversive falls with contraversive spontaneous nystagmus, rotational vertigo, and nausea	Acute unilateral peripheral vestibular loss (vestibular neuritis; MS plaque or lacunar infarctions at root entry zone of eighth nerve)
Paroxysmal loss of postural tone with unexpected falls without impaired consciousness	Labyrinths (vestibular drop attacks, Menière's disease)
Paroxysmal lateral and forward falls with rotational vertigo and nystagmus elicited by head extension or lateral head tilt	Posterior semicircular canal ipsilateral to the direction of fall (benign paroxysmal positional vertigo)
Episodic vertigo with postural imbalance, nystagmus, nausea, tinnitus, and fluctuating hearing loss	Labyrinth (Menière's disease)
Frequent spells of postural instability, dizziness, tinnitus, and hearing loss elicited or modulated by changes in head position	Neurovascular cross-compression of the eighth nerve (vestibular paroxysmia; disabling positional vertigo)
Central vestibular system	
Paroxysmal vertigo and/or ataxia with ocular motor deficiencies (also in the attack-free interval) and associated headache	Brainstem, cerebellum, labyrinth (basilar migraine)
Paroxysmal ataxia and dysarthria	Brainstem (paroxysmal attacks in MS)
Paroxysmal lateral or rotational falls with vertigo (nystagmus) and impaired consciousness	Parieto-insular vestibular cortex (vestibular epilepsy)
Episodic familial ataxia (with or without vertigo) with nystagmus or myokymia	Brainstem, cerebellum (familial episodic ataxias)
Fore-aft instability with vertical nystagmus	Ponto-medullary or ponto-mesencephalic-brainstem, or bilateral floccular lesions (downbeat/upbeat nystagmus)
Lateral instability or falls with tilts of perceived vertical and ocular skew deviation (without vertigo, paresis, or cerebellar ataxia)	Ponto-medullary or ponto-mesencephalic brainstem, midbrain tegmentum, vestibular thalamus, vestibular cortex (lateropulsion in Wallenberg's syndrome, or in vestibular cortex lesions, thalamic astasia)

and thalamic astasia (4). A predominantly fore-aft instability is observed in bilateral vestibulopathy, benign paroxysmal positioning vertigo, as well as in downbeat or upbeat nystagmus syndrome. Falls can be diagonally forward (or backward) and toward or away from the side of the lesion, depending on its site (the ocular tilt reaction is ipsiversive in medullary lesions, but contraversive in mesencephalic lesion; and on whether vestibular structures are excited or inhibited (2,5).

Although the majority of vestibular syndromes with imbalance of posture and gait are caused by a lesion-induced dysfunction, a considerable proportion result from pathological excitation of various structures (Table 16.3). Examples are otolith Tullio phenomenon, vestibular paroxysmia (cross-compression of the eighth nerve, disabling positional vertigo), paroxysmal dysarthria, and ataxia in multiple sclerosis or vestibular epilepsy. The particular pathological mechanisms that provoke postural instability and may cause vestibular falls differ greatly, because they can result from changes in otolith or in horizontal or vertical semicircular canal function.

Central vestibular syndromes can manifest with the complete syndrome of vertigo, nystagmus, postural imbalance, and nausea if lesions of the root entry zone of the eighth nerve or the vestibular nuclei cause them. Other lesions of the central vestibular pathways may induce different combinations of vertigo, perceived tilt, ocular motor disorders, unsteadiness, or vestibular falls. Central vestibular disorders are also frequently associated with nonvestibular syndromes, such as cerebellar brainstem, thalamic, or cortical signs. Table 16.3 lists typical constellations of signs and symptoms that should suggest either a peripheral or central vestibular origin for disorders of posture and gait that are not explained by paresis, sensory loss, or cerebellar dysfunction.

YOU ARE BETTER OFF RUNNING THAN WALKING WITH ACUTE VESTIBULOPATHY

Our recent finding that patients with acute vestibular disorders balance better when running than walking slowly led us to suggest that the automatic spinal locomotor program suppresses destabilizing vestibular input (6).

If an acute unilateral peripheral vestibular failure causes a distressing vestibular tone imbalance, the afflicted subjects move slowly, grasp searchingly for support, or must be guided in order to correct for their deviating gait and lateral falls. Slow motion is commonly believed to be much safer for these patients than fast motion. When walking slowly, the area of foot support is larger (both feet on the ground) than when running (one foot on the ground at a time). Thus, one would expect balance control to rely more on the actual vestibular input during running.

A chance observation of a dog, however, with acute left unilateral vestibular failure showed us that running is safer (6). After awakening one day, the dog suddenly showed a severe postural imbalance and repeatedly fell to the left. When she stood still, head movements caused the falls. When walking slowly, she veered to the left, staggered about in counterclockwise circles, and repeatedly fell. Surprisingly, once the dog was outside and began to trot, she was suddenly able to move without deviating from her course and obviously felt better and more confident as her raised, wagging tail indicated. However, as soon as she stopped trotting and began to slowly walk, she again showed the severe tendency to deviate from her intended path and fell to the left.

Neurological examination of the dog revealed a spontaneous nystagmus to the right and an ocular tilt reaction to the left (7,8). The high frequency head rotation test revealed a defective vestibulo-ocular reflex, best explained by an acute unilateral vestibular failure (9).

This observation prompted us to video record the balance during walking and running of patients with acute unilateral vestibulopathy and healthy volunteers with a postrotatory transient vestibular tone imbalance (6). Four patients (all women, aged 57 to 67 years) had a confirmed diagnosis of vestibular neuritis. Three to 5 days after the onset of the condition, they were requested to close their eyes and slowly walk or run 10 m through a 2.5-m wide corridor. All touched the wall for support two to four times during the 10-m stretch. In contrast, when running slowly, they maintained their direction for over 10 m and felt much more secure (Fig. 16.2). Increased walking speed also had a clearly stabilizing influence on their balance.

Ten blindfolded, healthy physical therapists (five women; mean age 26.5 [SD 3.7] years) were suddenly stopped after ten rotations in a chair at a constant angular velocity of 360 degrees/sec. They were then asked to either walk slowly or run straight ahead for 10 m. There was a mean deviation when they walked of 52.6 (12.4) degrees over 10 m (Fig. 16.3). In contrast, the mean deviation was 14.6 (9.2) degrees when they ran. All volunteers also felt it was easier to maintain their balance while running. There was, however, no difference in mean deviations for walking or running when the patients or subjects walked or ran in place without locomotion.

AUTOMATIC SPINAL LOCOMOTOR PATTERN LARGELY INDEPENDENT OF ACTUAL VESTIBULAR INPUT

All three observations of dog, patients, and volunteers after body rotation demonstrate that an acute vestibular tone imbalance has less effect

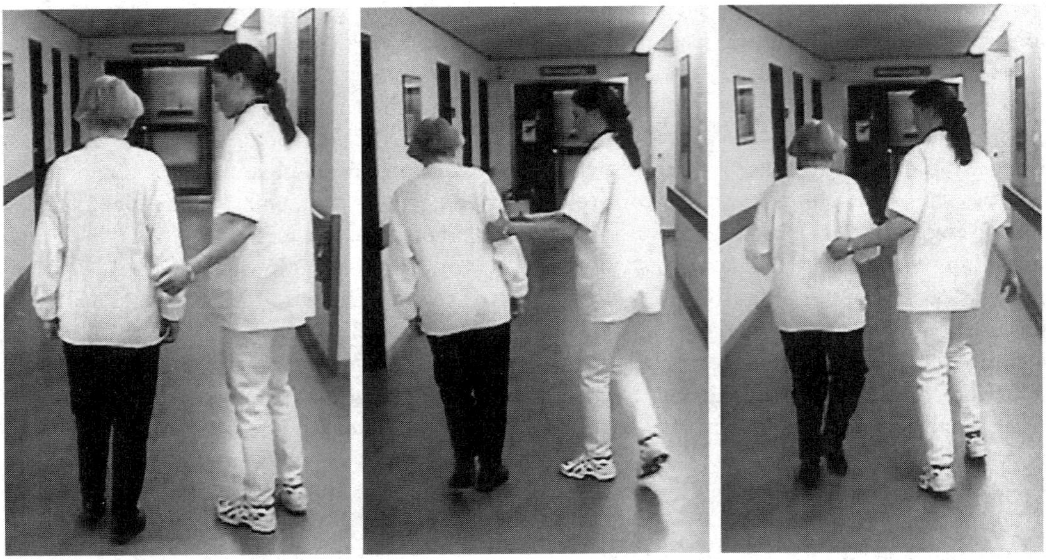

FIG. 16.2. Posture and gait of a 66-year-old patient on day 4 after an acute vestibular neuritis of the left ear (taken from a video sequence). With her eyes closed, she was able to maintain balance by increasing her body sway **(left)**. If she tried to walk in a straight line, her gait showed a marked deviation toward the affected ear and there were lateral falls **(middle)**. She found it easier to run straight ahead with eyes closed without touching the wall **(right)**.

on balance and the direction of locomotion if the individual runs rather than slowly walks. This apparent paradox is unlikely to have a simple explanation such as increased speed causes a mechanical stabilization of balance ("gyrocompass phenomenon"). Moreover, the same difference in balance and direction during walking or running was observed regardless of whether the subjects swung their arms spontaneously, which should aid balance, or held them close to the body. All three examples also show that locomotion is largely independent of the actual control of the vestibular system, especially active linear path integration.

Earlier reports in the literature also demonstrate that the actual control of the vestibular system can be bypassed. For example, blindfolded patients with bilateral vestibular failure are able to perform linear goal-directed locomotion toward memorized targets (10). Automatic locomotor patterns have been found in the chronic spinal cat and in paraplegic patients whose body weight was partially unloaded during suspension from a parachute harness connected to an overhead crane while walking on a moving treadmill (11,12). This spinal locomotor activity was induced only after signs of spinal shock had disappeared, and it was distinct from spinal stretch reflex activity (13).

A functional interpretation of the observation that you are better off running than walking with acute vestibulopathy would argue that an automatic spinal program of locomotion triggers the inhibition of descending vestibular sensory inflow. This explanation would agree with the recently proposed concept of sensory down-and-up channeling for multisensory postural control. According to this theory, the vestibular organ is the body's sensor of position, that is, it receives the "body-in-space" signals (down channeling), and the somatosensory system measures the joint angles, that is, it receives the "support-in-space-tilt" signals (up channeling) (14). In our examples, the ascending rather than the descending signals would define the desired value for the joints to control posture. A misleading vestibular signal could thus be suppressed via down-and-up channeling.

Further evidence in the literature supports this functional interpretation. Like the vestibular

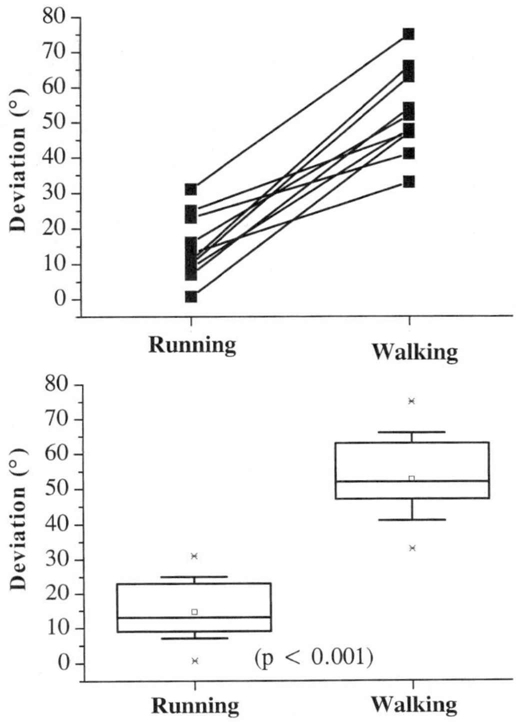

FIG. 16.3. Deviation of gait during running versus walking in volunteers with a transient physiological vestibular tone imbalance. Ten healthy blindfolded subjects were asked to either slowly walk or run 10 m straight ahead after being suddenly stopped out of a constant velocity body rotation of 360 degrees/sec. Individual deviation in degrees was consistently less when running **(top)**; mean deviation when running was 14.6 ± 9.2 degrees and when walking 52.6 ± 12.4 degrees (paired *t*-test, $P < 0.001$). *Open square,* mean; *horizontal lines of the box,* 25th, 50th, and 75th percentiles; *error bars above and below the boxes,* 5th and 95th percentiles; *crosses,* range. (Modified from Brandt T et al., 1999.)

system, the somatosensory system can also be inhibited. Monosynaptic stretch reflex responses in the human leg, for example, are suppressed and spinal pathways of group I afferents are blocked during gait (15). Moreover, muscular sense was reported to be attenuated when humans move (16). This finding is consistent with a general attenuation of sensory feedback, which occurs during movement and locomotion.

The multisensory–sensorimotor interaction necessary for postural control is, thus, not a simple fusion, but rather a complex of different processes that are fine-tuned by repetition and learning. How they interact is influenced not only by the pattern of actual motion stimulation, but also by the particular postural and locomotor tasks. This is reflected by the differential effects of an actual vestibular tone imbalance on slow walking and running as well as on walking and running in place without locomotion. Control of slow walking obviously depends on afferent and reafferent sensory input to a larger extent than does fast walking or running. It makes sense to suppress the vestibular (or somatosensory) input once a highly automatic motor pattern of fast walking or running has been initiated. Otherwise, the reafferent sensory stimulations caused by head and joint motion during locomotion would interfere, acting like adverse feedback, and modify an already optimized automatic program.

These findings on the differential effects of an acute vestibulopathy on walking or running may have important consequences for the physical therapy and rehabilitation of patients with vestibulopathic gait.

REFERENCES

1. Brandt T, Dieterich M. Vestibular falls. *J Vestib Res* 1993;3:3–14.
2. Brandt T, Dieterich M. Vestibular syndromes in the roll plane: topographic diagnosis from brainstem to cortex. *Ann Neurol* 1994;36:337–347.
3. Bjerner K, Silfverskiöld BP. Lateropulsion and imbalance in Wallenberg's syndrome. *Acta Neurol Scand* 1968;44:91–100.
4. Masdeu JC, Gorelick PB. Thalamic astasia: inability to stand after unilateral thalamic lesions. *Ann Neurol* 1988;23:596–603.
5. Lueck CJ, Hamlyn P, Crawford TJ, et al. A case of ocular tilt reaction and torsional nystagmus due to direct stimulation of the midbrain in man. *Brain* 1991;114:2069–2079.
6. Brandt T, Strupp M, Benson J. You are better off running than walking with acute vestibulopathy. *Lancet* 1999;354:746.
7. Westheimer G, Blair SM. *Synkinese der Augen- und Kopfbewegungen bei Hirnstammreizungen am wachen Macacus-Affen. Exp Brain Res* 1975;24:89–95.
8. Brandt T. *Vertigo: its multisensory syndromes*, 2nd ed. London: Springer, 1999.
9. Halmagyi GM, Curthoys IS. A clinical sign of canal paresis. *Arch Neurol* 1988;45:737–739.
10. Glasauer S, Amorim M-A, Vitte E, et al. Goal-directed

linear locomotion in normal and labyrinthine-defective subjects. *Exp Brain Res* 1994;98:323–335.
11. Grillner S. Control of locomotion in bipeds, tetrapeds, and fish. In: Brookhart M, Mountcastle M, eds. *Handbook of physiology. The nervous system II*. Washington, DC: American Physiological Society, 1981:1179–1235.
12. Dietz V, Colombo G, Jensen L. Locomotor activity in spinal man. *Lancet* 1994;344:1260–1263.
13. Dietz V, Wirz M, Curt A, et al. Locomotor pattern in paraplegic patients: training effects and recovery of spinal cord function. *Spinal Cord* 1998;36:380–390.
14. Mergner T, Rosemeier T. Interaction of vestibular, somatosensory and visual signals for postural control and motion perception under terrestrial and microgravity conditions—a conceptual model. *Brain Res Brain Res Rev* 1998;28:118–135.
15. Dietz V. Afferent and efferent control of posture and gait. In: Bles W, Brandt TH, eds. *Disorders of posture and gait*. Amsterdam: Elsevier, 1986:69–81.
16. Collins DF, Cameron T, Gillard DM, et al. Muscular sense is attenuated when humans move. *J Physiol (Lond)* 1998;508:635–643.

Gait Disorders. Advances in Neurology, Vol. 87,
edited by E. Růžička, M. Hallett, and J. Jankovic.
Lippincott Williams & Wilkins, Philadelphia © 2001.

17
Postural Ataxia Related to Somatosensory Loss

Fay B. Horak

Neurological Sciences Institute, Oregon Health Sciences University, Beaverton, Oregon 97006

ATAXIA OF POSTURE AND GAIT RELATED TO SOMATOSENSORY LOSS

Sensory-motor mechanisms responsible for postural and gait ataxia in patients with loss of somatosensory information are not well understood. The ataxic movements themselves have not been well quantified and the role of somatosensory information for balance, spatial orientation, and locomotion is controversial (1,2). Ataxia can result from sensory neuropathy that distorts, delays, and/or eliminates somatosensory information from proprioceptors in muscles and joints and from superficial and deep cutaneous receptors (3,4). This chapter summarizes studies of postural responses during stance in patients with loss of somatosensory information that reveal the importance of somatosensory information for: (a) triggering postural responses to external perturbations, (b) scaling responses to the magnitude of perturbations, (c) activating anticipatory postural adjustments specific to voluntary movements, and (d) limiting postural sway in stance.

Despite the important contribution of somatosensory information to normal balance and gait, many patients with sensory neuropathy compensate well enough to allow independent stance and ambulation, although falls are 23 times higher than in healthy controls (5,6). Recent studies in our laboratory show that postural compensation for somatosensory loss involves increased use of predictive mechanisms, substitution of haptic information from a hand in contact with a stable surface, and increased sensitivity to vestibular information for postural control (7–10). This chapter reviews studies from our laboratory of patients who have abnormal and diminished somatosensory information in the legs and trunk because of viral, generalized polyneuropathy, diabetic peripheral neuropathy, and multiple sclerosis (MS) to demonstrate the importance of somatosensory information for postural control and to show how patients compensate for their somatosensory loss to control balance in stance.

SOMATOSENSORY INFORMATION IS CRITICAL FOR TRIGGERING THE ONSET AND SCALING THE MAGNITUDE OF POSTURAL RESPONSES

Although vision and vestibular information make important contributions to control of posture, proprioception is the first line of defense in responding to unexpected external perturbations. Thus, loss of somatosensory, but not visual or vestibular, information results in significant delays and/or reduction of postural responses (2). Initial postural responses are normally triggered in a distal-to-proximal pattern in leg muscles at 70 to 120 ms after the onset of a surface perturbation in standing, healthy subjects (11). Figure 17.1A shows the normal EMG responses in gastrocnemius, hamstrings, and paraspinal muscles in a representative healthy subject to forward sway induced by a backward surface translation.

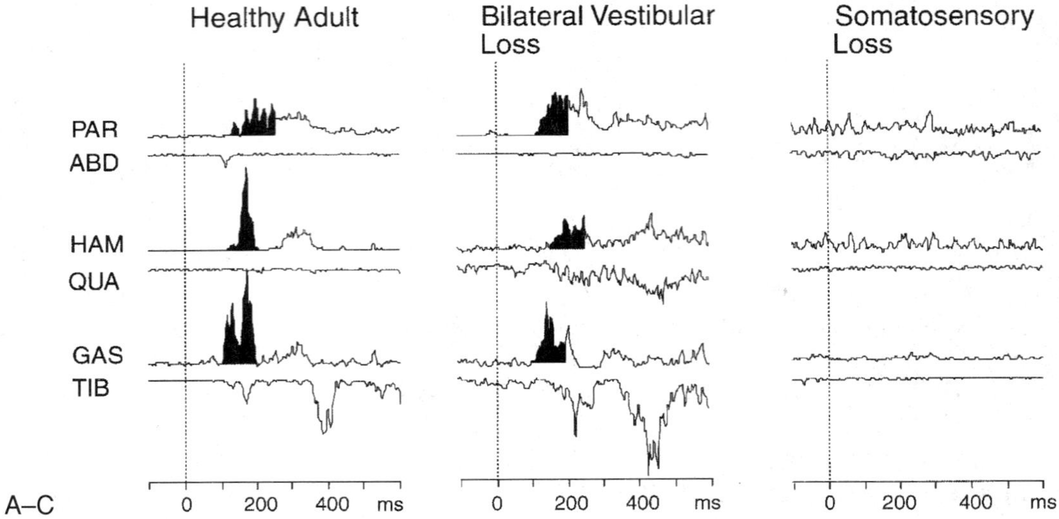

FIG. 17.1. Normal postural response in a healthy control subject **(A)** and a subject with profound, bilateral loss of vestibular function **(B)** compared with absent postural response in a subject with total body somatosensory loss **(C)**. Average of five trials of electromyographic responses in gastrocnemius (*GAS*), hamstrings (*HAM*), lumbar paraspinal (*PAR*) tibialis anterior (*TIB*), quadriceps (*QUA*), and rectus abdominus (*ABD*) muscles in response to a 6-cm backward surface translation at 15 cm/sec with eyes closed and hearing masked.

Eliminating vestibular information (and/or vision) does not significantly affect the early postural responses to surface translations (2,12–14). Although patients with vestibular dysfunction often show ataxia of gait and instability in stance, studies have shown that vestibular information is not required for triggering a normal spatial-temporal pattern of ankle, knee, and hip muscle activity in response to surface translations (12,15). Figure 17.1B shows a normal pattern of leg muscle activation in response to forward sway perturbations in a patient with profound, bilateral loss of vestibular information. This patient had bilaterally absent caloric responses, vestibulo-ocular reflex gains less than 0.01, absent ocular-counter-rolling, and free-fall on a compliant surface with eyes closed, but showed normal medium-latency postural responses. Other studies, however, show abnormal magnitudes of muscle activation to surface rotations and of neck muscle activation in patients with vestibular loss (16–18).

Thus, ataxia of gait in patients with vestibular loss is not owing to slowed sensory feedback for responding to unexpected disturbances of balance. Vestibular ataxia is more likely owing to poor control of the head and trunk in space, which results in excessive motion of the body's center of mass. This must be compensated for by irregular foot placement during stepping. Because the greatest challenge to balance during gait is from control of the trunk in the lateral direction, compensatory stepping to correct balance during gait is often in the lateral direction (19). In fact, vestibular patients often report veering into doorjambs and other obstacles as they stagger during quick head and trunk rotations.

Unlike the normal postural response latencies in patients with profound vestibular loss, a subject with total body loss of somatosensory function shows absent postural responses to surface perturbations, even with eyes open and adequate vestibular function (7,20). Figure 17.1C shows the lack of postural muscle electromyographic (EMG) bursts in response to the same backward surface perturbation as the control and vestibular loss subjects in Figure 17.1A,B. The subject in Figure 17.1C lost touch and proprioceptive sensation from the earlobes down to the feet but retained sensation of temperature and pain as well as normal strength following two bouts of viral polyneuropathy that destroyed all large fiber afferents 14 years ago. Bilateral sural nerve biopsies showed loss of all afferent fibers greater than 6 μm (21).

Ataxia was so severe in this patient, with total body, generalized somatosensory loss, that she was unable to stand or walk independently. She learned to stand in the laboratory for up to 30 seconds by using visual feedback from a mirror to prevent her knees from buckling. With eye closure, she immediately collapsed to the floor. She also reported that she was unable to detect whether she was standing, sitting, or lying down when in the dark. Her gait ataxia consisted of extremely large, lateral trunk leans over a very narrow stance width with visual attention focused on foot placement. Postural ataxia during stance involved excessive, uncoordinated intersegmental motion that may be related to inability to compensate for interactive joint torques (22). This lack of postural responses and inability to balance during gait occurred despite the presence of visual and vestibular information, which suggests that visual and vestibular information are not sufficient for stance and gait. Postural and gait ataxia associated with this generalized, total body somatosensory loss resulted from complete inability to control segmental and body center of mass equilibrium.

Partial somatosensory loss, primarily in the distal lower extremities, delays the onset of postural responses, whereas total body, generalized somatosensory loss eliminates postural responses. The delays in automatic postural responses are proportional to the conduction times in peripheral or central somatosensory pathways. For example, we evaluated postural responses to surface translations in nine subjects with symmetric lower extremity peripheral neuropathy associated with 15 to 44 years of diabetes (23). These subjects with peripheral neuropathy all had significantly increased vibration, joint position, and light-touch sensation thresholds at the toes and ankles with absent or significantly delayed sural nerve conduction. Figure 17.2A shows the averaged EMG responses to a backward surface translation from a representative

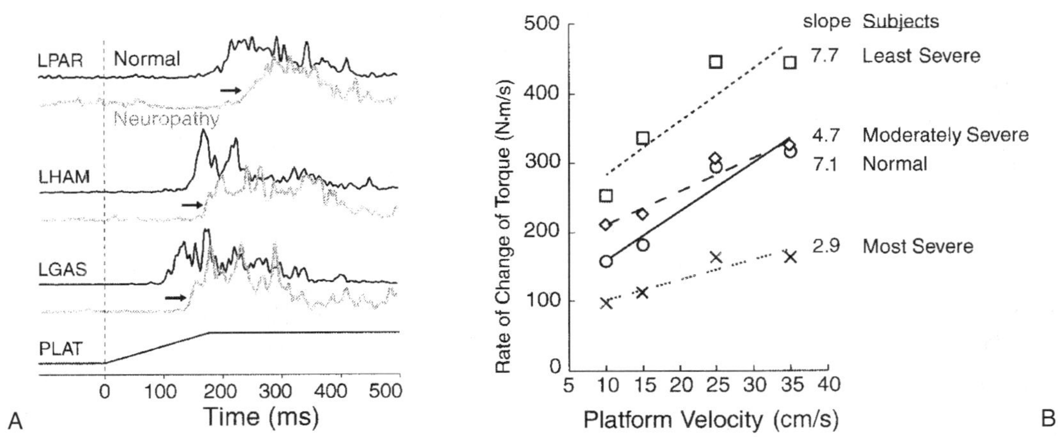

FIG. 17.2. A: Delayed postural responses from a subject with somatosensory loss from diabetic peripheral neuropathy (*bottom traces*) compared with age-matched control subject (*top traces*). *Vertical line* marks the beginning of the platform translation and the *arrows* indicate the delays in electromyographic latencies in the subject with neuropathy for each muscle. Electromyographic responses are averaged from five backward surface translations of 6 cm at 35 cm/sec. *LPAR,* left paraspinals; *LHAM,* left hamstrings; *LGAS,* left gastrocnemius. **B:** Scaling of earliest postural torque responses to four platform velocities in three subjects with the most severe neuropathy (absent sensory and motor conduction bilaterally), three subjects with moderately severe neuropathy (absent sensory conduction bilaterally), and three subjects with least severe neuropathy (sensory and motor conduction abnormal but present in at least one limb) compared to ten healthy control subjects (**A** is adapted from, Fig. 1, Inglis JT, et al. The importance of somatosensory information in triggering and scaling automatic postural responses in humans. *Exp Brain Res (Berlin)* 1994;101:159–164, with permission).

diabetic subject superimposed on responses from a typical healthy control subject. The onset of muscle responses in the subject with neuropathy were each delayed by about 20 ms at the ankle, thigh, and trunk, despite the typical distal-to-proximal severity of neuropathy in these diabetic subjects (Fig. 17.1A, *arrows*) (23). The onset of gastrocnemius postural response occurred at 116 ± 10 ms in the normals compared with 133 ± 20 ms in the diabetic subjects. Delays were similar in hamstring muscles (154 ± 25 ms compared with 174 ± 27 ms) and paraspinal muscles (173 ± 28 ms compared with 202 ± 22 ms). The similar delay of the entire postural synergy is consistent with a delay in triggering a centrally organized, multisegmental response. If local, segmental reflexes controlled automatic postural responses, delays would be larger in distal segments where the neuropathy was most severe (2,4).

Delayed conduction of somatosensory information in the spinal cord also leads to delays in automatic postural responses that contribute to posture and gait ataxia in subjects with MS. The latencies of postural responses to backward surface translations in patients with prolonged spinal somatosensory conduction owing to MS were delayed by approximately 44 ms (e.g., gastrocnemius latencies were 161 ± 31 ms instead of 117 ± 13 ms) (9). Significant delays in postural response latencies were seen in all subjects with MS who had significant, bilateral delays in spinal somatosensory evoked potentials recorded at C-7 from stimulation of the sural nerve. These delayed postural response latencies correlated significantly ($R = 0.69$; $P = 0.005$) with delayed spinal sensory conduction times but did not correlate ($R - 0.20$; $P = 0.21$) with delays in corticospinal motor conduction times evoked by magnetic coil stimulation (9). These correlations suggest that spinal somatosensory pathways are critical for triggering postural responses that do not likely include a corticospinal pathway. Unilateral delays in spinal somatosensory pathways were not associated with delayed postural responses, suggesting that sensory information from one leg is sufficient to trigger the earliest postural responses. Thus, although many patients with MS suffer neurological impairment in many central pathways important for posture and gait, delayed and distorted somatosensory conduction up the spinal cord resulting in delays in postural responses make an important contribution to their ataxia.

PREDICTIVE MECHANISMS FOR POSTURAL CONTROL PARTIALLY COMPENSATE FOR SOMATOSENSORY LOSS

Somatosensory information is not only responsible for triggering the onset of postural responses but also for scaling postural response magnitude based on the characteristics of the perturbing stimulus. For example, the magnitude of postural EMG responses and their resulting torque at the surface are proportional to the velocity of a surface translation (24). Loss of somatosensory information from diabetic peripheral neuropathy interferes with this scaling in reaction to the velocity of postural perturbations. Figure 17.2C shows that the severity of neuropathy was related to the ability to scale postural responses to surface translation velocity. The subjects with the most severe neuropathy (absent sural and plantar sensory and peroneal motor nerve conduction bilaterally) had the poorest postural response scaling.

When the characteristics of the stimulus are not completely known at the time of the postural response at 100 ms, prediction, using prior experience, can be used to scale postural response magnitude (25). For example, healthy subjects use prediction to scale the magnitude of their postural responses based on the amplitude of surface translations in immediately preceding trials (26). When the amplitude of surface translations is unpredictable, subjects cannot scale responses proportionately to surface amplitude, but produce a constant response magnitude either midrange between the maximum and minimum or near the maximum (25).

This ability to use sensory information from experience with previous trials to scale the size of postural responses appears to depend on an intact cerebellum because studies with patients with anterior lobe cerebellar ataxia show they are unable to scale their postural responses with translation amplitude (27,28). Unlike patients with peripheral or spinal sensory neuropathy, however, cerebellar patients show normal postural response latencies and scaling to feedback from perturbation velocity (27,28). In addition to the inability to use predictive scaling, the magnitudes of postural responses are extremely variable and hypermetric in patients with cerebellar ataxia. The hypermetric postural responses in subjects with midline cerebellar disorders often result in falls in the opposite direction of their external postural perturbation because it is their own postural responses that are destabilizing their equilibrium. Thus, gait and postural ataxia in patients with midline cerebellar disorders may be associated with inability to use prediction to accurately scale postural responses as well as with hypermetric postural and other movements. Specifically, the variable, wide-based foot placement in cerebellar gait may be a postural compensation for a primary problem of hypermetric, variable stepping force resulting in hypermetric, variable lateral center of mass motion as well as of an inability to appropriately scale the magnitude of proactive postural adjustments.

Postural and gait ataxia in patients with MS have often been attributed to cerebellar involvement. However, studies in our laboratory have shown that ataxic subjects with MS did not show the hypermetric or variable magnitude of postural responses seen in subjects with cerebellar ataxia (9). In fact, unlike cerebellar ataxia, subjects with postural and gait ataxia owing to MS showed an increased, rather than decreased, ability to use predictive mechanisms to scale postural responses.

Subjects with MS appear to compensate for their slowed somatosensory nerve conduction by relying on predictive mechanisms more than healthy subjects. Figure 17.3A shows the results from ten subjects with MS who showed steeper than normal scaling of postural response magnitude with predicted amplitudes of surface translations ataxia (9). The mean slope of the regression between initial surface reactive torque and surface translation amplitude was 8.4 ± 1.9 in the group with MS compared to 4.9 ± 1.2 in the control group ($P < 0.05$). In contrast, subjects with anterior lobe cerebellar ataxia did not scale the magnitude of their postural

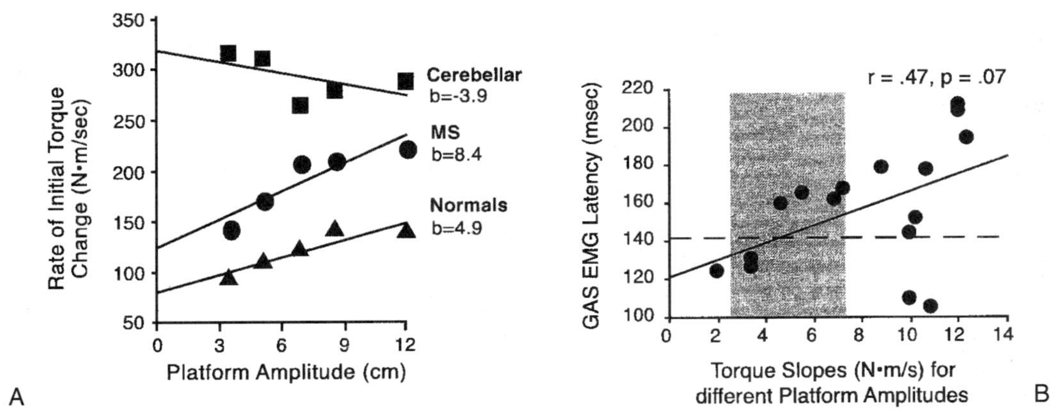

FIG. 17.3. A: Steeper than normal slope for scaling initial postural torque responses to predictable surface translation amplitudes in patients with somatosensory loss compared from multiple sclerosis (*MS*). In contrast, patients with anterior lobe cerebellar dysfunction showed absent predictive scaling. Means for ten subjects in each group are shown with their linear regressions. [Data from Horak FB, Diener HC. Cerebellar control of postural scaling and central set in stance. *J Neurophysiol (Bethesda, MD)* 1994;72:479–493.] **B:** Significant correlation between latencies of gastrocnemius latency to backward surface translations and slopes for predictive scaling of postural responses to translation amplitudes in patients with multiple sclerosis. The *dashed line* indicates the upper limit of normal EMG latency (mean + 2 SD) and the *shaded box* indicates the normal range of predictive scaling slopes.

responses at all based on prediction of platform amplitude (mean slope −3.9).

In addition, the MS subjects with the longest postural latencies showed the largest use of prediction (e.g., the steepest slopes of predictive scaling). Figure 17.3B shows the significant correlation between gastrocnemius response latencies and slopes of predictive scaling for the subjects with delayed spinal somatosensory pathways. This correlation suggests that MS subjects with the largest delays in equilibrium responses owing to slowed somatosensory conduction show the most powerful predictive scaling. This allows for larger postural response magnitudes when subjects fall further before an equilibrium response is initiated. Thus, when loss of somatosensory information becomes severe, subjects show a shift from online, feedback control to predictive, feedforward control of postural response magnitude. However, predictive, feedforward control depends on the availability of predictable stimuli, which are not always available in real world situations when trying to avoid a fall in response to unexpected postural perturbations.

The subject with total body somatosensory loss from Figure 17.1C was also able to compensate for her lack of somatosensory information by using predictive mechanisms. When the direction of the postural perturbation could be predicted, based on prior experience, she was able to trigger late, but functional, postural responses. Although postural responses were delayed between 20 and 500 ms and quite variable in latency from trial to trial, postural muscle activity occurred in the appropriate muscles for each direction of surface perturbation (7,20). For example, gastrocnemius was the first muscle active in response to a backward surface translation, whereas tibialis was the first muscle activated in response to a toes-up rotation. Auditory cues associated with onset of platform movement were apparently used to trigger these responses because postural responses were absent when hearing was masked. Availability of visual information from the ambient environment was not sufficient to trigger these postural responses when hearing was masked. Prediction of platform perturbation direction was necessary for direction-specific postural responses because auditory cues indicating platform onset were nonspecific for direction. Although remarkably rapid, these direction-specific postural responses were likely voluntarily triggered because they required intention by the subject as well as auditory cues and predictability of perturbation characteristics.

HAPTIC INFORMATION CAN HELP COMPENSATE FOR SOMATOSENSORY LOSS IN THE LOWER EXTREMITIES

Somatosensory information is such a powerful influence on postural control that even somatosensory information limited to cutaneous information from a fingertip (haptic) together with proprioceptors in the arm, can significantly improve postural stability (29,30). Recent studies have shown that the magnitude and velocity of postural sway in stance can be reduced more from somatosensory information from light touch of a fingertip on an earth-stationary reference than by vision when opening the eyes (29–31). Clinicians have long observed that postural steadiness in patients with ataxia benefit from using canes or by tracing fingertips along walls during gait. Currently, we are quantifying the extent to which subjects with somatosensory loss in the legs because of diabetic peripheral neuropathy can use somatosensory information from a fingertip on a stable reference to improve their balance (32).

Figure 17.4 compares anterior/posterior CoP sway under the feet of a subject with diabetic distal peripheral neuropathy while standing on a very slowly rotating platform (0.1 Hz) under three conditions: eyes closed, eyes open, and fingertip contact with eyes closed. With eyes closed and no touch, the subject swayed in proportion with the platform rotation. With eyes open and no touch, sway amplitude and velocity were moderately reduced. However, allowing less than 100 g of vertical fingertip touch on an earth-stable surface, even with eyes closed, greatly decreased postural sway. During quiet stance on a firm or foam surface, the CoP sway amplitude and sway velocity is larger in patients with diabetic peripheral neuropathy

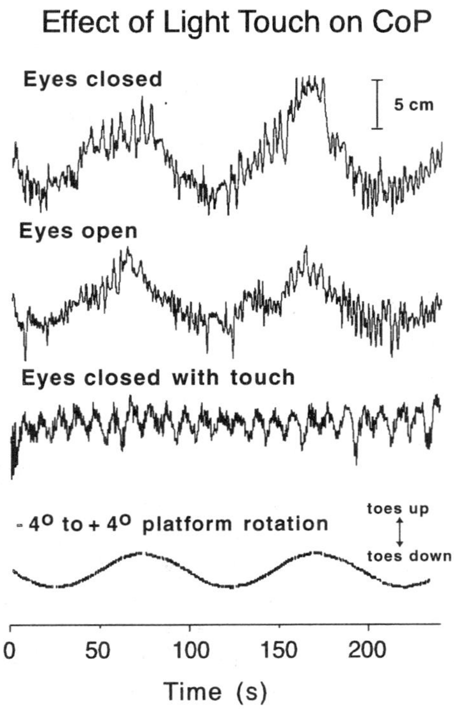

FIG. 17.4. Light touch of a fingertip on an earth-stationary support during sinusoidal platform rotations was more effective than vision in decreasing postural sway in a subject with somatosensory loss from diabetic peripheral neuropathy. Anterior/posterior center of pressure (*CoP*) from single trials without touch or vision, with vision alone, and with fingertip touch alone are shown.

than in age-matched control subjects, especially with closed eyes ($P < 0.05$) (33–35). Adding fingertip touch significantly reduces peak CoP and sway velocity in subjects with neuropathy even more than in control subjects ($P < 0.01$) (32). In fact, light touch of less than 100 g was just as helpful as self-determined heavy touch (averaging 1,000 g) in reducing postural sway (32).

Current studies are investigating whether light touch from a fingertip could also provide adequate sensory information for scaling the magnitude of postural responses to the velocity of platform perturbations. The reduced scaling of postural responses to platform translation velocities in patients with diabetic neuropathy suggests that normally, proprioceptive information from feet and leg muscles are responsible for this reactive scaling (Fig. 17.2C) (2,23). Recent results from ten subjects with diabetic peripheral neuropathy suggest that, although very light touch (50 to 150 N) did not improve velocity scaling, moderate touch (150 to 300 N) did significantly improve velocity scaling. These higher touch forces may be necessary because of mild upper extremity neuropathy in these patients and because higher forces may increase the contribution of proprioceptive information from arm muscles and joints, as well as from cutaneous information. Steeper slopes for scaling postural responses to platform velocity in subjects with neuropathy suggests that slip information from a fingertip or joint and muscle information from the arm in contact with a stable surface may be substituted for leg somatosensory information to interpret the velocity of postural disturbance.

VESTIBULOSPINAL SENSITIVITY INCREASES TO COMPENSATE FOR SOMATOSENSORY LOSS

Besides increased use of prediction and substitution of haptic cues from a fingertip to compensate for loss of somatosensory information in the legs, patients can also compensate by increasing the sensitivity of remaining senses for postural control. Recent studies suggest that subjects with somatosensory loss caused by diabetic peripheral neuropathy increase the sensitivity of their vestibulospinal responses to compensate for reduced gain of their somatosensory system for posture (10). When ten healthy subjects were exposed to incremental stimulus intensities of galvanic current, they swayed proportionately farther with increasing stimulus intensity with a linear slope of 1.5 cm of sway per mA galvanic current. However, when seven patients with severe diabetic somatosensory loss were exposed to similar increments of galvanic current intensities, the slope of their stimulus-response curve was steeper than normals, suggesting a higher sensitivity of the vestibulospinal sensitivity for posture. Three patients with mild neuropathy (e.g., with measurable, although delayed, sural nerve activity in sensory nerve conduction testing) did not show this compensatory increase in vestibulospinal gain. To determine whether this increase in stimulus-response slope could be due to decreased gain of somatosensory information alone, we compared the results of subjects with neuropathy with a computer simulation from a linear control, negative feedback model of vestibular-somatosensory interaction (36). The simulation showed that an increase gain of response to galvanic stimulation could be reproduced only when compensatory vestibulospinal gain increased as somatosensory gain decreased.

It is unlikely that the increase in vestibulospinal sensitivity in the patients was owing to long-term plasticity because similar increased sensitivity to galvanic current was also seen in healthy subjects standing on compliant foam or a moving platform (10). The increased vestibulospinal sensitivity in patients with diabetic peripheral neuropathy likely results from adaptive reweighing of reliance on vestibular information when support surface information is interpreted as unstable or unreliable. McCollom and coworkers hypothesized that healthy subjects readily increase or decrease their reliance on visual, vestibular, and somatosensory information as the environmental context regarding usefulness of sensory information for postural control changes (37). For example, when subjects stand on a support surface which is rotated in proportion to body sway ("sway-referenced"), subjects decrease reliance on somatosensory information that is no longer well correlated with body sway and toward increased reliance on vestibular and visual information. Horak and colleagues found support for this sensory weighting hypothesis by showing that leg muscle responses to head perturbations were enhanced when healthy subjects stood on a sway-referenced platform (38). In fact, sway-referencing the support surface or nulling ankle angle motion with rotations combined with translations makes healthy subjects respond like subjects with peripheral neuropathy with delayed latencies of postural responses (39). Thus, ataxia owing to somatosensory loss may be partially compensated for by an adaptive increase in reliance on and an increased sensitivity to vestibular information for postural control. Neuropathy may be interpreted by the nervous system as an "unstable surface" such that subjects use the normal adaptive mechanisms to reweigh reliance away from somatosensory and onto vestibular information.

CONCLUSION

One of the important contributions to postural and gait ataxia owing to loss of somatosensory information, whether from distal peripheral neuropathy, generalized total body polyneuropathy, spinal cord or demyelination, is slowing of important feedback pathways for control of balance and sensory orientation. These delays in feedback for equilibrium control result in increased body sway amplitude and sway energy in stance, which translate into excessive center of body mass displacement during gait. Postural stability in gait relies on somatosensory feedback to control automatic postural responses for foot placement and trunk alignment as well as on predictive mechanisms (40). Studies have shown that ataxic patients with somatosensory loss rely on a variety of compensatory mechanisms to maintain balance, including predictive mechanisms, sensory substitution with haptic information, and increased sensitivity to remaining sensory systems such as vestibular information.

Somatosensory information consists of the integration of information from a variety of receptors, each of which plays several roles in control of posture and gait. For example, cutaneous and deep pressure information contributes to detection of center of pressure under the feet, limits of stability over base of support, and surface characteristics. Muscle proprioceptive information may be important for rapidly triggering muscle synergies that recover body center of mass in response to external mechanical perturbations. Joint information combined with muscle proprioceptive information may be used to monitor body geometric alignment and as feedback for body sway. Force information from Golgi tendon organs may be used as loading information to scale the magnitude of postural responses (41). Somatosensory information from many sensory systems is integrated closely with vestibular information to allow the nervous system to determine surface orientation in space as well as the relation of the trunk to the surface and gravitational vertical (42). Further studies are needed to identify how each type of somatosensory information contributes to postural function and dysfunction.

Studies are also needed to better understand how balance deficits caused by somatosensory loss contribute to gait ataxia. New models suggest that balance disturbances, such as excessive center of mass motion, during gait are corrected by altering lateral step placement (19). Thus, it is not clear whether the irregular step placements associated with gait ataxia are owing to a direct effect of loss of somatosensory control of the stepping leg or to a normal, compensatory postural stepping strategy to recover balance. In order to understand the different causes for somatosensory-related ataxia, the variety of roles of different types of somatosensory information in control of balance and gait must be better understood.

ACKNOWLEDGMENT

This work was supported by NIH grants from NIA and NIDCD.

REFERENCES

1. Nutt JG, Horak FB. Gait and balance disorders. In: Watts R, Koller W, eds. *Movement disorders: neurologic principles and practice*. New York: McGraw–Hill, 1996:649–660.
2. Horak FB, Macpherson JM. Postural orientation and equilibrium. In: Smith JL, ed. *Handbook of physiology: exercise: regulation and integration of multiple systems*. New York: Oxford University Press, 1996:255–292.
3. Brown MJA. Diabetic neuropathy. *Ann Neurol* 1984;15:2–12.
4. Dyck PJ, Thomas PK, Asbury AK, et al. *Diabetic neuropathy*. Philadelphia: W.B. Saunders, 1987.
5. Richardson JK, Ching C, Hurvitz EA. The relationship between electromyographically documented peripheral neuropathy and falls. *J Am Geriatr Soc* 1992;40:1008–1012.
6. Richardson JK, Ashton-Miller JA. Peripheral neuropathy: An often-overlooked cause of falls in the elderly. *Periph Neurop* 1996;99:161–180.
7. Horak FB, LamarreY, Macpherson JM, et al. Postural control associated with total body somatosensory loss. *Soc Neurosci Abstr* 1996;22:1632.
8. Inglis JT, Shupert CL, Hlavacka F, Horak FB. Effect of galvanic vestibular stimulation on human postural responses during support surface translations. *J Neurophys* 1995;73:891–901.
9. Pratt CA, Horak FB, Herndon FM. Differential effects of somatosensory and motor system deficits on postural dyscontrol in multiple sclerosis patients. In: Woollacott M, Horak F, eds. *Posture and gait: control mechanisms*. Eugene, OR: University of Oregon Books, 1992:118–121.
10. Shupert CL, Hlavacka F, Horak FB. Somatosensory loss increases responses to galvanic vestibulospinal stimulation. *Soc Neurosci Abstr* 1998;24:152.
11. Horak FB, Nashner LM. Central programming of postural movements: adaptation to altered support surface configurations. *J Neurophys* 1986;55:1369–1381.
12. Horak FB, Nashner LM, Diener HC. Postural strategies associated with somatosensory and vestibular loss. *Exp Brain Res* 1990;82:167–177.
13. Macpherson JM, Inglis JT. Stance and balance following bilateral labyrinthectomy. *Prog Brain Res* 1993;97:219–228.
14. Diener HC, Dichgans J, Guschlbauer B, et al. Role of visual and static vestibular influences on dynamic posture control. *Hum Neurobiol* 1986;5:105–113.
15. Horak FB, Shupert CL. Role of the vestibular system in postural control. In: Herdman SJ, ed. *Vestibular rehabilitation*. Philadelphia: F.A. Davis, 1994:22–46.
16. Shupert CL, Horak FB, Black FO. Effect of peripheral vestibular disorders on head-trunk coordination during postural sway in humans. In: Berthoz A, Graf W, Vidal P, eds. *The head-neck sensory motor system*. New York: Oxford University Press, 1992:607–610.
17. Shupert CL, Horak FB. Effects of vestibular loss on head stabilization in response to head and body perturbations. *J Vestib Res* 1996;6:1–15.
18. Allum JHJ, Honegger F, Schicks H. The influence of a bilateral peripheral vestibular deficit on postural synergies. *J Vest Res* 1994;4:49–70.
19. Prince F, Winter DA, Stergiou P, et al. Anticipatory control of upper body balance during human locomotion. *Gait Post* 1994;2:19–25.
20. Horak FB, Lamarre Y, Macpherson JM, et al. Postural control in a patient with total body somatosensory loss. *Int Soc Posture Gait* 1997;June.
21. Nougier VB, Fleury C, Tesdale M, et al. Control of single-joint movements in deafferented patients: evidence for amplitude coding rather than position control. *Exp Brain Res* 1996;109:473–482.
22. Bastian A, Martin TA, Keating JG, et al. Cerebellar ataxia: abnormal control of interaction torques across multiple joints. *Neurophysiology* 1996;76:492–509.
23. Inglis JT, Horak JT, Shupert CL, et al. The importance of somatosensory information in triggering and scaling automatic postural responses in humans. *Exp Brain Res (Berlin)* 1994;101:159–164.
24. Mummel P, Timmann D, Krause UW, et al. Postural responses to changing task conditions in patients with cerebellar lesions. *J Neurol Neurosurg Psychiatry* 1998;65:734–742.
25. Horak FB, Adaptation of automatic postural responses. In: Bloedel J, Ebner TJ, Wise SP, eds. *Acquisition of motor behavior in vertebrates*. Cambridge, MA: MIT Press, 1996:57–85.
26. Horak FB, Diener HC, Nashner LM. Influence of central set on human postural responses. *J Neurophysiol (Bethesda, MD)* 1989;62:841–853.
27. Horak FB, Diener HC. Cerebellar control of postural

scaling and central set in stance. *J Neurophysiol (Bethesda, MD)* 1994;72:479–493.
28. Timmann D, Horak FB. Prediction and set-dependent scaling of early postural responses in cerebellar patients. *Brain* 1997;120:327–337.
29. Jeka JJ, Lackner JR. Fingertip contact influences human postural control. *Exp Brain Res (Berlin)* 1994;100:495–502.
30. Lackner JR, DiZio P, Jeka J, et al. Precision contact of the fingertip reduces postural sway of individuals with bilateral vestibular loss. *Exp Brain Res* 1999;126:459–466.
31. Jeka J, Easton RD, Bentzen BL, et al. Haptic cues for orientation and postural control in sighted and blind individuals. *Percep Psychophys* 1996;58:409–423.
32. Dickstein R, Shupert C, Horak FB. Finger touch improves postural stability in patients with peripheral neuropathy. *Gait and Posture*, 2000, in press.
33. Simoneau GG, Ulbrect JS, Derr JA, et al. Postural instability in patients with diabetic sensory neuropathy. *Diab Care* 1994;17:1411–1421.
34. Uccioli L, Giocomini PG, Monticone G, et al. Body sway in diabetic neuropathy. *Diab Care* 1995;18:339–344.
35. Shupert CL, Dickstein R, Horak FB, et al. Surface sway-referencing and peripheral neuropathy disrupt somatosensory information for postural stability in stance. *Gait Posture* 1999;9:S51.
36. Retka RJ. Simple model of sensory interaction in human postural control. In: Mergner TH, ed. *Multisensory control of posture.* New York: Plenum Press, 1995:281–288.
37. McCollum G, Shupert C, Nashner L. Organizing sensory information for postural control in altered sensory environments. *J Theor Biol* 1996;180:257–270.
38. Horak FB, Shupert CL, Dietz V, et al. Vestibular and somatosensory contributions to responses to head and body displacements in stance. *Exp Brain Res* 1994;100:93–106.
39. Allum JH, Honegger F. Interactions between vestibular and proprioceptive inputs triggering and modulating human balance-correcting responses differ across muscles. *Exp Brain Res* 1998;12(4):478–494.
40. Patla AE. Visual control of human locomotion. In: Patla AE, ed. *Adaptability of human gait.* Amsterdam: Elsevier, 1991:55–97.
41. Dietz V, Gollhofer A, Kleiber M, et al. Regulation of bipedal stance: dependency on “load” receptors. *Exp Brain Res (Berlin)* 1992;89:229–231.
42. Mergner T, Rosemeier T. Interaction of vestibular, somatosensory and visual signals for postural control and motion perception under terrestrial and microgravity conditions: a conceptual model. *Brain Res Rev* 1998;28:118–135.

Gait Disorders. Advances in Neurology, Vol. 87,
edited by E. Růžička, M. Hallett, and J. Jankovic.
Lippincott Williams & Wilkins, Philadelphia © 2001.

18

Central Disequilibrium Syndromes

Joseph C. Masdeu

Department of Neurology, University of Navarre; and Department of Neurology, University Hospital of Navarre, Pamplona 31008, Spain

As understood in this chapter, disequilibrium refers to an unsteady stance or gait. It is a purely phenomenological concept, referring to the phenomenon appreciated in the course of the patients' examination or reported by them. In principle, it does not imply any mechanism. It needs further refinement even as a clinical phenomenon. For instance, should the examiner record whether the patient always tends to fall in the same direction? Or, is the unsteadiness present only when the patient is not paying attention to his or her gait? Above all, the mechanisms of disequilibrium need to be better understood. For this reason, it is important to describe conditions that may cause disequilibrium, beyond the well-known cerebellar and vestibular syndromes. Eventually, the anatomy of these disorders may lead to an understanding of their biochemistry and hopefully, to therapies. Central disequilibrium was one of the categories of gait disorder proposed in a thoughtful classification of gait disorders (1). Central disequilibrium refers purely to the phenomenon of unsteadiness, but likely to have a causation in the brain, rather than in the spinal cord or peripheral nervous system.

In addition to lesions of the vestibular system and cerebellar vermis, Parkinson's disease (PD) and progressive supranuclear palsy (PSP) are well-known causes of disequilibrium of central origin. Parkinson's disease is a particularly good example of a disorder: Understanding the anatomy helped to clarify the biochemistry; this in turn led to efficacious therapies. This chapter contains a description of lesions of other brain structures that may result in disequilibrium.

BASIS PONTIS

Kwa and coworkers studied 17 atherosclerotic patients who had pontine hyperintense lesions on magnetic resonance imaging (MRI) but no supratentorial white matter lesions (2). These patients were identified in an ongoing prospective cohort study of 229 atherosclerotic patients who presented initially with nondisabling ischemic stroke, myocardial infarction, or peripheral arterial disease. Controls were patients from the same cohort with neither pontine nor supratentorial white matter lesions. Disequilibrium was ascertained by a questionnaire that asked, "Did you suffer from dizziness or unsteadiness (on walking or standing) during the past year?" Twelve of the 17 patients (71%) with pontine lesions complained of disequilibrium, versus five of the 17 controls (29%); this difference was significant. There was a trend for abnormal tandem-walking tests to be more frequent in patients than they were in controls. Babinski signs were equally distributed between the two groups. In the disorder recorded by these authors, the disequilibrium was less severe than in some of the disorders discussed in the following.

As described by Kwa and coworkers, the lesions were foci of hyperintensity on T2-weighted images of the basis pontis (2). The lesions did not appear in the mesencephalon or medulla and tended to spare the tegmentum of the pons containing vestibular pathways. The disequilibrium could be explained by involvement of structures known to participate in balance mechanisms. Alternatively, the finding may uncover new balance-mediating structures. Abnormal areas in the basis pontis overlapped the pontine nuclei, part of the fronto-ponto-cerebellar pathway. Infarcts in the basis pontis, particularly its anterolateral portion, can cause bilateral leg ataxia in addition to contralateral leg paresis (2,3). Because the lesions were likely to be ischemic, it is possible that, even in the absence of abnormal signal intensity on MRI, some of the vestibular structures were involved as well.

PEDUNCULOPONTINE NUCLEUS AREA

The laterodorsal region of the midbrain contains the mesencephalic locomotor region, which plays an important role in locomotion in animals (4). Stimulation of this region in the cat induces rapid walking, followed by running. This area contains the nucleus cuneiformis and the cholinergic pedunculopontine nucleus. In humans, loss of neurons in the pedunculopontine nucleus has been found in PSP and PD, but not in patients with Alzheimer's disease (AD), perhaps implying a role of this nucleus in ambulatory mechanisms. A patient with a small hemorrhage in this region had the acute onset of inability to walk, without hemiparesis or sensory loss (5). She was able to draw a circle with either leg when sitting down, but could not generate regular stepping movements with her feet. Holding on to a walker and stooped forward, she could walk with short, shuffling, irregular steps. Her base of ambulation was only minimally wide. Regular stepping was not initiated either in attempted walking or in response to loss of her balance. There was no cadence or rhythm to this patient's gait. The deficit of gait observed in this patient bears striking resemblance to the idiopathic gait failure experienced by many elderly individuals, which in most cases does not have a clear anatomic correlate (1). Interestingly, lesions in the midbrain may cause the lack of postural tone characteristic of asterixis (6,7).

BASAL GANGLIA

A tendency to fall despite good strength was recorded by Labadie and coworkers in patients with acute lesions in the basal ganglia (8). Bilateral lesions of the globus pallidus can also result in disequilibrium (9,10). Gait impairment is a prominent component of many degenerative disorders of the basal ganglia, including Cockayne's disease (11). However, unilateral chronic lesions of the putamen in young individuals seldom lead to disequilibrium, at least of a clinically relevant degree (12). Lesions in other areas of the brain confound studies of bilateral basal ganglia lesions in older individuals. The lesions of subcortical arteriosclerotic encephalopathy are often bilateral, but are accompanied by white matter lesions, which can cause gait unsteadiness by themselves (13,14). Unlike in the case of the globus pallidus, massive bilateral lesions of the striatum are rare with vascular disease (15). Smaller lesions are likely to cause a transient disorder, easily overlooked (8). Better clinicoradiologic correlation studies are needed to understand the role of the striatum in the genesis of central disequilibrium. The availability of functional studies with positron emission spectroscopy (PET) and single photon emission computed tomography (SPECT) may help this process.

THALAMUS

Inability to stand or walk despite minimal weakness has been recorded acutely with thalamic infarction (16–18) and hemorrhage, particularly when the superior portion of the ventrolateral nucleus or suprathalamic white matter were involved (18–20). It has also been reported in patients with lesions in the internal capsule or corona radiata who had the syndrome of unilateral ataxia and crural paresis (ataxic hemiparesis) (21–24). Alert, with normal or near normal strength on isometric muscle testing and a variable degree of sensory loss, these patients could not stand and some with larger lesions could not even sit up unassisted. They fell backward or toward the side contralateral to the lesion. These patients appeared to have a deficit of overlearned motor activity of an axial and postural nature. In the vascular cases, the deficit improved in a few days or weeks. However, these patients had a tendency to sustain falls during the rehabilitation period. It is important to note that this syndrome is transient. Chronic stroke patients with bilateral thalamic lesions severe enough to cause permanent astasia would be too hypokinetic to carry on volitional motor activity.

It is reasonable to ask whether the term originally used for this syndrome, *thalamic astasia,* is still appropriate. It may be objected that this term has often been used to indicate psychogenic imbalance. However, Gorelick and the present author refrained from using more classical neurologic terms, like ataxia, because the disturbance differs from cerebellar ataxia in that the gait is not broad-based or lurching (18). It resembles the marked balance impairment of patients with vestibulo-cerebellar disease. The term *astasia* is derived from the Greek negative particle *a* and the word *stasis,* meaning station. *Dorland's Medical Dictionary* defines astasia as "motor incoordination with inability to stand (25)." It seems appropriate to apply this term to the syndrome displayed by our patients. Regarding psychogenic imbalance, DeJong remarked, "the term *astasia–asbasia* has been given to the type of gait disturbance which is sometimes observed in hysterical individuals. These words, however, actually mean 'inability to stand and walk,' and it is better to use the term *hysterical dysbasia* . . ." when referring to psychogenic disturbances of gait (26).

Some of the discussion of the original article on *thalamic astasia* that continues to be current is reproduced in the following (18). This syndrome differs from pyramidal weakness because of corticospinal tract damage. Mild to moderate pyramidal damage is generally accompanied by distal weakness but enough extensor tone of the lower extremity to allow for safe station and ambulation. In contrast, the proximal muscles are less prone to be used in patients with thalamic astasia. With corticospinal tract damage, voluntary movements tend to be most affected. By contrast, on command our patients used limbs that seemed paralyzed when performing actions that required automatic synergistic movements, such as pushing themselves up in bed (18).

It could be asked whether thalamic astasia is caused by motor neglect affecting the lower limbs, or leg akinesia. Thalamic akinesia has been reported in patients with right thalamic (16,17,27) or left thalamic lesions (28,29). This deficit of motor control differs from nondominant parietal neglect, resulting in hemispatial neglect, anosognosia, tactile allesthesia, topographic disorientation, and hemiasomatognosia, which is often present to a mild degree in patients with right thalamic lesions. Similarly, a language disturbance is present in those with left thalamic lesions. Lateralizing manifestations of thalamic disease reflect the diverse specialization of the cortex and subcortical structures targeted by fibers originating in the thalami or coursing through them. These lateralizing findings confound the analysis and interpretation of the akinesia associated with thalamic astasia, a finding that is probably common to lesions of either thalamic nuclear complex.

Thalamic akinesia may be partially related to damage of pallido-thalamic and thalamostriatal connections. Bilateral pallidal damage causes akinesia (9,10). Some of the clinical findings in patients with thalamic astasia mimic the deficits resulting from basal ganglia disease, namely, proximal hypokinesia, poverty in the performance of automatic associated movements, and impairment in postural reflexes. They also share with parkinsonian patients a tendency to keep their hips and knees flexed. However, patients with thalamic astasia, like some of the patients with the so-called "lower-body parkinsonism," have greater instability than patients with PD (30).

It is also relevant to ask whether severe proprioceptive loss from damage to the lemniscal pathways in the ventroposterolateral thalamus could not be responsible for thalamic astasia. Inability to stand despite minimal weakness has been described with severe bilateral peripheral sensory loss (31,32). Zoll attributed to proprioceptive loss the impairment of balance after thalamotomy (33). Some of our patients with protracted inability to stand had moderate to severe proprioceptive loss (patients 2 and 6), but others did not (patients 1, 3, and 7) (18). Sensory loss correlated with involvement of the ventral-posterior nucleus. If present, sensory loss aids in the localization of the lesion. The presence of corticospinal tract or cerebellarlike findings and sensory loss on the same side renders a cerebellar localization unlikely and should suggest thalamic or suprathalamic involvement in patients with astasia.

Brandt and Dieterich postulated involvement of vestibular pathways to explain the syndrome of thalamic astasia (34). They documented an ocular tilt reaction, ocular torsion, and tilts of the perceived visual vertical in a study of 35 patients with thalamic infarction (35). Interestingly, only five patients had "ataxia," and they belonged to the group of 17 patients with posterolateral infarcts. The lesions were smaller and more caudally located than in the patients we described with thalamic astasia. Vestibular eye findings were most prominent in patients with paramedian thalamic infarction, likely from involvement of important vestibulo-ocular structures at the thalamo-mesencephalic junction. By contrast, patients with thalamic astasia tended to have lesions in the latero-dorsal thalamus, involving the ventrolateral nucleus and suprathalamic white matter (18). The unsteadiness of thalamic astasia certainly resembles vestibular unsteadiness. However, from the study of Dieterich and Brandt and from the observation that thalamic astasia is accompanied by an array of nonvestibular findings, such as proximal akinesia, this author suspects that the vestibular contribution to the syndrome is not critical (35).

The lesions in patients with thalamic astasia tended to cluster in the ventrolateral nucleus (18). The ventrolateral nucleus of the thalamus consists of two portions (36,37). The smaller anterior portion (VLa) receives projections from the medial globus pallidus via the thalamic fasciculus and projects to area 6 of the frontal cortex. The larger posterior portion (VLp) receives cerebellar, spinothalamic, and vestibular afferents and projects in a somatotopic fashion to area 4 of the precentral gyrus. Medial neurons project to the lateral part of the precentral gyrus, whereas latero-superior neurons project to the medial portion of the precentral gyrus, where the trunk and leg are represented. Fibers destined for the leg region course in the posterior limb of the internal capsule and then ascend in the more medial portion of the corona radiata, near the wall of the lateral ventricle. These fibers were probably involved in previously reported capsular cases of ataxic hemiparesis (21–24). Impairment of gait in the elderly with periventricular white matter disease might be related to involvement of this pathway (38). Through the fastigial projection, VLp receives information from the vestibulocerebellum (39). Bilateral representation of this projection, affected in our patients at the level of the thalamus, may be one of the factors explaining the transient nature of thalamic astasia.

Studies of cerebral perfusion in patients with thalamic astasia have shown decreased perfusion of the lesioned thalamus, but also of the ipsilateral frontal lobe and contralateral cerebellum (J. Masdeu, unpublished observations, 1990). In some cases, cerebellar perfusion was specifically decreased in the vermian and paravermian cerebellar cortex. These studies suggest that the thalamus plays a major role in the activation of frontal cortex, particularly regarding activities that are carried out in the background, without the need for the individual to directly attend to them. This is the case with gait. When normal individuals walk, they do not pay attention to the act of walking, but to other activities. Walking is carried out by an "automatic pilot" that is impaired in patients with thalamic astasia. For this reason, as these patients recover, they can appear quite normal in the constrained framework of a doctor's examination, because they compensate for their deficit by paying attention to their gait. It is in the familiar context of their daily life, when they switch back to using the "automatic pilot," that they tend to sustain falls.

Other disorders of postural stability have been described with thalamic lesions. Hyperekplexia, the sudden loss of postural tone caused by startling stimuli, was exacerbated by a superimposed thalamic infarction (40). Unilateral asterixis, which occurred in four of our patients with thalamic astasia, has been reported with lesions in the ventrolateral nucleus, but is not restricted to thalamic lesions (41–43). Both asterixis and thalamic astasia are manifestations of disordered postural tone. However, their relationship will remain unclear until more is known about the mechanisms underlying sustained muscle contraction in humans.

SUPRATHALAMIC WHITE MATTER

Disorders of gait were pronounced among 41 well-documented cases of progressive arteriopathic white matter disease described with histology since 1978 (males = 23; females = 18; mean age of onset: 60 ± 9.7 years; mean length of illness: 5.8 ± 4.2 years) (44–51). Impairment of ambulation preceded cognitive impairment in 43% of the cases, whereas in only 17% dementia developed before gait impairment; in 20% they evolved simultaneously, and in 20% insufficient data precluded timing of gait abnormality versus dementia. Comparing demented elderly subjects with controls for dementia, several authors failed to find a significant correlation between white matter disease and dementia, but white matter disease correlated with gait impairment (52,53). Periventricular white matter changes were present in cases of "lower body parkinsonism" (54,55). In controlled studies of older adults who are prone to falling, impaired gait and balance correlated with the presence of white matter disease on CT or MRI (38,56–63).

White matter changes are very frequent in older people on CT or MRI, the same population who has a high prevalence of gait disorders (64). Some degree of white matter change is present on MRI in about 30% of subjects over the age of 65 (65). Areas of the periventricular white matter hypodense on CT appear markedly hyperintense on T2-weighted images, and hypointense on T1-weighted images (66). However, high intensity areas on T2-MR are often undetected on CT. On T2-MR images, it may be difficult to differentiate areas of increased water content because of dilation of perivascular spaces with normal aging or transependymal cerebrospinal fluid absorption from areas of tissue damage because both have increased intensity values (67–69). For this reason it seems preferable to make the diagnosis of significant white matter changes only when the abnormalities are visible on T1-weighted images (70).

REFERENCES

1. Nutt J, Marsden C, Thompson P. Human walking and higher-level gait disorders, particularly in the elderly. *Neurology* 1993;43:268–279.
2. Kwa VI, Zaal LH, Verbeeten B Jr, et al. Disequilibrium in patients with atherosclerosis: relevance of pontine ischemic rarefaction. Amsterdam Vascular Medicine Group. *Neurology* 1998;51:570–573.
3. Fisher CM. Ataxic hemiparesis. *Arch Neurol* 1978;35:126–128.
4. Garcia-Rill E. The pedunculopontine nucleus. *Prog Neurobiol* 1991;36:363–389.
5. Masdeu J, Alampur U, Cavaliere R, et al. Astasia and gait failure with damage of the pontomesencephalic locomotor region. *Ann Neurol* 1994;35:619–621.
6. Bril V, Sharpe JA, Ashby P. Midbrain asterixis. *Ann Neurol* 1979;6:362–364.
7. Tarsy D, Lieberman B, Chirico-Post J, et al. Unilateral asterixis associated with a mesencephalic syndrome. *Arch Neurol* 1977;34:446–447.
8. Labadie E, Awerbuch G, Hamilton R, et al. Falling and postural deficits due to acute unilateral basal ganglia lesions. *Arch Neurol* 1989;261:492–496.
9. Rabitsch W, Brugger SA, Pirker W, et al. Symmetrical necrosis of globus pallidus with severe gait disturbance in a patient with myelodysplastic syndrome given allogeneic marrow transplantation. *Ann Hematol* 1997;75:235–237.
10. Haaxma R, van Boxtel A, Brouwer WH, et al. Motor function in a patient with bilateral lesions of the globus pallidus. *Mov Disord* 1995;10:761–777.
11. Ozdirim E, Topcu M, Ozon A, et al. Cockayne syndrome: review of 25 cases. *Pediatr Neurol* 1996;15:312–316.
12. Inagaki M, Koeda T, Takeshita K. Prognosis and MRI after ischemic stroke of the basal ganglia. *Pediatr Neurol* 1992;8:104–108.
13. Yamanouchi H, Nagura H. Neurological signs and frontal white matter lesions in vascular parkinsonism. A clinicopathologic study. *Stroke* 1997;28:965–969.
14. Chang CM, Yu YL, Ng HK, et al. Vascular pseudoparkinsonism. *Acta Neurol Scand* 1992;86:588–592.
15. Feve AP, Fenelon G, Wallays C, et al. Axial motor disturbances after hypoxic lesions of the globus pallidus. *Mov Disord* 1993;8:321–326.
16. Cambier J, Elghozi D, Strube E. *Lésions du thalamus droit avec syndrome de l'hémisphre mineur. Discussion du concept de négligence thalamique. Rev Neurol* 1980;136:105–116.
17. Laplane D, Escourolle R, Degos J, et al. *La négligence motrice d'origine thalamique. A propos de deux cas. Rev Neurol (Paris)* 1982;138:201–211.
18. Masdeu J, Gorelick P. Thalamic astasia: inability to stand after unilateral thalamic lesions. *Ann Neurol* 1988;23:596–603.
19. Jenkyn L, Alberti A, Peters J. Language dysfunction, somasthetic hemi-inattention, and thalamic hemorrhage in the dominant hemisphere. *Neurology* 1981;31:1202–1203.
20. Verma A, Maheshwari M. Hypesthetic-ataxic-hemiparesis in thalamic hemorrhage. *Stroke* 1986;17:49–51.
21. Fisher CM, Cole M. Homolateral ataxia and crural paresis; a vascular syndrome. *J Neurol Neurosurg Psychiatry* 1965;28:48–55.
22. Huang C, Lui F. Ataxic-hemiparesis, localization and clinical features. *Stroke* 1984;15:363–366.
23. Iragui V, McCutchen C. Capsular ataxic hemiparesis. *Arch Neurol* 1982;39:528–529.
24. Sage J, Lepore F. Ataxic hemiparesis from lesions of the corona radiata. *Arch Neurol* 1983;40:449–450.

25. Friel J. *Dorland's illustrated medical dictionary*, 25th ed. Philadelphia: W.B. Saunders, 1974.
26. DeJong R. Case taking and the neurologic examination. In: Baker A, Joynt R, eds. *Clinical neurology*. Hagerstown, MD: Harper & Row, 1985:48.
27. Watson R, Valenstein E, Heilman K. Thalamic neglect. Possible role of the medial thalamus and nucleus reticularis in behavior. *Arch Neurol* 1981;38:501–506.
28. Velasco F, Velasco M. A reticulothalamic system mediating proprioceptive attention and tremor in man. *Neurosurgery* 1979;4:30–36.
29. Bogousslavsky J, Miklossy J, Deruaz J, et al. Unilateral left paramedian infarction of thalamus and midbrain: a clinico-pathological study. *J Neurol Neurosurg Psychiatry* 1986;49:686–694.
30. Trenkwalder C, Paulus W, Krafczyk S, et al. Postural stability differentiates "lower body" from idiopathic parkinsonism. *Acta Neurol Scand* 1995;91:444–452.
31. Sobue G, Senda Y, Matsuoka Y, et al. Sensory ataxia. A residual disability of Guillain-Barré syndrome. *Arch Neurol* 1983;40:86–89.
32. Albin R, Albers J, Greenberg H, et al. Acute sensory neuropathy–neuronopathy from pyridoxine overdose. *Neurology* 1987;37:1729–1732.
33. Zoll J. Transient anosognosia associated with thalamotomy; is it caused by proprioceptive loss? *Confin Neurol* 1969;31:48–55.
34. Brandt T, Dieterich M. Vestibular syndromes in the roll plane: topographic diagnosis from brainstem to cortex. *Ann Neurol* 1994;36:337–347.
35. Dieterich M, Brandt T. Thalamic infarctions: differential effects on vestibular function in the roll plane (35 patients). *Neurology* 1993;43:1732–1740.
36. Jones EG, Steriade M, McCormick DA. *The thalamus*. New York: Elsevier, 1997.
37. Van Buren J, Borke R. *Variations and connections of the human thalamus*. New York: Springer Verlag, 1972.
38. Masdeu J, Wolfson L, Lantos G, et al. White matter disease in the elderly prone to falling. *Arch Neurol* 1989;46:1292–1296.
39. Asanuma C, Thach W, Jones E. Distribution of cerebellar terminations and their relation to other afferent terminations in the thalamic ventral lateral region of the monkey. *Brain Res Rev* 1983;5 237–265.
40. Fariello R, Schwartzman R, Beall S. Hyperexplexia exacerbated by occlusion of posterior thalamic arteries. *Arch Neurol* 1983;40:244–246.
41. Calzetti S, Gemignani F, Salati M, et al. Unilateral asterixis due to thalamic tumor. Case report. *Ital J Neurol Sci* 1983;1:87–90.
42. Donat J. Unilateral asterixis due to thalamic hemorrhage. *Neurology* 1980;30:83–84.
43. Young R, Shahani B. Asterixis: one type of negative myoclonus. *Adv Neurol* 1986;43:137–156.
44. Caplan L, Schoene W. Clinical features of subcortical arteriosclerotic encephalopathy (Binswanger disease). *Neurology* 1978;28:1206–1215.
45. Goto K, Ishii N, Fukasawa H. Diffuse white-matter disease in the geriatric population: a clinical, neuropathological, and CT study. *Radiology* 1981;141:687–695.
46. Dubas F, Gray F, Roullet E, et al. Leucoencéphalopathies artériopathiques (17 cas anatomo-cliniques). *Rev Neurol (Paris)* 1985;141:93–108.
47. Dupuis M, Brucher J, Gonsette R. *Obsevation anatomo-clinique d'une encéphalopathie sous-corticale artérioscléreuse ("maladie de Binswanger") avec hypodensité de la substance blanche au scanner cérébral. Acta Neurol Belg* 1984;84:131–140.
48. Gray F, Dubas F, Roullet E, et al. Leukoencephalopathy in diffuse hemorrhagic cerebral amyloid angiopathy. *Ann Neurol* 1985;18:54–59.
49. Huang K, Wu L, Luo Y. Binswanger's disease: progressive subcortical encephalopathy or multi-infarct dementia? *Can J Neurol Sci* 1985;12:88–94.
50. Janota I. Dementia, deep white matter damage and hypertension: 'Binswanger's disease.' *Psychol Med* 1981;11:39–48.
51. Rosenberg G, Kornfeld M, Stovring J, et al. Subcortical arteriosclerotic encephalopathy (Binswanger): computerized tomography. *Neurology* 1979;29:1102–1106.
52. George A, de Leon M, Gentes C, et al. Leukoencephalopathy in normal and pathologic aging: CT of brain lucencies. *Am J Neurol Res* 1986;7:561–566.
53. Hendrie H, Farlow M, Austrom M, et al. Foci of increased T2 signal intensity on brain MR scans of healthy elderly subjects. *Am J Neurorad* 1989;10:703–707.
54. Thompson P, Marsden CD. Gait disorder of subcortical arteriosclerotic encephalopathy: Binswanger's disease. *Mov Disord* 1987;2:1–8.
55. FitzGerald P, Jankovic J. Lower body parkinsonism: evidence for vascular etiology. *Mov Disord* 1987;4:249–260.
56. Baloh RW, Yue Q, Socotch TM, et al. White matter lesions and disequilibrium in older people. I. Case-control comparison. *Arch Neurol* 1995;52:970–974.
57. Hennerici MG, Oster M, Cohen S, et al. Are gait disturbances and white matter degeneration early indicators of vascular dementia? *Dementia* 1994;5:197–202.
58. Tell GS, Lefkowitz DS, Diehr P, et al. Relationship between balance and abnormalities in cerebral magnetic resonance imaging in older adults. *Arch Neurol* 1998;55:73–79.
59. van Zagten M, Lodder J, Kessels F. Gait disorder and parkinsonian signs in patients with stroke related to small deep infarcts and white matter lesions. *Mov Disord* 1998;13:89–95.
60. Kerber KA, Enrietto JA, Jacobson KM, et al. Disequilibrium in older people: a prospective study. *Neurology* 1998;51:574–580.
61. Brooks WM, Wesley MH, Kodituwakku PW, et al. 1H–MRS differentiates white matter hyperintensities in subcortical arteriosclerotic encephalopathy from those in normal elderly. *Stroke* 1997;28:1940–1943.
62. Briley DP, Wasay M, Sergent S, et al. Cerebral white matter changes (leukoaraiosis), stroke, and gait disturbance. *J Am Geriatr Soc* 1997;45:1434–1438.
63. Sohn YH, Kim JS. The influence of white matter hyperintensities on the clinical features of Parkinson's disease. *Yonsei Med J* 1998;39:50–55.
64. Waite LM, Broe GA, Creasey H, et al. Neurological signs, aging, and the neurodegenerative syndromes. *Arch Neurol* 1996;53:498–502.
65. Fazekas F, Niederkorn K, Schmidt R, et al. White matter signal abnormalities in normal individuals: correlation with carotid ultrasonography, cerebral blood flow measurements, and cerebrovascular risk factors. *Stroke* 1988;19:1285–1288.

66. Kinkel W, Jacobs L, Polachini I, et al. Subcortical arteriosclerotic encephalopathy (Binswanger's disease). Computed tomographic, nuclear magnetic resonance, and clinical correlations. *Arch Neurol* 1985;42:951–959.
67. Awad I, Johnson P, Spetzler R, et al. Incidental subcortical lesions identified on magnetic resonance imaging in the elderly. II. Postmortem pathological correlations. *Stroke* 1986;17:1090–1097.
68. Kirkpatrick J, Hayman L. White-matter lesions on MR imaging of clinically healthy brains of elderly subjects: possible pathologic basis. *Radiology* 1987;162:509–511.
69. Zimmerman R, Fleming C, Lee B, et al. Periventricular hyperintensity as seen by magnetic resonance: prevalence and significance. *Am J Radiol* 1986;146:443–450.
70. Gass A, Oster M, Cohen S, et al. Assessment of T2- and T1-weighted MRI brain lesion load in patients with subcortical vascular encephalopathy. *Neuroradiology* 1998;40:503–506.

Gait Disorders. Advances in Neurology, Vol. 87,
edited by E. Růžička, M. Hallett, and J. Jankovic.
Lippincott Williams & Wilkins, Philadelphia © 2001.

19

Freezing of Gait

Clinical Overview

Nir Giladi

Movement Disorders Unit, Department of Neurology, Tel Aviv Medical Center, Tel Aviv University, Tel Aviv, Israel 64239

Freezing of gait (FOG) is a unique gait disturbance associated with parkinsonism (1–3). Freezing of gait refers to transient episodes, usually lasting seconds, in which a patient is unable to initiate or continue locomotion, occurring on a background of relatively good ability to move (3). Freezing of gait is highly variable in appearance and severity, influenced by attention and sensory input, and usually responds to tricks of all types (4–6). Freezing of gait is best described by patients as a unique feeling that their "feet get glued to the ground." It is a midline symptom affecting both legs, but in asymmetric parkinsonism, unilateral or asymmetric freezing has been observed. Freezing of gait is a classical disturbance of locomotion and gait initiation (start hesitation) (Table 19.1). It typically appears when a patient is forced to change his or her normal, automatic gait pattern or speed (at tight quarters, reaching destination) or when responding to stressful situations, such as the ringing of a telephone or the doorbell, in elevators, or when one has to cross the street at the green light. One of the classical features of freezing episodes is its dramatic and continuous response to different motor or behavioral tricks (4–6). Moderate emotional stress (e.g., being in the doctor's office) frequently improves FOG, in contrast to being at home, where 75% of the patients experienced the worst freezing (Giladi, unpublished data, 1999). Stress associated with timing is especially difficult in freezers.

Freezing of gait is a common phenomenon in parkinsonism, but its frequency in the various parkinsonian syndromes is highly variable (Table 19.2) (2). Freezing of gait was most commonly reported in pathologically proven progressive supranuclear palsy (PSP) and vascular parkinsonism. Pure freezing syndrome, where FOG is the predominant and sometimes the only symptom, is also a variant of PSP and further supports the high prevalence of FOG in PSP (7,8). Freezing of gait is common in Parkinson's disease (PD), with increasing prevalence as the disease progresses (1,9). Surprisingly, FOG has not been reported in pathologically proven multiple system atrophy (MSA) cases, but it is common clinically (Giladi, unpublished data, 2000). Freezing of gait also is rare in neuroleptic-induced parkinsonism (NIP) (10). Hassin-Bear et al. have recently confirmed the rare appearance of FOG in NIP when they assessed 75 consecutive psychiatric patients with NIP (11). Based on the wide range of parkinsonian syndromes that are associated with FOG and its tight relationship with the extrapyramidal system, Fahn has recently added FOG as the fifth cardinal symptom of parkinsonism (Table 19.3) (12).

Freezing of gait is part of the general slowness of movement (bradykinesia) seen in

TABLE 19.1. *Freezing of gait and locomotion*

At gait initiation
Start hesitation
In locomotion
On open runway
While adjusting to circumstances
Reaching destination
At doorway
On turns

TABLE 19.3. *Cardinal features of parkinsonism*

Rest tremor
Bradykinesia/hypokinesia
Rigidity
Abnormal postural reflexes
Locomotion gait disturbances—FOG

FOG, freezing of gait.

parkinsonism; it is more precisely related to abnormal execution of complex motor tasks such as repetitive, simultaneous, or sequential motor acts (13,14). It is suggested that the primary underlying abnormality is related to the inability to deliver (execute) or hold a preprogrammed, continuous, complex motor act in response to an established and correct internal plan of action (13). Freezing episodes classically appear in complex, highly synchronized, automatic motor tasks, such as gait and speech. Freezing episodes usually can be overcome by switching from a task governed by internal queues to one driven by external queues. For example, stepping over lines on the floor, using a metronome, or following an external command will improve gait and decrease the severity of FOG.

ASSESSMENT OF FREEZING OF GAIT

Assessment of FOG with objective measures, either on neurological examination during an office visit or using sophisticated gait laboratory, is very difficult. One of the most typical features of FOG is the tendency of parkinsonian "freezers" not to freeze while examined. As a result, one should rely on historical information collected from the patient as well as from the caregivers. Table 19.4 summarizes the points one should look at when assessing FOG while taking the history. Several attempts have been made to develop a questionnaire specifically for FOG, taking into an account the variability and subjective nature of this symptom; however, none of these scales has been validated (15–17). A recent questionnaire for quantified assessment of FOG was found to be highly reliable (Cronbach alpha = 0.94) and with good interrater agreement (Kappa values ranged between 0.53 and 0.74) (18). The Freezing of Gait Questionnaire is built out of six questions that were found to be easy to apply by movement disorder specialists as well as by nonneurologist physicians or medical students (Table 19.5). When the Freezing of Gait Questionnaire was compared to the FOG item of the activity of daily living (ADL) part of the Unified Parkinson's Disease Rating Scale (UPDRS) (19) there was only moderate correlation (alpha = 0.66 for "off" FOG and 0.77 for "on" FOG) (18). This difference is mainly because the FOG questionnaire does not assess falls and does not give higher scores for freezers who fall in relation to FOG.

TABLE 19.2. *Freezing of gait in parkinsonian syndromes*

Name of disease	Frequency
PSP (Pure freezing syndrome)	Very common
Vascular parkinsonism	Very common
NPH	Common
Parkinson's disease	Common
MSA (SND, SDS, OPCA)	Rare
Drug-induced parkinsonism	Very rare

MSA, multiple system atrophy; NPH, normal pressure hydrocephalus; OPCA, olivo-ponto cerebellar atrophy; PSP, progressive supranuclear palsy; SND, striatal nigral degeneration.

TABLE 19.4. *Assessment of freezing of gait—points to look at*

1. The degree of disability it causes
2. Type of FOG: start hesitation, turn, narrow space
3. Frequency of episodes
4. Duration of typical FOG
5. Relation to "on" or "off"
6. Response to levodopa or other therapeutic intervention
7. Response to tricks
8. The association with falls

FOG, freezing of gait.

TABLE 19.5. *Freezing of gait questionnaire (FOG-Q)*

1. During your *worst* state—Do you walk: ☐
- 0 Normally
- 1 Almost normally—somewhat slow
- 2 Slow but fully independent
- 3 Need assistance or walking aid
- 4 Unable to walk

2. Are your gait difficulties affecting your daily activities and independence? ☐
- 0 Not at all
- 1 Mildly
- 2 Moderately
- 3 Severely
- 4 Unable to walk

3. Do you feel that your feet get glued to the floor while walking, making a turn or when trying to initiate walking (freezing)? ☐
- 0 Never
- 1 Very rarely—about once a month
- 2 Rarely—about once a week
- 3 Often—about once a day
- 4 Always—whenever walking

4. How long is your *longest* freezing episode? ☐
- 0 Never happened
- 1 1–2 seconds
- 2 3–10 seconds
- 3 11–30 seconds
- 4 Unable to walk for more than 30 seconds

5. How long is your *typical start hesitation* episode (freezing when initiating the first step)? ☐
- 0 None
- 1 Takes longer than one second to start walking
- 2 Takes longer than 3 seconds to start walking
- 3 Takes longer than 10 seconds to start walking
- 4 Takes longer than 30 seconds to start walking

6. How long is your *typical turning hesitation* (freezing when turning)? ☐
- 0 None
- 1 Resume turning in 1–2 seconds
- 2 Resume turning in 3–10 seconds
- 3 Resume turning in 11–30 seconds
- 4 Unable to resume turning for more than 30 seconds

From Giladi N, Shabtai H, Simon E, et al. Freezing of gait in Parkinson's disease: scale construction. *Mov Disord* 1998;13:104.

FREEZING OF GAIT IN PARKINSONS DISEASE

Charcot appears to have been the first to describe the freezing phenomenon—both start hesitation and freezing when reaching destination—in 1877 in patients with parkinsonism (20). Fifty years later, in 1927, Wechsler gave the first detailed description of start hesitation in a parkinsonian patient. During the next 40 years, in the pre–L-Dopa period, freezing was mentioned by several authors as part of parkinsonian akinesia (6,21,22). However, because of the poor differentiation between the different etiologies for parkinsonism in the pre–L-Dopa period, it is impossible to know the real frequency of FOG in patients with PD at that period. Barbeau and Ambani and Van Woert were the first to notice a significant increase in FOG frequency starting about 1 year after the introduction of high dosage of L-Dopa treatment. They related this increment to long-term exposure to L-Dopa (23–25).

Freezing of gait is rarely the presenting symptom of PD, and if so it is very brief, mild, and has minor impact on quality of life or activities of daily living (ADL). If a patient is experiencing significant FOG at the very early stage of the disease it is most likely PSP or vascular parkinsonism and not PD. Generally, one can look at FOG in patients with PD as a symptom of the advanced stage of the disease. At that stage it becomes a major symptom that can cause significant disability (Table 19.6).

Freezing of gait in patients with PD is closely related to disease progression or antiparkinsonian treatment. In spite of the tight association between the two, it is practical to separate them from the pathophysiologic and therapeutic point of view. There are several pieces of evidence that progression of the disease is a major contributing factor for the development of FOG. One way to link the two is to look at the frequency of FOG in the pre–L-Dopa period or in untreated

TABLE 19.6. *Freezing of gait in relation to clinical stages of Parkinson's disease*

Early stages	
	Brief episodes (seconds)
	Minor interference with ADL
	No need for tricks
Advanced stages	
	Can last seconds to minutes
	Major influence on quality of life
	Part of the "on/off" phenomenon
	Heavily dependent on tricks

ADL, activities of daily living.

patients with PD. Freezing of gait has been experienced by about 7% of untreated parkinsonian patients (1,26) and 16% of patients prior to the introduction of L-Dopa (9). Support for the contribution of disease progression to the development of FOG came from analysis of data collected prospectively in the deprenyl and tocophenol treatment on Parkinson's disease (DATATOP) study. Eight hundred naive parkinsonian patients included in the study were randomly assigned into four arms and were treated with selegiline, vitamin E, or placebo (27). After a mean of 14 ± 2 months of treatment, all patients were taken off study medications and were assessed after a washout period of 30 to 60 days without any antiparkinsonian medication. There was a significant increase in FOG frequency at the end of the washout in comparison to baseline. Twenty-four percent of the patients experienced FOG at the end of the washout period with a very significant association between the development of FOG and disease progression, as reflected on the UPDRS score as well as Hoehn and Yahr (H&Y) clinical stage (26,28). The association between FOG and higher stage of H&Y was also observed in patients with more advanced disease who were treated with L-Dopa (1,29). However, because of the retrospective nature of those studies it was difficult to differentiate between the contribution of the primary degenerative process of the nigrostriatal dopaminergic pathway and the long-term treatment with L-Dopa in the advanced stages.

Duration of L-Dopa treatment has become a major contributing factor for the appearance of FOG (1,9,29). Interestingly, it seems that L-Dopa is contributing to the appearance of FOG mainly in the younger symptom onset subgroup (less than 59 years old) and not nearly as much in the older onset patients (59 or more years old) (29). Several studies have suggested that treatment with dopamine agonist drugs might also contribute to the appearance of FOG (29–31), but these relationships should be evaluated further in prospective studies.

There are basically two types of FOGs seen in patients with PD who are taking L-Dopa. The most common is an "off"-related FOG, which can be improved with L-Dopa or dopaminergic treatment such as apomorphine (32,33). Infrequently, one can see a patient with "on"-freezing that does not improve with L-Dopa treatment. "Off"-freezing is easy to diagnose when it is seen during an "off" state, when the patient is bradykinetic and rigid, and experiencing the parkinsonian symptoms that will go away when L-Dopa takes effect. However, one should differentiate between "off"- and "on"-freezing when FOGs appear at a time when the patient is relatively free of parkinsonian symptoms. There is no clinical characteristic that will differentiate between the two other than the response to higher doses of L-Dopa. "Off"-freezing improves by increasing the L-Dopa dose. In contrast, "on"-freezing is characterized by a worsening of symptoms as the dose of L-Dopa is increased and improvement as the dose is decreased. Patients who experience "on" FOGs frequently report that they walk better before the first morning dose of L-Dopa or at their "off" state. One can look at "off" FOG as a symptom of the hypodopaminergic state and "on" FOG as symptom-induced and exacerbated by L-Dopa.

The most common type of FOG in patients with PD is start hesitation, which was experienced by 86% of 318 patients who reported the presence of FOG and by 87% out of 60 patients with PD who were studied by Lamberti et al. (1,9). Other types of FOG, such as occur in doorways, on open runways, in stressful situations, or in turns have been reported less frequently; however, about 50% of freezers experience those in conjunction with start hesitation (1,9). Classically, FOG affects gait symmetrically but in asymmetric or unilateral parkinsonism, rarely only the affected leg freezes and freezing on turns is commonly worsened when turning to one direction and improved when turning to the opposite direction (personal experience). These observations suggest some laterality in freezing pathophysiology.

At the DATATOP study there was an increased risk for FOG if initial motor symptoms were on the left side of the body or if gait difficulties, balance problems, or speech disturbances were the initial motor symptoms (26). Lamberti et al. observed higher frequency of FOG among women with PD (9). The risk to develop FOG was significantly decreased if the initial motor symptom of PD was tremor (26); it increased if a patient had the akinetic-rigid type of parkinsonism (9). At the more advanced stages of the disease, FOG is strongly associated with the presence of L-Dopa–induced dyskinesia as well as early morning dystonia (1,29). One can speculate from this association with dystonia and dyskinesia as well as from earlier reports about the coactivation of antagonist muscles in the legs during a freezing episode that FOG is the result of involuntary, nonsynchronized, overactivation of leg muscles in an attempt to walk (34). Furthermore, the dramatic effect of sensory or motor tricks and their appearance in a specific gait pattern suggest some pathophysiologic similarities with dystonic gait.

TREATMENT OF FREEZING OF GAIT

Freezing of gait is a very complex symptom that should be treated using behavioral, medical, and surgical approaches; choose the right strategy on an individual basis (Table 19.7). Tricks of all kinds are very effective therapeutic approaches in overcoming FOG. Stern et al. were the first to report details of tricks, dividing them into: (a) gait modification by the patient alone or with the assistance of another person, and (b) assistance by auditory, verbal, or visual stimuli (35). The use of any trick is highly recommended because of its effectiveness, safety, and availability.

TABLE 19.7. *Treatment of freezing of gait*

Behavioral approach
Strips on the floor
Inverted cane
Change of gait pattern
Increase of attention
Metronome
Avoid narrow/tight spaces at home
Medical approach
Selegiline
Levodopa
Apomorphine
L-threo-DOPS
Dopa agonists?
SSRIs—Serotonin reuptake inhibitors
Botulinum toxin?
Physical intervention
Pallidotomy
Bilateral high frequency subthalamic nucleus stimulation
Fetal cell grafts to the putamen

Selegiline is the only drug that has been specifically reported to decrease the frequency and risk of gait freezing in the early stages of PD (26). This effect was purely symptomatic and disappeared when selegiline was stopped. Furthermore, patients who were on the selegiline arms of treatment in the DATATOP study did not have any long-term benefit in comparison to the placebo group (36). If anything, the selegiline-treated group had a tendency to freeze more at follow-up visits. A recent, retrospective assessment of patients with advanced PD did not find any effect for the duration of selegiline treatment on the frequency of FOG (29). One can conclude that selegiline has a short-term symptomatic effect on FOG but no protective effect. The mechanism of selegiline action on freezing is poorly understood and theoretically can be explained by its known dopaminergiclike activity, the amphetaminergic activity of its metabolite, or an undefined nonaminergic/nonmonoamine oxidase-B inhibitory effect.

Amantadine has been suggested as an effective drug in selected cases. In a retrospective analysis of the association between FOG and duration of amantadine treatment, Shabtai et al. recently reported a trend toward decreased frequency of FOG in the amantadine-treated group (29). Considering the retrospective nature of this study and the loss of that association when a multivariate analysis was implied, great caution should be exercised interpreting this observation. Only a controlled, prospective study will give a reliable answer to the actual effect of amantadine as well as other drugs on such a difficult symptom to assess as FOG.

L-threo DOPS (a chemical precursor of norepinephrine) has been reported to be of moderate symptomatic effect for freezing, mainly in those patients who had "pure freezing syndrome" in Japan (37). A similar study in patients with PD in United States reported a complete disappearance of freezing in two patients, an improvement that lasted 3 weeks and disappeared without any additional response even to higher dosages of L-threo-DOPS (38). Two additional patients had transient subjective improvement for 4 weeks. Another two studies at Columbia Presbyterian Medical Center in New York and Queen Square Medical Center in London did not find any benefit from L-threo-DOPS treatment for freezing in advanced PD (Fahn, personal communication) (39). The role of L-threo-DOPS for FOG in parkinsonian patients is still controversial, but it seems to help only patients with pure freezing syndrome for a short period of time.

Botulinum toxin type A (BTX-A) was reported to improve FOG when injected to the leg muscles of a patient with PD with foot dystonia and severe FOG (40). This observation was the basis for a pilot study performed by the same group. Ten parkinsonian patients (seven with PD, one with vascular parkinsonism, one with gait ignition failure, and one with Parkin mutation EO-AR parkinsonism) who suffered from severe and disabling FOG, were injected with 175 to 300 units of BTX-A (Allergan, US) to the calf muscles. Out of 20 sessions of injections, 12 gave moderate or marked improvement of FOG started after a mean of 7 days from the time of injection and lasting for a mean of 6.6 weeks (41). This preliminary observation should be followed by a double-blind study to further assess the approach.

Stereotactic neurosurgery has become an increasingly common approach to the treatment of patients with advanced PD. Deep brain stimulation of the subthalamic nucleus (STN) has been shown to be highly effective for alleviation of parkinsonian gait as well as "off"-freezing with marked decrease of antiparkinsonian medications. For further details and a review of the effect of DBS, pallidotomy, or fetal cell grafts please refer to Chapters 12, 28, and 30.

REFERENCES

1. Giladi N, McMahon D, Przedborski's, et al. Motor blocks in Parkinson's disease. *Neurology* 1992;42:333–339.
2. Giladi N, Kao R, Fahn S. Freezing phenomenon in patients with parkinsonian syndromes. *Mov Disord* 1997;12:302–305.
3. Giladi N, Fahn S. Freezing phenomenon, the fifth cardinal sign of parkinsonism. In: Fisher A, Hanin I, Yoshida M, eds. *Progress in Alzheimer's and Parkinson's diseases*. New York: Plenum, 1998:329–335.
4. Stern GM, Lander CM, Lees AJ. Akinetic freezing and trick movements in Parkinson's disease. *J Neural Transm Suppl* 1980;16:137–141.
5. Dietz M, Goetz C, Stebbins G. Evaluation of a modified inverted walking stick as a treatment for parkinsonian freezing episodes. *Mov Disord* 1990;5:243–247.
6. Martin J. Disorder of locomotion associated with disease of the basal ganglia. In: Anonymous, ed. *The basal ganglia and posture*. Philadelphia: J.B. Lippincott, 1967:24–35.
7. Narabayashi H, Imai H, Yokochi M. Cases of pure akinesia without rigidity and tremor and with no effect by L-Dopa therapy. In: Birkmyer W, Horniekiewicz O, eds. *Advances in parkinsonism*. Basel: Roche, 1976: 335–342.
8. Imai H, Narabayashi H, Sakata E. "Pure akinesia" and the later added supranuclear ophthalmoplegia. *Adv Neurol* 1987;45:207–212.
9. Lamberti P, Armenise S, Castaldo V, et al. Freezing gait in Parkinson's disease. *Eur Neurol* 1997;38:297–301.
10. Giladi N, Kao R, Fahn S. Freezing phenomenon in patients with parkinsonian syndromes. *Mov Disord* 1997;12:302–305.
11. Hassin-Baer S, Sirota P, Treves A, et al. Clinical characteristics of neuroleptic induced parkinsonism. *Mov Disord* 1998;13:185–185.
12. Fahn S. Parkinsonism. In: Rowland L, ed. *Merritt's textbook of neurology*. Philadelphia: Lea & Febiger, 1994.
13. Marsden C. Slowness of movement in Parkinson's disease. *Mov Disord* 1989;4:S26–S37.
14. Schwab R, England A, Peterson E. Akinesia in Parkinson's disease. *Neurology* 1959;9:65–72.
15. Achiron A, Ziv I, Goren M, et al. Primary progressive freezing gait. *Mov Disord* 1993;8:293–297.
16. Tohgi H, Abe T, Takahashi S, et al. Concentrations of serotonin and its related substances in the cerebrospinal fluid of Parkinsonian patients and their relations to the severity of symptoms. *Neurosci Letts* 1993;150: 71–74.
17. Narabayashi H. Clinical analysis of akinesia. *J Neural Transm* 1980;16:129–136.
18. Giladi N, Shabtai H, Simon E, et al. Freezing of gait in Parkinson's disease: scale construction. *Mov Disord* 1998;13:104.
19. Fahn S, Elton R, Members of the UPDRS development committee. Unified Parkinson's Disease Rating Scale. In: Fahn S, Marsden C, Calne D, et al., eds. *Recent developments in Parkinson's disease*. Florham Park, NJ: Macmillan, 1987:153–163.
20. Charcot J. *Clinical lectures on disease of the nervous system*. London: New Sydenham Society, 1877:145–146.
21. Luria A. *The nature of human conflicts*. New York: Liveright 1932;153.
22. Schwab R, Chafetz ME. Control of two simultaneous voluntary motor acts in normals and in parkinsonism. *Arch Neurol Psychiatry* 1954;72:591–598.
23. Barbeau A. Long term appraisal of levodopa therapy. *Neurology* 1972;22:22–24.
24. Barbeau A. Six years of high level levodopa therapy in severely akinetic parkinsonian patients. *Arch Neurol* 1976;33:333–338.
25. Ambani L, Van Woert M. Start hesitation—a side effect of long-term levodopa therapy. *N Engl J Med* 1973;1113–1115.
26. Giladi N, McDermott M, Fahn S, et al. Freezing of gait in Parkinson's disease. *Neurology* 1996;46:A377.
27. Parkinson Study Group. Effect of deprenyl on the progression of disability in early Parkinson's disease. *N Engl J Med* 1989;321:1364–1371.

28. Hoehn MM, Yahr MD. Parkinsonism: onset, progression, and mortality. *Neurology* 1967;17:427–442.
29. Giladi N, Treves TA, Simon ES, et al. Freezing of gait in patients with advanced Parkinson's disease. *J Neural Transm* 2001, in press.
30. Ahlskog J. Dopamine agonist treatment of fluctuating parkinsonism. D-2 (controlled release MK-458) vs combined D-1 and D-2 (pergolide). *Arch Neurol* 1992;49:560–568.
31. Weiner WJ, Factor SA, Sanchez RJ, et al. Early combination therapy (bromocriptine and levodopa) does not prevent motor fluctuations in Parkinson's disease. *Neurology* 1993;43:21–27.
32. Camicioli R, Oken BS, Sexton G, et al. Verbal fluency task affects gait in Parkinson's disease with motor freezing. *J Geriatr Psychiatry Neurol* 1998;11:181–185.
33. Linazasoro G. The apomorphine test in gait disorders associated with parkinsonism. *Clin Neuropharmacol* 1996;19:171–176.
34. Andrews CJ. Influence of dystonia on the response to long-term L-dopa therapy in Parkinson's disease. *J Neurol Neurosurg Psychiatry* 1973;36:630–636.
35. Stern G, Lander C, Lees A. Akinetic freezing and trick movements in Parkinson's disease. *J Neural Transm* 1980;16(Suppl.):137–141.
36. Parkinson Study Group USA. Impact of deprenyl and tocopherol treatment on Parkinson's disease in DATATOP subjects not requiring levodopa. *Ann Neurol* 1996;39:29–36.
37. Narabayashi H, Kondo T, Nagatsu T, et al. DL Threo-3,4-Dihydoxyphenylserine for freezing symptom in parkinsonism. In: Hassler R, Christ J, eds. *Advances in neurology*. New York: Raven, 1984:497–552.
38. Oribe E, Kaufman H, Yahr M. Freezing phenomena in Parkinson's disease: clinical features and effect of treatment with L-threo-DOPS. In: Narabayashi H, Mizuno Y, eds. *Norepinephrine deficiency and its treatment with L-threo DOPS in Parkinson's disease and the related disorders*. New York: Parthenon, 1993:89–96.
39. Quinn N, Perlmutter J, Marsden CD. Acute administration of DL-threo DOPS does not affect the freezing phenomenon in parkinsonian patients. *Neurology* 1984;34:149.
40. Giladi N, Honigman S. Botulinum toxin injections to one leg alleviate freezing of gait in a patient with Parkinson's disease. *Mov Disord* 1997;12:1085.
41. Gurevich, T, Simon, ES, Paleacu D, et al. *Treatment of parkinsonian gait with botulinum toxin injections to the calf muscles*. International Symposium on Gait Disorders. Prague, Czech Republic, Sept. 1999,146.

Gait Disorders. Advances in Neurology, Vol. 87,
edited by E. Růžička, M. Hallett, and J. Jankovic.
Lippincott Williams & Wilkins, Philadelphia © 2001.

20

Pathophysiology of Frozen Gait in Parkinsonism

*†Nobuo Yanagisawa, ‡Ryoichi Hayashi, and §Hiroshi Mitoma

**Chubu National Hospital, National Institute for Longevity Sciences, Morioka, Obu-shi, Aichi 474-8511, Japan; †Department of Medicine (Neurology), Shinshu University School of Medicine; ‡Division of Clinical Neurophysiology, School of Allied Medical Sciences, Shinshu University, Matsumoto 390-8621, Japan; §Mitoma Neurological Clinic, Toshima, Tokyo 171-0022, Japan*

A unique disorder in gait appears in advanced stages of Parkinson's disease (PD) or in cerebral infarction affecting the frontal lobe and the basal ganglia. It is characterized by difficulty in stepping forward caused by trembling of the legs and an inability to lift the foot from the floor. This gait disorder in patients with frontal lobe tumors was first called apaxia by Gerstmann and Schilder (1) in order to differentiate it from what Bruns (2) called frontal ataxia, which is characterized by disequilibrium and retropulsion. The disorder does not meet the classical criteria of "apraxia" (3) because it only appears in locomotion, which requires the equilibrium and highly organized neural mechanisms phylogenetically developed in humans with bipedal locomotion (4). Instead, frozen gait, freezing gait, or lower half Parkinsonism have been used to designate the condition (5–7).

HISTORICAL REVIEW

Gerstmann and Schilder characterized apraxia of gait by: (a) rooting of the feet in effort of walking, (b) marked disequilibrium, falling backward, and (c) maintenance of voluntary motion of extremities (1). They attributed its causative lesions to the medial-basal part of the prefrontal lobe. Denny-Brown called the rooting of the feet in gait effort the "slipping clutch syndrome" (8) and evaluated foot grasp reflex as an important factor in the condition and attributed the inability to lift the foot to "magnetic apraxia" or positive supporting reaction. Meyer and Baron, students of Denny-Brown, also stressed the importance of foot grasp response; they observed clumsiness of voluntary limb movement in free space and considered neural mechanisms as "transcortical innervatory paralysis" (9). Petrovici observed persistent tonic EMG activity and difficulty in initiation of stepping in muscles of the lower extremities (10). Petrovici attributed this difficulty to a disorder of the "postural set." Andrews stressed disorders in reciprocal innervation in leg muscles (11). Ueno described a patient who developed a unique disorder of locomotion that met the classic criteria of apraxia as defined by Liepmann: The gait was different from frozen gait in clinical features, and the patient showed difficulty in shift of interests and perseveration of daily life activities (3,12).

METHODS

Various novel instruments and classic methods to detect analysis of gait have been employed:

- Floor reaction forces using force plate
- Pressure at different parts of foot sole
- Trace of body parts with position sensor
- Joint angle displacement with goniometer
- Electromyography (EMG)
- Accelerometer
- Video

Floor reaction forces exerted by feet in each step of forward locomotion are measured in three directions (fore-aft, Y; lateral, X; vertical, Z), which provide valuable information for the pathophysiology of gait disturbance (5).

In our study, a floor 4 m in length and 80 cm in width with four force plates was installed in the walkway at the same level as the rest of the floor. In order to record parkinsonism gait, the position of the center of the body pressure on the floor (gravity), cadence, the distance between the left and right foot in the lateral direction, the patterns of foot pressure in the z-axis (vertical), the z-y (vertical/fore-aft) vector of foot pressure, and the on and off periods of the feet from the floor were measured for forward locomotion over either 10 sec or a 4-m walk from the starting point. Surface EMG of flexors and extensors of the thigh and lower leg gave information on activities of functionally different muscle groups semiquantitatively. Phases of stepping in forward locomotion are divided into four: (a) step in, (b) stance, (c) kick off, and (d) swing. Integrated EMG at each phase represents tension produced by contraction of the concerned muscles semiquantitatively (13). Reciprocity between activities of antagonists is particularly important in locomotion.

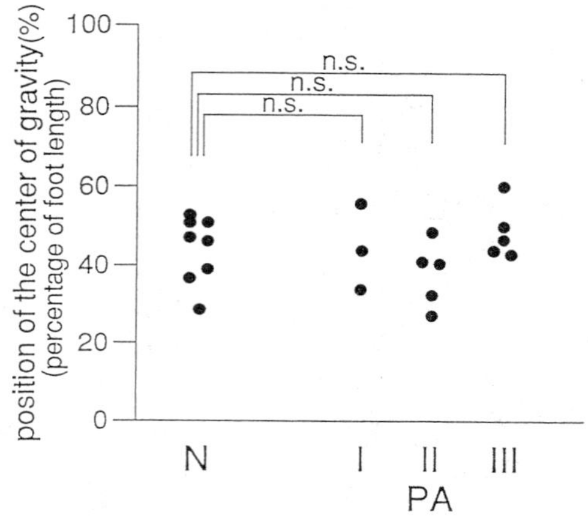

FIG. 20.1. Position of center of foot pressure on natural standing in normals (*N*) and different stages of Parkinson's disease (*PA*). *I, II, III* showed stages of illness by Hoehn and Yahr. Ordinate shows COP from the top of the big toe by percentage of foot length.

POSSIBLE FACTORS AND ABNORMALITIES

Equilibrium

Since Gerstmann and Schilder, it has been shown that disequilibrium or disorders in postural reflexes, irrespective of underlying diseases, tumors in the frontal lobe, PD, or multiple cerebral infarction (MCI), are characteristics of frozen gait (1). Postural reflexes, as examined by pushing the shoulder or chest, are commonly disturbed in PD from the early stages of illness. Typical forward bending of the upper half of the body in PD does not produce forward shift of center of foot pressure (COP) on the floor. Center of foot pressure with natural standing was not different in patients with PD from normals, although a slight tendency to shift backward was observed as motor disturbances become more severe (Fig. 20.1). The maximal voluntary shift of COP without falling was smaller in patients with PD than normals (14). A typical posture in patients with PD is that of forward bent upper body with slight flexion at the knee, which is employed to prevent the patient from falling back. This is similar to the posture of natural gait in normal subjects who are walking on a slippery floor or skiing downhill. Parkinsonism with MCI does not necessarily show forward bending posture, even in patients with frozen gait (5). Patients with MCI may show upright posture with a wider step width between the left and right foot, but easy falling or stepping out similar to patients with PD is observed by pushing the chest (12).

Foot Grasp

Foot grasp or tonic foot response was claimed as an important sign in apraxia of gait (8,9). We observed it in 85% of patients with frozen gait and 100% of patients with MCI (5). It is elicited by stroke stimuli on the sole along radius of toes; the toes flex as if to grasp the floor on standing. The grasp reflex of toes with positive supporting reaction of lower extremities would likely hinder smooth locomotion (8).

Floor Reaction Forces

Floor reaction forces of the feet during forward locomotion represent characteristics of

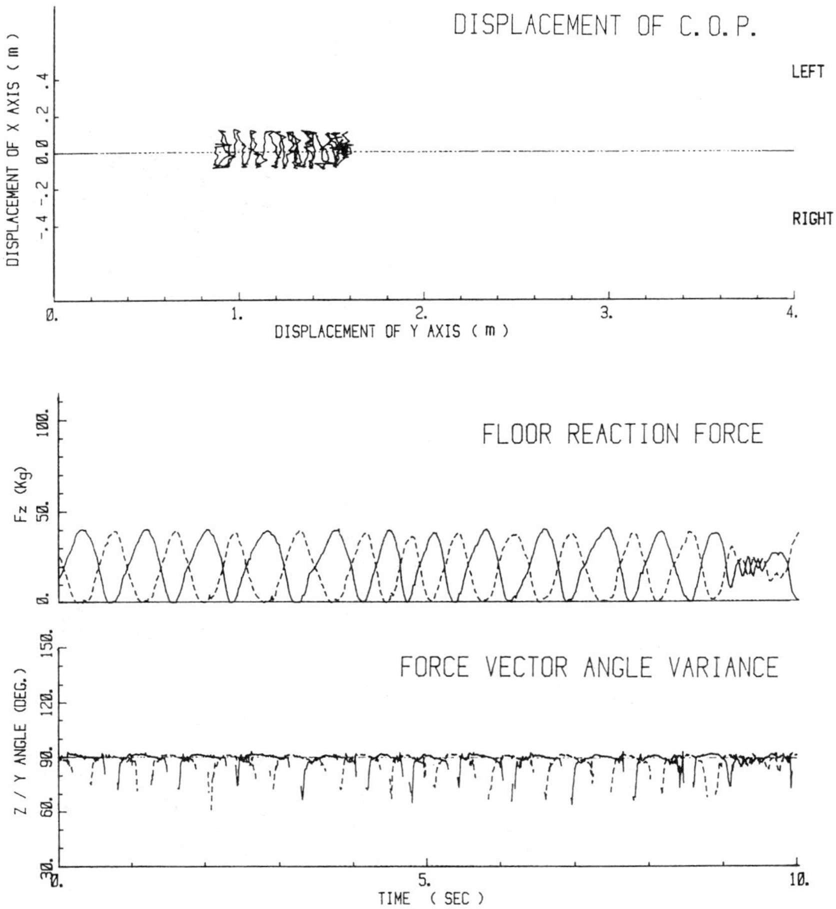

FIG. 20.2. Traces of locomotion and floor reaction forces in shuffling and frozen gait in a patient with Parkinson's disease. **Upper Record:** Displacement of the center of pressure (*C.O.P.*) for 10 seconds shows shuffling gait with little forward movement in most of the record and cessation of locomotion near the end, shown by dark tracings. **Middle Record:** Vertical component of floor reaction forces. Solid line shows trace of pressure on the right foot and dotted line on the left. In shuffling gait, both vertical pressure on stepping and zero phase in swing phases showed narrow single peaks at frequencies higher than normal. In freezing with no progression, which is shown in the last part of the record, the rate of alternate shift became higher and the range of foot pressure became smaller and a complete shift of body weight onto one foot was no longer observed. **Lower Record:** z-y force vector shows frequent step-in forces (below 90 degrees), but little kick-off power (above 90 degrees) was observed even during shuffling gait. (From Yanagisawa N, Ueno E, Takami M. Frozen gait of Parkinson's disease and parkinsonism: a study with floor reaction forces and EMG. In: Shimamura M, Grillner S, Edgerton VR, eds. *Neurophysiological basis of human locomotion*. Tokyo: Japan Scientific Societies Press, 1991:291–304, with permission.)

short-stepped or shuffling gait and frozen gait (5,15).

Traces of Center of Pressure

Traces of COP showed alternating shifts of body pressure on the left and right foot in the shuffling gait, but the size of forward displacement was small and the trace was a zigzag pattern (Fig. 20.2) (5). Detailed measurement of displacement of COP in forward gait disclosed hesitation at both step-in and kick-off phases of stance even in natural gait in patients with PD (Fig. 20.3). Forward displacement in frozen gait does not occur without lifting the foot from the floor at the swing phase (Fig. 20.2).

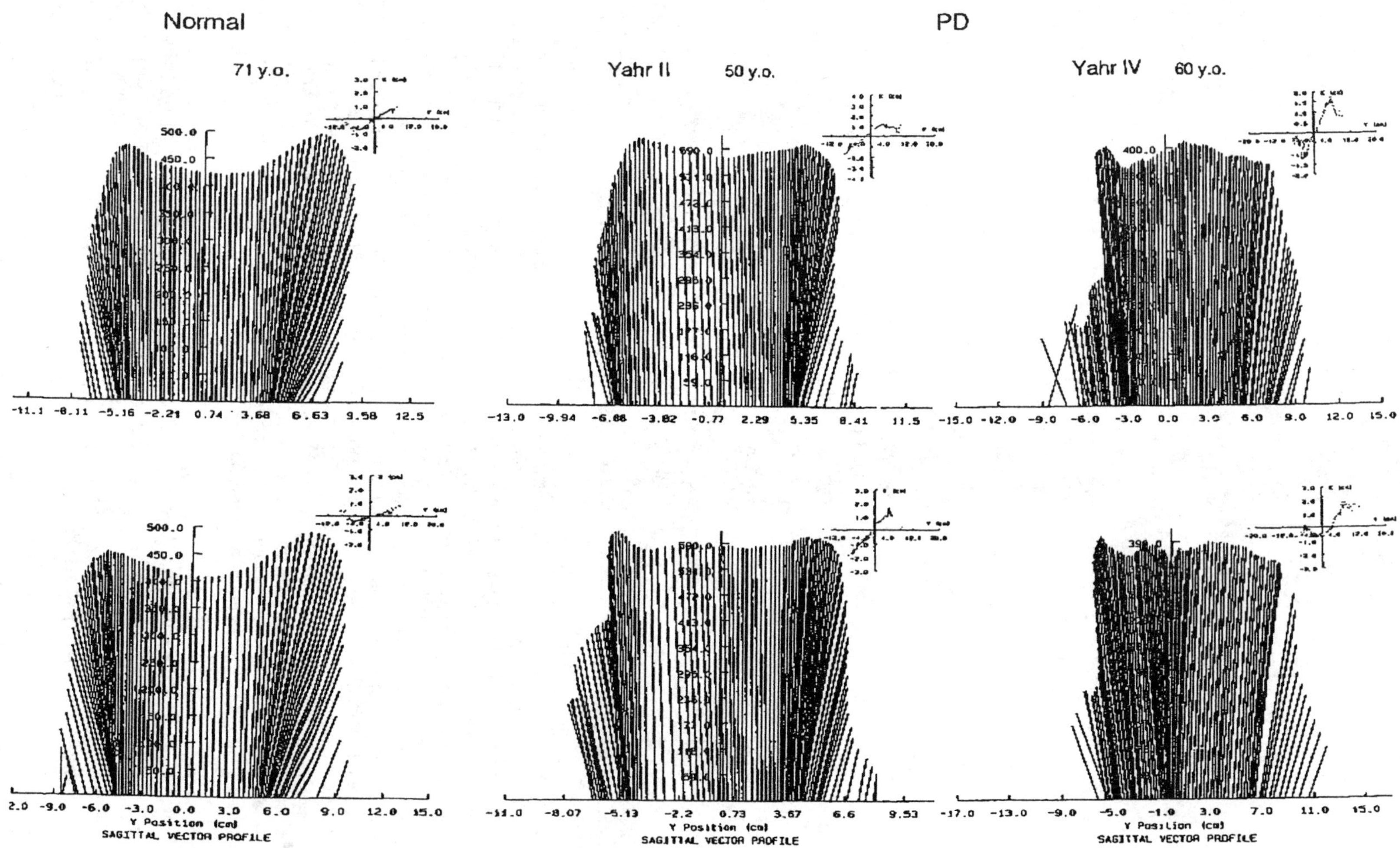
Normal
PD
71 y.o.
Yahr II
50 y.o.
Yahr IV
60 y.o.
Y Position (cm)
SAGITTAL VECTOR PROFILE
Y Position (cm)
SAGITTAL VECTOR PROFILE
Y Position (cm)
SAGITTAL VECTOR PROFILE

Stepping Rhythm

The cadence or one cycle of stepping rhythm is nearly 1.0 Hz for young adults; it gradually decreases to 0.83 Hz at 80 years of age in normals. It does not exceed 1.1 Hz (16). In patients with PD, cadence is normal in short-stepped or shuffling gait (0.9 ± 0.3 Hz), but in patients with MCI it is 1.5 ± 0.3 Hz. In frozen gait, the rhythm is 4.6 ± 0.8 Hz in patients with PD and 2.3 ± 0.6 Hz in those with MCI (15). Other than average rhythm, there was obvious divergence between patients with PD and those with MCI in transition from shuffling gait to freezing. In patients with PD, the rhythm of stepping suddenly jumped into high frequency, similar to the rhythm of resting tremor in patients with PD, whereas the rhythm of stepping gradually increased and reached a point where freezing and stopping locomotion occurred in those with MCI. This causes an inability in lift the foot from the floor (Fig. 20.4) (15).

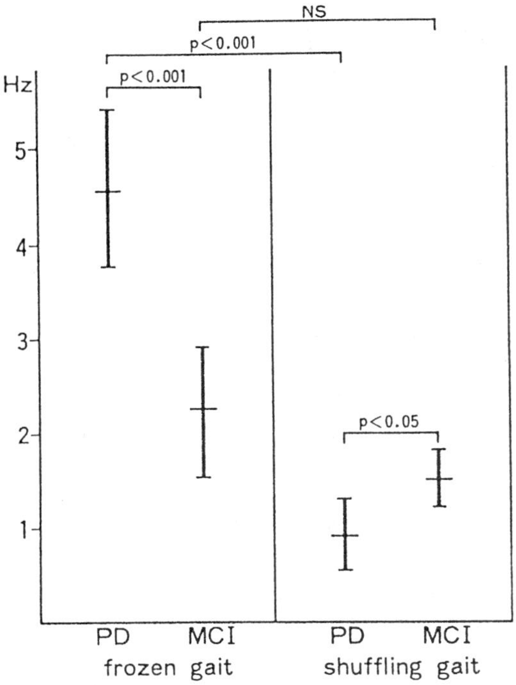

FIG. 20.4. Rhythm of steps in shuffling and frozen gait in patients with Parkinson's disease (*PD*) and multiple cerebral infarction (*MCI*). In frozen gait, the frequency of rhythm of one walking cycle in patients with PD was significantly greater than in patients with MCI. In shuffling gait, rhythm in patients with PD was within normal range, but patients with MCI showed faster rhythm. (From Ueno E, Yanagisawa N, Takami M. Gait disorders in parkinsonism. A study with floor reaction forces and EMG. In: Narabayashi H, Nagatsu T, Yanagisawa N, et al., eds. *Parkinson's disease. From basic research to treatment.* New York: Raven Press, 1993:414–418, with permission.)

Step Width

Step width or stance between the left and right foot was different between patients with MCI and those with PD. The mean of step width in patients with MCI was 24.3 ± 6.9 cm, 17.2 ± 3.3 in patients with PD, and 13.6 ± 3.4 in normal control subjects. Step width in patients with MCI was significantly larger than in those with PD or controls, which coincides well with clinical observation (15).

Driving Forces in Forward Locomotion

Foot pressure in the vertical direction in a step during forward locomotion in normal subjects showed two peaks corresponding to the increase in pressure on stepping-in and kicking-off from the floor. During these two peaks, the pressure of the other foot was zero as it was on the swing phase. In contrast, shuffling gait showed changes

←

FIG. 20.3. Traces of vectors of vertical pressure in fore-aft direction were shown in the natural gait of normal controls and patients with Parkinson's disease (*PD*) with Hoehn and Yahr's stage *II* and *IV*. Two samples of one right footstep for each subject was shown in the **upper** and **lower** records. Higher density at step-in (left) and kick-off (right) in records of PD showed that longer time was required for stance phase. Vector angles at these dense areas were more vertical than normal, and they showed less step-in and kick-off forces than normal. (Sample time of a bar, 5 msec.)

in patterns: (a) The two peaks of vertical pressure in one step were replaced by a narrow, single peak. (b) The duration of the zero pressure phase was much shorter. In frozen gait, changes in foot pressure in alternating stepping behavior were smaller than those in the shuffling gait, and complete shift of the center of pressure from one foot to the other was not observed (Fig. 20.2). The force vector angle variance in z/y (vertical/fore-aft) direction shows angles to step-in and kick-off from the floor in forward locomotion. Vector angles exceeding 90 degrees showed the angle of kickback on the floor by the foot. The maximum of vector angle variance at the point of toe-off was 114.1 ± 6.5 degrees in normal subjects, 94.9 ± 3.2 degrees in patients with PD, and 90.9 ± 3.3 degrees in patients with MCI (15) in shuffling or frozen gait.

The direction of kickback was nearly vertical and progression force was small in shuffling gait. In contrast, vector angle in step-in direction is shown by values below 90 degrees, which was obviously smaller in shuffling gait than normal (Fig. 20.2). The direction of step-in was an acute angle to the floor, probably owing to the small foot lift-up (Fig. 20.3).

Electromyography

Electromyography was recorded from hip flexor (adductor femoris) and extensor (gluteus medius), thigh flexor (biceps femoris) and extensor (vastus lateralis), and leg flexor (tibialis anterior) and extensor (gastrocnemius) simultaneously in natural gait in patients with PD.

Thigh flexor and extensor showed significantly higher amount of EMG continuously at step-in, stance, and kickoff phases and a lower amount in the tibialis anterior in step-in phase in patients with PD than in normals. These were more marked in advance stages of illness.

This lack of change in EMG at different phases of stepping coincides with results of Petrovici (10).

Reciprocity of EMG between antagonists is worth mentioning. Andrews and Ohi et al. claimed that disturbance in reciprocal innervation was crucial in the development of apraxia of gait (17,18).

In our study, thigh flexors and extensors contracted synchronously in some instances in frozen gait, but it was not a constant finding (Fig. 20.5). Instead, phases of EMG activity between antagonists throughout freezing disclosed reciprocal contraction between leg flexors and extensors (5). Thus, it is reasonable not to attribute a cause of apraxia of gait or frozen gait to disturbance in reciprocity in activities in leg muscles.

ESSENTIAL FEATURES

Responsible Lesion Sites

Pathology of patients showing apraxia of gait or frozen gait suggests that frontal white matter and the basal ganglia are essential sites of lesions. The appearance of frozen gait in patients with PD suggests the importance of the basal ganglia. On the other hand, the development of typical frozen gait was observed in a young patient who suffered from occlusion of an anterior cerebral artery after a subarachnoid hemorrhage, in which case the lesion was confined to the deep white matter in the unilateral frontal lobe. Recent neuroimaging techniques do not necessarily demonstrate hypoperfusion in the frontal lobe in patients showing frozen gait, which suggests that structural destruction is not mandatory (12,19).

The possible involvement of the noradrenergic system should be mentioned. Narabayashi and colleagues found that a synthesized noradrenaline precursor L-threo-DOPS improves frozen gait and other gait disorders in patients with PD (20). Tohgi et al. found that norepinephrine (NE) and its metabolites in cerebrospinal fluid (CSF) decreased but dopamine did not in patients showing frozen gait, and degree of decrease in NE level correlated with severity of frozen gait (21).

Neurologic Features

Disequilibrium and tonic foot response seem essential for development of frozen gait. Short steps, loss of sufficient swing phase, or little kick-off power, which are observed in both patients with PD and those with MCI, may be attributable to disequilibrium.

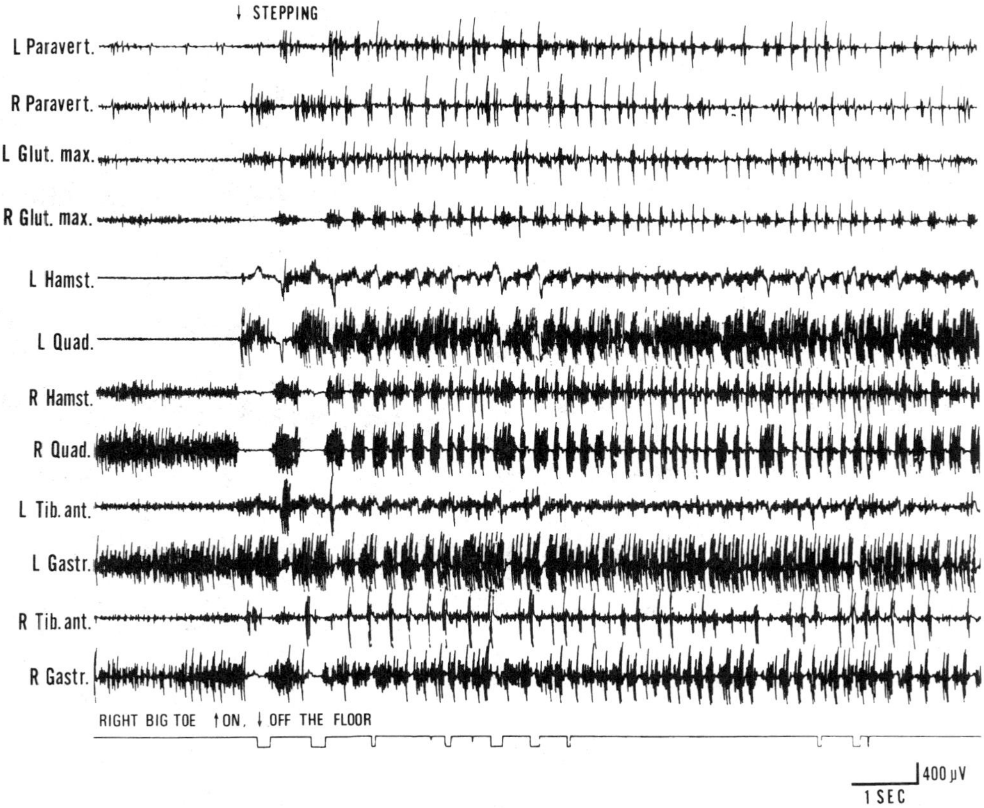

FIG. 20.5. Electromyogram (EMG) of frozen gait. From the top downward, EMG left (*L*) and right (*R*): paravertebral (*Paravert.*), gluteus maximus (*Glut. max.*), hamstrings (*Hamst.*), quadriceps (*Quad.*), tibialis anterior (*Tib. ant.*) and gastrocnemius (*Gastr.*) muscles. The lowest record showed a period of touching (*on*) or lifting up (*off*) from the floor of the plantar surface of the right big toe. On stepping, grouping of muscular contractions at rates of 4 to 6 Hz developed after initial normal steps, corresponding to trembling of the legs and freezing of steps. (From Yanagisawa N, Ueno E, Takami M. Frozen gait of Parkinson's disease and parkinsonism: a study with floor reaction forces and EMG. In: Shimamura M, Grillner S, Edgerton VR, eds. *Neurophysiological basis of human locomotion.* Tokyo: Japan Scientific Societies Press, 1991:291–304, with permission.)

Electromyographic Abnormalities

Tonic activity in thigh muscles and inability to switch from active to inactive patterns in lower limb muscles in various phases of stepping may result from postural reactions to disequilibrium or postural responses to forward bending, knee-semiflexed characteristic posture in patients with PD. This tonic background EMG activity may be a factor in gait disorders including frozen gait. However, tonic activities in quadriceps and leg muscles, as exemplified in Figure 20.6, were common on standing in patients with PD, but they did not necessarily hinder smooth gait in those with PD.

The role of disturbance in reciprocal innervation in leg muscles is a matter of conjecture. Our findings in patients with PD were inconsistent in appearance of nonreciprocal contraction in extensors and flexors. Diffuse activation of flexors and extensors is a normal postural response in standing. Inability to switch over to gait pattern from standing may be an important factor in locomotion in patients with PD.

Stepping Frequency

Increase in step rhythm seems an important factor for development of frozen gait. Hastening is

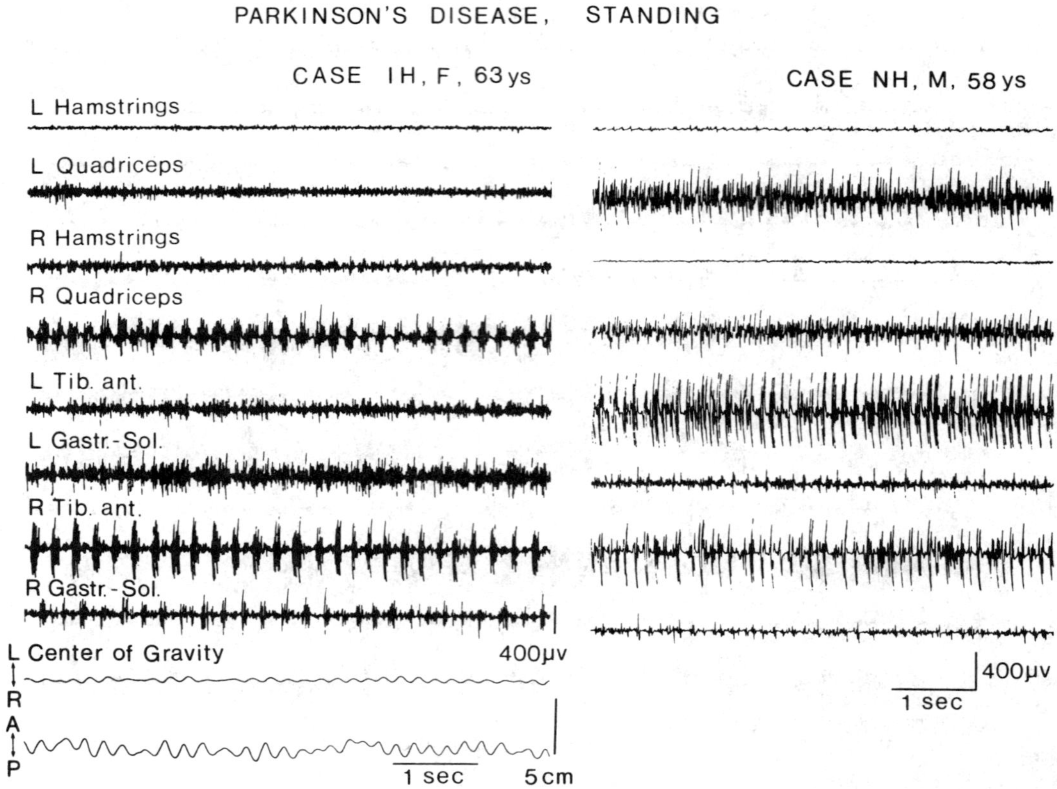

FIG. 20.6. Electromyogram of leg muscles on standing in two patients with Parkinson's disease. Simultaneous recordings from thigh flexors and extensors and leg flexors and extensors were made. The lowermost two records on the left showed the center of pressure in the lateral and fore-aft directions. Rates of grouping discharges in left record (4 to 5 Hz) demonstrate resting tremor, whereas those in the right record (8 Hz) show postural tremor. *L*, left; *R*, right; *A*, anterior; *P*, posterior; *M*, male; *F*, female.

characteristic in repetitive movements in PD. It is observed in alternating pronation and supination of hand, finger tapping, and stuttering of speech in ordinary clinical examination. These repeating motions rapidly decrease in amplitude with consecutive motions and lead to freezing. Nakamura and colleagues disclosed that rhythm of repetitive motion falls in certain frequencies in freezing in patients with PD (22). A sudden increase to a characteristic rhythm was observed in the frozen gait of patients with PD. It coincided with that of resting tremor. However, presence of tremor in the leg on standing is not a risk factor for frozen gait. Figure 20.6 demonstrates electromyographies of tremors in the lower extremities of two patients with PD. The patient on the left showed 4.0 Hz grouping in the lower leg muscle and 5.0 Hz in the thigh of the right side. The patient on the right showed 8 Hz grouping in tibialis anterior muscles. The rhythm of tremor in the legs on standing may result from the frequency of either resting or postural tremor, as shown in Figure 20.6. These patients did not show freezing on gait. Electromyographic patterns of leg muscles in freezing and tremor are different from each other (Figs. 20.5 and 20.6).

On the other hand, a gradual increase in step rhythm was observed in patients with MCI. A higher frequency of stepping is crucial for the development of freezing, and the rhythm in EMG on freezing is that of stepping and is not related to tremor itself on standing.

Kinesie Paradoxale

Recovery from freezing by looking at striped visual markers on the floor or listening to acoustic stimuli at a rate of normal stepping is a unique observation at early to middle stages of frozen gait, called kinesie paradoxale. There are diverse locomotion centers in hierarchical fashion in mammals and humans in spinal cord, brainstem, thalamus, basal ganglia, and frontal lobe (23). Straight gait was produced in rabbits by lesions in the caudate nuclei, but the basal ganglia and frontal lobe seem to be higher locomotion centers phylogenetically developed in humans (24). Different centers are considered to control different types of gait, such as reflex, automatic, and conscious (23). Each of these appears to be innervated by a center located from the lower to the higher levels of the central nervous system. Kinesie paradoxale is considered the result of shifting from innervation by malfunctioned automatic gait centers to intact centers for conscious gait driven by external cues. In advanced stages, external cues may no longer shift centers for action from diseased to intact ones. Further studies on this issue are needed.

REFERENCES

1. Gerstmann J, Schilder P. *Uber eine besondere Gangstorung bei Stirnhirnerkrankung. Wien Med Wschr* 1926;26:97–102.
2. Bruns L. *Über Störung des Gleichgewichtes bei Stirnhirntumoren. Dtsh Med Wochenshr* 1892;18:138–140.
3. Liepmann H. *Das Krankheitsbild der Apraxie (motorischen Asymbolie). Mtschr Psychiat* 1900;8:15–44, 102–132, 182–197.
4. Geschwind N. Disconnexion syndromes in animals and man. *Brain* 1965;88:237–294, 585–644.
5. Yanagisawa N, Ueno E, Takami M. Frozen gait of Parkinson's disease and parkinsonism: a study with floor reaction forces and EMG. In: Shimamura M, Grillner S, Edgerton VR, eds. *Neurophysiological basis of human locomotion*. Tokyo: Japan Scientific Societies Press, 1991:291–304.
6. Achiron A, Ziv I, Goren M, Goldberg H, et al. Primary progressive freezing gait. *Mov Disord* 1993;8:293–297.
7. Elble RJ, Cousins R, Leffler K, et al. Gait initiation by patients with lower-half parkinsonism. *Brain* 1996;119:1705–1716.
8. Denny-Brown D. The nature of apraxia. *J Nerv Ment Dis* 1958;126:9–33.
9. Meyer JS, Barron DW. Apraxia of gait: a clinicophysiological study. *Brain* 1960;83:261–284.
10. Petrovici I. Apraxia of gait and of trunk movements. *J Neurol Sci* 1968;7:229–243.
11. Andrews CJ. Influence of dystonia on the response to long term L-dopa therapy in Parkinson's disease. *J Neurol Neurosurg Psychiatry* 1973;36:630–636.
12. Ueno E. Clinical and physiological study of apraxia of gait and frozen gait. *Clin Neurol* 1989;29:275–283.
13. Yanagisawa N, Hashimoto T. Quantification of involuntary movements with electromyography. In: Clifford Rose F, ed. *Parkinson's disease and the problems of clinical trials*. London: Smith-Gordon, 1992:131–142.
14. Hayashi R, Tokuda T, Takou K, et al. Impaired modulation of tonic muscle activities and H-reflexes in the soleus muscle during standing in patients with Parkinson's disease. *J Neurol Sci* 1997;153:61–67.
15. Ueno E, Yanagisawa N, Takami M. Gait disorders in parkinsonism. A study with floor reaction forces and EMG. In: Narabayashi H, Nagatsu T, Yanagisawa N, et al., eds. *Parkinson's disease. From basic research to treatment*. New York: Raven Press, 1993:414–418.
16. Takami M, Fukui K. Force-plate study of normal walking. *Rehabil Med* 1987;24:93–101.
17. Andrews CJ. Influence of dystonia on the response to long-term L-DOPA therapy in Parkinson's disease. *J Neurol Neurosurg Psychiatry* 1973;36:630–636.
18. Ohi T, Shibasaki H, Kato M, et al. Gait apraxia improved by the rhythmical visual input: report of three cases. *Clin Neurol (Tokyo)* 1976;16:551–557.
19. Fabre N, Brefel C, Sabatini U, et al. Normal frontal perfusion in patients with frozen gait. *Mov Disord* 1998;13:677–683.
20. Narabayashi H, Kondo T, Yokochi F, et al. Clinical effects of L-threo-3, 4-dihydroxyphenylserine in cases of parkinsonism and pure akinesia. In: Yahr MD, Bergman KJ, eds. *Parkinson's disease*. New York: Raven Press, 1986:593–602.
21. Tohgi H, Abe T, Takahashi S, et al. Cerebrospinal fluid dopamine, norepinephrine, and epinephrine concentrations in Parkinson's disease correlated clinical symptoms. In: Streifler MB, Korczyn AD, Melamed E, et al., eds. *Parkinson's disease: anatomy, pathology, and therapy*. New York, Raven Press, 1990:277–282.
22. Nakamura R, Nagasaki H, Narabayashi H. Disturbances of rhythm formation in patients with Parkinson's disease. Part 1. Characteristics of tapping response to the periodic signals. *Percept Mot Skills* 1978;46:63–75.
23. Mori S, Takakusaki K. Integration of posture and locomotion. In: Ambland B, Berthoz A, Clarac F, eds. *Posture and gait*. Amsterdam: Elsevier, 1988:341–354.
24. Martin JP. *The basal ganglia and posture*. London: Pitman Medical, 1967:33–35.

Gait Disorders. Advances in Neurology, Vol. 87,
edited by E. Růžička, M. Hallett, and J. Jankovic.
Lippincott Williams & Wilkins, Philadelphia © 2001.

21

Postural Instability and Falls in Parkinson's Disease

*†Bastiaan R. Bloem, ‡Jeroen P.P. van Vugt, and §Dennis J. Beckley

**Department of Neurology, University Hospital Nijmegen, 6500 HB Nijmegen, The Netherlands; †MRC Human Movement and Balance Unit, Institute of Neurology, London WC1N 3BG, United Kingdom; ‡Department of Neurology, Leiden University Medical Centre, 2300 RC Leiden, The Netherlands; and §Human Balance Laboratory, Neurology Services, Veteran's Administration Medical Centre, Martinez, California 94553*

Postural instability is regarded as one of the most disabling signs of Parkinson's disease (PD). In his classic *Essay on the Shaking Palsy,* James Parkinson already stressed that "the utmost care is necessary to prevent falls" (1). In early PD, patients complain mostly about tremor, but as the disease progresses, instability and immobility become increasingly significant (2). Although balance impairment may be the presenting symptom in occasional patients, postural difficulties typically emerge in patients with more advanced PD (3). Recurrent falls occur, on average, 10 years after onset of the disease (4). Early occurring and pronounced postural instability or falls should alert the clinician that the patient does not have idiopathic PD. Patients with postural instability as the very first symptom most likely have progressive supranuclear palsy (PSP). Others may have multiple system atrophy, corticobasal degeneration, or vascular parkinsonism.

Many patients with PD have static postural problems, as evidenced by their characteristically stooped posture. However, most postural problems are reflected mainly during dynamic activities, such as walking or standing up from a chair. Other postural difficulties emerge while lying in a recumbent position, resulting in an inability to turn in bed at night. Gait disturbances are closely intertwined with the postural abnormalities. The typical parkinsonian gait is characterized by a shuffling and short-stepped gait, a reduced arm swing (often asymmetrically), and slow turns that are executed en bloc. In more advanced stages of the disease, patients may speed up during a walk by taking rapid sequential steps (festination). Several years after onset of the disease, many patients experience freezing (a sudden "gluing" of the feet to the floor) at the initiation of gait, during walking or while making turns (5).

EPIDEMIOLOGY OF FALLS

Epidemiologic information on falls in PD is limited and obtained mostly retrospectively; sometimes only using mailed questionnaires (6). According to these studies, the proportion of patients who fall at least once averages 40% to 50%, compared to about 30% in healthy ambulatory subjects over 60 years of age (6–9). Weekly and often even daily falls occurred in 13% of patients (7). In one retrospective and autopsy-confirmed survey, recurrent falls occurred in no less than 91% of patients with PD since the time of diagnosis (4). Bloem and coworkers have recently completed a prospective survey of falls in PD and found that almost 60% fell at least once during a 6-month period (10). Even though our patients were relatively mildly affected (mean

Hoehn and Yahr stage 2.3), 33% had multiple falls during this period. Most falls occurred when patients were in their best clinical condition ("on"), with or without dyskinesias. We believe this reflects the increased mobility when symptoms are well controlled.

REDUCED QUALITY OF LIFE

Contrary to common belief, the absolute number of falls may not be the most important consequence of balance impairment in PD. We speculate that falls are most common in moderately affected patients who are not only unstable, but also sufficiently mobile to actually fall. This is illustrated schematically in Figure 21.1. In later stages of the disease, when patients become more aware of their balance problems, compensatory strategies help limit the falling frequency. For example, patients may try to prevent falls by stiffening their body during quiet stance (11). Furthermore, patients can purposely adopt a cautious gait, characterized by a slow walking speed with small, careful steps (12). This strategy augments the typical parkinsonian gait disorder that is inherent to the disease itself. Other patients may actively assume a stooped (but rarely wide-based) posture that can help prevent falls (13,14). In addition, recurrent falls often induce a fear of future falls that forces patients to reduce their physical activities (7,8). Some patients may even develop a fall phobia and become virtually socially isolated. This immobilization does solve the falling problem, because a limited ambulatory status is associated with fewer falls; however, the lost ability to participate in many aspects of social life is a grave consequence of postural instability that must not be overlooked.

Such adaptive processes may benefit patients in early stages of the disease, but the disease process eventually overcomes these compensatory strategies. Because of increasing postural instability, patients become progressively immobilized and fall incidence drops (Fig. 21.1). Some patients lose their independence and are admitted to nursing homes. Indeed, postural instability and hip fractures are important risk factors for nursing home admission in PD (15,16). However, it is rare for patients with PD to become entirely bedridden or permanently confined to a wheelchair (17). In such patients, alternative diagnoses must be considered, such as PSP or multiple system atrophy.

Needless to say, the quality of life is progressively reduced in the course of this process (Fig. 21.1). Indeed, patients with PD often report that gait impairment, falls, loss of mobility, and reduction of social activities negatively influence

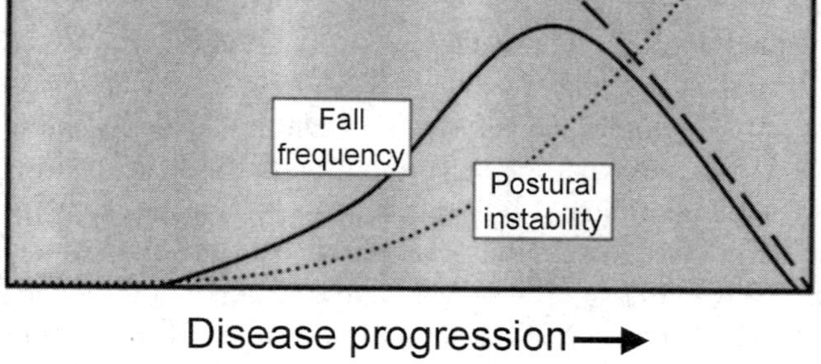

FIG. 21.1. Hypothetical model of postural instability and falls in Parkinson's disease. The absolute number of falls may be highest in moderate stages of the disease. In later stages, the falling frequency levels off owing to compensatory strategies (partially stirred by a fear of falling) and, eventually, progressive immobilization. At this point, a reduced quality of life becomes increasingly significant.

their quality of life (18,19). Quality of life (in terms of regained mobility and independence), therefore, should be an important outcome measure in trials that investigate preventive or therapeutic strategies. After all, a reduced frequency of falls at the end of such a trial might simply reflect an increased awareness of balance problems that led patients to reduce their activities.

POSTURAL INSTABILITY: AN OMINOUS SIGN

Postural instability marks the onset of severe disability for several reasons (Fig. 21.2). Recurrent falls constitute an eminent risk factor for fractures or other injuries. Hip fractures are particularly common in patients with PD (9,20). Some 25% of all patients have suffered a hip fracture within 10 years after diagnosis of the disease (21). The incidence of wrist fractures appears considerably lower, perhaps because of the absence or slow activation of protective arm movements (9,21). Hip fractures in patients with PD are an ominous sign because they are associated with a higher-than-normal morbidity and mortality (22,23). The resultant immobilization promotes development of osteoporosis, together with a vitamin D deficiency, which further increases the fracture risk (9). Loss of activity also leads to muscle weakness, which is a risk factor for further falls.

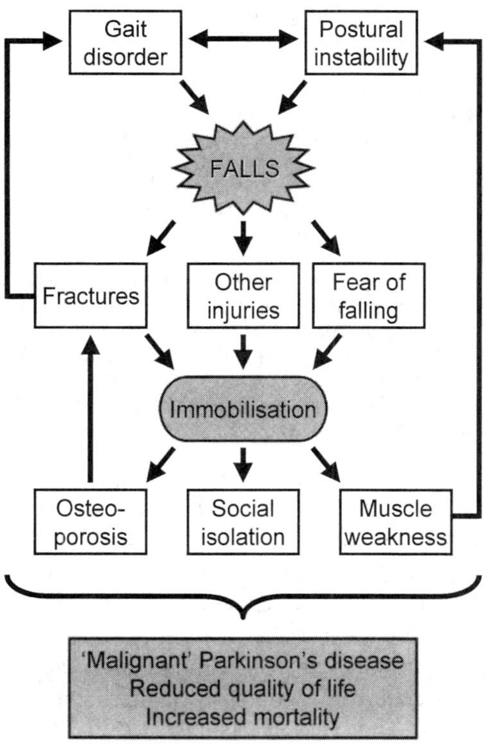

FIG. 21.2. The vicious circle of postural instability and falls in Parkinson's disease.

Other injuries can be life threatening, such as subdural or epidural hematomas. However, most soft-tissue injuries, such as bruises or lacerations, attract clinical attention less easily; however, when carefully monitored, their incidence far exceeds that of bone fractures (10). All injuries may lead to a fear of falling and thus contribute to the immobilization of patients.

Once present, balance impairment often heralds the onset of progressive physical and sometimes mental decline. Patients who develop prominent postural instability are often considered to have a form of "malignant" parkinsonism, associated with rapid disease progression, severe disability, and development of cognitive impairment (24). As mentioned earlier, these patients probably do not have idiopathic PD, but a different parkinsonian syndrome with reduced survival and poor responsiveness to L-Dopa therapy (17).

An increased mortality risk is another important concomitant of postural instability in PD. Parkinson patients with gait or balance disorders have a reduced survival, compared to patients who walk normally (25,26). Average survival is reduced to about 7 years, once recurrent falls are present (4). This association is partially explained by the reduced cardiovascular fitness of immobile patients, which increases their risk of myocardial infarction or stroke. In addition, unstable patients may suffer fatal injuries owing to accidental falls. Finally, many patients are unable to get up without help after a fall and may die from exhaustion, dehydration, or decubitus. Patients with advanced PD are thus saddled with a vicious circle of recurrent falls, immobilization and progressive weakness that jointly contribute to a reduced quality of life and, eventually, to an increased mortality (Fig. 21.2).

CLINICAL ASSESSMENT OF POSTURAL INSTABILITY

History Taking

Postural instability should always be assessed during routine neurological investigation of patients with PD because of these severe implications. The physician must actively ask for balance impairment and its consequences because elderly patients often forget or fail to volunteer their falls. Careful history taking should never be omitted, but is notoriously unreliable when patients are asked about the number of recent falls, in particular if patients suffer from cognitive impairment (27). The Mini Mental State Examination can be used to screen for cognitive dysfunction and as a rough estimate for the reliability of the interview. Interviewing the spouse or caretaker may provide valuable additional information. Special fall-diaries can be informative in some patients. Use of standardized questionnaires assures that most aspects of gait, posture, and falls are discussed with patients (8). It is very important to determine whether falls always occur under comparable circumstances, because this opens ways for prevention. Asking for consequences of falls can unveil a pathological fear of falling.

TABLE 21.1. *Physical examination in patients with postural instability*

Quiet stance
Feet apart or together
Tandem stance
Self-initiated movements
Functional reach
External perturbations
Retropulsion test
Lateropulsion and propulsion
Functional tasks
Walking
Tandem gait
Turning around
Standing up and sitting down
Lifting up objects
Climbing stairs
Dual and multiple tasks
"Stops walking when talking"[a]
Obstacle course
The Multiple Task Test
Standardized rating scales
Tinetti Mobility Index[b]
Sit-stand-walk test
Rating Scale for Gait Evaluation in Parkinson's Disease[c]
Leg strength
Orthostatic hypotension
Cognition
Vision

Adapted from Smithson F, Morris ME, Iansek R. Performance on clinical tests of balance in Parkinson's disease. *Phys Ther* 1998;78:577–592.

[a]Data from Lundin-Olsson L, Nyberg L, Gustafson Y. "Stops walking when talking" as a predictor of falls in elderly people. *Lancet* 1997;349:617.

[b]Data from Tinetti ME. Performance-oriented assessment of mobility problems in elderly patients. *J Am Geriatr Soc* 1986;34:119–126.

[c]Data from Martinez-Martin P, Gil-Nagil A, Morlan Gracia L, et al. Unified Parkinson's Disease Rating Scale characteristics and structure. *Mov Disord* 1994;9:76–83.

Physical Examination

The pathophysiology of balance impairment in PD is complex, and multiple causes usually contribute to falls. Not surprisingly, there is no single clinical test that can probe the entire spectrum of balance abnormalities in patients with PD. In fact, most clinical tests have (by themselves) a poor predictive capacity for actual falls in daily life (10). A combination of different tests is usually most informative (Table 21.1). Most tests are included in standardized rating scales (8,28). Whenever possible, patients should be examined both during optimal response to treatment and in a practically defined off-state.

Postural instability is usually assessed by determining the response to a sudden and unexpected pull at the shoulders, exerted by the examiner standing behind the patient ("retropulsion test" or "pull test"). This test is also termed sternum push because some clinicians prefer to push the patient, rather than pull from behind. The term retropulsion test more aptly describes the procedure as used in the Unified Parkinson's Disease Rating Scale (UPDRS) (29). Normal subjects resist this pull from behind with a corrective trunk movement and only a few corrective steps backward. Unstable patients require more corrective steps and may even have to be caught by the examiner to prevent a fall. The retropulsion test is more often abnormal in fallers than nonfallers, and the intrarater and interrater reliability are good (30–32). Many clinicians make therapeutic decisions based on outcome of this test. However, the retropulsion test has important shortcomings. First, the test is difficult to standardize across subjects of differing height, weight, and degree of postural instability. Second, there is no consensus regarding execution of the test. Many clinicians prepare the patient by one or two practice trials (29). However, the response to the first shoulder pull is probably most informative because patients adapt to the test (10,15). In addition, the postural perturbation can be administered unexpectedly or after a warning signal (15,30,33). These two variants yield different responses (10). Theoretically, the first response to an unexpected pull without prior notice is most representative for falls in daily life, which are also sudden and unpredictable. Third, different scoring systems have been described. Some regard the test as mildly abnormal when one corrective step is taken, whereas others feel that three corrective steps is still normal (29,30). Fourth, the retropulsion test does not correlate well to presumably more objective measures of postural instability, obtained with dynamic posturography (34). Finally, and perhaps most important, the outcome of the retropulsion test (irrespective of how it is executed) does not predict actual falls in daily life (10).

We prefer to administer functional tests, such as standing up from a chair, climbing stairs or picking up objects from the floor, as these provide insight into the relevance of postural instability for daily life. More complicated tests, such as the sharpened Romberg test, the functional reach test or single-legged stance, may be sensitive techniques, but are typically neither specific nor relevant for routine daily activities (30). The Romberg test is usually unremarkable. Gait assessment may provide valuable insight into the patient's postural instability and falling risk. Judgment of step height (a risk factor for trips over obstacles on the floor) and trunk stability while turning around are usually most informative. It is also worthwhile to have the patient execute a second task while walking, such as answering questions or starting a routine conversation. Indeed, it is well appreciated that patients with PD have difficulty executing two different motor tasks simultaneously or shortly after each other. This is apparently also true if standing or walking is one of the two tasks. Thus, patients execute arm movements more slowly while standing than sitting, or have difficulty talking while walking (35,36). Conversely, unrelated motor tasks might be properly executed only at the expense of adequate postural control, resulting in balance impairment or falls. Although such a dual-task design seems particularly helpful for prediction of falls in older adults, in our prospective study the predictive value for falls in patients with PD was disappointing (37,37a). However, preliminary results from our group suggest that simultaneous performance of multiple tasks (e.g., walking, talking, avoiding obstacles, and carrying a tray at the same time) is very sensitive to postural abnormalities in PD. Details of this Multiple Task Test are presented elsewhere (37b).

Measuring strength in the legs can indicate whether patients are capable of standing up after a fall. Finally, although prominent orthostatic hypotension is rare in patients with idiopathic PD, it is suitable to measure the blood pressure and pulse rate in a recumbent position and after a prolonged period of standing.

PATHOPHYSIOLOGY OF POSTURAL INSTABILITY

Patients with PD cannot cope with the many balance threats they encounter every day (Fig. 21.3A). However, the precise mechanisms underlying postural instability in PD remain unclear. Studies using posturography (quantitative assessment of posture and balance) have increased our insights into these mechanisms. A summary of the most relevant causes of postural instability is presented in Figure 3B.

Static Posturography

Static posturography (assessment of spontaneous body sway during quiet stance) has yielded

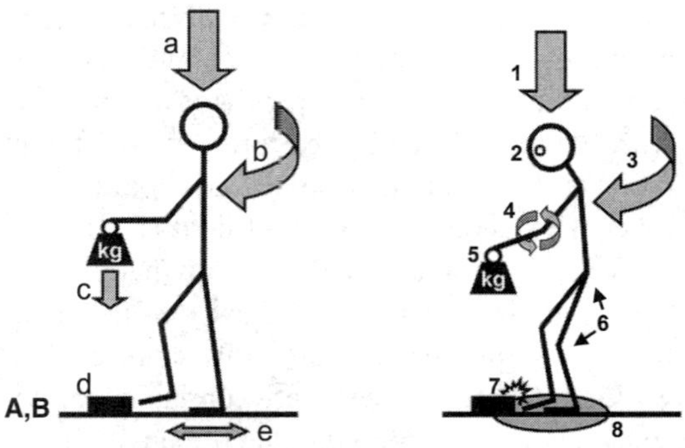

FIG. 21.3. A: Postural threats, encountered in daily life. *a,* gravity; *b,* external postural perturbations; *c,* self-generated movements; *d,* moving or slippery support surface; *e,* obstacles. **B:** Schematic illustration of postural abnormalities in Parkinson's disease. *1,* orthostatic hypotension and abnormal graviception; *2,* visual and oculomotor disturbances; *3,* impaired automatic (peripherally triggered) postural responses; *4,* dyskinesias; *5,* abnormal anticipatory postural responses; *6,* stiffness; *7,* reduced step height and abnormal stepping responses (both reactive and centrally initiated); *8,* narrowed limits of stability.

several interesting observations. Static body sway seems reduced early in the course of PD, possibly because patients actively cocontract their muscles and stiffen the body owing to a fear of falling (11,38). The muscle rigidity that is inherent to the disease itself, an increase of tonic stretch reflexes, and secondary changes in muscles or joints may further contribute to this stiffness (39,40). It is possible that patients consciously switch to this stiffening strategy to keep their center of gravity within their narrowed limits of stability (11,38,41). Patients may also adopt this strategy to compensate for their abnormal automatic postural corrections. Postural stiffness as measured during static stance indeed correlates with postural instability (42). However, although such conscious postural strategies may improve sway under fairly static conditions, it is potentially dangerous under dynamic conditions because voluntary postural corrections are initiated later than automatic postural corrections. Furthermore, the stiffening strategy reduces the viscoelastic properties of the body, which normally form the first line of defense against postural perturbations. Consequently, destabilizing perturbations are not effectively absorbed. Postural control in patients with PD thus starts to resemble a toy soldier who stands motionless when unperturbed, but falls like a log when pushed (11).

Dynamic Posturography

Dynamic posturography involves analysis of either self-generated postural movements or postural corrections to standardized external perturbations of upright stance. This technique is generally considered to be more informative than static posturography. Studies using dynamic posturography have revealed a host of abnormalities in patients with PD.

Afferent Sensory Information

There is little evidence that afferent sensory information is disturbed in PD. Except for an unconfirmed report of a subclinical polyneuropathy in young-onset PD, afferent proprioceptive information seems intact (43). The weight of the evidence suggests that labyrinthine function is normal in PD and, significantly, postural responses induced by vestibular stimulation are normal (44). Visual feedback is impaired because of oculomotor disturbances, an inability to suppress inappropriate visual information, or incorrect central processing of visual information (6,45,46). These abnormalities could lead to flawed perception of the environment, resulting in selection of inadequate postural corrections. However, the contribution of visual disturbances to falls in daily life remains unclear. Finally, a decreased sensitivity of extensor load mechanisms may contribute to impaired gait and posture in PD (47).

These different modes of afferent information must be centrally weighted, integrated, and consequently transformed into an appropriate postural response. This central weighting process seems largely intact in PD (11,48). However, central processing of kinesthetic feedback seems impaired, resulting in hypometric movements and, possibly, underscaling of postural corrective movements (49,50). It would be interesting to investigate if this faulty kinesthetic feedback loop could underlie the directional preponderance of falls in a backward direction.

Automatic Postural Corrections

The corrective postural responses that normally counteract a destabilizing external perturbation (a moving support surface or push to the body) are faulty at several levels. Automatic postural corrections normally constitute the second line of defense against perturbations. The term automatic encompasses anything ranging from the early occurring and pure reflexes to the longer latency responses (also termed long-loop reflexes or balance-correcting responses); the term peripherally triggered is also used to indicate that these responses react to external perturbations.

Many investigators have shown that automatic postural responses are abnormal in PD. Thus, amplitudes of destabilizing responses are increased, whereas posturally stabilizing responses are decreased (39,51–55). The response to the very first postural perturbation seems most abnormal, and this may underlie falls that occur with the unexpected postural perturbations encountered in daily life (56). These response abnormalities result in weaker stabilizing forces about the ankle joint (51,55,57). More important, however, is the fact that the abnormally sized automatic postural responses are inflexible, that is, patients cannot modulate the response magnitude according to the demands of the actual postural task at hand. Thus, patients are always saddled with fixed postural responses, irrespective of their body position, the environmental conditions, or the actual postural task at hand (11,54,58). This may well be one of the most important reasons why patients with PD have so much difficulty coping with the constantly changing environment. The activation sequence of automatic postural responses is also altered, with earlier than normal activation occurring in proximal leg muscles (57,59). This early activation of proximal muscles is unfavorable because it causes cocontraction and joint stiffness that interfere with the rapid corrective movements needed to prevent falls. Indeed, only patients with clinically rated balance impairment appear to resort to this strategy (59). Finally, a delayed initiation of automatic postural responses in the legs has been described (39,51,52). It is conceivable that a delayed onset of stabilizing responses contributes to postural instability because it causes destabilizing movements at the knee and hip.

Automatically triggered stepping movements are an important defensive strategy against postural perturbations, and should be distinguished from the feet in place reactions described in the preceding. Compensatory steps appear to be the preferred strategy when subjects are free to decide how they maintain balance, and are certainly necessary when large perturbations occur. In PD, reactive stepping movements following external perturbations are slowed and too small (60).

Voluntary Postural Corrections

Voluntarily (or centrally) initiated postural corrections constitute the third line of postural defense against external perturbations. Impaired feedforward programming and poor coordination of voluntary movement (akinesia and bradykinesia) likely result in absent, delayed, or inappropriate voluntary postural responses. Furthermore, the stiffness mentioned earlier may superimpose on bradykinesia and cause a biomechanical delay of voluntary postural responses. Bradykinesia and voluntary weight shifts indeed seem related to clinically rated balance impairment (7,13,41). Centrally initiated stepping movements and voluntary rises to the toes are weaker and prolonged in patients with PD (57,60). Sudden freezing of voluntary movements may also interfere with execution of voluntary postural adjustments. Freezing while walking in narrow spaces such as doorways is particularly associated with falls (5).

Anticipatory Postural Responses

Patients with PD also have difficulties making appropriate anticipatory postural adjustments prior to self-initiated movements (35,61). The general activation pattern seems preserved, suggesting that the observed deficits are quantitative in nature, rather than qualitative (62,63). Poor postural anticipation could reflect problems with feedforward planning and use of predictive motor actions. Impaired anticipatory postural responses may well contribute to falls occurring during everyday activities, such as lifting up objects.

Other Factors Contributing to Postural Instability and Falls

Several factors may increase body sway in patients with PD, and thereby heighten the risk of exceeding the already narrow limits of stability. Thus, dyskinesias (owing to an overshoot effect of antiparkinson medication) may cause excessive body sway and result in a fall (6). The typical shuffling gait creates a risk of tripping over small obstacles, particularly in a dimly lighted environment because patients require visual control to improve their gait (64). En bloc turning, as well as retropulsion, lateropulsion, and propulsion, are also risk factors for falls.

Both isotonic and isometric muscle strength are reduced in PD (65,66). As in the general population, muscle weakness is a risk factor for falls in patients with PD. Weakness in leg muscles can also keep patients from standing up after a fall to the floor.

Many patients with PD eventually manifest some form of (subcortical) cognitive impairment. This cognitive impairment is another risk factor for falls, perhaps because patients engage in dangerous activities that they can no longer handle.

Finally, autonomic disturbances may lead to orthostatic hypotension and thus contribute to postural instability. However, symptomatic autonomic disturbances are rarely severe in true PD (17,67). Furthermore, orthostatic hypotension did not correlate with postural instability and falls in two studies, suggesting that autonomic disturbances do not play a major role in balance impairment in patients with PD (7,13).

TREATMENT OF POSTURAL INSTABILITY

Postural instability is generally difficult to treat, and falls are equally difficult to prevent; however, several approaches may be fruitful (Table 21.2).

TABLE 21.2. *Treatment of postural instability and prevention of falls in Parkinson's disease*

Pharmacotherapy[a]
Stereotaxic neurosurgery
Lesions or chronic electrical stimulation?
Unilateral or bilateral procedures?
Thalamus, globus pallidus, or subthalamic nucleus?
Transplantation of dopaminergic grafts
Physical therapy
Gait training
Exercise therapy
Improve strength
Safer transfers
Orthostatic maneuvers
Reduce fear of falling
Supportive measures
Reduce domestic hazards
High chairs and beds
Handrails
Proper footwear
Ankle braces for trips
Walking aids
Electronic warning system
Reduce orthostatic hypotension[b]
Arrest osteoporosis (pro-Vitamin D; alendronate)
Protective pads

[a] See Fig. 21.4.

[b] See Nutt JG, Hammerstadt JP, Gancher ST. *Parkinson's disease: 100 maxims.* London: Edward Arnold, 1992; Mathias CJ, Kimber JR. Treatment of postural hypotension. *J Neurol Neurosurg Psychiatry* 1998;65:285–289 for further details.

Pharmacotherapy

Postural instability and falls respond poorly to treatment with dopaminergic drugs (55,68,69). Dopaminergic medication is also ineffective for other axial motor problems, such as turning in bed (70), voluntary head rotation and gait disorders (68,72), including "on-period" freezing (5,73). This dopa-resistance of postural instability may be caused by three mechanisms, and each requires a different approach (Fig. 21.4). First, postural instability may partially reflect the progressive loss of dopamine producing cells in the substantia nigra. Indeed, in controlled experiments, some postural abnormalities improved with antiparkinson medication (in particular the centrally initiated responses), but usually not to normal levels (41,55,57,60). Other postural abnormalities were present not only in PD, but also in patients with selective hypodopaminergic syndromes, such as MPTP-induced parkinsonism

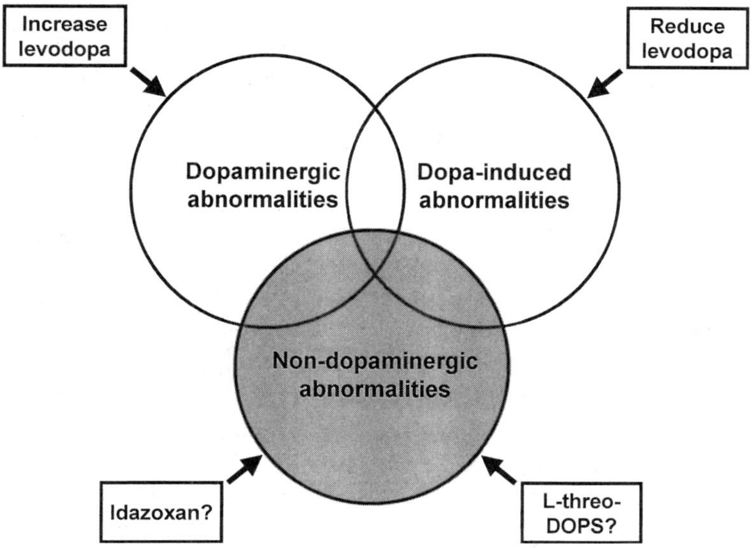

FIG. 21.4. Pharmacologic treatment of postural instability in Parkinson's disease. *Dopaminergic abnormalities* (e.g., centrally initiated postural corrections) require an increase of dopaminergic drugs, whereas the opposite is necessary for postural abnormalities that may be *dopa-induced* (e.g., "on-period" freezing or orthostatic hypotension). The residual abnormalities are conceivably related to "extranigral" lesions and may require correction of *nondopaminergic* neurotransmitter deficits. However, unequivocally effective nondopaminergic treatments are not yet available. Treatment is particularly complex for signs that receive a contribution from multiple domains, such as freezing, which can be both a dopaminergic and a dopa-induced feature.

(74). Therefore, increasing dopaminergic therapy should always be considered and is sometimes effective (7,75).

This approach is not without risks, however. In some patients, dopaminergic medication may paradoxically increase falls and fractures because the reduction of rigidity and bradykinesia improves mobility without reducing postural instability. In addition, dopaminergic treatment can cause dyskinesias, "on-period" freezing, and orthostatic hypotension, thus leading to falls (67,76). In such patients, reducing the dosage or number of antiparkinson drugs may improve postural control (Fig. 21.4).

A third possibility is that nondopaminergic lesions play a role in the pathophysiology of postural instability and falls (7,55,68,69). Indeed, both postural instability and nondopaminergic lesions typically emerge (and thus coincide) in advanced PD. Furthermore, dynamic posturography studies suggest that several balance problems (mainly the reactive automatic postural responses) in PD are not primarily dopamine-dependent (39,77). Therefore, pharmacotherapy of postural instability ideally should aim at correction of both dopaminergic and nondopaminergic deficits. The nature of the underlying nondopaminergic lesions remains obscure. However, based on the hypothesis that the noradrenergic locus ceruleus might be involved, several investigators have studied the effects of the synthetic norepinephrine precursor L-threo-dihydroxyphenylserine (DOPS). Quinn et al. found no improvement of freezing in a single-dose, placebo-controlled study of DOPS in six patients (78). However, in a prospective, double-blind and placebo-controlled study, 6 weeks of oral DOPS led to improved clinical scores for gait, retropulsion, and festination (73). Others also reported mild improvement of clinically rated gait impairment and freezing in patients with longstanding PD, but these studies were not placebo-controlled (79,80). Finally, a preliminary report mentioned a reduction of orthostatic hypotension in patients with PD who were treated with DOPS (81).

Idazoxan also is able to increase central norepinephrine levels. Treatment with idazoxan led to both objective and subjective improvement of postural instability in patients with PSP, but its effect on postural instability has thus far not been tested in patients with PD (82). Correction of other nondopaminergic deficiencies, such as the central serotonin deficit, did not correct balance impairment in PD (83). Unfortunately, none of the preceding studies ascertained balance changes objectively using dynamic posturography or standardized electrophysiologic gait assessment. Furthermore, the effect on actual falls in daily life was not studied. Therefore, although theoretically plausible, the evidence available to date is insufficient to support a role for nondopaminergic drugs in the treatment of postural instability.

Finally, it is always necessary to try to reduce any concomitant medication, psychoactive drugs such as benzodiazepines in particular, because these are important risk factors for falls in older adults, including patients with PD (10a).

Neurosurgery

The disappointing effects of pharmacotherapy underscore the importance of alternative therapeutic approaches, including surgery. Stereotaxic neurosurgery aimed at the thalamus was originally developed to provide symptomatic relief of tremor particularly. In occasional patients, electrical stimulation of the nucleus ventralis intermedius of the thalamus may improve postural control, apparently via a reduction of tremor in the legs and trunk (84). Unilateral lesions in the thalamus may result in minor, short-lasting amelioration of balance impairment in up to 30% of all patients (85). However, thalamic procedures generally provide little relief of postural instability or gait (86,87). After long-term follow-up, balance has deteriorated in most patients because of progression of the underlying disease. Bilateral operations in fact may aggravate balance impairment in a substantial number of patients (88).

Better results likely can be achieved using stereotaxic neurosurgical approaches that aim to restore the normal function of the basal ganglia by blocking the function of the internal globus pallidus or subthalamic nucleus. Lesions or chronic electrical stimulation can achieve this. The rationale behind this treatment is that degeneration of the nigrostriatal pathway in PD leads to disinhibition of the internal globus pallidus and subthalamic nucleus. The resultant hyperactivity of these nuclei is probably responsible for at least part of the symptoms of the disease.

The first results of these novel therapeutic approaches are promising. Pallidal and subthalamic surgery can markedly alleviate tremor, rigidity, bradykinesia, and drug-induced dyskinesias, but the effects on postural instability and falling have thus far received relatively little attention (89). The outcome measures were often limited to fairly coarse clinical measures such as the retropulsion test. Only few studies incorporated more objective measures, obtained with quantified gait analysis or dynamic posturography (Chapter 12) (90,91).

Although balance may deteriorate in occasional patients, the global impression is that deep brain surgery leads to sometimes impressive improvements in postural instability (92). Unilateral procedures can ameliorate clinically rated gait and balance, but most investigators feel that bilateral procedures are required for optimal improvement of axial signs such as postural instability (93–95). The best results can be expected in patients with postural instability that was at least partially dopa-responsive preoperatively. The effects also depend on the exact site of the lesion (96). Direct comparisons between statistically meaningful patient populations with either lesions or stimulators are not yet available. Subthalamic stimulation may be more effective than pallidal stimulation for some features of the disease (including freezing of gait), but it remains unclear whether the globus pallidus or the subthalamic nucleus is the optimal target for patients with postural instability (89,92). Significantly, elderly patients with prominent and dopa-resistant postural instability are not good candidates for deep brain surgery, unless significant effects on other incapacitating features of the disease are expected.

Transplantation of dopamine producing cells (in particular fetal mesencephalic grafts) has also gained considerable interest over the past decade. Several investigators reported a reduction of postural instability following transplantation of dopaminergic neuronal grafts (97,98). Balance is most likely to improve if dopamine-producing cells are transplanted bilaterally over larger areas of the striatum (99). However, prominent postural instability is, by itself, not a good indication for this type of surgery.

Surgery for Fractures

Operating hip fractures in patients with PD is a challenge, but appears preferable over conservative treatment, provided special care is given before, during, and after surgery (23). Particular attention must be paid to avoid bronchopneumonia, which is the leading cause of death in these patients. Similar measures are probably necessary in patients treated for other types of major fractures that cause immobilization.

Physical Therapy

Several trials have shown the efficacy of physical therapy and strength training for balance impairment in the elderly, but no controlled studies have determined their effectiveness and cost:benefit ratio in PD. Several investigators found no improvement of posture after physical therapy (100,101), whereas others reported subjective improvement (102,103). Physical therapy may improve some postural disturbances, such as walking, turning over in bed, and standing up from a sitting position (102,103). Other potentially useful approaches include strength training and assistance in learning to make safer transfers to or from beds, chairs, and toilets. Physical therapists can also teach patients specific maneuvers to reduce orthostatic hypotension, such as standing with legs crossed and muscles contracted (104). Finally, exercise therapy will increase physical fitness and help reduce both cardiovascular morbidity and development or progression of osteoporosis. The beneficial effects seem to wane if physical therapy is abandoned, suggesting that prolonged treatment programs are required (103).

The intrinsic effects on balance impairment and the tendency to fall remain to be clarified. Clearly, physical therapy will not cure postural instability, but may teach patients how to cope with a given degree of balance impairment. Perhaps most important, physical therapists may help patients to reduce their fear of falling, allowing them to participate more in social activities.

Other Supportive Measures

A multidisciplinary intervention can help prevent falls in older adults, but no controlled studies have been specifically directed toward patients with PD. However, it seems reasonable to assume that similar measures will also benefit patients with PD. Thus, occupational therapists can help reduce home accidents caused by domestic hazards such as loose rugs, slippery floors, or insufficiently lighted rooms. High chairs and beds may reduce the risk of falling during transfers. Handrails might prevent some falls (e.g., bathrooms), provided the patient can make rapid corrective arm movements (which is not always the case). Patients should wear sturdy shoes with leather soles (to avoid accidental slips) and heightened heels (to reduce backward falls and retropulsion). Ankle braces can be recommended to patients who trip by catching their toe (15). Many patients benefit from the use of walking aids (cane, quadripod, or frame). Patients who merely carry (rather than use) their walking aids should use a wheeled rollator. Several specific designs are available for patients with PD, such as a walking stick with a small horizontal bar just above the ground to overcome freezing (105). Some patients with freezing benefit from the use of a laser pointer, which can be aimed at the floor in front of the subject (106). An interesting anecdotal report suggested that freezing might also improve with botulinum toxin injected into the legs, but this observation requires confirmation (107). Patients who are unable to stand up after a fall must wear an electronic warning system around the neck or wrist. Patients with marked orthostatic hypotension should avoid precipitating circumstances, such as rapid changes in posture or prolonged recumbence. Some can be treated with compression stockings, sodium chloride tablets, or pharmacologically using fludrocortisone and sympathicomimetics such as midodrine (104). Progression of osteoporosis can be arrested using the oral provitamin 1α-hydroxyvitamin D3, resulting in a lower incidence of fractures (even in fallers) (9). Alendronate also halts progression of osteoporosis and reduces fractures, but its effects have not been studied in patients with PD (108). Finally, in patients who continue to fall despite all these measures, wearing protective hip, knee, or elbow pads may help reduce injuries (15,108a).

FUTURE OBJECTIVES

One important future goal is to develop clinical screening tests that can help predict falls in individual patients. As mentioned, most can be expected from functional tests that mimic everyday activities and use of a multiple task design. More objective techniques, such as dynamic posturography, also may be helpful. However, although posturography remains interesting as a research tool, it appears to be only a crude measure of clinically relevant instability, at least as it is presently used. Indeed, the abnormalities found with dynamic posturography may be clearly present in patients with PD as a group, but none has proved to be a valuable tool for diagnostic purposes in individual subjects (48,109). This may be owing to shortcomings in the study designs. Most previous reports focused largely on postural responses in the lower legs, induced by serial perturbations in one direction (mostly the pitch plane). We are presently investigating whether analysis of trunk motion and activation of trunk muscles will yield an increased diagnostic utility for balance problems in patients with PD. In addition, we are now studying postural responses to random perturbations in multiple directions, because these may be more relevant to falls in daily life. These new techniques may prove helpful in longterm follow-up of patients with PD, for example, to assist in evaluating the efficacy of antiparkinson medication and neurosurgical techniques.

A second important goal is to identify which central lesions in patients with PD are responsible for postural instability. This could serve as a guide for development of new and more effective treatment programs, both pharmacologic and surgical. One approach would be to further evaluate the effect of nondopaminergic drugs, using both objective assessment of posture and gait (e.g., dynamic posturography) and the frequency of actual falls in daily life as outcome measures. Stereotaxic neurosurgery is another promising strategy. Future studies should determine which technique (stimulation or lesions; unilateral or bilateral procedures) and which target (thalamus, globus pallidus, or subthalamic nucleus) is most effective for treatment of balance disorders. It would also be interesting to evaluate whether patients with prominent balance impairment as the dominant sign could be candidates for surgery. Patients with implanted deep brain stimulators have the major advantage over patients with destructive surgery in that balance can be evaluated with the stimulator "on" or "off," allowing for a direct comparison of postural performance across different disease states. Finally, the results of the ongoing placebo-controlled trial of fetal transplants should reveal whether this is a useful option for patients with postural instability (110).

There is an urgent need to evaluate the benefits of individually tailored physical therapy for treating balance disorders. It is necessary to compare different treatment programs, distill the most effective elements, and evaluate what the optimal frequency and duration of these treatment programs should be. Is a brief training period sufficient, or do patients have to comply with a lifelong treatment program? Can a physical therapist provide patients with simple exercise programs that, after practice, can be executed independently at home? Again, such studies should include the actual falling frequency in daily life as an outcome measure. Some studies may have showed statistically significant improvements in well-practiced variables such as duration stance on one leg, but the clinical relevance of this outcome for the unexpected falls in daily life is unclear.

Finally, new treatment programs should evaluate the effect on the patient's quality of life. A reduction in falling frequency is only meaningful if patients actually regain mobility and functional independence. With the recommendations made in this chapter, better treatments for balance impairment in PD hopefully will become available in the near future.

ACKNOWLEDGMENT

We thank professor R.A.C. Roos for his critical comments.

REFERENCES

1. Parkinson J. *An essay on the shaking palsy.* London: Sherwood, Neely and Jones, 1817.
2. Wendell CM, Hauser RA, Nagaria MH, et al. Chief complaints of patients with Parkinson's disease. *Neurology* 1999;52:A90–A91.
3. Klawans HL, Topel JL. Parkinsonism as a falling sickness. *JAMA* 1974;230:1555–1557.
4. Wenning GK, Litvan I, Jankovic J, et al. Natural history and survival of 14 patients with corticobasal degeneration confirmed at postmortem examination. *J Neurol Neurosurg Psychiatry* 1998;64:184–189.
5. Lamberti P, Armenise S, Castaldo V, et al. Freezing gait in Parkinson's disease. *Eur Neurol* 1997;38:297–301.
6. Paulson GW, Schafer K, Hallum B. Avoiding mental changes and falls in older Parkinson's patients. *Geriatrics* 1986;41:59–67.
7. Koller WC, Glatt S, Vetere-Overfield B, et al. Falls and Parkinson's disease. *Clin Neuropharmacol* 1989;2:98–105.
8. Martinez-Martin P, Urra DG, Quijano TD, et al. A new clinical tool for gait evaluation in Parkinson's disease. *Clin Neuropharmacol* 1997;20:183–194.
9. Sato Y, Manabe S, Kuno H, et al. Amelioration of osteopenia and hypovitaminosis D by 1 alpha-hydroxyvitamin D3 in elderly patients with Parkinson's disease. *J Neurol Neurosurg Psychiatry* 1999;66:64–68.
10. Bloem BR, Grimbergen YAM, Cramer M, et al. Prospective assessment of falls in Parkinson's disease. *Mov Disord* 1998;10:147.

10a. Willemsen MD, Grimbergen YAM, Slabbekoorn M, et al. Vallen bij de ziekte van Parkinson: vaker door houdingsinstabiliteit dan door omgevingsfactoren. *Ned Tijdschr Geneeskd* 2000;144:2309–2314.

11. Horak FB, Nutt JG, Nashner LM. Postural inflexibility in parkinsonian subjects. *J Neurol Sci* 1992;111:46–58.
12. Elble RJ, Thomas SS, Higgins C, et al. Stride-dependent changes in gait of older people. *J Neurol* 1991;238:1–5.
13. Charlett A, Weller C, Dobbs SM, et al. What makes a faller in early Parkinsonism? *Eur Neurol* 1997;38:312–314.
14. Bloem BR, van Dijk JG, Beckley DJ. Are automatic postural responses in patients with Parkinson's disease abnormal due to their stooped posture? *Exp Brain Res* 1999;124:481–488.
15. Nutt JG, Hammerstadt JP, Gancher ST. *Parkinson's disease: 100 maxims.* London: Edward Arnold, 1992.
16. Hely MA, Morris JGL, Traficante R, et al. The Sydney multicentre study of Parkinson's disease: progression and mortality at 10 years. *J Neurol Neurosurg Psychiatry* 1999;67:300–307.
17. Quinn NP. Parkinsonism—recognition and differential diagnosis. *Br Med J* 1995;310:447–452.
18. de Boer AGEM, Wijker W, Speelman JD, et al. Quality of life in patients with Parkinson's disease: development of a questionnaire. *J Neurol Neurosurg Psychiatry* 1996;61:70–74.
19. Martinez-Martin P. An introduction to the concept of "quality of life in Parkinson's disease." *J Neurol* 1998;245:S2–S6.
20. Grisso JA, Kelsey JL, Strom BL, et al. Risk factors for falls as a cause of hip fracture in women. *N Engl J Med* 1991;324:1326–1331.
21. Johnell O, Melton ILJ, Atkinson EJ, et al. Fracture risk in patients with parkinsonism: a population based study in Olmsted County, Minnesota. *Age Ageing* 1992;21:32–38.
22. Coughlin L, Templeton J. Hip fractures in patients with Parkinson's disease. *Clin Orthop Rel Res* 1980;148:192–195.
23. Eventon I, Moreno M, Geller E, et al. Hip fractures in patients with Parkinson's syndrome. *J Trauma* 1983;23:98–101.
24. Jankovic J, McDermott M, Carter J, et al. Variable expression of Parkinson's disease: a base-line analysis of the DATATOP cohort. *Neurology* 1990;40:1529–1534.
25. Bennett DA, Beckett LA, Murray AM, et al. Prevalence of parkinsonian signs and associated mortality in a community population of older people. *N Engl J Med* 1996;334:71–76.
26. Ebmeier KP, Calder SA, Crawford JR, et al. Mortality and causes of death in idiopathic Parkinson's disease: results from the Aberdeen whole population study. *Scott Med J* 1990;35:173–175.
27. Cummings SR, Nevitt MC, Kidd S. Forgetting falls. The limited accuracy of recall of falls in the elderly. *J Am Geriatr Soc* 1988;36:613–616.
28. Tinetti ME. Performance-oriented assessment of mobility problems in elderly patients. *J Am Geriatr Soc* 1986;34:119–126.
29. Lang AE. Clinical rating scales and videotape analysis. In: Koller WC, Paulson G, eds. *Therapy of Parkinson's disease.* New York: Marcel Dekker, 1995:21–46.
30. Smithson F, Morris ME, Iansek R. Performance on clinical tests of balance in Parkinson's disease. *Phys Ther* 1998;78:577–592.
31. Hely MA, Chey T, Williamson PM, et al. Reliability of the Columbia Scale for assessing signs of Parkinson's disease. *Mov Disord* 1993;8:466–472.
32. Martinez-Martin P, Gil-Nagil A, Morlan Gracia L, et al. Unified Parkinson's Disease Rating Scale characteristics and structure. *Mov Disord* 1994;9:76–83.
33. Sudarsky L. Geriatrics: gait disorders in the elderly. *N Engl J Med* 1990;322:1441–1446.
34. Bloem BR, Beckley DJ, van Hilten JJ, et al. Clinimetrics of postural instability in Parkinson's disease. *J Neurol* 1998;245:669–673.
35. Bazalgette D, Zattara M, Bathien N, et al. Postural adjustments associated with rapid voluntary arm movements in patients with Parkinson's disease. *Adv Neurol* 1986;45:371–374.
36. Nisipeanu P, Inzelberg R. Falls in elderly people. *Lancet* 1997;349:1180.
37. Lundin-Olsson L, Nyberg L, Gustafson Y. "Stops walking when talking" as a predictor of falls in elderly people. *Lancet* 1997;349:617.

37a. Bloem BR, Grimbergen YAM, Cramer M, et al. "Stops walking when talking" does not predict falls in Parkinson's disease. *Ann Neurol* 2000;48:268.

37b. Bloem BR, Valkenburg VV, Slabbekoorn M, et al. The

Multiple Tasks Test. Strategies in Parkinson's disease. *Exp Brain Res*, in press.
38. Schieppati M, Hugon M, Grasso M, et al. The limits of equilibrium in young and elderly normal subjects and in parkinsonians. *Electroenceph Clin Neurophysiol* 1994;93:286–298.
39. Dietz V, Berger W, Horstmann GA. Posture in Parkinson's disease: impairment of reflexes and programming. *Ann Neurol* 1988;24:660–669.
40. Hayashi R, Tokuda T, Tako K, et al. Impaired modulation of tonic muscle activities and H-reflexes in the soleus muscle during standing in patients with Parkinson's disease. *J Neurol Sci* 1997;153:61–67.
41. Beckley DJ, Panzer VP, Remler MP, et al. Clinical correlates of motor performance during paced postural tasks in Parkinson's disease. *J Neurol Sci* 1995;132:133–138.
42. Lauk M, Chow CC, Lipsitz LA, et al. Assessing muscle stiffness from quiet stance in Parkinson's disease. *Muscle Nerve* 1999;22:635–639.
43. Taly AB, Muthane UB. Involvement of peripheral nervous system in juvenile Parkinson's disease. *Acta Neurol Scand* 1992;85:272–275.
44. Pastor MA, Day BL, Marsden CD. Vestibular induced postural responses in Parkinson's disease. *Brain* 1993;116:1177–1190.
45. Bronstein AM, Hood JD, Gresty MA, et al. Visual control of balance in cerebellar and parkinsonian syndromes. *Brain* 1990;113:767–779.
46. Bronstein AM, Yardley L, Moore AP, et al. Visually and posturally mediated tilt illusion in Parkinson's disease and in labyrinthine defective subjects. *Neurology* 1996;47:651–656.
47. Dietz V, Colombo G. Influence of body load on the gait pattern in Parkinson's disease. *Mov Disord* 1998;13:255–261.
48. Waterston JA, Hawken MB, Tanyeri S, et al. Influence of sensory manipulation on postural control in Parkinson's disease *J Neurol Neurosurg Psychiatry* 1993;56:1276–1281.
49. Klockgether T, Borutta M, Rapp H, et al. A defect of kinesthesia in Parkinson's disease. *Mov Disord* 1995; 10:460–465.
50. Demirci M, Grill S, Mcshane L, et al. A mismatch between kinesthetic and visual perception in Parkinson's disease. *Ann Neurol* 1997;41:781–788.
51. Allum JHJ, Keshner EA, Honegger F, et al. Disturbance of posture in patients with Parkinson's disease. In: Amblard B, Berthoz A, Clarac F, eds. *Posture and gait: development, adaptation and modulation.* Amsterdam: Elsevier, 1988:245–257.
52. Schieppati M, Nardone A. Free and supported stance in Parkinson's disease. *Brain* 1991;114:1227–1244.
53. Bloem BR, van Dijk JG, Beckley DJ, et al. Correction for the influence of background muscle activity on stretch reflex amplitudes. *J Neurosci Meth* 1993;46:167–174.
54. Bloem BR, Beckley DJ, Remler MP, et al. Postural reflexes in Parkinson's disease during "resist" and "yield" tasks. *J Neurol Sci* 1995;129:109–119.
55. Bloem BR, Beckley DJ, van Dijk JG, et al. Influence of dopaminergic medication on automatic postural responses and balance impairment in Parkinson's disease. *Mov Disord* 1996;11:509–521.
56. Bloem BR, van Vugt JPP, Beckley DJ, et al. Habituation of lower leg stretch reflexes in Parkinson's disease. *Electroenceph Clin Neurophysiol* 1998;109: 73–77.
57. Horak FB, Frank JS. Three separate postural systems affected in parkinsonism. In: Stuart DG, Gurfinkel VS, Wiesendanger M, eds. *Motor control*, vol 7. Tucson, AZ: Motor Control Press, 1996:343–346.
58. Beckley DJ, Bloem BR, Remler MP. Impaired scaling of long latency postural reflexes in patients with Parkinson's disease. *Electroenceph Clin Neurophysiol* 1993;89:22–28.
59. Beckley DJ, Bloem BR, van Dijk JG, et al. Electrophysiological correlates of postural instability in Parkinson's disease. *Electroenceph Clin Neurophysiol* 1991;81:263–268.
60. Burleigh-Jacobs A, Horak FB, Nutt JG, et al. Step initiation in Parkinson's disease: influence of levodopa and external sensory triggers. *Mov Disord* 1997;12:206–215.
61. Traub MM, Rothwell JC, Marsden CD. Anticipatory postural reflexes in Parkinson's disease and other akinetic-rigid syndromes and in cerebellar ataxia. *Brain* 1980;103:393–412.
62. Dick JP, Rothwell JC, Berardelli A, et al. Associated postural adjustments in Parkinson's disease. *J Neurol Neurosurg Psychiatry* 1986;49:1378–1385.
63. Aruin AS, Neyman I, Nicholas JJ, et al. Are there deficits in anticipatory postural adjustments in Parkinson's disease? *Neuroreport* 1996;7:1794–1796.
64. Azulay JP, Mesure S, Amblard B, et al. Visual control of locomotion in Parkinson's disease. *Brain* 1999;122:111–120.
65. Koller WC, Kase S. Muscle strength testing in Parkinson's disease. *Eur Neurol* 1986;25:130–133.
66. Yanagawa S, Shindo M, Yanagisawa N. Muscular weakness in Parkinson's disease. *Adv Neurol* 1990;53:259–269.
67. van Dijk JG, Haan J, Zwinderman K, et al. Autonomic nervous system dysfunction in Parkinson's disease: relationships with age, medication, duration, and severity. *J Neurol Neurosurg Psychiatry* 1993;56:1090–1095.
68. Bonnet AM, Loria Y, Saint-Hilaire MH, et al. Does long-term aggravation of Parkinson's disease result from nondopaminergic lesions? *Neurology* 1987;37:1539–1542.
69. Klawans HL. Individual manifestations of Parkinson's disease after ten or more years of levodopa. *Mov Disord* 1986;1:187–192.
70. Lakke JPWF. Axial apraxia in Parkinson's disease. *J Neurol Sci* 1985;69:37–46.
71. Weinrich M, Koch K, Garcia F, et al. Axial versus distal motor impairment in Parkinson's disease. *Neurology* 1988;38:540–545.
72. Blin O, Ferrandez AM, Pailhous J, et al. Dopa-sensitive and dopa-resistant gait parameters in Parkinson's disease. *J Neurol Sci* 1991;103:51–54.
73. Narabayashi H, Kondo T, Yokochi F, et al. Clinical effects of L-threo-3,4-dihydroxyphenylserine in cases of parkinsonism and pure akinesia. *Adv Neurol* 1987;45:593–602.
74. Bloem BR, Beckley DJ, van Vugt JPP, et al. Long latency postural reflexes are under supraspinal dopaminergic control. *Mov Disord* 1995;10:580–588.
75. Rogers MW. Disorders of posture, balance, and gait in Parkinson's disease. *Clin Geriatr Med* 1996;12:825–845.

76. Giladi N, Kao R, Fahn S. Freezing phenomenon in patients with parkinsonian syndromes. *Mov Disord* 1997;12:302–305.
77. Bloem BR, Beckley DJ, van Dijk JG, et al. Medium latency stretch reflexes in young-onset Parkinson's disease and MPTP-induced parkinsonism. *J Neurol Sci* 1994;123:52–58.
78. Quinn NP, Perlmutter JS, Marsden CD. Acute administration of DL-threo-DOPS does not affect the freezing phenomenon in parkinsonian patients. *Neurology* 1984;34:149.
79. Teelken AW, van den Berg GA, Muskiet FA, et al. Catecholamine metabolism during additional administration of DL-threo-3,4-dihydroxyphenylserine to patients with Parkinson's disease. *J Neural Transm Park Dis Dement Sect* 1989;1:177–188.
80. Tohgi H, Abe T, Takahashi S. The effects of L-threo-3,4-dihydroxyphenylserine on the total norepinephrine and dopamine concentrations in the cerebrospinal fluid and freezing gait in parkinsonian patients. *J Neural Transm Park Dis Dement Sect* 1993;5:27–34.
81. Hasegawa Y, Mukai E, Matsusoka Y, et al. Effect of oral L-threo-3,4-dihydroxyphenylserine (L-DOPS) on orthostatic hypotension in Parkinson's disease. *Mov Disord* 1997;12:88.
82. Ghika J, Tennis M, Hoffman E, et al. Idazoxan treatment in progressive supranuclear palsy. *Neurology* 1991;41:986–991.
83. Klein P, Lees A, Stern G. Consequences of chronic 5-hydroxy-tryptophan in parkinsonian instability of gait and balance and in other neurological disorders. In: Yahr MD, Bergmann KJ, eds. *Advances in neurology.* New York: Raven Press, 1986:603–604.
84. Burleigh AL, Horak FB, Burchiel KJ, et al. Effects of thalamic stimulation on tremor, balance, and step initiation: a single subject study. *Mov Disord* 1993;8:519–524.
85. Speelman JD. *Parkinson's disease and stereotaxic neurosurgery.* Thesis. Amsterdam, 1991.
86. Benabid AL, Pollak P, Gao D, et al. Chronic electrical stimulation of the ventralis intermedius nucleus of the thalamus as a treatment of movement disorders. *J Neurosurg* 1996;84:203–214.
87. Defebvre L, Blatt JL, Blond S, et al. Effect of thalamic stimulation on gait in Parkinson disease. *Arch Neurol* 1996;53:898–903.
88. Pollak P, Benabid AL, Limousin P, et al. Chronic intracerebral stimulation in Parkinson's disease. *Adv Neurol* 1997;74:213–220.
89. Quinn NP, Bhatia K. Functional neurosurgery for Parkinson's disease. Has come a long way, though much remains experimental. *Br Med J* 1998;316:1259–1260.
90. Masterman D, Desalles A, Baloh RW, et al. Motor, cognitive, and behavioral performance following unilateral ventroposterior pallidotomy for Parkinson disease. *Arch Neurol* 1998;55:1201–1208.
91. Melnick ME, Dowling GA, Aminoff MJ, et al. Effect of pallidotomy on postural control and motor function in Parkinson disease. *Arch Neurol* 1999;56:1361–1365.
92. Krack P, Pollak P, Limousin P, et al. Subthalamic nucleus or internal pallidal stimulation in young onset Parkinson's disease. *Brain* 1998;121:451–457.
93. Iacono RP, Lonser RR. Reversal of Parkinson's akinesia by pallidotomy. *Lancet* 1994;343:418–419.
94. Samuel M, Caputo E, Brooks DJ, et al. A study of medial pallidotomy for Parkinson's disease: clinical outcome, MRI location and complications. *Brain* 1998;121:59–75.
95. Ondo WG, Jankovic J, Lai EC, et al. Assessment of motor function after stereotactic pallidotomy. *Neurology* 1998;50:266–270.
96. Gross RE, Lombardi WJ, Lang AE, et al. Relationship of lesion location to clinical outcome following microelectrode-guided pallidotomy for Parkinson's disease. *Brain* 1999;122:405–416.
97. Allen GS, Burns RS, Tulipan NB, et al. Adrenal medullary transplantation to the caudate nucleus in Parkinson's disease. Initial results in 18 patients. *Arch Neurol* 1989;46:487–491.
98. Jankovic J, Grossman R, Goodman C, et al. Clinical, biochemical, and neuropathologic findings following transplantation of adrenal medulla to the caudate nucleus for the treatment of Parkinson's disease. *Neurology* 1989;39:1227–1234.
99. Sawle GV, Bloomfield PM, Björklund A, et al. Transplantation of fetal dopamine neurons in Parkinson's disease: PET [F]6-L-fluorodopa studies in two patients with putaminal implants. *Ann Neurol* 1992;31:166–173.
100. Gibberd FB, Page NGR, Spencer KM, et al. Controlled trial of physiotherapy and occupational therapy for Parkinson's disease. *Br Med J* 1981;282:1196.
101. Szeleky BC, Kosanovich NN, Sheppard W. Adjunctive treatment in Parkinson's disease: physical therapy and comprehensive group therapy. *Rehab Lit* 1982;43:72–76.
102. Banks MA, Caird FI. Physiotherapy benefits patients with Parkinson's disease. *Clin Rehabil* 1989;3:11–16.
103. Palmer SS, Mortimer JA, Webster DD, et al. Exercise therapy for Parkinson's disease. *Arch Phys Med Rehabil* 1986;67:741–745.
104. Mathias CJ, Kimber JR. Treatment of postural hypotension. *J Neurol Neurosurg Psychiatry* 1998;65:285–289.
105. Pearce JMS. A walking aid for parkinsonian patients. *Lancet* 1993;342:62.
106. Zhang L, Siddiqui A, Counihan T, et al. A novel treatment for transient freezing in Parkinson's disease: application of a laser pointer. *Neurology* 1999;52:A222.
107. Giladi N. Botulinum toxin injections to one leg alleviate freezing of gait in a patient with Parkinson's disease. *Mov Disord* 1997;12:1085–1086.
108. Cummings SR, Black DM, Thompson DE, et al. Effect of alendronate on risk of fracture in women with low bone density but without vertebral fractures. Results from the fracture intervention trial. *JAMA* 1998;280:2077–2082.
108a. Kannus P, Parkkari J, Niemi S, et al. Prevention of hip fracture in elderly people with use of a hip protector. *N Engl J Med* 2000;343:1506-1513.
109. Bloem BR, Beckley DJ, van Dijk JG, et al. Are medium and long latency reflexes a screening tool for early Parkinson's disease? *J Neurol Sci* 1992;113:38–42.
110. Fahn S, Greene PE, Tsai W-Y, et al. Double-blind controlled trial of human embryonic dopaminergic tissue transplants in advanced Parkinson's disease: clinical outcomes. *Neurology* 1999;52:A405.

Gait Disorders. Advances in Neurology, Vol. 87,
edited by E. Růžička, M. Hallett, and J. Jankovic.
Lippincott Williams & Wilkins, Philadelphia © 2001.

22

Somatoform Phobic Postural Vertigo and Psychogenic Disorders of Stance and Gait

Marianne Dieterich, Siegbert Krafczyk, Veronika Querner, and Thomas Brandt

Department of Neurology, Grosshadern Clinic, Ludwig Maximilians University, 81377 Munich, Germany

Somatoform *phobic postural vertigo* (PPV) and *psychogenic disorders of stance and gait* (PSG) differ greatly in how patients experience and represent their conditions. Patients with PPV tend to hide their problem and usually continue working, although they suffer enormously from impending failure. Patients with PSG, on the contrary, openly show their obvious disability, usually do not work, and seem to suffer less.

PHOBIC POSTURAL VERTIGO

This is the third most common cause of vertigo, and is distinguishable from agoraphobia and acrophobia as well as from the fear of falling, cautious gait, and psychogenic disorders of stance and gait. Somatoform PPV is characterized by the combination of dizziness and a subjective disturbance of balance at upright position and during locomotion frequently in the form of brief postural vertigo attacks (1). The diagnosis is based on the following six characteristic features (2,3):

1. Dizziness and subjective disturbance are experienced during upright static stance and during gait despite normal clinical balance tests.
2. Postural vertigo is described as fluctuating unsteadiness, often in the form of attacks (seconds to minutes) or sometimes the perception of illusionary body perturbation for mere fractions of seconds.
3. These attacks occur spontaneously as well as in association with particular constellations of perceptual stimuli (e.g., bridges, staircases, empty rooms, streets, driving a car) or social situations (e.g., store, restaurant, cinema, concert, meeting, reception) from which the patient has difficulty withdrawing and that are recognized as provoking factors. There is a tendency for rapid conditioning, generalization, and avoidance behavior to develop.
4. Anxiety and distressing vegetative symptoms often (57%), but not always, accompany the vertigo attack. Its symptoms have to be elicited by direct questioning. Most patients experience these attacks both with and without excess anxiety.
5. Typically, a person with an obsessive–compulsive type personality (48%) is found to have affective liability and mild reactive (to the subjective vertigo) depression.
6. The onset of the condition frequently occurs after the patient has experienced an illness (37%), usually a vestibular disorder (21%), or after important psychosocial stress and psychodynamic conflicts (93%).

FOLLOW-UP OF PATIENTS WITH PHOBIC POSTURAL VERTIGO

Forty-two patients with PPV took part in a recent neurologic and psychiatric follow-up study

(4). The aim of the study was twofold: (a) to specify the diagnostic nature of the neurologic syndrome of *phobic postural vertigo* from a perspective of the *Diagnostic and Statistical Manual*, 3rd ed. (DSM III-R), and (b) to trace the course of illness with respect to the leading neurootologic syndrome and other concomitant psychopathologic syndromes. During the follow-up time of about 2.5 years the neurologic diagnosis remained stable. PPV could be assigned to various psychiatric categories according to DSM-III-R. The psychiatric diagnosis assessment according to SCID (DSM III-R) revealed that the syndrome of PPV on first admission to the Dizziness Unit had to be classified as a depressive disorder in four patients, as a generalized anxiety disorder in six patients, and as a panic disorder in 14 patients (with agoraphobia in 12 patients). Eighteen patients suffered from recurrent monosymptomatic attacks of vertigo, which were *not* accompanied by physical symptoms that occur in panic states (Table 22.1.) None of these 18 patients complained of subjective feelings of anxiety or even panic during the attacks. With recurring attacks of vertigo, however, 15 patients developed a phobic avoidance pattern that finally could be classified as agoraphobia. In one case an acrophobic behavior was also recorded. Thus, although an association with anxiety disorders was evident, not all patients presented with symptoms of anxiety or panic during attacks of vertigo; on the contrary they (42%) developed a disabling phobic avoidance pattern with recurrent vertigo attacks but without anxiety disorder (4).

The majority of patients (N = 20) showed features of an obsessive-compulsive personality type. Other personality traits (narcissistic, histrionic, dependent, avoidant, passive-aggressive) prevailed in some patients (Table 22.1). The course of illness varied depending on the neurologic syndrome of vertigo, on the one hand, and the concomitant psychopathologic syndromes, on the other. Despite a considerable improvement rate of 72% (22% became symptom-free), which confirmed the findings of an earlier study, the group of patients with phobic postural vertigo as a whole presented with significant psychopathologic problems at follow-up term (74%) (2). They required specific psychiatric and/or psychotherapeutic interventions. Dependent or avoidant personality traits, a pronounced somatic concept of illness, and hypochondria were prognostic of a more negative course of illness. Distressing psychosocial influences could be identified during the first manifestation of vertigo symptoms in all but three patients. Above all, stressors in personal relationships (N = 22), family (N = 16), and professional surroundings (N = 21) had to be evaluated as factors either directly releasing or mediating the onset of PPV. The majority of patients (N = 30) had to deal with serious midlife problems under duress.

TABLE 22.1. *Diagnostic classification of the syndrome of phobic postural vertigo*[a]

Axis I: DSM III-R diagnosis	N	Axis II: Personality features	N
Major depressive episode	2	Compulsive	20
Dysthymic disorder	2	Narcissistic	7
		Dependent	3
Generalized anxiety disorder	6	Histrionic	2
Panic disorder	14	Avoidant	6
With agoraphobia (complete)	8	Passive-aggressive	4
With agoraphobia (partial)	4		
PPV (monosymptomatic)	18		
With agoraphobia	15		

[a] According to structured clinical interview (SCID) at onset of condition and prevailing personality features (DSM III-R). PPV, phobic postural vertigo. From Kapfhammer HP, Mayer C, Hock U, et al. Course of illness in phobic postural vertigo. *Acta Neurol Scand* 1997;95:23–28, with permission.

POSTUROGRAPHIC EVALUATION OF PATIENTS WITH PHOBIC POSTURAL VERTIGO

The dissociation of subjective postural instability and objectively maintained balance skills is a typical feature of all nonorganic disorders. As a rule, routine otoneurologic and balance tests (e.g., electro-oculography with caloric irrigation, Romberg test, tandem walking) do not reveal any pathology. Moreover, objective quantitative balance tests do not provide any positive findings for most of these somatoform or psychogenic disorders. In an initial study on 12 patients with PPV we quantitatively analyzed the postural sway during upright stance in comparison to an age-matched control group of 12 healthy volunteers by means of a stabilometer platform (Kistler Type 9281, Winterthur, Switzerland), a device that transduces force changes exerted on the foot support (5). Changes of the center of pressure were measured in fore-aft (Y) and right-left (X) directions. Patients were instructed to remain upright and refrain from any voluntary movements during the recording. In order to make balancing more difficult, a slab of foam rubber was placed under the rigid foot support. This reduces the somatosensory contribution to postural control and therefore enhances the particular weight of afferent visual and vestibular cues. Recordings were made under three different conditions with the eyes open and closed: when standing on a foam rubber pad with the head upright, turned 30 degrees to the right or left, or during 1-Hz horizontal oscillations. Postural sway analysis included calculations of sway path, root mean square values (RMS) of sway, and power spectrum of sway in fore-aft and lateral directions.

The patients with PPV showed a significant increase in sway activity, which was spread across the frequency range 3.5 to 8 Hz but did not impair objective postural stability (Fig. 22.1). This increase in the middle and higher frequency range was found in lateral and fore-aft directions under all conditions tested. In a larger

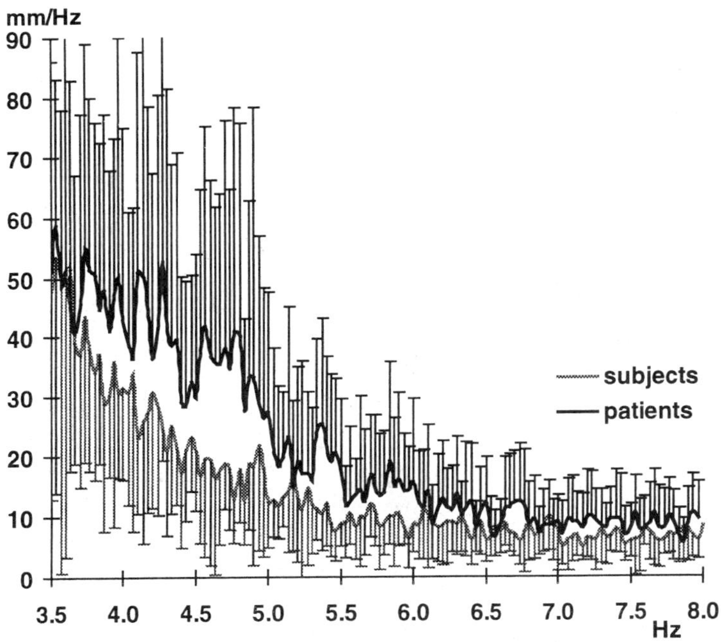

FIG. 22.1. Average of the frequency spectrum of the y body sway in 12 patients (*black line*) and 12 normal controls (*gray line*) for the frequency range 3.5 to 8 Hz (eyes closed, standing on foam rubber). Patients with phobic postural vertigo showed increased activity in this frequency range.

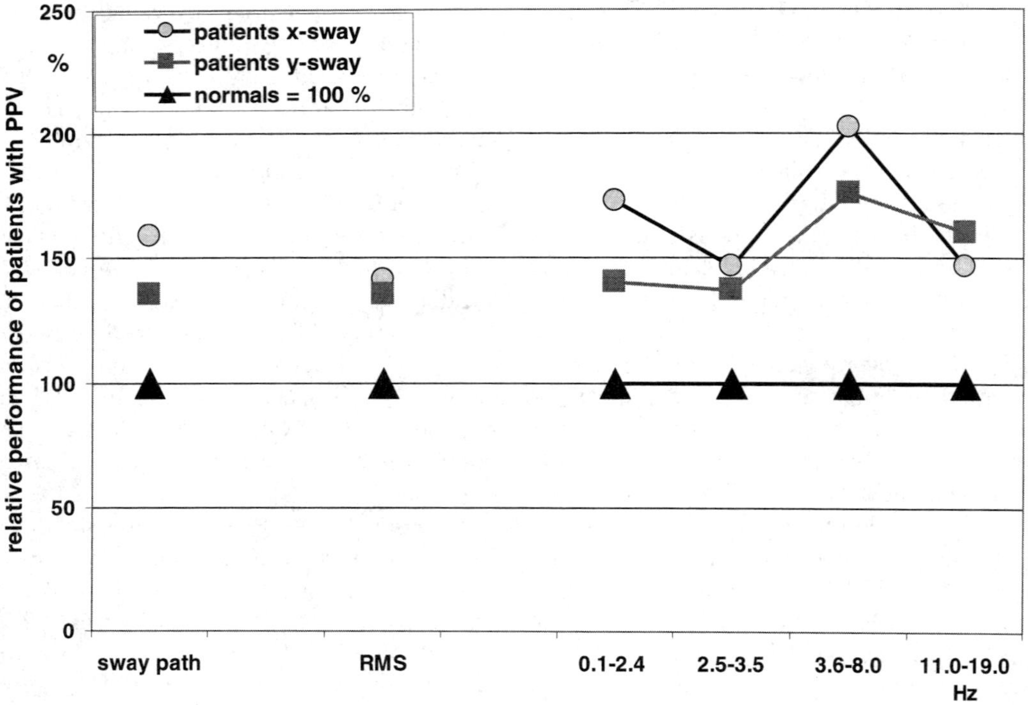

FIG. 22.2. Sway path, root mean square values of body sway and body sway activity in lateral (X, *circles with black lines*) and fore-aft (Y, *squares with gray lines*) directions of 17 patients with phobic postural vertigo (PPV) compared to 15 normals (*triangles with black lines*) in four frequency ranges (0.1 to 2.4 Hz; 2.5 to 3.5 Hz; 3.6 to 8.0 Hz; 11 to 19 Hz) under the condition eyes closed, standing on foam rubber with the head upright. Sway activity of normals was set to 100%. Patients with PPV showed increased activity in all frequency bands with a peak up to 200% in the range 3.6 to 8.0 Hz.

group of patients (N = 17) it turned out that sway activity was increased in all frequency ranges with the largest amount between 3.5 and 8 Hz (Fig. 22.2; Table 22.2). The sway pattern in patients with PPV was clearly distinguishable from that in patients with orthostatic tremor who typically show an additional narrow peak in the high frequency range of 14 to 18 Hz (Figs. 22.3 and 22.4) (6). It was also distinguishable from that in patients with cerebellar postural tremor owing to alcoholic cerebellar atrophy, who show—consistent with the literature—a distinct peak in the frequency band around 3 Hz (7, 8). Other sway parameters such as sway path or RMS of body sway did not differ significantly from those of normal subjects. The increased sway activity may simply reflect a change in postural strategy rather than a sensorimotor dysfunction because postural stability was not impaired (5).

This finding raised the question of whether the increase in body sway activity is related to an objective impairment of balance or not. Therefore, a second posturographic study was conducted on the differential effects of a more demanding balance task on balance (9). Tandem stance on a piece of foam rubber placed on the force measuring platform was chosen, a condition under which even normal subjects have difficulties maintaining balance with eyes closed. Body sway was analyzed in 17 patients with PPV and 15 control subjects for normal upright stance and tandem stance, with the eyes open or closed for each condition. During the most difficult task (tandem stance with the eyes closed) body sway activity and sway path values did not differ between patients and controls, whereas during normal upright stance patients with PPV again showed a significantly increased body sway

TABLE 22.2. *Sway path, body sway, and sum activity of body sway*[a]

	P-value
Sway path	
R/L	**0.017**
A/P	**0.008**
Body sway	
R/L	0.099
A/P	0.081
Sum activity	
0.1–2.4 Hz, R/L	**0.039**
A/P	**0.025**
2.5–3.5 Hz, R/L	**0.044**
A/P	**0.034**
3.5–8.0 Hz, R/L	**0.002**
A/P	**0.005**
11–19 Hz, R/L	**0.003**
A/P	**0.002**

[a] For fore-aft (A/P) and lateral (R/L) body sway during the condition eyes closed, standing on foam rubber with the head upright.

P-values of group differences between normal subjects and patients with PPV (student's *t*-test).

Significant differences ($P < 0.05$) in bold.

Note that significant differences were predominantly found for sum activity in the higher frequency range.

activity between 0.1 and 8 Hz (Table 22.2). Thus, objective balance skills were not impaired in patients with PPV during demanding balance tasks at the limits of postural control. These results reveal a feature that was also described in patients with other psychogenic balance disorders: The more difficult the task, the better the balance performance in these patients (10).

CHANGE IN POSTURAL STRATEGY BECAUSE OF ANXIOUS BALANCE CONTROL

The increased body sway activity observed in nonchallenging normal upright stance could reflect a cocontraction of antigravity muscles. This is a postural strategy that normal subjects adopt only for demanding balance conditions. As to the underlying mechanism, we favor a change in postural strategy owing to anxious balance control rather than a sensorimotor dysfunction. In normal subjects, maintenance of balance is achieved unconsciously. Conscious control is required only in unusual and therefore unadapted balance tasks (e.g., when walking on slippery ground or a beam). In the latter situation, the normal reciprocal activation pattern of the anterior tibial and the soleus muscles during treadmill walking is replaced by a pattern dominated by cocontraction (11). Increased coactivation of antagonistic muscles occurs when learning a new motor task, in situations when unpredictable perturbations may be encountered, and when uncertainty exists about the required task (12,13). As to biometric aspects, cocontraction stabilizes joints and reduces their mechanical sensitivity to external perturbation, thereby shortening the settling time of the system (13,14). Coactivation of antigravity muscles may be responsible for the increased higher-frequency and low-amplitude sway of patients with PPV. It reflects the unnecessary application of a postural strategy of caution.

This view is further supported by patients' reports of continuously controlling their stance even on firm ground, and by the obsessive-compulsive personality ascertained in the majority of patients with PPV by psychiatric evaluation (4). Two follow-up studies showed that subjective instability is reversible in the majority of patients (2,4). The therapeutic regimen mainly consists of relieving patients of their fear of an occult organic disease by providing them with a detailed explanation of the causative mechanism and factors provoking phobic reactions. Afterward, self-desensitization (by repeated exposure to situations that evoke the condition) within the context of behavioral therapy is recommended. Behavioral therapy causes more improvement when a functional rather than an organic mechanism is involved.

PSYCHOGENIC DISORDERS OF STANCE AND GAIT

The most common psychogenic movement disorders are tremor, dystonia, and gait disturbances, which account for more than 75% of psychogenic movement disorders (15). Among 405 patients presenting with psychogenic disorders, 47 were diagnosed with PPV and 52 with psychogenic disorders of stance and gait (PSG) (16). Phobic postural vertigo and psychogenic disorders of stance and gait accounted for about 1% each

(text continued on page 232)

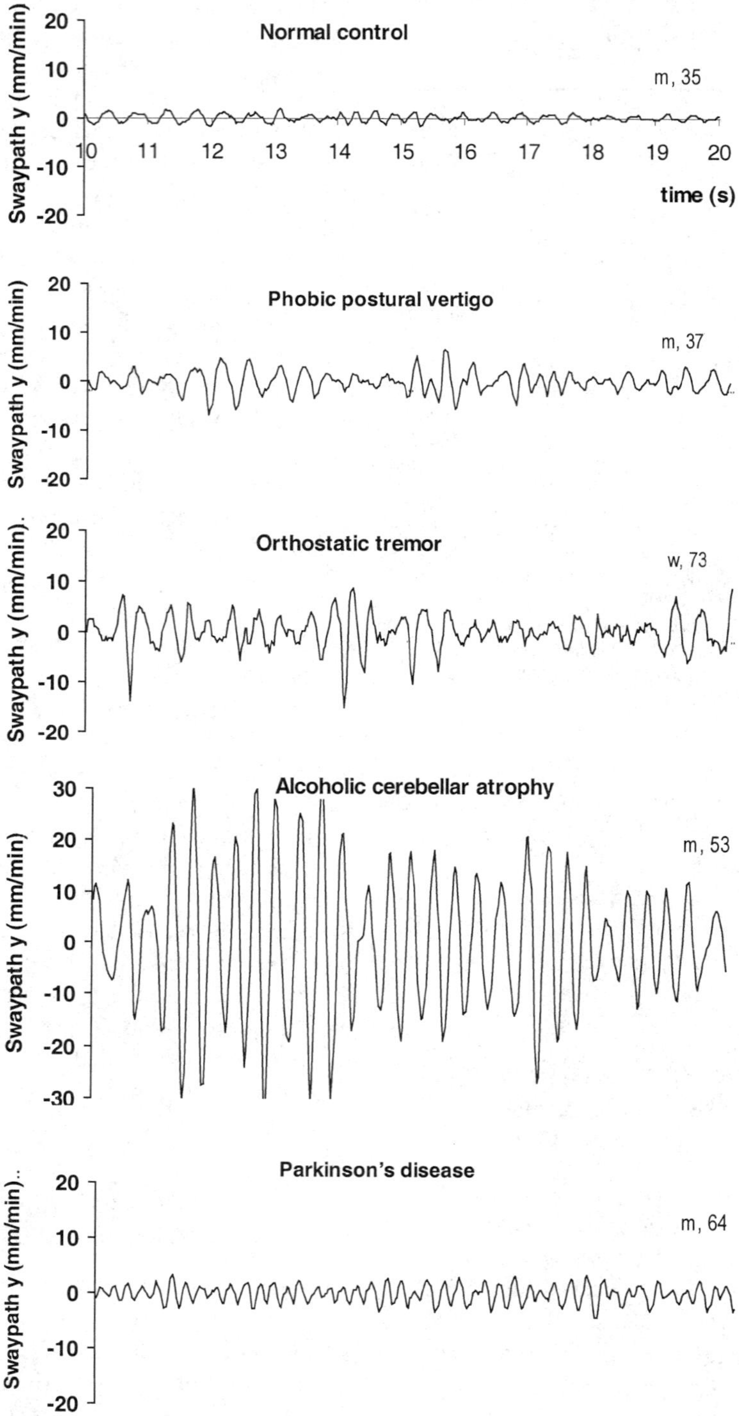

FIG. 22.3. Fore-aft (*Y*) body sway of single patients with different diseases compared to a normal control (**top**) under the eyes-closed condition and while standing on foam rubber with the head upright. Sway activity between 2 and 20 Hz is shown after frequencies of 0 to 2 Hz were erased by Fourier transformation and the spectra were then transformed back into the time domain. Compared to normals, the patient with phobic postural vertigo shows increased sway activity in the frequency range up to 20 Hz, which was also observed in the other patients.

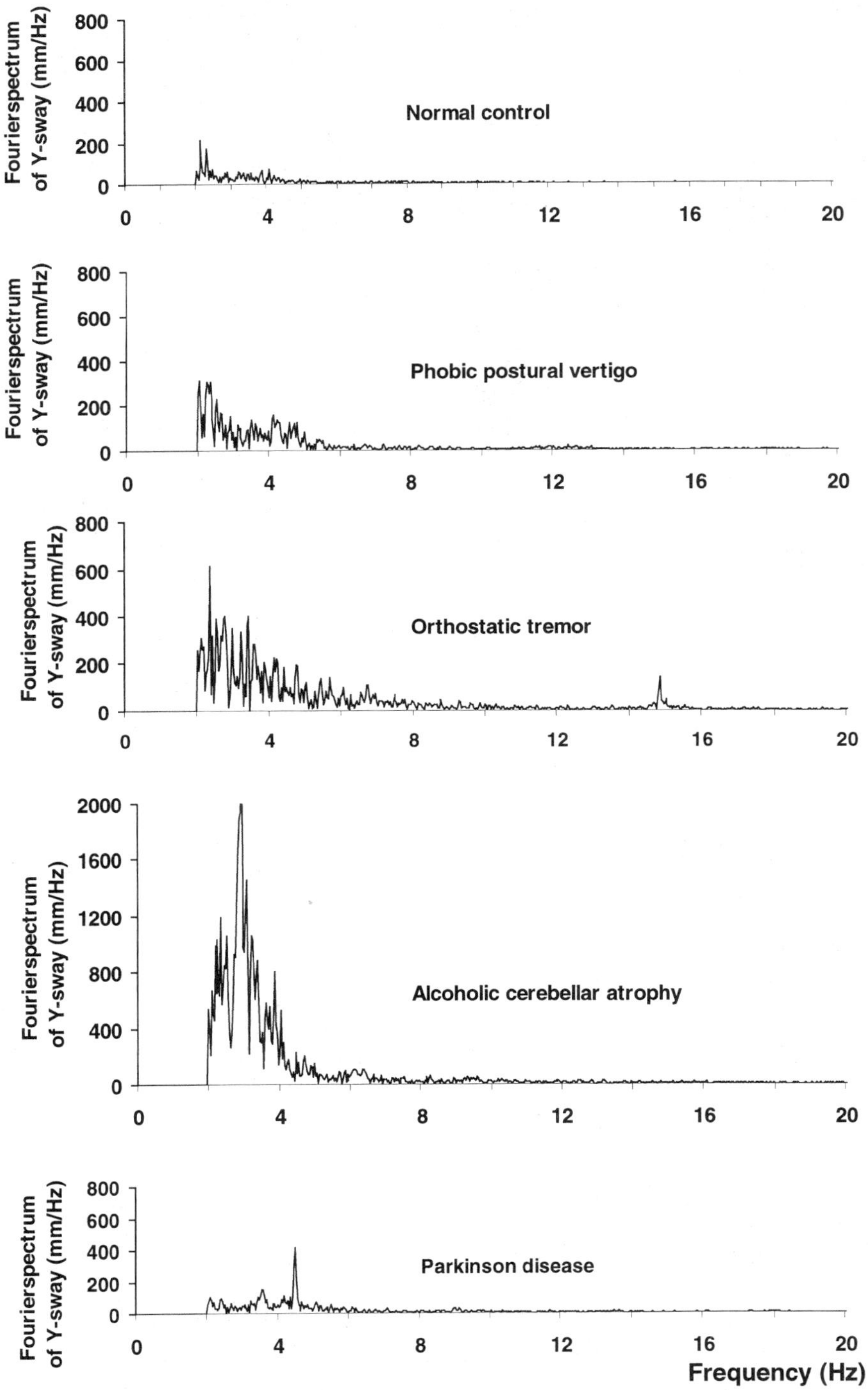

FIG. 22.4. Fourier analysis spectra of Y body sway in the frequency range 2 to 20 Hz of the same individuals under the same conditions as in Figure 22.3 after erasing the lower frequencies 0 to 2 Hz. Fourier analysis discloses increased sway activity in the patients and allows differentiation. The patient with phobic postural vertigo shows a broader increase, particularly in the frequency range 3.5 to 8.0 Hz, whereas patients with orthostatic tremor show an additional peak at 15 Hz (range, 14 to 18 Hz), patients with alcoholic cerebellar atrophy a peak at 3 Hz, and patients with Parkinson's disease a peak between 4 and 6 Hz.

of the diagnoses in our inpatients. We tried to establish diagnostic criteria for PSG as previous authors have done for psychogenic seizures because the importance and frequency of PSG are not reflected in recent textbooks and literature (17).

Thirty-seven patients with PSG were clinically evaluated, video recorded, and examined with regard to clinical phenomenology. The latter was done to determine if phenomenologic differentiation alone is practical for diagnosis. Normal findings on neurologic evaluation are a precondition for the diagnosis of purely PSG. Psychiatric findings were heterogeneous and included conversion disorder and depression.

Six clinical features proved more valuable for the diagnosis because they occurred alone or in combination in more than 90% of our 37 tested patients (17):

1. Momentary fluctuations of stance and gait, often in response to suggestion (N = 19)
2. Excessively slow (N = 13) or hesitating (N = 6) locomotion incompatible with neurologic disease
3. Psychogenic Romberg test showing increased sway amplitudes after latency or improvement during distraction (N = 12)
4. Uneconomic postures with wastage of muscle energy (N = 11)
5. The "walking on ice" gait pattern (N = 11), characterized by small cautious steps with fixed ankle joints
6. Sudden buckling of knees, usually without falls (N = 10)

Less frequent features included astasia (N = 4) and vertical shaking tremor (N = 3).

Encouragement and distraction by certain tasks, such as finger-nose testing or walking on tiptoe considerably improved the disturbance. Furthermore, additional signs suggesting a psychogenic disorder occurred in 73% of our patients (e.g., pseudoataxia, sudden sidesteps, bizarre tremors, continuous flexion or extension of the toes). The similarity of manifestations was striking in some patients. The overall variability, however, was large, and classification into characteristic subtypes was not useful, because predominant features varied from patient to patient and occurred in various combinations.

The use of posturographic measurements has been proposed as a means of differentiating malingerers from vertiginous patients, but the sensitivity and specificity of this measure are limited and clearly inferior to clinical experience (18). Therefore, we prefer the phenomenologic approach to psychogenic dysfunction of stance and gait, because it is direct, effective, and avoids unnecessary and potentially harmful diagnostic procedures.

ACKNOWLEDGMENTS

The authors thank Judy Benson for critically reading the manuscript. This work was supported by the Deutsche Forschungsgemeinschaft, SFB 462, A5.

REFERENCES

1. Brandt Th, Dieterich M. *Phobischer Attacken-Schwankschwindel. Ein neues Syndrom. Münch Med Wochenschr* 1986;128:247–250.
2. Brandt Th, Huppert D, Dieterich M. Phobic postural vertigo, a first follow-up. *J Neurol* 1994;241:191–195.
3. Brandt Th. *Vertigo. Its multisensory syndromes*, 2nd ed. London: Springer, 1999.
4. Kapfhammer HP, Mayer C, Hock U, et al. Course of illness in phobic postural vertigo. *Acta Neurol Scand* 1997;95:23–28.
5. Krafczyk S, Sclamp V, Dieterich M, et al. Increased body sway at 3.5–8 Hz in patients with phobic postural vertigo. *Neurosci Lett* 1999;259:149–152.
6. McManis PG, Sharbrough FW. Orthostatic tremor: clinical and electrophysiologic characteristics. *Muscle Nerve* 1993;16:1254–1260.
7. Dichgans J, Mauritz KH, Allum JHJ, et al. Postural sway in normals and ataxia patients. *Agressologie* 1976;17: 15–24.
8. Dichgans J, Diener HC. Different forms of postural ataxia in patients with cerebellar diseases. In: Bles W, Brandt Th, eds. *Disorders of posture and gait.* Amsterdam: Elsevier, 1986:207–215.
9. Querner V, Krafczyk S, Dieterich M, et al. Patients with somatoform phobic postural vertigo: the more difficult the balance task, the better the balance performance. *Neurosci Lett* 2000; 285:21–24.
10. Cevette MJ, Puetz B, Marion MS, et al. Aphysiologic performance on dynamic posturography. *Otolaryngol Head Neck Surg* 1995;112:676–688.
11. Llewellyn M, Yang YF, Prochazka A. Human H-reflexes are smaller in difficult beam walking than in normal treadmill walking. *Exp Brain Res* 1990;83:22–28.

12. De Luca CJ, Mambrito B. Voluntary control of motor units in human antagonist muscles: coactivation and reciprocal activation. *J Neurophysiol* 1987;58:525–542.
13. Smith AM. The coactivation of antagonistic muscles. *Can J Physiol Pharmacol* 1981;59:733–747.
14. Chou PC, Hannaford B. Study of human forearm posture maintenance with the physiologically based robotic arm spinal level neural controller. *Biol Cybernet* 1997;76:285–298.
15. Williams DT, Ford B, Fahn S. Phenomenology and psychopathology related to psychogenic movement disorders. In: Wiener WJ, Lang AE, eds. *Behavioral neurology movement disorders.* New York: Raven Press, 1995:231–257.
16. Lempert Th, Dieterich M, Huppert D, et al. Psychogenic disorders in neurology: frequency and clinical spectrum. *Acta Neurol Scand* 1990;82:335–340.
17. Lempert Th, Brandt Th, Dieterich M, et al. How to identify psychogenic disorders of stance and gait. A video study in 37 patients. *J Neurol* 1991;238:140–146.
18. Allum JHJ, Huwiler M, Honegger F. Identifying cases of non-organic vertigo using dynamic posturography. *Gait Posture* 1996;4:52–61.

Gait Disorders. Advances in Neurology, Vol. 87,
edited by E. Růžička, M. Hallett, and J. Jankovic.
Lippincott Williams & Wilkins, Philadelphia © 2001.

23

Gait Disorders Accompanying Diseases of the Frontal Lobes

Philip D. Thompson

University Department of Medicine and Department of Neurology, Royal Adelaide Hospital and University of Adelaide, Adelaide, South Australia 5000

Disease of the frontal lobes and interruption of the subcortical circuits connecting the frontal lobes, basal ganglia, cerebellum, and brainstem interferes with several aspects of normal gait. The clinical features of the gait abnormalities in frontal lobe disease are complex and vary considerably. The mechanisms underlying them are poorly understood. Accordingly, the nomenclature and classification of frontal gait disorders remains the subject of debate (1). Of the various pathologies responsible for frontal gait disorders, diffuse cerebrovascular disease and hydrocephalus are among the most common causes (Table 23.1). Collectively, these conditions are estimated to account for 20% to 30% of cases of significant walking difficulties in older adults (1,2). Frontal gait disorders may occur at any age but are most common in older adults.

CLINICAL SIGNS OF FRONTAL GAIT DISORDERS

The core clinical elements of frontal gait disorders can be summarized as an akinetic, hypokinetic, rigid gait with ataxia, impaired postural reflexes, and a tendency to fall. Patients commonly present with a combination of these clinical signs, each of which may vary in severity. The characteristics that assist in differentiating cerebellar ataxia, the hypokinesia of Parkinson's disease and the gait of frontal lobe disease are listed in Table 23.2. The combination of an ataxic and hypokinetic gait along with impairment of postural reflexes provides an important clue to the presence of a frontal gait disorder. These findings along with the upright posture of the trunk are characteristic of the early stages of a frontal gait disorder and are illustrated in the cartoon figures shown in Figure 23.1.

Early in the evolution of a frontal gait disorder the stance is slightly wide-based and the posture of the trunk and neck is upright. Leg movements are stiff and steps are short and shuffling. The initiation of walking is hesitant, with a series of short shuffling steps (start hesitation). Once walking is underway, freezing (sudden cessation of stepping), or a burst of small shuffling steps are common. Freezing and shuffling may reappear on turning a corner, encountering an obstacle, or with distraction and diversion of attention away from the task of walking. During walking the normal rhythmic flow of trunk and limb motion is lost. Arm swing is normal or even exaggerated. The combination of exaggerated arm swing and the upright posture of the trunk has been referred to as a "military two-step" gait. In

TABLE 23.1. *Causes of a frontal gait disturbance*

Multiple lacunar infarcts (Binswanger's disease)
Anterior cerebral artery infarction
Hydrocephalus
Frontal lobe tumors (glioma, meningioma)
Demyelination (multiple sclerosis)
Corticobasal degeneration
Subdural hematoma
Frontotemporal dementia

TABLE 23.2. *Summary of the main clinical features of gait in Parkinson's disease, cerebellar ataxia, and accompanying frontal lobe disease*

Feature	Parkinson's disease	Cerebellar ataxia	Frontal gait disorder
Trunk posture	Stooped flexed trunk	Stooped, leans forward	Upright
Stance	Narrow	Wide-based	Wide-based
Initiation of gait	Start hesitation	Normal	Start hesitation
Stepping	Shuffles	Staggers, lurches	Shuffles
Stride length	Short	Variable	Short
Speed	Slow	Normal, slow	Very slow
Festination	Common	Absent	Rare
Leg movement	Stiff rigid	Variable, ataxic	Stiff, rigid
Arm swing	Reduced, absent	Normal, exaggerated	Exaggerated
Heel-toe	Normal	Unable	Unable
Turning corners	Freezes	Veers away	Freezes, shuffles
Romberg's test	Negative	±	±
Heel-shin test	Normal	Abnormal	Normal
Postural reflexes	Preserved (until late disease)	±	Impaired, absent
Falls	Late	Uncommon	Common

±, May be abnormal.

contrast to the lower body, facial expression, and upper limb movement are normal. Upper motor neuron signs are often also evident.

The ataxia and parkinsonism become more pronounced with progression of the underlying condition. The initiation of stepping becomes increasingly difficult. Start hesitation may manifest as repetitive small shuffling foot movements that fail to initiate a step (the slipping clutch phenomenon) and progress to a complete inability to move the feet that are seemingly glued to the floor (the magnetic foot). Exaggerated upper

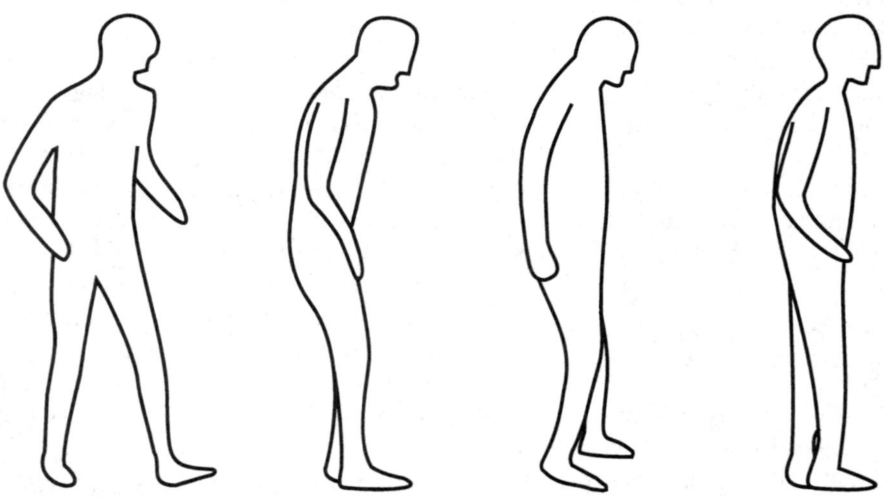

A–D

FIG. 23.1. Cartoon figures traces from videotape records of patients with cerebellar ataxia **(A)**, Parkinson's disease (PD) **(B)**, subcortical arteriosclerotic encephalopathy **(C** and **D)**. In cerebellar ataxia **(A)**, the stance is wide-based, steps are of variable length, and direction and associated upper-limb movement during the walking cycle is preserved. In PD **(B)**, the trunk adopts a posture of flexion, steps are small and shuffling, and there is a lack of associated arm swing during the walking cycle. In subcortical arteriosclerotic encephalopathy, the wide stance base **(C)**, upright trunk posture, and short shuffling steps **(D)** are accompanied by an awkward rigid appearance of the upper body motion and arm swing during walking, with loss of the normal fluidity and interplay of movement between body segments.

body movement may be employed to shift the body weight toward one side to free the opposite foot to swing forward and initiate walking. Postural and righting reactions are impaired causing unsteadiness while standing and walking leading to falls. The patient may require support and assistance to take a step. The slightest perturbation, such as when first standing up from a seated position, when attempting to initiate the first step or on encountering an unexpected obstacle when walking may lead to a fall. Once underway shuffling becomes even more pronounced. Postural corrections may be inappropriate or absent. Festination, as seen in Parkinson's disease (PD), is unusual. A few steps of propulsion or retropulsion prompt the patient to seek support and sit down or they may fall.

A fear of falling may lead to additional slowness and caution when walking. The patient may seek support of nearby objects and become afraid to venture into open spaces or busy crowded areas (cautious gait) (1).

In contrast with the difficulty walking, patients may be capable of moving their legs with greater facility when seated or lying supine (3). Stepping movements of the legs may be possible when lying but not when standing. Other leg movements such as bicycling movements may appear relatively preserved in comparison with the difficulty encountered when walking. On close examination, however, a number of abnormalities of leg movement are evident when the patient is seated or supine. For example, there may be a loss of the ability to perform repetitive sequences of movement, particularly those that involve both legs during bilateral alternating movements of the legs and feet. Simple leg movements describing the outline of a number on the floor with the foot or kicking an imaginary ball often are performed poorly. The initiation of movement is slow and movement execution is clumsy (4). There may also be a degree of heel-shin ataxia.

Postural responses and locomotor patterns are increasingly disrupted with further progression. The disorder of truncal balance progresses and falls are common. Although the patient is still able to stand, it is evident that stepping has also become disorganized. In the advanced stages, truncal ataxia and loss of truncal mobility become increasingly severe, making standing and walking impossible. Patients may be unable to sit in a chair or turn over when lying in bed.

Signs of frontal lobe disease, including a general slowing of cognitive and motor function, rigidity or gegenhalten, grasp reflexes, perseveration, difficulty initiating and maintaining repetitive movements of the upper as well as the lower limbs, and urinary incontinence also may be evident on clinical examination.

CAUSES OF FRONTAL GAIT DISORDERS

Two of the most common conditions causing this pattern of gait disturbance are subcortical arteriosclerotic encephalopathy (Binswanger's disease) and hydrocephalus. The gait disturbance in these conditions can be very similar (5). Clinical recognition of the underlying cause of a frontal gait disorder is greatly simplified by imaging of the brain, but also requires careful evaluation of the history and neurologic examination.

Subcortical Arteriosclerotic Encephalopathy

The typical features of Binswanger's disease include a history of stroke, a stepwise evolution and accumulation of neurologic deficits with upper motor neuron signs and a pseudobulbar palsy in addition to the disturbance of gait. Descriptions of this clinical picture include *marché à petit pas* (attributed to Dejerine), arteriosclerotic parkinsonism, lower half parkinsonism, parkinsonian ataxia, and lower body parkinsonism (Table 23.3) (5–7).

This pattern of gait is frequently misinterpreted as a sign of PD. However, facial expression and upper limb function are relatively preserved (in comparison to the gait disorder) and tremor is uncommon. The absence of resting tremor, the disparity between upper and lower body involvement, the presence of upper motor neuron signs (including a pseudobulbar palsy) and the failure to respond to L-Dopa distinguish this syndrome from PD (Table 23.2).

TABLE 23.3. *Terms used to describe the clinical features of gait in frontal lobe disease*

Descriptive terms	Clinical signs
Magnetic apraxia	Start hesitation, freezing, unable to initiate step, "magnetic" feet, "feet glued to the floor"
Slipping clutch phenomenon	Start hesitation, freezing, shuffling foot movements ineffective in initiation stepping
Marche a petits pas	Start hesitation, freezing, small shuffling steps, wide base, mild ataxia
Arteriosclerotic parkinsonism	Start hesitation, freezing, small shuffling steps, wide base, mild ataxia
Lower body parkinsonism	Start hesitation, freezing, small shuffling steps, wide base, mild ataxia
Lower half parkinsonism	Start hesitation, freezing, small shuffling steps, wide base, mild ataxia
Parkinsonian ataxia	Start hesitation, freezing, small shuffling steps, wide base, mild ataxia
Frontal ataxia	Start hesitation, freezing, small shuffling steps, impaired postural reflexes, very unsteady
Gait apraxia	Start hesitation, freezing, small shuffling steps, impaired postural reflexes, unsteady May need support to stand Slowness of all movements, frontal lobe signs
Trepidant abasia (Petren's gait)	Fear of walking, cautious gait
Astasia–abasia	Inability to stand, or move legs to walk while standing in the absence of leg weakness

Hydrocephalus

The presentation of hydrocephalus with a gait disturbance is well recognized; gait may be affected before cognitive changes or incontinence develop. Evolution of the gait disturbance with progression of hydrocephalus may be striking (8). Initially, the gait appears ataxic and hypokinetic. Later, increasing difficulty initiating stepping and "magnetic feet" appear accompanied by loss of truncal balance. The latter may become so severe that the patient is unable to sit. Early intervention with ventricular drainage and shunting may reverse these features.

With advancing hydrocephalus, the clinical deficits may extend beyond a gait disorder to include soft speech and a marked reduction in spontaneous movement with a loss of normal facial expression. Mutism (akinetic mutism) and other frontal lobe release signs are often associated features (9).

In several descriptions of the parkinsonism that may accompany hydrocephalus, upper body parkinsonism with typical resting tremor, have been described in addition to the ataxia, apraxia, and lower half parkinsonism (10,11). In some cases, the parkinsonism has been L-Dopa–responsive, suggesting additional structural or functional disruption of the nigrostriatal system (10,11).

Other Causes of Frontal Gait Disorders

The gait disorder of corticobasal degeneration, which may be a presenting feature of this disease, has many of the characteristics of a frontal gait disorder. Frontal lobe tumors also may present with a frontal gait disturbance. Indeed, many of the descriptions of the "parkinsonism" accompanying frontal tumors are based on the hypokinetic elements of a frontal gait disorder. However, as with hydrocephalus, L-Dopa responsiveness, a rest tremor, and upper body parkinsonism suggests indirect involvement of the nigrostriatal system in some cases.

Fragments of the clinical picture of a frontal gait disorder may be observed in some patients without defined anatomic or pathologic evidence of frontal lobe disease. Isolated gait ignition failure or primary progressive freezing gait refer to syndromes in which start hesitation and freezing are accompanied by normal stepping, once walking is underway, and preservation of balance and postural reflexes (12,13). Occasionally, this clinical picture is the presenting feature of hydrocephalus or Binswanger's disease.

The *senile gait disorders* are also characterized by a wide-based, unsteady stance with an upright posture, start hesitation, freezing, and shuffling steps (14). In many cases, there is no anatomic or pathologic evidence of an underlying abnormality and a frontal lobe disorder has also been postulated for these conditions.

QUANTITATIVE ANALYSIS OF FRONTAL GAIT DISORDERS

Detailed analyses of gait kinematics in subcortical arteriosclerotic encephalopathy and lower body parkinsonism reaffirm most of these clinical observations. In a study of gait initiation, Elble and colleagues demonstrated abnormalities of the early postural shifts that are necessary to allow the stepping or stride limb to swing into motion (15). Transfer of weight toward the supporting leg was more variable in amplitude and direction than in normal (elderly age-matched) subjects. Tonic muscle activity recorded in gastrocnemius, vastus lateralis, and hamstrings obscured the normal phasic changes in muscle activation at the initiation of gait, perhaps consistent with the slightly flexed "stiff" posture and restricted movement of the legs. Activation of tibialis anterior, which heralds the shift of body weight as gait begins, also was more variable. These effects lead to a delay in the transition from standing to walking. The abnormal postural shifts also were accompanied by several unsuccessful attempts to start walking, with interruption of the sequence perhaps reflecting voluntary attempts to compensate for faulty postural mechanisms and prevent a possible fall. These authors concluded that impaired postural contol was a significant factor in the delayed gait initiation (15).

Slow walking speeds and short steps, with increased variability in step timing and amplitude, were observed in patients with subcortical arteriosclerotic encephalopathy, emphasizing the ataxic elements in addition to the hypokinetic stepping in this condition (16).

Patients with hydrocephalus also walk slowly with short steps, postural instability, and increased body sway (17–19). All measures, particularly the latter, improved after ventricular drainage.

NOMENCLATURE OF FRONTAL GAIT DISORDERS

Many descriptions of the gait accompanying frontal lobe disease are recorded in the literature. There was a tendency for these descriptions to focus on specific but different elements of the complex gait disturbance (Table 23.3). Early descriptions of frontal gait syndromes emphasized the ataxic elements (referred to as frontal ataxia); involvement of frontopontocerebellar pathways was considered the most likely mechanism. Subsequently, the relative preservation of leg movements when lying or sitting, in contrast to the difficulties walking, prompted the designations apraxia and truncal apraxia (14,20,21). Denny Brown postulated that mesial frontal lobe disease released grasp reflexes in the feet and "tonic innervation," resulting in the feet being glued to the floor (magnetic apraxia) (3). Meyer and Barron defined gait apraxia as, "the loss of ability to properly use the lower limbs in the act of walking which cannot be accounted for by demonstrable sensory impairment or motor weakness" (4). They also emphasized the combination of ataxia, slow shuffling steps, rigidity (gegenhalten), and brisk reflexes as the essential features of gait apraxia. The finding of slow small leg movements and rigidity distinguished gait apraxia from cerebellar ataxia. These authors viewed apraxia of gait as a failure of the normal mechanisms of initiation of movement (4). This difficulty was compounded by the basic requirement of coordinated action of both legs in bilateral simultaneous movement during walking and provided an explanation for the improvement in the performance of leg movements when seated or lying down using only one limb at a time. In their cogent review, Meyer and Barron concluded that frontal lobe disease produced a striking disorder of gait but were careful to not to draw any anatomic correlations because their cases and many of those in the literature had diffuse cerebral disease (4).

There are several reservations about the use of the term apraxia in the context of gait disorders. First, the term does not take into account the many different elements that are critical for the performance of normal gait, including for example, the requirement to stand, maintain an upright posture, negotiate the postural adjustments to initiate stepping, then maintaining a rhythmic stepping action of both legs. Second, leg movements are not normal when performing other tasks when seated or lying, yet gait is abnormal under all circumstances. Finally, the term apraxia overlooks the role of the frontal lobes in organizing and maintaining repetitive sequences of movement and interlimb coordination.

MECHANISMS OF FRONTAL GAIT DISORDERS

The proposed mechanism for the predominant lower body involvement is selective involvement of long corticospinal fibers controlling leg movement as they descend close to the lateral ventricles. Periventricular pathology in both hydrocephalus and Binswanger's disease is common and corticospinal fibers controlling leg function are vulnerable in this location (21,22). The ataxia and disturbance of equilibrium are thought to be related to the involvement of frontocerebellar fibers and frontal projections to brainstem centers concerned with postural control. Such projections would also follow a similar periventricular trajectory. Interruption of the reciprocal connections between the basal ganglia and supplementary motor area also may be interrupted and contribute to the akinetic elements of the gait disturbance (1,13).

Several observations suggest a functional or structural disruption of the nigrostriatal system when generalized parkinsonism with a resting tremor appear as signs of hydrocephalus and frontal tumors. The appearance of parkinsonism is accompanied by pretectal signs indicating rostral midbrain compression in young adults with aqueduct stenosis and secondary hydrocephalus (11). This observation supports the notion of an associated disruption of nigrostriatal function perhaps as a consequence of the rostral midbrain compression (10,11,23). Finally, normal pressure hydrocephalus in older adults may be accompanied by idiopathic PD in some cases (10,24,25).

CONCLUSION

The anatomic basis for the individual components of frontal gait disorders are unknown, reflecting the incomplete understanding of the neural substrates of human locomotion. The term gait apraxia frequently is used to describe the gait of frontal lobe disease and is virtually synonymous with the gait disorder accompanying hydrocephalus and older adults with Binswanger's disease. However, the designation apraxia in the context of gait disorders remains the subject of debate (1). The combination of lower body akinesia, hypokinesia, impaired balance, lower limb ataxia, and poor postural control in disease of the frontal lobes and frontal-subcortical connections has tentatively been explained by interruption of the connections between frontal (motor, premotor, and supplementary motor cortex) and subcortical (cerebellum, basal ganglia, and brainstem) motor areas. The spectrum of gait abnormalities associated with frontal lobe disease, therefore, may represent a breakdown of higher-order motor control of complex sequential and simultaneous interlimb and truncal movements during gait, involving the initiation and maintenance of rhythmic bilateral leg movement during locomotion, truncal posture, and balance (1). It is suggested that many of the previous terms used to describe the patterns of gait associated with frontal lobe disease have focused on a specific aspect. An alternative approach is to consider a spectrum of clinical pictures reflecting the variable combinations of the core elements of limb hypokinesia and ataxia, and impaired postural reflexes.

REFERENCES

1. Nutt JG, Marsden CD, Thompson PD. Human walking and higher level gait disorders, particularly in the elderly. *Neurology* 1993;43:268–279.
2. Sudarsky L, Ronthal M. Gait disorders among elderly patients: a survey of 50 patients. *Arch Neurol* 1983;40:740–743.
3. Denny Brown D. The nature of apraxia. *J Nerv Ment Dis* 1958;126:9–31.

4. Meyer JS, Barron D. Apraxia of gait: a clinicopathological study. *Brain* 1960;83:61–84.
5. Thompson PD, Marsden CD. Gait disorder of subcortical arteriosclerotic encephalopathy: Binswanger's disease. *Mov Disord* 1987;2:1–8.
6. Critchley M. Arteriosclerotic parkinsonism. *Brain* 1929;52:23–83.
7. Fitzgerald PM, Jankovic J. Lower body parkinsonism: evidence for a vascular aetiology. *Mov Disord* 1989; 4:249–260.
8. Messert B, Baker NH. Syndrome of progressive spastic ataxia and apraxia associated with occult hydrocephalus. *Neurology* 1966;16:440–452.
9. Messert B, Henke TK, Langheim W. Syndrome of akinetic mutism associated with obstructive hydrocephalus. *Neurology* 1966;16:635–649.
10. Curran T, Lang AE. Parkinsonian syndromes associated with hydrocephalus: case reports, a review of the literature and pathophysiological hypotheses. *Mov Disord* 1994;9:508–520.
11. Zeidler M, Dorman PJ, Ferguson IT, et al. Parkinsonism associated with obstructive hydrocephalus due to idiopathic aqueductal stenosis. *J Neurol Neurosurg Psychiatry* 1998;64:657–659.
12. Atchison PR, Thompson PD, Frackowiak RSJ, et al. The syndrome of isolated gait ignition failure: a report of six cases. *Mov Disord* 1993;8:285–292.
13. Achiron A, Ziv I, Goren M, et al. Primary progressive freezing gait. *Mov Disord* 1993;8:293–297.
14. Critchley M. On senile disorders of gait, including the so-called "senile paraplegia." *Geriatrics* 1948;3:364–370.
15. Elble R, Cousins R, Leffler K, et al. Gait initiation by patients with lower-half parkinsonism. *Brain* 1996;119: 1705–1716.
16. Ebersbach G, Sojer M, Valldeoriola F, et al. Comparative analysis of gait in Parkinson's disease, cerebellar ataxia and subcortical arteriosclerotic encephalopathy. *Brain* 1999;122:1349–1355.
17. Sorensen, PS, Jansen EC, Gjerris F. Motor disturbances in normal pressure hydrocephalus. Special reference to stance and gait. *Arch Neurol* 1986;43:34–38.
18. Sudarsky L, Simon S. Gait disorder in late-life hydrocephalus. *Arch Neurol* 1987;44:267–267.
19. Knutsson E, Lying-Tunell U. Gait apraxia in normal pressure hydrocephalus: patterns of muscle activation. *Neurology* 1985;35:155–160.
20. Gerstmann J, Schilder P. *Uber eine besondere gangstorieng bei stirnhirnerkankhungen. Wien Med Wschr* 1926; 76:97–107.
21. Yakovlev PI. Paraplegias of hydrocephalus. *Am J Ment Defic* 1947;51:561–576.
22. Ishii N, Nishihara Y, Imamura T. Why do frontal lobe symptoms predominate in vascular dementia with lacunes? *Neurology* 1986;36:340–345.
23. Jankovic J, Newmark M, Peter P. Parkinsonism and acquired hydrocephalus. *Mov Disord* 1986;1:59–64.
24. Lobo Antunes J, Fahn S, Cote L. Normal pressure hydrocephalus and Parkinson's disease. *J Neural Transm* 1983;19:225–231.
25. Krauss JK, Regel JP, Droste DW, et al. Movement disorders in adult hydrocephalus. *Mov Disord* 1997;12: 53–60.

Gait Disorders. Advances in Neurology, Vol. 87,
edited by E. Růžička, M. Hallett, and J. Jankovic.
Lippincott Williams & Wilkins, Philadelphia © 2001.

24

Imbalance of Attentional and Sensory Inputs on Gait

*Serge Mesure, *Axel Darmon, and *†Olivier Blin

**CPCET and UPRES 2199, CHU la Timone; †Department of Clinical Pharmacology, Timone University Hospital UMR CRNS Universite Mediteranee, F-13385 Marseille, France*

Several studies have shown that sensory and attentional stimuli play important roles in gait. For example, attentional tasks during a motor undertaking provoke the subject to perform poorer than previously (1–3). Attention in this situation acts as a distractor. Yet we know that the prefrontal and sensory cortices are closely interrelated, and both are connected to the amygdala and limbic system, which mediate cognitive and emotional inputs. Both sensory information and planned movement commands converge in the superior colliculus; therefore, sensory inputs can interact on motor programming via the sensory cortex, whereas cognitive inputs can interact on the drive representation via the amygdala (4–9). The general model we propose is represented in Figure 24.1. This theoretical model allows us to address: (a) the role of arousal and attention on gait, and (b) the possible imbalance between sensory inputs and attention. In order to document this model, we will use data obtained in normal subjects, elderly subjects, and patients with Parkinson's disease (PD).

Several examples of gait disorders possibly related to the imbalance between sensory inputs, attention, and motor execution can be stressed before going into more details. Hyperarousal provoked by music and complex motor programming (dance) might lead to motor blockade in normal people. In the same way, divided attention degrades more obstacle avoidance abilities in elderly subjects than in young controls. This phenomenon is also observed in pathologic conditions.

An example of underarousal can be found in PD when patients have to divide their attention to perform a motor task: Patients with PD experience great trouble in dividing attention and perform very poorly. On the other hand, patients with PD are still able to intentionally modulate their gait velocity; the increase in gait velocity is greater than that caused by L-Dopa administration. The opposite example is found when a patient hears the telephone ringing (excess in auditory inputs), or when passing through a doorway (excess in visual inputs). The excess of attention required for performing the task, or the hyperarousal provoked by the unexpected stimulus, induces a hypoexcitability that can be manifested by motor blockade. This model also explains how sensory or attentional stimuli can help patients to better perform motor tasks: The excitability is greatest and the performance of patients improves when the threshold is neither too low nor too high. External cues have been described to trigger motor tasks, such as walking toward a goal or on a striped pathway. Thus, in this chapter we will try to explain the modulatory effect of attentional and visual cues at the light of volitional and motivational theories.

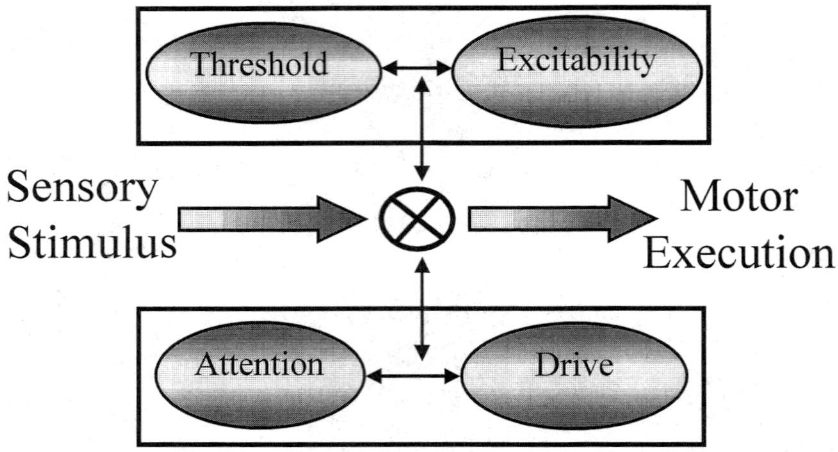

FIG. 24.1. Hypothetical block diagram of interaction between sensory stimulus and motor execution.

A THEORETICAL MODEL LINKING ATTENTIONAL DEMAND AND PERFORMANCE

Motor execution and especially gait is controlled first by sensory inputs such as vision, audition, proprioception, and second by cognitive processes. Among these processes, arousal, volition, adaptation to immediate circumstances, and insight for adaptation to personal goals should be distinguished. These factors modify the threshold and the excitability of the system. A neural model proposed by Grossberg links arousal with motor behavior, with a bell-shape curve (10,11). It consists of a series of filtering, competitive end-cooperative stages (11–13). This model was elaborated first to understand how the visual system integrates visual inputs, and more precisely the visual information about motion. It is interesting to interpolate this model of general sensory integration and motor execution on the attentional demands process. Following this model, when the subjects are underaroused, they are hyperexcitable, with an increased threshold; therefore, they are hypersensitive to the stimuli. On the other hand, when they are hyperaroused, they become hypoexcitable, with a decreased threshold; therefore, they become hyposensitive. A hypothetical neural model derived from those proposed by Grossberg links the attention with the motor response (Fig. 24.2). There is a level of attention that allows an optimal motor response, but with higher or lower attention, the motor response faints. However, the level of attention is related to a suboptimal motor performance in a rest situation (the Neutral point).

Experimental data in healthy subjects, elderly patients, and patients with PD support this model. Most of these results are driven from data obtained with a dual-task methodology, for example, asking subjects to perform a reaction time task (RT) during walking. In this case, we consider that the overall attentional demand is the sum of the attentional demand related to RT and those related to walking. Therefore, during simultaneous tasks, if the RT performance decreases, the attentional cost for walking is increased.

In his 1994 report, Kurosawa measured the reaction time of 13 normal male subjects when walking at different velocities (14). The mean RT value was shortest at the walking velocity of 4 km/h that corresponded to the spontaneous preferred velocity of the subjects. The interpretation of the author was that, "walking at the optimum velocity calls for extremely low demands for attention and walking at velocities higher or lower requires more attention." When transposed on our model, we can say that starting from the Neutral point, walking at a higher velocity increases the attentional demand for walking and then leads to a worsening in RT response. Walking at a lower speed is a voluntary motor task that requires a lot of attention and then also leads to a worsening in RT. In this case we can

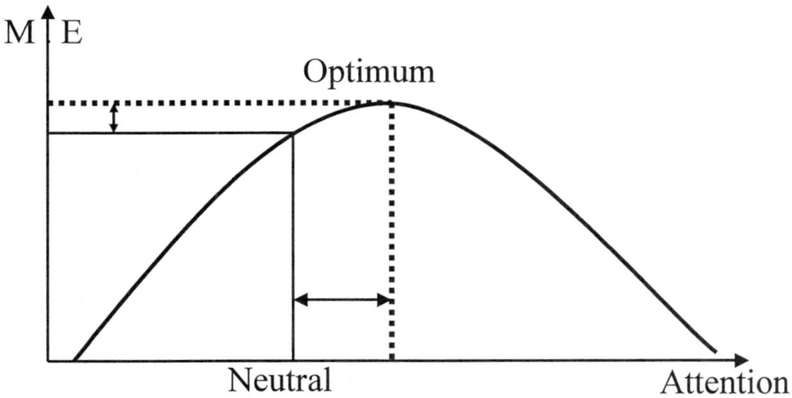

FIG. 24.2. Imbalance between attention and motor execution (*ME*). The *solid line* indicates that, in rest condition, the level of attention leads to a suboptimal motor performance. The *dotted line* represents maximum motor performance obtained for increased attention.

hypothesize that attentional demand for walking slowly is more important than for walking at a higher velocity. This may be explained by the fact that at a low walking speed, balance demands require a greater proportion of attentional resources and constant vigilance is required to prevent reverting to more automatic control mechanisms. On the contrary, adding a low attentional demand (such as thinking) could lead in certain circumstances to an increase in walking velocity.

Other results using dual-task methodology led to comparable results: Lajoie showed in six young volunteers that the attentional cost for walking is significantly higher than for standing, and that the single-support phase of walking induces more attentional demand than the double-support phase (15). These results suggest that attentional demands of a postural task increase with an increase in balance requirements. Ebersbach demonstrated on 10 healthy volunteers that double-support time increases when a memory-retention task (digit span) and fine motor task (buttoning) were performed simultaneously during walking (16). The conclusion was that attentional demand of concurrent cognitive and motor tasks appears to force subjects to modulate their gait strategy to ensure control of balance.

It is important to determine if there is a deficit and/or a modification in the allocation of the attentional resources necessary for balance, gait, and daily activities control in normal aging. Chen et al. showed in 16 young adults (mean age, 24 years) and 16 elderly adults (mean age, 72 years) that abilities to avoid stepping on an obstacle that appears suddenly were decreased in elderly subjects when they were asked to perform an RT simultaneously (2). Performance was poorer in elderly subjects (corresponding to a decrease in the optimum performance on our curve) and dividing attention-degraded obstacle avoidance abilities of the old significantly more than it did in the young (corresponding to a shift of our curve to the right). Lajoie showed that elderly subjects adopt a slower speed than young persons, with a shorter stride length in order to produce a more secure gait (also confirming a decrease in the optimum performance) and that, even so, they responded to the probe RT task with greater delays than young adults (15). Their conclusion was that normal aging requires that a greater proportion of attentional resources be allocated to walking and postural task demands (corresponding to an attenuation of our bell-shaped curve for high level of attention). Comparing 19 elderly subjects to 19 young controls, Maylor and Wing observed that age differences in postural stability were increased by concomitant cognitive tasks requiring use of the visuospatial sketchpad component of working memory (17).

We can therefore figure that the optimum is shifted to the right in elderly subject, that is, elderly subjects require more attention to reach the optimum level of motor performance. Furthermore, the overall motor performance

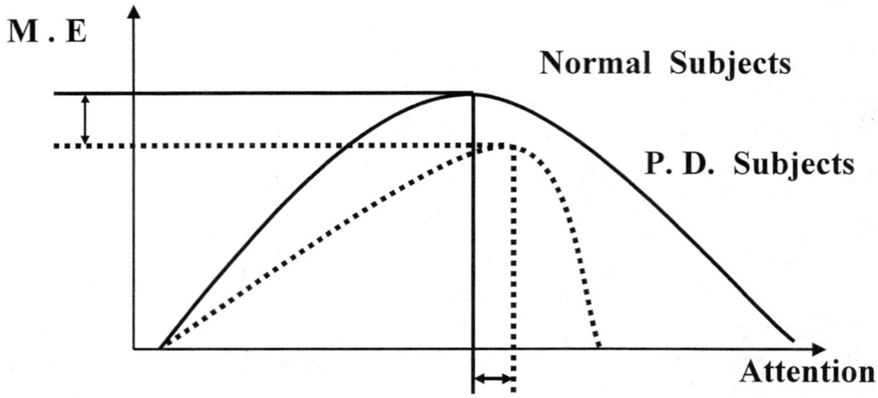

FIG. 24.3. Imbalance between attention and motor execution (*M.E*) for the normal population and elderly subjects. *P.D.,* Parkinson's disease. *Solid lines* represent the relationship between attention and ME in normal subjects. *Dotted lines* indicate that, in patients with PD, a poorer performance is obtained for higher attention levels.

decreases. Finally, there is an attenuation of the curve for a very high level of attention; thus, the attentional cost for walking is higher than in young subjects (Fig. 24.3).

Gait disorders observed in PD can also fit into our theoretical model to some extent. Walking is known to be impaired in PD (18–22). One study has shown that patients with PD (when "off") walk more slowly with shorter strides and a longer duration of stance and double-support phase (corresponding to a lower level of performance on our curve) (23). However, intentional modulations remain possible. When the patients were asked to walk as quickly as possible to a goal, they increased their velocity by about 50% (from 0.4 to 0.6 m/sec). This suggests that the Neutral point is at the left of the optimum because the ability to generate a normal stepping pattern is not lost in PD. Gait hypokinesia could reflect a difficulty in activating the locomotor control system in this population. However, the improvement was smaller in patients with PD than in controls, suggesting that optimal motivation and attention do not allow them to reach the same improvement (corresponding to a shift to the right of the optimum point of our curve). Patients with PD also never reach the control walking velocity, suggesting that attentional and motivational processes do not completely reverse their deficit.

Generally speaking, simultaneous cognitive task performance, as well as simultaneous motor acts are impaired in PD. Malapani et al. showed that "off" patients had normal performance in separate auditory and visual choice RT tasks, but demonstrated significant deficit when performing simultaneous and concurrent choice RT tasks (24). Thus, patients with PD are impaired in their ability to process simultaneous cognitive information. Furthermore, they tend to neglect the auditory modality in the dual task, suggesting a priority of visual over nonvisual signals for this population. Camicioli also demonstrated that verbal fluency task affects the gait of freezing patients and that patients increase the number of steps required to complete the walk (25). This author concluded that this pathology is characterized by a greater dependence on attention for walking and that this result is linked to the degree of severity of the disease. Behrman and colleagues showed that patients improve and tend to normalize their gait parameters according to the stimulation and degree of attention (26). The instructional set can aid in the normalization of parkinsonian gait, although its benefits may depend on the stage of disease progression and the difficulty of and the degree of attention to instructions. These results tend to confirm the importance of stimulation and drive on motor activity. An increase in stimuli can involve a better driving answer, but performance decreases beyond the threshold (Fig. 24.4).

Morris showed, in a study of 27 PD patients and 27 age-controlled subjects, that attentional

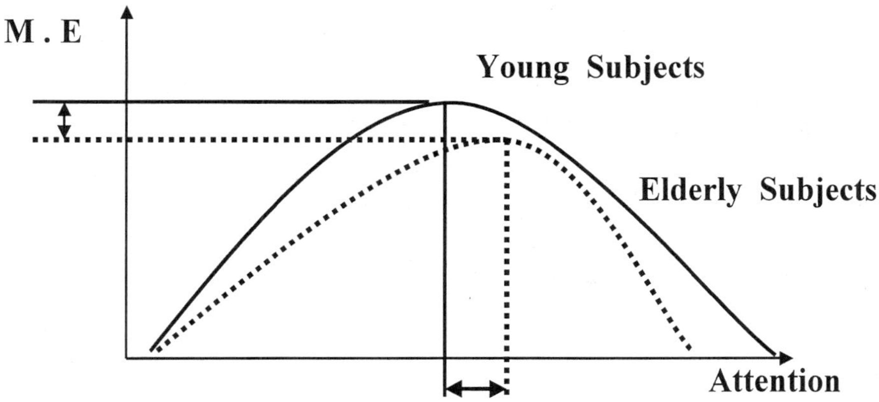

FIG. 24.4. Imbalance between attention and motor execution (*M.E*) for the normal population and parkinsonian subjects. *Solid lines* represent the relationship between ME and attention for young subjects. *Dotted lines* indicate that, in elderly subjects, a higher level of attention is required to achieve a poorer motor response.

strategies and visual cues result in normal stride length in patients with PD (27). (In the condition used in this experiment, they used visual floor markers at a distance equivalent of the mean stride length of each PD subject's matched control or a mental picture of the appropriate stride length.) The normal movement size could be achieved in patients with PD given the appropriate condition, for example, when provided visual cues (27). Therefore, one hypothesis postulates that visual stimulation acts as an attentional stimulus. In accord with this hypothesis, Martin (18) asked his patients to reach a ball on the floor, whereas Forssber et al. report the case of a patient with PD who dropped small paper balls to start walking (28). Bagley et al. showed that small obstacles on the walkway could stimulate the walking pattern (29). The authors noted the stimulating effect of the obstacles when they were removed, suggesting that they were acting as attentional stimuli.

Moreover, Morris et al. showed a very similar pattern of deterioration in gait parameters that was graded according to the level of attention required for the secondary task performance (visual cues recognition and attentional strategy task) (27). It seems plausible that use of a secondary task removes attentional mechanisms from the most automatic movement (e.g., gait) and directs them to the attention-requiring (e.g., cognitive) task. This may explain the decrease of temporal and spatial gait parameters for the experimental double-task situation.

We suggest that there is a decrease in optimum performance in PD that is not reversed by attention. The Neutral point remains to the left of the optimum. Training strategies, verbal instructions, and cues can improve walking in patients with PD; however, the optimum might be to the right of controls—patients might need greater attention to achieve the same level of performance. Moreover, the slope of the bell-shaped curve is very stiff. When increasing stimulation beyond the optimum point, subjects with PD demonstrate a rapid degradation in their performance. In other words, as soon as the attentional demand increases, the walking performance decreases. This might be owing to the difficulty in apprehending excessive information and can lead to motor blockades.

We summarize the different hypothetical curves obtained by young and elderly normal subjects and patients with PD in Figure 24.5.

ROLE OF SENSORY INPUTS ON GAIT

We also added sensory inputs to our theoretical model. Motor activity, upright standing, and walking—the most common motor tasks—require the integration of several sources of

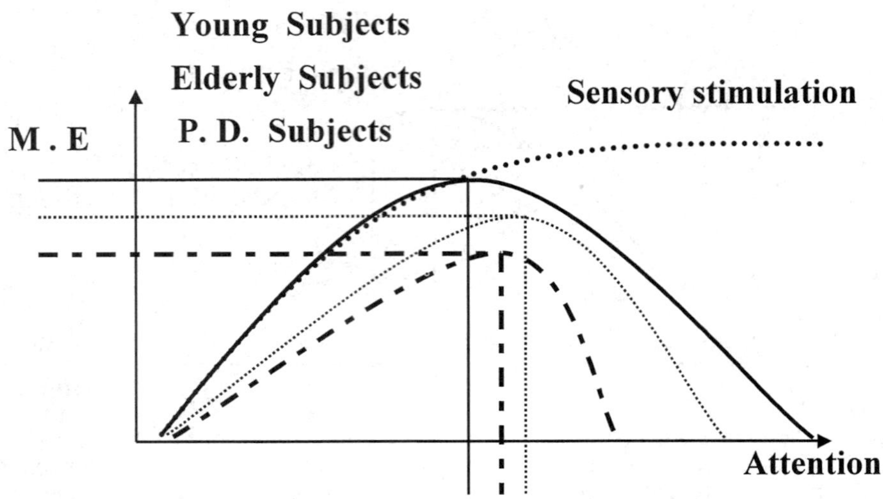

FIG. 24.5. Imbalance between attention and motor execution (*M.E*) for the different populations. *P.D.,* Parkinson's disease. *Solid lines* represent young subjects, *dashed lines* represent elderly subjects, and *squared lines* represent subjects with PD.

sensory information. In a normal and highly predictable environment, locomotor synergies involving several muscles may take place at lower spinal levels. However, when ongoing regulation of motor activity is necessary, supraspinal involvement is required to perform movement adapted to the environment. In this case, driving and sensory data processing must be carried out simultaneously. This operation requires an obligatory attentional demand. This attentional demand is clearly evaluated by the classic dual-task methodology.

Sensory stimulation (visual, auditory, and proprioceptive) can be progressively increased up to a plateau (Fig. 24.5). Perception of sensory stimuli decreases with age and/or in some pathologic conditions; however, it might be compensated for by increased attention and/or stimulation. Focusing on patients with PD, there is a clear decrease in sensory inputs. We previously showed a defect in the visual perception of contrasts and especially of movement sensitivity; abnormalities of auditory evoked potentials have been reported, and proprioceptive perception also might have been impaired (30,31). Therefore, there is a deficit in the sensory stimuli available for motor control and execution (corresponding on our curve to a difference between normal and PD curves). In the literature, some references tried to show the sensory stimulation effects on motor behavior.

Auditory Stimulation

Nagasaki et al. studied 1,134 elderly adults (32). They were asked to fingertap in time to the sound of a 4-Hz metronome. Hastening tapping or finger festination occurred in 17% of subjects (30% of patients in their eighties) and was accompanied by an increased step rate. Ebersbach et al. also have shown that performing fast fingertapping during walking led to an increase in step rate in 10 normal elderly subjects (1).

Rhythmic auditory stimulation has been shown to induce sensorimotor facilitation in patients with PD (e.g., an increase in gait spatiotemporal parameters such as cadence, stride length, and symmetry in gait patterns). However, rhythmic auditory stimulation training improves gait parameters in patients with PD after only 3 weeks of training (33). In a recent study of patients with PD and control subjects, Ebersbach et al. showed that they were equally able to adapt their cadence to an external stimulus (16). This is in accordance with the observation of Morris et al., who showed that patients with PD can entrain their stepping rate to that of control subjects when provided with a metronome signal (34).

Proprioceptive Stimulation

Personal clinical observation of a patient with PD, who put a ring around each ankle to improve his gait and elicit stepping when he experienced motor blocks, suggests that proprioceptive stimulation is a sensorimotor-based technique that is clinically useful for gait facilitation.

Burleigh-Jacobs et al., in studying anticipatory postural adjustments associated with step initiation, showed that normal subjects increased force and velocity of movement when an external cutaneous stimulus was used as a GO (start) signal (35). They also showed that an external stimulus (cutaneous cue-triggered step) improves the deficient force production, timing, and velocity of movement in patients with PD. They observed that both patients with PD and normal subjects execute the anticipatory postural adjustments for step rapidly, when voluntarily initiating step in response to a small backward surface translation, which produces a slight forward sway of the body and then promotes a more forceful and longer step; however, patients with PD failed to increase force in order to execute push-off more rapidly. The findings also suggested that force production during the postural adjustment phase of self-generated, but not externally triggered, step initiation is influenced by dopaminergic pathways. This was consistent with the fact that movements driven by external stimuli employ different pathways from those driven by internal decisions (36,37).

Visual Stimulation

Visual stimuli can improve the gait in patients with PD. For example, Martin used stripes on the walkway and assessed that only the parallel transversal stripes, separated by 18 inches (44.1 cm) were able to improve parkinsonian gait (18). On the other hand, diagonal, longitudinal, or other transverse lines did not improve parkinsonian gait. Later, other authors found the same results with a width of 30 cm (38–40).

A recent study addressed the effect on gait of placing parallel lines on the walking surface in patients with PD and controls in two visual conditions [normal lighting and stroboscopic lighting (3 Hz)] (41). Whereas with normal light, the subjects could use both static and dynamic visual information, stroboscopic light was used to suppress dynamic visual cues and retain position visual abilities only. The authors did not observe any significant changes in gait parameters when 16 control elderly subjects were asked to walk on stripes or with stroboscopic illumination. However, it should be noticed that Prokop et al. observed that optic flow modulates walking velocity in normal subjects (42). Visual cues from the lines on the walking surface induced significant improvement in gait velocity and stride length in patients with PD under normal lighting. With stroboscopic illumination and without lines, patients with PD demonstrated a decrease in stride length and velocity, whereas the controls indicated a greater dependence on dynamic visual information. When stroboscopic light was used with stripes on the floor, the improvement in gait caused by the stripes was suppressed in patients with PD. These results indicate that the perceived motion of stripes induced by a patient's walking is essential to improve gait parameters (and thus favors the hypothesis of a specific visual-motor pathway). However, excessive visual sensory stimulation can lead to motor blockades. It can occur in patients with PD, for example, when passing a door. This could explain the increase in sensory stimulation on our curve, which corresponds to a decrease in motor performance. Consequently, when patients with PD are confronted with external cues (e.g., visual stimuli), their ability to cope with stimulation is more easily overloaded than in normal subjects.

Motor activity is the result of a constant interaction between sensory stimulation and attentional demand. The imbalance between these two components plays an essential role on action. All experimental study designs, interpretation of results, or rehabilitation processes should take into account the relative weight of each of these factors.

REFERENCES

1. Ebersbach G, Dimitrijevic MR, Poewe W. Influence of concurrent tasks on gait: a dual-task approach. *Percept Mot Skills* 1995;81:107–113.
2. Chen H-C, Schultz AB, Ashton-Miller JA, et al. Stepping over obstacles: dividing attention impairs performance of old more than young adults. *J Gerontol A Biol Sci Med Sci* 1996;51A:M116–M122.

3. Taylor RA, Marshall PH, Dunlap RD, et al. Knee position error detection in closed and open kinetic chain tasks during concurrent cognitive distraction. *J Orthop Sports Phys Ther* 1998;28:81–87.
4. Mountcastle VB, Anderson RA, Motter BC. The influence of attentive fixation upon the excitability of the light-sensitive neurons of the posterior parietal cortex. *J Neurosci* 1981;1:1218–1235.
5. Wurtz RH, Goldberg ME, Robinson DL. Brain mechanisms of visual attention. *Sci Am* 1982;246:124–135.
6. Maylor EA, Hockey R. Inhibitory components of externally controlled covert orienting in visual space. *J Exp Psychol Hum Percept Perform* 1985;11:777–787.
7. Fisher B. The role of attention in the preparation of visually guided eye movements in monkey and man. *Psychol Res* 1986;48 251–257.
8. Fisher B, Breitmeyer B. Express saccades and visual attention revealed by saccadic eye movement. *Neuropsychologia* 1986;25 73–83.
9. Rizzolatti G, Riggio L, Dascola I, et al. Re-orienting attention across the horizontal and vertical meridians. *Neuropsychologia* 1987;25:31–40.
10. Grossberg S. How does the cerebral cortex work? Learning, attention, and grouping by the laminar circuits of visual cortex. *Spat Vis* 1999;12:163–185.
11. Grossberg S, Mingolla E, Ross WD. A neural theory of attentive visual search: interactions of boundary, surface, spatial, and object representations. *Psychol Rev* 1994;101:470–489.
12. Grossberg S. Cortical dynamics of three-dimensional form, color, and brightness perception I: monocular theory. *Percept Psychophys* 1987;41:97–116.
13. Grossberg S, Mingolla E, Todorovi D. A neural network architecture for preattentive vision. *IEEE Trans Biomed Eng* 1989;36:65–84.
14. Kurosawa K. Effects of various walking speeds on probe reaction time during treadmill walking. *Percept Mot Skills* 1994;78:768–770.
15. Lajoie Y, Teasdale N, Bard C, et al. Attentional demands for static and dynamic equilibrium. *Exp Brain Res* 1993;97:139–144.
16. Ebersbach G, Heijmenberg M, Kindermann L, et al. Interference of rhythmic constraint on gait in healthy subjects and patients with early Parkinson's disease: evidence for impared locomotor pattern generation in early Parkinson's disease. *Mov Disord* 1999;14:619–625.
17. Maylor EA, Wing AM. Age differences in postural stability are increased by additional cognitive demands. *J Gerontol* 1996;51B:143–154.
18. Martin JP, Locomotion and basal ganglia. In: Martin JP, ed. *The basal ganglia and posture.* London: Pittman, 1967:20–35.
19. Knutsson E, Mårtenson A. Quantitative effects of L-DOPA on different types of movements and muscle tone in parkinsonian patients. *Scand J Rehabil Med* 1971;3:121–130.
20. Knutsson E. An analysis of Parkinsonian gait. *Brain* 1972;95:475–486.
21. Murray MP, Sepic SB, Gardner GM, et al. Walking patterns of men with Parkinsonism. *Am J Phys Med Rehabil* 1978;57:278–294.
22. Blin O, Ferrandez A-M, Serratrice G. Quantitative analysis of gait in Parkinson patients: increased variability of stride length. *J Neurol Sci* 1990;98:91–97.
23. Ferrandez A-M, Blin O. A comparison between the effect of intentional modulations and the action of L-DOPA on gait in Parkinson's disease. *Behav Brain Res* 1991;45:177–183.
24. Malapani C, Pillon B, Dubois B, et al. Impaired simultaneous cognitive task performance in Parkinson's disease: a dopamine-related dysfunction. *Neurology* 1994;44:319–326.
25. Camicioli R, Oken BS, Sexton G, et al. Verbal fluency task affects gait in Parkinson's disease with motor freezing. *J Geriatr Psychiatry Neurol* 1998;11:181–185.
26. Behrman AL, Teitelbaum P, Cauraugh JH. Verbal instructional sets to normalise the temporal and spatial gait variables in Parkinson's disease. *J Neurol Neurosurg Psychiatry* 1998;65:580–582.
27. Morris ME, Iansek R, Matyas TA, et al. Stride length regulation in Parkinson's disease. Normalization strategies and underlying mechanisms. *Brain* 1996;119:551–568.
28. Forssberg H, Johnels B, Steg G. Is parkinsonian gait caused by a regression to an immature walking pattern? *Adv Neurol* 1984;40:375–379.
29. Bagley S, Kelly B, Tunnicliffe N, et al. The effect of visual cues on the gait of independently mobile Parkinson's disease patients. *Physiotherapy* 1991;77:415–420.
30. Mestre D, Blin O, Serratrice G, et al. Spatiotemporal contrast sensitivity differs in human aging and Parkinson's disease. *Neurology* 1990;40:1710–1714.
31. Fradis M, Samet A, Ben-David J, et al. Brainstem auditory evoked potentials to different stimulus rates in parkinsonian patients. *Eur Neurol* 1988;28:181–186.
32. Nagasaki H, Itoh H, Hashizume K, et al. Walking patterns and finger rhythm of older adults. *Percept Mot Skills* 1996;82:435–447.
33. Thaut MH, McIntosh GC, Rice RR, et al. Rhythmic auditory stimulation in gait training for Parkinson's disease patients. *Mov Disord* 1996;11:193–200.
34. Morris ME, Iansek R, Matyas TA, et al. Ability to modulate walking cadence remains intact in Parkinson's disease. *J Neurol Neurosurg Psychiatry* 1994;57:1532–1534.
35. Burleigh-Jacobs A, Horak FB, Nutt JG, et al. Step initiation in Parkinson's disease: influence of levodopa and external sensory triggers. *Mov Disord* 1997;12:206–215.
36. Goldberg G. Supplementary motor area: structure and function: review and hypotheses. *Behav Brain Sci* 1985;8:567–615.
37. Passingham RE, Chen YC, Thaler D. Supplementary motor cortex and self-initiated movement. In: Ito M, ed. *Neural programming.* Basel: Karger 1989:13–24.
38. Dietz MA, Goetz CG, Stebbins GT. Evaluation of a modified inverted walking stick as a treatment for parkinsonian freezing episodes. *Mov Disord* 1990;5:243–247.
39. Glickstein M, Stein J. Paradoxical movement in Parkinson's disease. *Trends Neurosci* 1991;14:480–482.
40. Azulay J-P, van den Brand CL, Mestre D, et al. *Analyse cinématique de la marche du Parkinsonien: effets de la lévodopa et de stimulation visuelles. Rev Neurol (Paris)* 1996;152:128–134.
41. Azulay J-P, Mesure S, Amblard B, et al. Visual control of locomotion in Parkinson's disease. *Brain* 1999;122:111–120.
42. Prokop T, Schubert M, Berger M. Visual influence on human locomotion. Modulation to changes in optic flow. *Exp Brain Res* 1997;114:63–70.

Gait Disorders. Advances in Neurology, Vol. 87,
edited by E. Růžička, M. Hallett, and J. Jankovic.
Lippincott Williams & Wilkins, Philadelphia © 2001.

25
Psychogenic Gait Disorders

Kailash P. Bhatia

University Department of Clinical Neurology, Institute of Neurology and National Hospital for Neurology, London WC1N 3BG, United Kingdom

Psychogenic movement disorders fall in a domain between neurology and psychiatry, and these patients often pose a discomforting challenge for the neurologist. An abnormal gait may be the presenting or even the sole manifestation of a psychogenic disorder. On the other hand, when faced with a diagnostic dilemma, the recognition of the abnormal gait as "psychogenic" among a multitude of clinical features may clarify the situation and provide a *diagnostic epiphany,* as Keane pointed out in his 1989 review of the subject (1).

There was considerable interest in psychogenic (or "hysterical" as they were called) gait disorders around the turn of the last century. The French school headed by Charcot was particularly interested in classifying these disorders (Table 25.1) (2,3). New terms such as "astasia–abasia" appeared in the medical literature. This paradoxical ability to use the legs normally except when standing (astasia) or walking (abasia) was described by Jaccoud in 1860 (4). Gait disorders such as *camptocormia,* or the bent back syndrome, almost assumed epidemic proportions in the World War I armed forces. Typically, a soldier would develop a forward stooped posture and an unusual gait (or inability to walk), usually after a spell of heavy shelling, and would have to be removed from the frontlines (5). Investigations were normal and typically after a few weeks in a hospital (away from the front) he would recover without any specific treatment, suggesting the psychological nature of the condition (6). Although psychogenic gait disorders are not uncommon (see the following), there has been scant literature about this in recent times. The focus of this chapter is on the clinical aspects and phenomenology of psychogenic gaits, which may help with its diagnosis.

FREQUENCY OF THE PROBLEM

In 1986, Marsden estimated that psychogenic (hysterical) disorders comprised 1% of all UK hospital admissions (7). This may well be an underestimate. Factor et al. reported in 1995 that 28 (3.3%) of their movement disorder patients out of 842 had a psychogenic condition (8). This figure is similar to that estimated by Fahn in their population of 3,700 movement disorder patients, of whom 2.1% were believed to have a psychogenic condition (9). Of these, psychogenic gait disorders accounted for 9% of all psychogenic movement disorders (9). However, in one report, 26% (60 of 228) of all patients admitted to a neurologic service with "functional neurological disorders" over a 10-year period had a hysterical gait disorder (1). Hysterical gait disorders also accounted for 1.5% (68 of 4,470) of neurologic admissions to the Munich University Clinic, over a 3-year period (10); thus, psychogenic gait disorders appear to be common.

CLINICAL ASPECTS AND PHENOMENOLOGY

It is necessary for the clinician to glean clues from the history and clinical phenomenology as

TABLE 25.1. *French school classification of hysterical gait disorders*

Charcot and Tourette	Roussy and Lhermitte
Astasia-abasia	Astasia–abasia
Paralysis	Pseudotabetic
Choreiform	Pseudopolyneurotic
Trepidant	Tightrope walker
	Robot
	Limping
	Choreic
	As on sticky surface

From Keane JR. Hysterical gait disorders: 60 cases. *Neurology* 1989;39:586–589, with permission.

well as any other associated features that may be present in order to arrive at the diagnosis of psychogenic gait disorder.

Clues from the History

An abrupt onset of a gait disorder is unusual and may suggest a psychogenic cause. Vascular or demyelinative disorders can be fairly acute but appropriate physical signs would be present in such cases. Variability of the gait with periods of normality should also arouse suspicion. Possible secondary gain, for example, pending litigation relating to accidental trauma could be a factor. Past history should be investigation, particularly multiple previous medical consultations, and investigations may suggest a somatization disorder or Briquet's syndrome. Lastly, a sudden resolution of the problem almost always suggests a psychogenic disorder.

Clues by Clinical Phenomenology

The clinical phenomenology suggestive of a psychogenic gait is remarkably similar in the different reviews of large series of patients with psychogenic gaits disorders (1,10,11). Keane reported 60 patients with hysterical gait disorders seen over a 10-year period. There were 37 women and 23 men (1.6:1). The female-to-male preponderance has been noted in other studies and is generally true of psychogenic disorders overall (9). However, in a recent study of nonorganic motor disorders Crimlisk et al. found an almost equal male-to-female ratio (12). Interestingly, in this study, subjects with negative motor symptoms [e.g., unexplained (nonorganic) hemiplegia or paraplegia] were more likely to be men, whereas women more commonly had positive motor symptoms such as tremor or dystonia (12). The mean age of presentation of patients with psychogenic gait was 36.3 years in the study by Keane with a range from 19 to 80 years (1). Psychogenic disorders are rare in very young children and very elderly adults (13).

Some patients present with a very bizarre gait that does not resemble that seen in any neurologic condition and can be recognized quite easily as psychogenic in character. Quite often, however, the gait resembles that caused by an organic neurologic condition. In the series of 60 patients reported by Keane, the most common psychogenic gaits seen (some patients had more than one type of gait disturbance) were most commonly ataxic (38%), followed by hemiparetic (20%), paraparetic (16%), and trembling (14%). Others have noted similar presentations (11). Why these presentations are psychogenic is usually suggested by the absence of other relevant signs, as pointed out by Hayes et al. (11). Examples include the absence of hyper-reflexia or weakness in the hemiparetic gait; rigidity or bradykinesia in the parkinsonian gait; nystagmus, dysarthria, and intention tremor in the ataxic gait; and so on (11). On the other hand, giveway weakness and sensory loss in a nonanatomic pattern can also occur in these patients (11). It is this discrepancy in the signs that makes the diagnosis of a psychogenic gait disorder likely.

In another series of psychogenic gait disturbances, 37 patients seen at the Munich University Clinic over 9 years (1980 to 1989), were video analyzed (22 prospectively and 15 retrospectively) for the purposes of establishing diagnostic criteria and to determine if a diagnosis of psychogenic gait disturbance was possible on phenomenologic grounds alone (10). In this series, the features that are characteristic of psychogenic gaits included: (a) hesitation (16.2%), (b) excessive slowness of movements (35%), (c) fluctuations in the gait impairment with "uneconomic" postures and wasting of muscle energy (51%), (d) a trepidant "walking on ice" gait (30%), and (e) a "psychogenic Romberg" test

(32%). The authors suggested that a diagnosis of a psychogenic gait disturbance could be made on phenomenologic grounds alone with over 90% certainty if one or more of these features were present (10). Other features included sudden knee buckling (27%); however, over 80% of patients did not fall despite this feature. Eleven percent of patients had astasia and vertical shaking tremor was present in 8% of cases. A suffering or strained facial expression was seen in 19 patients, associated in all with moaning, mannered posturing of hands, and grasping of the leg along with hyperventilation (10). Hayes et al. also remarked on the exaggerated effort, fatigue, or pronounced slowness of movements (11). Slowness is accentuated by novel tasks such as walking backward or tandem gait. Repetitive finger and foot taps also may be performed slowly, but muscle tone and stride length can be normal, unlike parkinsonism (11).

CLUES BY ASSOCIATED FEATURES

In our own experience and from reported series, the presence of other incongruent features may point to a diagnosis of a psychogenic disorder. Keane found that 43% of patients (26 of 60) had associated hysterical eye findings, including 13 with visual field cuts, six with decreased visual acuity, four with eye movement limitation, and three with monocular diplopia. Other "false" neurologic signs were present in 71% of patients (43 of 60); including unusual motor weakness, voice abnormalities, odd tremor, and abnormal finger-to-nose testing where three patients had either finger-to-eye or finger-to-cheek alterations. Other odd associated features present in 23 of 60 patients included a scissoring gait, knees giving way with quick recovery, posturing of an "arm-above-head" while walking, and ataxic (tandem) gaits that blended into trembling (10). Hayes et al. refer to this sort of trembling as "convulsive shaking" and have suggested that this is a strong indicator of a psychogenic disorder (11). Lempert et al. also noted very similar associated "hysterical" findings (10). The most common abnormalities included other motor disturbances in 53 (45%), which often added to the gait disorder. These included hemiparesis (23%), quadriparesis (13%), scissoring (9%), knee give-way with recovery (9%), assuming a tandem gait (9%), dragging a leg (7.5%), paraparesis (7.5%), and flailing of the arms (5%). Other associated findings included, bizarre tremors (12%), pseudoataxia (8%), and voice abnormalities (7%). Another associated feature that may be present in nonorganic disorders is the incongruous affect of the patient. The patient appears to be rather unconcerned (surprisingly) despite marked disability.

DIFFERENTIAL DIAGNOSIS

A bizarre gait may not necessarily be of psychogenic origin. Certain neurologic conditions can present with unusual gaits, including Huntington's disease and other forms of chorea. Additional clues should be evident by history or examination. Drug-induced movement disorders (e.g., tardive dystonia affecting the axial musculature) can look extremely odd. A good history of previous drugs is very important. Finally, rare disorders that the clinician may not have previously encountered (e.g., propriospinal myoclonus) often are called psychogenic. In this author's experience, patients with rare paroxysmal movement disorders may be initially misdiagnosed as hysterical because of the brevity of the episodes, and the fact that they are normal between attacks (14). Last, it should be kept in mind that the patient may have an underlying organic condition in addition to the nonorganic problem.

Management and Psychiatric Aspects

Fahn and Williams have noted that the definite diagnosis of a psychogenic disorder is made clear when psychotherapy, psychologic suggestion, or placebo achieve relief (15). Only a probable or possible diagnosis can be made in many instances (15). Obviously, the patient has to be thoroughly investigated to rule out an organic cause. Psychiatric consultation is important to reveal occult psychopathology; however, the diagnosis of a psychogenic disorder has to be made by the neurologist. Somatoform (conversion reaction) and factitious disorders are the most common psychiatric conditions in these patients;

malingering is less common. Close liaison with the psychiatrist and neurologist is important. Treatment, like in any other psychogenic condition, may require a combination of physiotherapy, psychotherapy, behavioral therapy, suggestion, and rarely psychopharmacology (16).

Outcome

In two influential reports in 1965, Slater drew attention to a group of patients whose initial symptoms were diagnosed to be psychogenic and subsequently over half of them were found to have developed major physical or psychiatric disease over time (17,18). These papers undoubtedly made clinicians (at least in the United Kingdom) somewhat wary of making a diagnosis of a nonorganic or conversion reaction (7). Thirty years later, there have been few recent studies with long-term follow-up of patients diagnosed with nonorganic disorders (12,19,20). The results suggest that and in this era of modern imaging there is a low incidence of a new physical or psychiatric diagnosis that could explain the patients' initial symptoms or signs deemed nonorganic or psychogenic (12,19). A new neurologic diagnosis was present only in three of 64 patients who were followed up (12). Nearly half of the patients in this study had a gait disorder (personal experience) (12). Overall long-term outcome in these patients was poor with regard the initial motor symptoms. Only 28% had resolution of their initial symptom, whereas there was improvement in 20%. However, 52% were either unchanged or worse. Factors associated with a good outcome were short length of initial symptoms (less than a year), comorbid psychiatric disorder, and interestingly, a change in marital status during follow-up (12).

CONCLUSION

Psychogenic gait disorders are common and may cause marked disability. Clues in the history, typical clinical phenomenology, as well as notable incongruity and absence of certain relevant signs may help make the diagnosis and avoid unnecessary investigations and treatments. Organic conditions may coexist. It is important to have close liaison with a psychiatrist for diagnosis and management of these patients, which can be difficult.

REFERENCES

1. Keane JR. Hysterical gait disorders: 60 cases. *Neurology* 1989;39:586–589.
2. Havens LL. Charcot and hysteria. *J Nerv Ment Dis* 1966;141:505–516.
3. Roussy G, Lhermitte J. The psychoneurosis of war. In: *Neurosis.* New York: D Appleton & Co., 1918:718–906.
4. Pasteur W. Thyssen on astasia-abasia *(Arch de Neurologie, t21).* Abstracts of British and foreign journals. *Brain* 1891;14:557–567.
5. Southhard EE. *Shell-shock and other neuropsychiatric problems.* Boston: WM Leonard, 1919.
6. Gavin H. *On feigned and factitious diseases, chiefly of soldiers and sailors, on the means used to simulate and produce them, and on the best modes of discovering imposters.* London: Churchill Livingstone, 1843.
7. Marsden CD. Hysteria: a neurologist's view. *Psychol Med* 1986;16:277–288.
8. Factor SA, Podskalny GD, Molho ES. Psychogenic movement disorders: frequency, clinical profile and characteristics. *J Neurol Neurosurg Psychiatry* 1995;59:406–412.
9. Fahn S. Psychogenic movement disorders. In: Marsden CD, Fahn S, eds. *Movement disorders 3.* Oxford: Butterworth Heinemann 1994:359–372.
10. Lempert T, Brandt T, Dieterich M, et al. How to identify psychogenic disorders of stance and gait. A video study in 37 patients. *J Neurol* 1991;238:140–146.
11. Hayes MW, Graham S, Heldorf P, et al. A video review of the diagnosis of psychogenic gait: appendix and commentary. *Mov Disord* 1999;14:914–921.
12. Crimlisk HL, Bhatia K, Cope H, et al. Slater revisited: 6 year follow up study of patients with medically unexplained motor symptoms. *Br Med J* 1998;316:52–56.
13. Thompson APJ, Sills JA. Diagnosis of functional illness presenting with a gait disorder. *Arch Dis Child* 1988;63:148–153.
14. Bhatia KP. The paroxysmal dyskinesias. *J Neurol* 1999;246:149–155.
15. Fahn S, Williams DT. Psychogenic dystonia. *Adv Neurol* 1988;50:431–455.
16. Ford B, Williams DT, Fahn S. Treatment of psychogenic movement disorders. In: Kurlan R, ed. *Treatment of movement disorders.* Philadelphia: J.B. Lippincott, 1995:475–485.
17. Slater E. Diagnosis of hysteria. *Br Med J* 1965;1:1395–1399.
18. Slater E, Glithero E. A follow up of patients diagnosed as suffering from hysteria. *J Psychosom Res* 1965;9:9–13.
19. Couprie W, Wijdicks EFM, Rooijmans HGM, et al. Outcome in conversion disorder: a follow up study. *J Neurol Neurosurg Psychiatry* 1995;58:750–752.
20. Mace CJ, Trimble MR. Ten year prognosis of conversion disorder. *Br J Psychiatry* 1996;169:282–288.

Gait Disorders. Advances in Neurology, Vol. 87,
edited by E. Růžička, M. Hallett, and J. Jankovic.
Lippincott Williams & Wilkins, Philadelphia © 2001.

26

The Pharmacologic Treatment of Gait Ignition Failure

[*‡]Olivier Rascol, [†§]Nelly Fabre, [*¶]Christine Brefel-Courbon, and [*¶]Jean-Louis Montastruc

Departments of [*]Clinical Pharmacology and [†]Neurology, Toulouse University, 31073 Toulouse, France; and [‡]Clinical Investigation Center and Departments of [§]Neurology and [¶]Pharmacology, Toulouse University Hospital, 31059 Toulouse, France

Gait ignition failure (GIF), also called "freezing when walking" or "frozen gait," where the foot feels "stuck" to the ground, is a well-described phenomenon seen when a patient initiates walking (1). Freezing is also common when a patient encounters a visible obstacle or turns. Gait ignition failure, which is commonly experienced by subjects suffering from idiopathic Parkinson's disease (IPD) and related disorders, remains a significant clinical problem for both patients and physicians because it includes a substantial risk of falls and it responds only partially and variably to currently available treatments.

The pharmacologic treatment of GIF is disappointing for several reasons. First, there is no current definite reliable scientific background to support a specific pharmacologic strategy. Gait ignition failure remains poorly understood. There are no reliable available specific animal models. Gait ignition failure is a symptom rather than a disease. It is common in IPD, but also in "Parkinson-plus" syndromes [e.g., progressive supranuclear palsy (PSP) and multiple system atrophy]; in many symptomatic parkinsonisms such as MPTP-induced, postencephalitic, or vascular parkinsonism; and in posthypoxic pallidal lesions or normal pressure hydrocephalus (2). Presently it is impossible to establish if the mechanisms leading to GIF in such different conditions share similar causes or are related to different contributing factors, which adds to the confusion in our understanding of this symptom.

Second, most published clinical trials designed to assess the response of GIF to various treatments suffer from methodologic shortcomings that markedly reduce the impact of their conclusions: lack of a validated method of assessment; insufficient numbers of patients; heterogeneous etiologic diagnoses; and lack of randomization and placebo control. Gait ignition failure is highly variable and unpredictable, and is influenced by a number of external (sensorial, psychological) factors that are extremely difficult to control in clinical situations.

GAIT IGNITION FAILURE AND DOPAMINERGIC MEDICATIONS

It is not surprising that the effects of most dopamine antiparkinsonian medications have been tested on frozen gait because GIF is frequently observed in patients suffering from IPD. The conclusions of these studies are rather contradictory.

On one hand, there are a number of clinical observations that suggest that GIF is, at least partly, related to the central deficit of dopamine pathways, and thus should be L-Dopa–responsive:

(a) GIF is observed in patients with IPD and MPTP-induced parkinsonism, (b) GIF can occur in IPD when L-Dopa is temporarily ineffective (so-called motor fluctuations or "offs"), in which case GIF is also often called "off-freezing," (c) GIF, and especially "off-freezing," can be relieved by dopaminergic treatments (3–6).

On the other hand, the following observations suggest that GIF is not necessarily directly linked to the central dopaminergic deficit:

1. Gait ignition failure is observed in diseases that do not involve dopamine systems (e.g., normal pressure hydrocephalus), and that are known to be resistant to L-Dopa therapy [e.g., corticobasal degeneration, multisystem atrophy, vascular parkinsonism, PSP, and "almost pure" freezing (also known as "pure akinesia," "gait ignition failure," or "primary progressive freezing gait")] (7–11).
2. Blocking the dopamine system at the receptor site does not appear to be enough to cause freezing episodes because there is a significantly low association between freezing and drug-induced parkinsonism (12).
3. Gait ignition failure is not an early feature of PD, but rather occurs later in the illness. Therefore it is significantly associated with a longer disease duration and higher Hoehn and Yahr stage, whereas such an association in advanced PD might be the result of pathology in nondopaminergic pathways (3,13).
4. Finally, GIF can appear in IPD during the "on" phase, called "on-freezing," at the time L-Dopa is effective; therefore, it will not respond to dopaminergic treatments, but can be made worse while increasing doses of L-Dopa (see the following).

Off-Freezing Response to Dopamine Medications in Idiopathic Parkinson's Disease

L-Dopa therapy often can be beneficial in IPD, when GIF is caused by the disease ("off-freezing") (2). This assumption is supported by a number of observations with a variety of dopaminergic medications.

L-Dopa

Quinn and colleagues described the case of a patient with typical L-Dopa-responsive "pure akinesia" and freezing of gait, whose brain showed the classical changes of Lewy body PD at postmortem examination (14). In this patient, frozen gait was clearly linked with "off" periods. It was improved by dopamine medications, disappearing during "on" periods, and there is no doubt about the dopa-responsiveness of GIF in this case.

Burleigh-Jacobs and colleagues studied the anticipatory postural adjustments contributing to gait initiation deficit in IPD subjects, before and after L-Dopa (15). They observed that L-Dopa improved the deficient force production for such anticipatory postural adjustments, suggesting that L-Dopa can improve this early component of gait. However, this deficient force production during self-generated step initiation is not sufficient to explain the phenomenon of freezing: although the subjects of this study were selected because of problems with freezing, GIF was seldom observed during the protocol. Only two of six subjects were unable to self-generate a step during two trials. In these trials, no anticipatory postural adjustment could be discerned. It is possible that the heightened level of attention and/or the instruction to step rather than walk may have contributed to fewer episodes of freezing in the experimental paradigm. This is a frequent problem when studying GIF. The total absence of any postural adjustments in the two trials with freezing suggests that GIF is related to lack of initiation of postural adjustments rather than to weak ineffective patterns.

Apomorphine

Apomorphine is a potent D_1 and D_2 agonist. Subcutaneous apomorphine acute tests are currently used to predict dopaminergic responsiveness in parkinsonian syndromes (16,17). Apomorphine challenges have also been used to assess the responsiveness of GIF to dopamine stimulation in some patients with PD.

A marked reduction in the number of freezing episodes was reported by Linazasoro following

TABLE 26.1. *Demographic characteristics of six patients with idiopathic Parkinson's disease who exhibit gait ignition failure*

Patient	Age (yr)	Disease duration (yr)	Hoehn and Yahr	"Off-freezing"	Freezing (UPDRS item 14)
1	69	9	III	YES	3
2	70	14	IV	YES	4
3	67	4	III	?(Stable patient with no "off" periods")	3
4	62	12	III	"On" and "off freezing"	3
5	60	9	IV	"On" and "off freezing"	2
6	64	5	II	?(Stable patient with no "off" periods)	2

UPDRS, Unified Parkinson's Disease Rating Scale.

apomorphine injections in nine patients suffering from IPD, whose GIF occurred exclusively during "off" periods (18). After a mean follow-up of 14 months, these patients clearly improved once the dopaminergic drug dosage was adjusted. Corboy and colleagues reported a similar observation in one patient (19).

We have personally studied six patients with IPD (20) and severe GIF (Table 26.1) and have assessed the dopaminergic responsiveness of these freezing episodes using acute apomorphine challenges and a subsequent chronic increase in antiparkinsonian treatments. The assessment of the acute apomorphine effects was performed in a crossover randomized placebo-controlled double-blind design. We performed the apomorphine test according to the description by Hughes et al. (16); however, the six patients were challenged in the morning, in addition to their usual antiparkinsonian treatment, rather than after a night of drug withdrawal. We did not intend to test the GIF dopaminergic responsiveness *per se,* but rather wanted to determine if supplementary dopamine stimulation would influence GIF positively or negatively. We also wanted to evaluate the correlation between the acute challenge results and the effects of chronic treatment adjustments. Such a strategy has already been discussed for other motor parkinsonian symptoms (17).

Freezing was evaluated at baseline and 20 minutes after the apomorphine or placebo subcutaneous injections. Each injection was separated by 90 minutes. We assessed freezing by measuring the time (seconds) taken by the patient to walk a 15-meter long circuit with several standardized obstacles. The freezing episodes (start hesitations, target hesitations, or turning hesitations) also were counted. Three consecutive assessments were repeated at 5-minute intervals 20 minutes after each drug challenge because freezing is a highly variable symptom. Some patients were not able to walk the full distance of the circuit in several assessments, because of severe freezing. The scores were infinite in this situation. For this reason, rather than comparing the means of the values obtained during the three successive assessments, we compared the range of the walking times and the range of the numbers of freezing episodes in each patient (Table 26.2). The test was considered positive if apomorphine induced a clear improvement on both parameters on the three consecutive assessments compared with placebo. The test was considered equivocal if a less clear benefit was observed. The test was considered negative if no improvement occurred. We also looked for deterioration. After this acute challenge assessment phase, patients entered an open chronic phase, when oral dopaminergic (L-Dopa and/or dopamine agonists) daily doses were increased for several months according to tolerance and response. Gait ignition failure was then assessed using item 14 (freezing when walking) of the Unified Parkinson's Rating Scale (UPDRS); a decrease of one score compared with baseline was considered an improvement. In two patients (patients 1 and 2), GIF was considered at baseline as "off-freezing," freezing episodes clearly being more severe during "off" periods. It was difficult to clearly determine if GIF corresponded to "off-freezing" or "on-freezing" in the four other

TABLE 26.2. *Response to acute subcutaneous injections in six patients with Parkinson's disease who exhibit gait ignition failure*

	Placebo			Apomorphine				
		Walking circuit				Walking circuit		
Patient	UPDRS	Time (sec)	Freezing episodes	Dose (mg)	UPDRS	Time (sec)	Freezing episodes	Test conclusion
1	10	40–∞	6–∞	5	8	23–30	2–2	Positive
2	17	∞	∞	1	12	25–41	2–4	Positive
3	7	34–52	4–8	5	8	40–∞	3–∞	Negative
4	4	30–46	4–12	5	4	26–40	3–10	Equivocal
5	6	20–∞	4–∞	3	6	25–∞	2–∞	Equivocal
6	7	30–35	2–2	5	6	28–39	2–3	Negative

Time, time in seconds needed by the patient to walk a 15-meter circuit with standardized obstacles.
Freezing episodes, number of motor blocks experienced by the patient while walking this circuit.
∞, the score was "infinite" because the patient could not finish one or more assessments as a result of severe freezing episodes.
Patients were assessed on three consecutive occasions following each injection of placebo and apomorphine. The results of these three consecutive assessments are given as ranges.
UPDRS, Unified Parkinson's Disease Rating Scale.

patients. Patients 3 and 6 had no motor fluctuations, but remained mildly akinetic all day. It was thus difficult to anticipate if these patients were "undertreated," and would benefit from increasing the dose of antiparkinsonian medications, or if they were already "fully" medicated, and were then suffering from "on-freezing," which is resistant to L-Dopa. Gait ignition failure was unpredictable in patients 4 and 5, occurring both in "off" and "on" periods. However, its at least partial responsiveness to dopamine treatments was suspected because a previous short (24-hour) drug holiday led to worsening of frozen episodes in both cases.

The apomorphine test was considered to be positive in two cases (patients 1 and 2), equivocal in two cases (patients 4 and 5), and negative in two cases (patients 3 and 6) (Table 26.2). No patient showed a clear deterioration of GIF after apomorphine. The

TABLE 26.3. *Gait ignition failure response to chronic increase in antiparkinsonian medications in six patients with idiopathic Parkinson's disease*

	Treatment daily dose				UPDRS (item 14 = Freezing when walking)		
Patient	Baseline		After adjustment	Follow-up	Baseline	After adjustment	Subjective assessment
1	L-Dopa Bromo	600 mg 60 mg	1,200 mg 60 mg	6 Months	3	1	Improved
2	L-Dopa Bromo Deprenyl	1,000 mg 20 mg 10 mg	1,600 mg 40 mg 10 mg	4 Months	4	2	Improved
3	L-Dopa	400 mg	1,200 mg	6 Months	3	3	No change in freezing, dyskinesia worse
4	L-Dopa	800 mg	800 mg Bromo 25 mg	4 Months	3	2	Improved
5	L-Dopa Bromo Deprenyl	800 mg 40 mg 10 mg	No change because of dose-limiting dyskinesia	6 Months	2	2	?
6	L-Dopa Bromo	400 mg 30 mg	1,000 mg 60 mg	6 Months	2	2	No benefit

Bromo, bromocriptine; UPDRS, Unified Parkinson's Disease Rating Scale.

subsequent increase in chronic dopaminergic treatments led to a substantial improvement of GIF in three patients (Table 26.3). This result had been predicted by the apomorphine test in two of the three patients (patients 1 and 2). Frozen episodes clearly improved after the adjunction of 25 mg of bromocriptine in the third patient (patient 4), although the results of the apomorphine test were considered equivocal. No benefit was observed on long-term follow-up in two patients. This negative result had been predicted from the apomorphine test (patients 3 and 6). No conclusion could be drawn on long-term follow-up in the last patient (patient 5) because the severity of dyskinesias prevented the significant increase of dopaminergic medications.

Taken together, these findings indisputably show a proportion of patients with IPD and GIF who can improve with dopaminergic treatment. In some cases, the fact that GIF is associated with "off" episodes is a good clinical predictor of its potential dopaminergic responsiveness. However, in several instances, it is more difficult to anticipate the effect of increasing the dose. This is so because some patients do not actually suffer from motor fluctuations (stable, possibly "undertreated" putative responders) or because frozen gait is present during both "off" and "on" periods, making difficult to clearly state if freezing occurs in a truly random way, or is relatively worse during "off" periods. The acute apomorphine challenge test may have partial predictability in these cases.

Selegiline

The DATATOP study suggested that another class of dopaminergic agents, monoamine oxidase-B (MAO-B) inhibitors, also improves GIF in IPD. During the initial 2 years of the trial, 193 (24.1%) of the DATATOP subjects developed GIF. Subjects assigned to selegiline showed a 53% reduction in the risk of developing freezing of gait compared with those receiving placebo [odds ratio, 0.47; 95% CI (0.34 to 0.66; $P < 0.0001$)]. This beneficial effect waned after withdrawal of experimental treatment, suggesting a symptomatic rather than a protective effect of the drug (21). This positive effect of selegiline has not always been reported in the literature (22).

Other dopaminergic replacement therapies (e.g., restoration of dopaminergic function with fetal mesencephalic cell grafting) have been reported to improve freezing in patients with IPD; however, such findings remain controversial (23).

"On-Freezing" Nonresponsive to Dopaminergic Medications in Idiopathic Parkinson's Disease

L-Dopa

There are indisputable examples of patients with GIF who respond well to L-Dopa; however, a number of patients fail to improve with dopamine treatments. In these cases, frozen gait usually occurs during "on" periods. Such "on-freezing" sometimes is worsened with higher doses of L-Dopa. Ambani and Van Woert and Barbeau first described this phenomenon; they reported the increased frequency of start hesitation shortly after the introduction of L-Dopa treatment (24,25). Although most clinicians empirically agree that GIF can worsen in some patients in response to excessive dopaminergic treatment, there are no recent published data on such cases. It will be interesting to reassess this question in the future.

Giladi and colleagues reported supportive data for the possible contribution of L-Dopa, rather than dopamine denervation, in the development of GIF (3). They found that 69 of 990 IPD patients in a retrospective survey experienced motor blocks only when "on." Such cases allow a direct relationship between high plasma levels of L-Dopa and the occurrence of GIF, which presents as a peak-of-dose side effect. The same authors also found a significant correlation between the presence of GIF and L-Dopa–induced dyskinesias, suggesting the existence of common pathophysiologic mechanisms between both syndromes. This reinforces the notion that some type of GIF can be seen as an L-Dopa–induced adverse event. This hypothesis, however, is not supported by more recent prospective data. We recently conducted a 5-year prospective double-blind

L-Dopa–controlled study in 287 patients with early PD who received ropinirole, a novel D_2 agonist, as the initial treatment (26). The early use of the dopamine agonist dramatically reduced the risk for dyskinesia, whereas it had no impact on the incidence of freezing when walking. This observation suggests that L-Dopa therapy has different effects on dyskinesia and GIF and that both symptoms were correlated in Giladi and colleagues' analysis because they are both more common in the advanced stages of the disease.

Apomorphine

Linazasoro reported that GIF appeared unpredictable during "on" and "off" periods in two of 11 patients with IPD (18). Both patients showed a remarkable improvement in motor function with low doses of apomorphine (1 to 3 mg) with no concomitant change in the severity of GIF. Such patients may correspond to patients 3 and 6 of our own series. These observations support the idea that GIF is far from being systematically sensitive to dopamine drugs, although no clinical feature, except its presence during "on" episodes, differentiates L-Dopa–responsive from L-Dopa–nonresponsive GIF. Interestingly, five of the nine patients described by Linazasoro as having "off-freezing" and a clear positive GIF response to subcutaneous apomorphine experienced a transient exacerbation of parkinsonism and GIF before they switched "on" soon after the apomorphine injection. This "super-off" phenomenon has previously been described for other motor parkinsonian symptoms, and is possibly explained by an inhibitory effect via the stimulation of presynaptic dopamine receptors (27). The same might then be true for GIF.

Other Dopamine Agonists

The adjunction of orally active dopamine agonists (e.g., bromocriptine, pergolide, or ropinirole) failed to significantly improve GIF in most published studies (22,26,28,29). This can be seen as an argument for the lack of responsiveness of GIF to dopamine medications, even in IPD. It is possible, however, that such negative results resulted from the fact that both "off-freezing" and "on-freezing" were assessed simultaneously in the same study, thus reducing the sensitivity of the analysis. It is also possible that oral dopamine agonists induced less potent dopaminergic stimulation than subcutaneous apomorphine or oral L-Dopa, which was insufficient to positively influence GIF.

Recently, Giladi and colleagues reported a positive correlation between the use of dopamine agonists and the prevalence of GIF (Chapter 19). This observation may be explained by two different hypotheses: either dopamine agonists cause or facilitate GIF, or both parameters (GIF and the use of dopamine agonists) are simply correlated because both are more frequently observed in more advanced stages of the disease. The results of our 5-year ropinirole–L-Dopa controlled study do not support the hypothesis that dopamine agonists by themselves cause or represent a risk factor for GIF (26). The risk of increase in freezing during walking after 5 years of treatment was similar in the ropinirole and the L-Dopa–treated patients (32% versus 25%, respectively; odds ratio, 0.71; CI, 0.40, 1.26; $P = 0.234$). It is likely that the observed correlation between the use of dopamine agonists and GIF in the survey by Giladi and colleagues was simply because they are both more frequent in the more advanced stages of the disease.

Not surprisingly, in Parkinson-plus syndromes, GIF, like most other aspects of the parkinsonian syndrome, is hardly benefited by L-Dopa and other dopaminergic treatments (18).

In summary, "off-freezing" is a frequent form of GIF observed in IPD. In this case, adequate therapeutic adjustments that can improve the "on-off" phenomenon (increasing L-Dopa dose, adjunction of dopamine agonists or MAO-B or COMT inhibitors) should be beneficial for freezing. However, physicians must be aware of the fact that GIF, and especially "on-freezing," may not respond to such adjustments in a proportion of patients, who might even benefit from a reduction of dopamine treatments in some instances. The reasons why some GIF syndromes should or should not respond to L-Dopa remain obscure. Moreover, when GIF actually responds to L-Dopa, it is impossible to understand how and where the drug is working. It could act at the striatal level to correct the dopaminergic nigrostriatal deficit that characterizes IPD, as is believed to be the case in other motor symptoms. It is impossible, however, to exclude the hypothesis that dopaminergic medications could act at "higher" levels, in the frontal cortex via the mesocortical dopamine pathways, or at "lower" levels, in the brainstem or even in the spinal cord.

GAIT IGNITION FAILURE AND NONDOPAMINERGIC MEDICATIONS

L-threo-DOPS

Narabayashi and colleagues described cases of pure akinesia or freezing without rigidity and tremor that are unresponsive to L-Dopa treatment as a new condition or specific form of parkinsonism (9). L-Dopa treatment, either alone (up to 3 g) or combined with C-Dopa, was not at all effective against the freezing symptom, and sometimes made it worse. A number of other clinical observations of this syndrome have been published (10,11,30). The relationship between this entity and PSP has been discussed on clinical, neuroimaging, and clinicopathologic findings (31–34).

The clinical hallmark of all these observations, apart from the almost pure GIF clinical presentation, at least in the early stages, is the constant absence of response to any dopaminergic treatments (10,11,30). Other treatments have been looked for because of the resistance to L-Dopa therapy.

L-threo-3,4-dihydrophenylserine (L-threo-DOPS), a synthetic noradrenaline (NA) precursor, was introduced in Japan as an agent specifically effective against GIF (Fig. 26.1) (9). The idea of the NA hypothesis for freezing came from the observation that the activity of the NA synthesizing enzyme, dopamine-β-hydroxylase, was more markedly lowered in the cerebrospinal fluid (CSF) of the late stages than in the early stages of IPD, whereas dopa-unresponsive GIF also appeared at the later stages of the disease. The efficacy of L-threo-DOPS on GIF remains a matter of controversy 20 years after the initial reports. The first observations emphasized the moderate to considerable improvement provided by the drug on GIF, both in "pure akinesia" and in the later stages of IPD (9,31,35–37). In Japan, L-threo-DOPS is now commercially available against freezing in parkinsonism (DROXIDOPA, Sumitomo Pharmaceuticals Co., Osaka, Japan). However, such positive results have been difficult to reproduce in western countries for unexplained reasons (2,38).

Recently, the effects of the long-term administration of L-threo-DOPS have been reported in one Japanese patient with "pure akinesia." Initially, this patient presented with a typical form of pure GIF (39). At this early stage, among several tested drugs, only DL-threo-DOPS and L-threo-DOPS were effective. However, this positive effect was only temporal and disappeared within a 16-month treatment period, whereas the clinical phenomenology of this patient resembled PSP (40).

Several factors could explain the conflicting data reported in the literature regarding the efficacy of L-threo-DOPS on GIF. As suggested by the observation of Yamamoto and colleagues, it is possible that the syndrome might respond differently at different stages of the disease (40). The effects of L-threo-DOPS might have been tested in patients in western countries who were too severely affected. It is also possible that the compound has not been titrated up to truly effective doses. For example, the negative data reported by Quinn and colleagues only concern the acute effects of L-threo-DOPS in response to a single dose of the drug (14). Chronic effects might be more positive. It is also possible that GIF is part of the spectrum of different etiologic entities, which have various therapeutic responses. In the absence of large enough clinicopathologic studies, it is impossible currently to definitely answer to this crucial question. Progressive supranuclear palsy is among these entities (31,32). It is particularly interesting to consider the effects of L-threo-DOPS and the possible relationship between pure GIF and PSP on the reported partial efficacy of imipraminic antidepressants in PSP, keeping in mind the fact that such antidepressants are supposed to act by NA reuptake inhibition (41). Another possible explanation for the discrepancies regarding

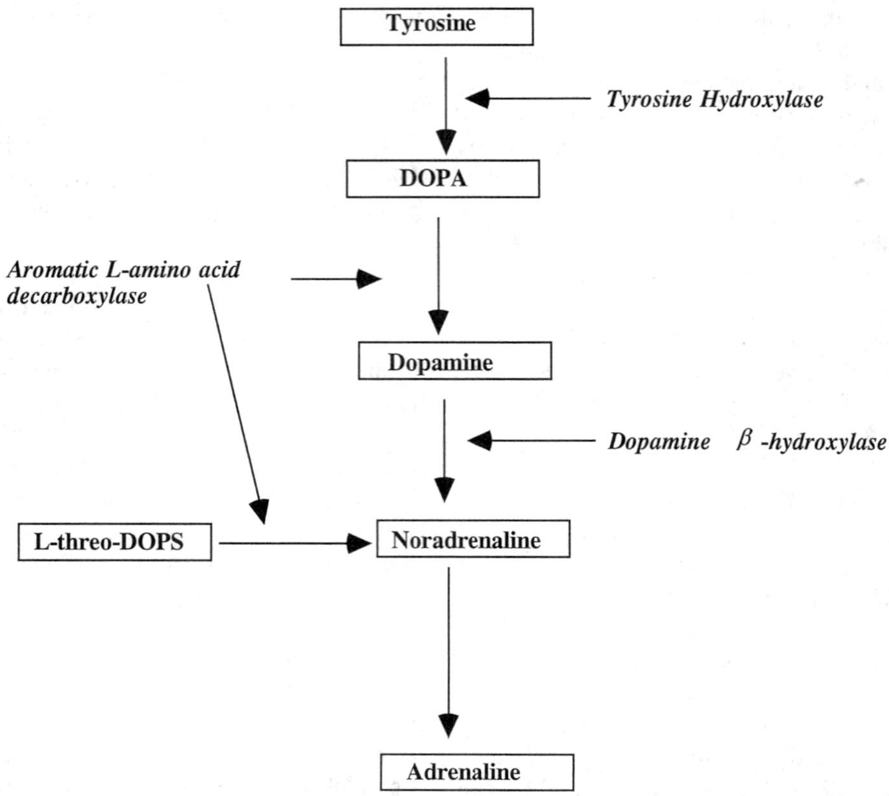

FIG. 26.1. Biosynthesis of noradrenaline from L-threo-3,4-dihydroxyphenylserine (*L-threo-DOPS*). *DOPA*, dihydroxyphenylalanine.

L-threo-DOPS effects might be the existence of different responses to this drug in Asian and Caucasian populations. There are several examples of such ethnic differences in the pharmacologic literature. For example, male Chinese subjects are more sensitive than male Caucasian subjects to the effects of propranolol on heart rate and blood pressure (42). Further large, placebo-controlled, prospective, long-term studies are justified before any definite conclusion may be drawn on the efficacy of L-threo-DOPS.

The mechanisms of action of L-threo-DOPS, especially at the central level, remain another matter of controversy (43,44). Inconsistent data on the increase in free NA content in the brain or in the CSF after administration of L-threo-DOPS have been reported in animal models and humans. However, the NA concentration has been reported to increase dose-dependently after administration of L-threo-DOPS in both L-Dopa/C-Dopa–pretreated and L-Dopa/C-Dopa–untreated patients (45). Other arguments for actual central effects of the drug are its effects on EEG and on mood, with the risk of drug-induced hypomania (39,36,43).

Other Nondopaminergic Treatments

A number of other drugs have been tested to try to improve GIF. Most of these studies (usually single case reports) are simply anecdotal, given that they have been conducted in an open way in very small numbers of heterogeneous patients. No significant improvement has been observed with several drugs acting on NA systems such as yohimbine, an α_2 antagonist, or maprotiline, a tetracyclic antidepressant with NA uptake inhibitory properties, although some positive results have been reported with this last compound and with tizanidine, an α_2 agonist (Montastruc, personal communication, 2000; Maertens de Noordhout and colleagues, Eleventh International Symposium on Parkinson's Disease, Rome, 1994) (18,39,40). Apart from the initial observation that β-hydroxylase was defective in the CSF of patients with advanced IPD, there is little evidence that the NA systems are particularly impaired in patients with GIF. We are aware of no available biochemical or pathologic data in this subset of patients. It would be interesting to look at this question in brain bank materials. Even in the absence of NA deficit, NA drugs could act indirectly via nonspecific mechanisms (e.g., increased vigilance or attention), because it has been speculated that the level of attention could influence the severity of gait deficits (Chapter 24).

Incidental therapeutic benefits have been reported in the Japanese literature with other drugs, such as amantadine or L-5-hydroxytryptamine (47,48). Negative results have been reported with clonazepam, citicoline, and nimodipine (18,39). A preliminary report has suggested that botulinum toxin injections might be useful in the treatment of GIF (Chapter 19) (49).

In conclusion, any recommendation on the pharmacologic treatment of GIF is hazardous because of the heterogeneity of GIF and the insufficient reliability of the available clinical trials. Empirically, clinicians must be aware of the fact that one patient with GIF can respond very differently to dopaminergic medications from another. It is thus quite important to carefully question and observe each individual patient with GIF, to assess as well as possible if he or she is complaining of "off-freezing" rather than "on-freezing." In the first case, increasing dopaminergic stimulation with dosage adjustments should improve GIF to the same extent as the "off" periods. Conversely, in the second case, L-Dopa usually fails to improve GIF, making it worse in some instances; therefore, lowering the dose may be justified in these patients. Patients with GIF will hardly benefit from L-Dopa therapy in conditions other than IPD. Nondopaminergic treatments, such as L-threo-DOPS, require further assessment, especially in the western population.

REFERENCES

1. Nutt JG, Marsden CD, Thompson PD. Human walking and higher-level gait disorders, particularly in the elderly. *Neurology* 1993;43:268–279.
2. Fahn S. The freezing phenomenon in Parkinsonism. In: Fahn S, Hallett M, Lüders HO, et al, eds. *Negative motor phenomena*. Philadelphia: Lippincott–Raven, 1995:53–63.
3. Giladi N, McMahon D, Przedborski S, et al. Motor blocks in Parkinson's disease. *Neurology* 1992;42:333–339.
4. Lamberti P, Armenise S, Castaldo V, et al. Freezing gait in Parkinson's disease. *Eur Neurol* 1997;38:297–301.
5. Ballard PA, Tetrud JW, Langston JW. Permanent human parkinsonism due to 1-methyl-4-phenyl-1,2,3,6-tetrahydropyridine (MPTP): seven cases. *Neurology* 1985;35:949–956.
6. Widner H, Tetrud J, Rehncrona S, et al. Bilateral fetal mesencephalic grafting in two patients with parkinsonism induced by 1-methyl-4-phenyl-1,2,3,6-tetrahydropyridine (MPTP). *N Engl J Med* 1992;327:1556–1563.
7. Lobo Antunes J, Fahn S, et al. Normal pressure hydrocephalus and Parkinson's disease. *J Neural Transm* 1983;19:S225–S231.
8. Abe K, Hashimoto T, Tamaru F, et al. Analysis of gait disturbance in a patient with corticobasal degeneration. *Rinsho Shinkeigaku* 1995;35:153–157.
9. Narabayashi H, Imai H, Yokochi M, et al. Cases of pure akinesia without rigidity and tremor and with no effect by L-Dopa therapy. In: Birkmayer W, Hornykiewicz O, eds. *Advances in parkinsonism*. Basel: Editions Roche, 1976:335–342.
10. Atchison PR, Thompson PD, Frackowiak RSJ, et al. The syndrome of gait ignition failure: a report of six cases. *Mov Disord* 1993;8:285–292.
11. Achiron A, Ziv I, Goren M, et al. Primary progressive freezing gait. *Mov Disord* 1993;8:293–297.
12. Giladi N, Kao R, Fahn S. Freezing phenomenon in patients with Parkinsonian syndromes. *Mov Disord* 1997;12:302–305.
13. Bonnet AM, Loria Y, Saint-Hilaire MH, et al. Does long-term aggravation of Parkinson's disease result from non-dopaminergic lesions? *Neurology* 1987;37:1539–1542.
14. Quinn NP, Luthert P, Honavar M, et al. Pure akinesia due to Lewy Body Parkinson's disease: a case with pathology. *Mov Disord* 1989;4:85–89.
15. Burleigh-Jacobs A, Horak FB, Nutt JG, et al. Step initiation in Parkinson's disease: influence of levodopa and external sensory triggers. *Mov Disord* 1997;12:206–215.
16. Hughes AJ, Lees AJ, Stern GM. Apomorphine test to predict dopaminergic responsiveness in parkinsonian syndromes. *Lancet* 1990;336:32–34.
17. Rascol O, Senard JM, Rascol A, et al. Apomorphine test in parkinsonian syndromes. *Lancet* 1990;336:518.
18. Linazasoro G. The apomorphine test in gait disorders associated with parkinsonism. *Clin Neuropharmacol* 1996;19:171–176.
19. Corboy DL, Wagner ML, Sage JI. Apomorphine for motor fluctuations and freezing in Parkinson's disease. *Ann Pharmacother* 1995;29:282–288.
20. Gibb WR, Lees AJ. The significance of the Lewy body in the diagnosis of idiopathic Parkinson's disease. *Neuropathol Appl Neurobiol* 1989;15:27–44.

21. Shoulson I and the Parkinson Study Group. DATATOP: a decade of neuroprotective inquiry. *Ann Neurol* 1998; 44:S160–S166.
22. Lander CM, Lees A, Stern G. Oscillations in performance in levodopa-treated parkinsonians: treatment with bromocriptine and L-deprenyl. *Clin Exp Neurol* 1979;16:197–203.
23. Iacono RP, Tang ZS, Mazziotta JC, et al. Bilateral fetal grafts for Parkinson's disease: 22 month's results. *Stereotact Funct Neurosurg* 1992;58:84–87.
24. Ambani LM, Van Woert MH. Start hesitation: side effect of long-term levodopa therapy. *N Engl J Med* 1973;288:1113–1115.
25. Barbeau A. Six years of high level levodopa therapy in severely akinetic parkinsonian patients. *Arch Neurol* 1976;33:333–338.
26. Rascol O, Brooks DJ, Korczyn AD, et al, on behalf of the 056 Study Group. A five-year study of the incidence of dyskinesia in patients with early Parkinson's disease who were treated with ropinirole or levodopa. *N Engl J Med* 2000 342:1484–1491.
27. Merello M, Lees AJ. Beginning-of-dose motor deterioration following the acute administration of levodopa and apomorphine in Parkinson's disease. *J Neurol Neurosurg Psychiatry* 1992;55:1024–1026.
28. Lang AE, Quinn N, Brincat S, et al. Pergolide in late-stage Parkinson disease. *Ann Neurol* 1982;12:243–247.
29. Jankovic J. Long-term study of pergolide in Parkinson's disease. *Neurology* 1985;35:296–299.
30. Imai H. Dopa-unresponsive pure akinesia or freezing. In: Nagatsu T, Narabayashi H, Yoshida M, eds. *Parkinson's disease. From clinical aspects to molecular basis.* Berlin: Springer–Verlag, 1991:157–166.
31. Matsuo H, Takashima H, Kishikawa M, et al. Pure akinesia: an atypical manifestation of progressive supranuclear palsy. *J Neurol Neurosurg Psychiat* 1991;54:397–400.
32. Imai H, Nakamura T, Kondo T, et al. Dopa-unresponsive pure akinesia or freezing. A condition within a wide spectrum of PSP? *Adv Neurol* 1993;60:622–625.
33. Riley DE, Fogt N, Leigh RJ. The syndrome of "pure akinesia" and its relationship to progressive supranuclear palsy. *Neurology* 1994;44:1025–1029.
34. Fabre N, Brefel-Courbon C, Sabatini U, et al. Normal frontal perfusion in patients with frozen gait. *Mov Disord* 1998;13:677–683.
35. Narabayashi H, Kondo T, Nagatsu T, et al. DL-Threo-3,4-Dihydroxyphenylserine for freezing symptom in parkinsonism. In: Hassler RG, Christ JF, eds. *Parkinson-specific motor and mental disorders. Role of pallidum: Pathophysiological, biochemical, and therapeutic aspects.* New York: Raven Press, 1984:497–502.
36. Narabayashi H, Kondo T, Yokochi F, et al. Clinical effects of L-threo-3,4-Dihydroxyphenylserine in cases of parkinsonism and pure akinesia. In: Yahr MD, Bergmann KJ, eds. *Parkinson's disease.* New York: Raven Press, 1986:593–602.
37. Ogawa N, Yamamoto M, Takayama H. L-threo-3,4-dihydroxyphenylserine treatment of Parkinson's disease. *J Med* 1985:16:525–534.
38. Quinn NP, Perlmutter JS, St Louis MO, Marsden CD. Acute administration of DL-Threo-DOPS does not affect the freezing phenomenon in parkinsonian patients. *Neurology* 1984;34:S149.
39. Yamamoto M, Ujike H, Ogawa N. Effective treatment of pure akinesia with L-threo-3,4-dihydroxyphenylserine (DOPS): report of a case, with pharmacological considerations. *Clin Neuropharmacol* 1985;8:334–342.
40. Yamamoto M, Fujii S, Hatanaka Y. Result of long-term administration of L-threo-3,4-dihydroxyphenylserine in patients with pure akinesia as an early symptom of progressive supranuclear palsy. *Clin Neuropharmacol* 1997;20:371–373.
41. Nieforth KA, Golbe LI. Retrospective study of drug response in 87 patients with progressive supranuclear palsy. *Clin Neuropharmacol* 1993;16:338–346.
42. Zhou HH, Koshakji RP, Silberstein DJ, et al. Racial difference in drug response. Altered sensitivity to and clearance of propranolol in men of Chinese descent as compared with American whites. *N Engl J Med* 1989;320:565–570.
43. Kondo T. L-*threo*-DOPS in advanced parkinsonism. In: Narabayashi H, Nagatsu T, Yanagisawa N, et al, eds. *Parkinson's disease: from basic research to treatment.* New York: Raven Press, 1993:660–665.
44. Freeman R, Landsberg L. The treatment of orthostatic hypotension with dihydroxyphenylserine. *Clin Neuropharmacol* 1991;14:296–304.
45. Tohgi H, Abe T, Takahashi S. The effects of L-threo-3,4-dihydroxyphenylserine on the total norepinephrine and dopamine concentrations in the cerebrospinal fluid and freezing gait in parkinsonian patients. *J Neural Transm* 1993;5:27–34.
46. Iwasaki S, Narabayashi Y, Takakusagi M, et al. Maprotiline therapy for freezing of Parkinson's disease. In: *Abstracts of Alzheimer's and Parkinson's disease.* Kyoto, 1989:144.
47. Kurihara T, Terao A, Araki S. Effective amantadine therapy for kinesie paradoxale. *Neurol Med* 1977;6:151–156.
48. Tokiguchi S, Natsukawa M, Kawase Y, et al. Pure akinesia with apraxia of lid-opening. *Clin Neurol* 1978;18:208–212.
49. Giladi N, Honigman S. Botulinum toxin injections to one leg alleviate freezing of gait in a patient with Parkinson's disease. *Mov Disord* 1997;12:1085–1086.

Gait Disorders. Advances in Neurology, Vol. 87,
edited by E. Růžička, M. Hallett, and J. Jankovic.
Lippincott Williams & Wilkins, Philadelphia © 2001.

27

Chemodenervation with Botulinum Toxin for Spasticity and Dystonia

The Effects on Gait

Christopher F. O'Brien

Department of Medical Affairs, Elan Pharmaceuticals, South San Francisco, California 94080

Can chemodenervation improve gait? This apparently simple question is deceptively complex. For the purposes of this chapter, three main issues are addressed: (a) the characterization of abnormal gait, (b) the selection of appropriate treatment goals, and (c) technical issues in chemodenervation.

Chemodenervation has been available in our therapeutic arsenal for many years. The basic concept of interrupting the nerve supply to a specific muscle is relatively straightforward. Whether such denervation is of clinical benefit depends on the actual biomechanical abnormality in the affected limb. Recently, increased interest in gait disorders along with more precise analytic techniques and improved chemodenervation agents have allowed focusing on patient physiology and more effective treatments for patients with spasticity or dystonia.

Case studies have shown dramatic results following chemodenervation in selected patients and variable results in clinical trials. Most convincing of the potential benefit of chemodenervation have been data from studies of children with spastic diplegia attributed to cerebral palsy (1). Smaller open-label series have demonstrated significant improvement in adults with specific gait abnormalities, clearly identified focal muscle over activity (e.g., excess plantar flexion owing to soleus overactivity) and effective denervation with botulinum toxin (BTX) (2). Although guidelines have been published, we have limited data regarding the optimal patient selection and treatment methods (3).

CHARACTERIZATION OF ABNORMAL GAIT: SPASTICITY AND DYSTONIA: CLASSIFICATION

Common descriptors used in clinic, such as "spastic" or "dystonic" gait, lack precision. We must often add specific details in order for better understanding of biomechanics, physiology, impairments, or disability. In this volume several classification schemes have been reviewed and it is hoped that more precise and meaningful approaches will become available. Some common patterns and associated clinical features are delineated in Table 27.1. Common clinical problems faced by the clinician include the following:

- Plantar flexion
- Foot inversion
- Thigh adduction ("scissoring")
- Hip–knee flexion
- Hip–knee extension
- Toe curling
- "Striatal toe"
- "Freezing" phenomena
- Truncal dystonia: distal effects

TABLE 27.1. *Common patterns and associated clinical features of abnormal gait*

Physical signs description	Associated signs
Hemiparetic gait	Extension and circumduction of one leg; weakness on the affected side; hyperreflexia; extensor plantar response; flexed arm
Paraparetic gait	Stiffness, extension, adduction, and scissoring of both legs; bilateral leg weakness, hyperreflexia, spasticity, and extensor plantar responses
Sensory gait	Unsteadiness of walking when visual input is withdrawn (positive Romberg sign); decreased position sense
Steppage gait	Weakness of foot dorsiflexors; foot-drop; excessive flexion of hips and knees when walking; short strides; unilateral of bilateral. Atrophy of distal leg muscles; decreased ankle reflex; possible sensory loss
Petits pas gait	Wide-based, cautious gait, small and shallow steps; hypokinesia; increased muscle tone; dementia
Apraxic gait	Difficulty initiating a step; freezing; feet almost stuck to floor; turn hesitation; shuffling gait; hypokinesia; muscular rigidity; grasp reflexes; possible resting tremor, dementia, or urinary incontinence
Pulsive or retropulsive gait	Body's center of gravity appears to be either in front or behind the patient, who is struggling to keep his or her feet up to center of gravity; festination; hypokinesia; muscular rigidity; postural instability
Ataxic gait	Wide-based gait; incoordination; staggering; decomposition of movements, dysmetria; dysdiadochokinesia; tremor; postural instability
Waddling gait	Wide-based gait; swaying; toe-walk; lumbar lordosis; symmetrical proximal muscle weakness of lower extremities
Dystonic gait	Sustained abnormal posture of the foot or leg; distorted gait; hyperflexion of hips. Action-related gait disturbance; atypical presentations
Choreic gait	Irregular, dancelike gait; slow and wide-based; spontaneous knee flexion and leg raising; autoerotic and choreic movements of the upper extremities
Intaglio gait	Limping; avoidance of bearing full weight on the affected leg; limitation of range of movement; pain in lower extremity aggravated by leg movement
Vertiginous gait	Unsteady gait; falling to one side; postural imbalance; vertigo; nausea; nystagmus
Psychogenic (hysteric) gait	Bizarre and nonphysiologic gait; different varieties; rare fall or injury; give-way weakness; Hoover's sign; other signs of conversion

Adapted from Jankovic J. *Gait disorders. Neurobase.* La Jolla, CA: Arbor Publishing, 1999, with permission.

Although lacking in precision, the terms listed in the preceding at least allow us to begin thinking about biomechanics and possible treatment options. Specifically, we can narrow down the choice of target muscles to consider for denervation in patients with one of these patterns.

Assessment tools for abnormal gait range from simple clinical rating scales to sophisticated laboratory techniques employing multichannel electromyography (EMG), force plates in the floor to record ground reaction forces, and computer analysis of multicamera video recordings. Increasingly, instrumented motion analysis and dynamic EMG are needed for good surgical outcome (5). Similar analysis can be used successfully for chemodenervation (6). This is especially true for postural abnormalities such as foot inversion and crouch gait. In the classic case of foot inversion with plantar flexion, one must determine to what extent hip flexors, hamstrings, soleus, gastrocnemius, and posterior tibialis are contributing to the abnormal gait. Multichannel EMG is quite useful in that regard.

On a practical level, impairment and outcome can be assessed using simple, noninstrumented methods. Some of the more common clinical tools include the "sit-stand-walk" test, the time–distance test, and the physician gait assessment, among others (7). Alteration of muscle contraction or joint kinemetics may not translate into change or improvement of clinical status. Typically, the clinician needs to employ measures of technical effect, biomechanical effect, and outcome, as discussed in the following.

APPROPRIATE GOAL SELECTION

"Patient selection" refers to the process of matching optimal treatment to individual patient needs. For abnormal gait, this typically includes identification of patients for whom reduction in focal muscle overactivity may be useful. Clearly, patients with profound weakness of the legs would not be considered for chemodenervation. Patients with fixed contractures may be candidates but often require additional intervention such as taping, serial casting, or surgical release (8,9).

The desired clinical outcome of treatment is often the ideal starting point for determination of short-term objectives that should logically translate into specific technical objectives. For example, a goal of safe, easy, and more rapid ambulation for a child with "scissoring" might include an alteration of hip–thigh biomechanics. The functional alteration might be reduction of thigh adductor overactivity (including the inappropriate cocontraction of antagonist, muscle shortening, spasms, and so on). The technical objective in this case would be denervation of some or all of the adductor muscles. Table 27.2 summarizes the hierachy of decision making. As with all spasticity management, a multidisciplinary team appears to be most effective.

Target muscle selection for chemodenervation is based on the clinical assessment and other analytic tools such as EMG. The treating clinician must have a good working knowledge of functional anatomy. The reader is referred to an introduction to this topic (10). There is no single treatment plan that is universally applicable for all patients. Table 27.3 lists some of the more common muscles for several frequently encountered gait problems.

CHEMODENERVATION: TECHNICAL ISSUES

The choice of agent for chemodenervation is limited to two at present: phenol or BTX. Some of their advantages and disadvantages are discussed further by Gracies (11). Phenol is technically difficult; very effective for "pure" motor nerves; and low cost; but carries a risk for causalgia, thrombosis, and fibrosis. Botulinum toxin is relatively simple to inject and low risk, but has a higher cost and a dose-dependent effect.

It must be emphasized that phenol denervation typically is used either for motor point block (with large volumes of phenol infused into the belly of the muscle) or motor nerve blocks. The latter requires precise isolation of a relatively pure motor nerve, such as the obturator, employing electrical stimulation and successive approximation. Only 0.25 to 0.50 mL of 5% to 6% phenol is needed to achieve complete denervation of the target muscle when done correctly. Unfortunately, this technique does not permit dose-dependent, controlled denervation and there are only a limited number of "pure" motor nerve supplied muscles common to spastic patients.

Localization techniques for placement of the denervating agent include use of surface landmarks, palpation, radiographic guidance, electrical stimulation, or EMG guidance (12). The clinician must use whichever method allows the greater precision at the least risk to the patient.

TABLE 27.2. *Hierarchy of decision making for chemodenervation*

Initial evaluation	Patient presents with spasticity that is disabling
Multidisciplinary team	Disability is assessed for specific impairments and biomechanical abnormalities
Focused assessment	Biomechanical abnormalities are clearly defined using assessment tools, EMG, gait lab, etc.
Functional anatomy	Potential target muscles are identified for denervation
Goal setting	Technical, functional, and clinical outcome goals are set and assessment tools are chosen
Dose calculation	Based on technical goal and guidelines

TABLE 27.3. *Common target muscles for denervation for abnormal gait patterns*

Abnormal gait pattern	Common target muscles
Flexed hip	Iliacus Psoas Rectus femoris
Flexed knee	Medial hamstrings Gastrocnemius (as knee flexor) Lateral hamstrings
Adducted thighs	Adductor brevis/longus/magnus
Stiff (extended) knee	Quadriceps
Equinovarus foot	Gastrocnemius medial/lateral Soleus Tibialis posterior Tibialis anerior Flexor digitorum longus/brevis Flexor hallucis longus
Striatal toe	Extensor hallucis longus

For most target muscles, electrical stimulation for phenol motor nerve block and EMG guidance for BTX are the usual methods.

Neurotoxin effects may be modified by altering dose, concentration and, perhaps, serotype of toxin. Type-A toxin has enjoyed the widest use because of its commercial availability and reliable effects. Several serotypes of BTX produce chemodenervation in human muscle. There are currently two type-A toxins available (Botox Allergan, Inc., Irvine, CA, U.S.A.; and Dysport, Ipsen, France) as well as a type-B toxin (Myobloc and Neurobloc, Elan Pharmaceuticals, South San Francisco, CA, U.S.A) nearing registration in several countries. These serotypes appear to have different potencies, diffusion properties, "stickiness" or binding affinity, and risk of producing secondary nonresponsiveness (resistance) (13–15). Studies are currently underway to determine if one serotype confers specific advantages in the treatment of spasticity and gait disorders (16).

The physical characteristics of toxin diffusion and binding to nerve terminals may be altered by increasing the volume of the diluent. In clinic, this may be adjusted for different target muscles. In our clinic, we have reduced diffusion by injecting very concentrated doses (e.g., 100 units of Botox in 0.5 mL of saline). We have maximized diffusion by injecting dilute solutions (e.g., 100 units of Botox in 4 mL of saline). The latter employed for calf muscles in diplegic children. Although some diffusion and denervation data are available from animal studies, further human trials are warranted (17).

The dose of BTX may be adjusted to produce mild or near-complete denervation of the target muscle. Early trials with CP children used 2 units of Botox/kg, a dose subsequently found to be insufficient for typical toe walking and scissoring. More recent trials have injected doses specific for target muscle using a "cap" of 10 to 12 units Botox/kg. A discussion of dose modifiers is available (18).

Activation of target muscles after BTX injection may improve toxin binding and potentially enhance clinical effect. Data for rat hemidiaphragm studies, adults with spastic hemiparesis, and forearm dystonia suggest that actively contracting muscles bind BTX more avidly (19–21). This may be a useful strategy for optimization of response in gait disorders. Studies are currently underway using electrical stimulation and voluntary activation of targeted muscles.

TREATMENT FAILURE

There are a variety of reasons for lack of benefit following chemodenervation. The most common include the following:

- Fixed contractures, which prevent full range of motion
- Wrong muscle injected, resulting in no effect or worsening of underlying problem
- Inadequate dose of neurotoxin producing insufficient effect
- Incomplete phenol block producing insufficient effect
- Excessive treatment effect producing new deficit
- Inappropriate goal selection

Inappropriate goal selection is the most troublesome cause of failure because it reflects poor communication among patient, physician, family, or therapists. Good team assessments and planning sessions are the best way to avoid such difficulties. Postinjection therapies must be tailored to individual patient needs (22). If in doubt, the team can have each member reiterate their perception and comparisons can be made.

RESEARCH ISSUES

Many issues remain regarding the role of chemodenervation in the treatment of gait disorders at each of the hierarchy levels described in the preceding. We need to better understand injection technique, especially as it relates to motor endpoint localization. We need to improve patient selection and goal setting. We need to clarify physiology of spasticity, particularly in regard to plasticity and recovery of function. The preliminary data on selective effects of botulinum toxin on intrafusal and extrafusal fibers need exploration. We need to further delineate the pharmacology of neurotoxins and how their beneficial effects may be extended. Clearly, there are opportunities for basic scientists and clinicians alike.

CONCLUSION

In summary, clinicians interested in modification of abnormal gait must be skilled at recognition and classification of the disorders. This volume is an important step in refinement of our lexicon and should help set standards for future communication and study. Once identified, the abnormal gait pattern should be defined as to specific biomechanical characteristics and appropriate treatment goals established. If focal muscle overactivity, incomplete relaxation or agonist–antagonist cocontraction is present, chemodenervation may indeed help improve abnormal gait.

REFERENCES

1. Wong V. Use of botulinum toxin injection in 17 children with spastic cerebral palsy. *Pediatr Neurol* 1998;18:124–131.
2. Hesse S, Reiter F, Konrad M, et al. Botulinum toxin type A and short-term electrical stimulation in the treatment of upper limb flexor spasticity after stroke: a randomized, double-blind, placebo-controlled trial. *Clin Rehabil* 1998;12:381–388.
3. Gormley ME, O'Brien CF, Yablon SA. A clinical overview of treatment decisions in the management of spasticity. *Muscle Nerve* 1997;20:S14–S20.
4. Jankovic J. *Gait disorders. Neurobase*. La Jolla, CA: Arbor Publishing, 1999.
5. Perry J. The use of gait analysis for surgical recommendation in traumatic brain injury. *J Head Trauma Rehabil* 1999;12:116–135.
6. Wilson DJ, Childers MK, Cooke DL, et al. Kinematic changes following botulinum toxin injection after traumatic brain injury. *Brain Inj* 1997;11:157–167.
7. Koman LA, Mooney JF, Smith BP, et al. Management of cerebral palsy with botulinum toxin A: preliminary investigation. *J Paediatr Orthop* 1994;14:229–303.
8. Corry IS, Cosgrove AP, Duffy CM, et al. Botulinum toxin A compared with stretching casts in the treatment of spastic equinus: a randomised prospective trial. *J Pediatr Orthop* 1998;18:304–311.
9. Reiter F, Danni M, Lagalla G, et al. Low-dose botulinum toxin with ankle taping for the treatment of spastic equinovarus foot after stroke. *Arch Phys Med Rehabil* 1998;79:532–535.
10. Gage JR. Gait analysis in cerebral palsy. *Clin Dev Med* 1991;121.
11. Gracies JM, Elovic E, McGuire J, et al. Traditional pharmacological treatments for spasticity part I: local treatments. *Muscle Nerve* 1997;20:SS61–S91.
12. O'Brien CF. Injection techniques for botulinum toxin using electromyography and electrical stimulation. *Muscle Nerve Suppl* 1997;6:S176–S180:
13. Doellgast GJ, Brown JE, Koufman JA, et al. Sensitive assay for measurement of antibodies to *Clostridium botulinum* neurotoxins A, B, and E: use of hapten-labeled-antibody elution to isolate specific complexes. *J Clin Microbiol* 1997;35:578–583.
14. Sankhla C, Jankovic J, Duane D. Variability of the immunologic and clinical response in dystonic patients immunoresistant to botulinum toxin injections. *Mov Disord* 1998;13:150–154.
15. Kessler KR, Skutta M, Benecke R. Long-term treatment of cervical dystonia with botulinum toxin A: efficacy, safety and antibody frequency. German Dystonia Study Group. *J Neurol* 1999;246:265–274.
16. O'Brien CF. Overview of clinical trials and published reports of botulinum toxin for spasticity. *Eur J Neurol* 1997;4:S11–S13.
17. Shaari CM, Sanders I. Quantifying how location and dose of botulinum toxin injections effect muscle paralysis. *Muscle Nerve* 1993;16:964–969.
18. Brin MF and the Spasticity Study Group. Dosing, administration and a treatment algorithm for the use of botulinum toxin A for adult-onset spasticity. *Muscle Nerve* 1997;6:S208–S220.
19. Hughes R, Walker BC. Influence of nerve-ending activity and of drugs on the rate of paralysis of rat diaphragm preparations by *Clostridium botulinum* type toxin A. *J Physiol* 1962;160:221–223.
20. Hesse S, Jahnke MT, Luecke D, et al. Short-term electrical stimulation enhances the effectiveness of botulinum toxin in the treatment of lower limb spasticity in hemiparetic patients. *Neurosci Lett* 1995;201:37–40.
21. Chen R, Karp BI, Goldstein SR, et al. Effect of muscle activity immediately after botulinum toxin injection for writer's cramp. *Mov Disord* 1999;14:307–312.
22. Albany K. Physical and occupational therapy considerations in adult patients receiving botulinum toxin injections for spasticity. *Muscle Nerve* 1997;20:S221–S231.

Gait Disorders. Advances in Neurology, Vol. 87,
edited by E. Růžička, M. Hallett, and J. Jankovic.
Lippincott Williams & Wilkins, Philadelphia © 2001.

28

Effects of Pallidotomy on Gait and Balance

*‡§Joseph Jankovic, *§Eugene C. Lai, *§William G. Ondo, **Deborah Roberts-Warrior, ¶Sharon L. Olson, ††Joachim K. Krauss, and †||Robert G. Grossman

*Departments of *Neurology and †Neurosurgery and ‡ Parkinson's Disease Center and Movement Disorders Clinic, Baylor College of Medicine; §Neurology Service and ||Neurosurgical Service, The Methodist Hospital; ¶School of Physical Therapy, Texas Woman's University, Houston, Texas 77030; **Department of Rehabilitation Sciences, University of Oklahoma Health Sciences Center, Oklahoma City, Oklahoma 73190; and ††Department of Neurosurgery, University Hospital Mannheim, Ruprecht Karls University Heidelberg, 68167 Mannheim, Germany*

Gait and postural control are typically impaired in patients with Parkinson's disease (PD), but, in contrast to other parkinsonian symptoms, these axial features respond poorly to dopaminergic therapy (1,2). Stereotactic surgery, particularly posteroventral pallidotomy (PVP), has become an important treatment alternative for patients whose symptoms cannot be adequately controlled with pharmacologic therapy. Posteroventral pallidotomy has been found to be beneficial in alleviating motor complications of chronic L-Dopa therapy as well as in the treatment of tremor, rigidity, and even bradykinesia, but its effects on gait and postural stability are unclear (3–14). Improvements in gait, postural stability, and other PD features after PVP have been documented by the Unified Parkinson's Disease Rating Scale (UPDRS) (15) and with timed tasks from the Core Assessment Program for Intracerebral Transplantation (CAPIT) (16). In addition, we have used a variety of quantitative measurements of gait and balance to assess aspects of ambulation in patients with PD. The purpose of this study was to investigate locomotion and postural control changes in patients with advanced PD before and after unilateral and bilateral PVP utilizing a variety of clinical, functional, and other quantitative measures of gait and balance.

METHODS

Patients were recruited from the Baylor College of Medicine Parkinson's Disease Center and Movement Disorders Clinic. All patients had moderately advanced PD and satisfied the following inclusion criteria: (a) Hoehn and Yahr stage III to V while "off," (b) L-Dopa responsiveness, (c) age 76 years or younger, and (d) absence of other neurologic disease including dementia, psychosis, autonomic dysfunction, or unstable medical illness. The total daily dose of L-Dopa equivalent was calculated as the regular dose of L-Dopa + (0.75× the dose of controlled-release L-Dopa plus C-Dopa) + (10× the dose of bromocriptine) + (100× the dose of pergolide) + (100× the dose of pramipexole) + (300× the dose ropinirole).

The surgical procedure used in our studies has been described in detail elsewhere (12–14). Briefly, after fixation of the Leksell G head frame to the patient's skull, stereotactic contiguous 1-mm axial computed tomography (CT) scans with reconstruction in coronal and sagittal planes were used to identify the anatomic locations of the anterior (AC) and posterior commissures (PC). A target in the posteroventral globus pallidus internum (GPi) was chosen 19 to 21 mm lateral to the midline, 4 to 5 mm below the

AC–PC line, and 2 to 3 mm anterior to the mid-commissural point. Microelectrode trajectories were planned at an angle of 40 to 45 degrees above the AC–PC line and parallel to the mid-sagittal line. The microelectrode was advanced via a stereotactically placed guiding cannula. Single unit recording was analyzed online and the firing pattern and frequency were used to confirm the location of the electrode using established criteria. The electrode was gradually advanced and the putamen, the globus pallidus externum (GPe), the laminar borders, and the GPi were mapped. GPi cells were characterized by high frequency discharges that could be modulated by passive joint movements. When the ventral border of the GPi was identified, the recording was supplemented by microstimulation at 3 to 4 mm below to identify the optic pathway. In the majority of patients one or two tracks were used, but in a few patients up to five tracks were necessary to adequately map the target area. A 1.1-mm diameter electrode with a 3-mm base tip was used for macrostimulation and to make the lesion. Two lesions were made along the same electrode trajectory, the second being made 2 mm above the first. Radiofrequency lesions were made at 75°C for 60 seconds. During lesioning, the strength and mobility of the contralateral arm, speech, and visual fields were monitored. Patients underwent MRI scanning of the brain within 3 days postoperatively and at 6 months.

Assessments

The patients were examined during their practically defined "off" state (in the morning at least 12 hours after their last dose of L-Dopa) and during their peak "on" state (typically, 1 hour after taking their first daily dose of L-Dopa). In addition to demographic information, L-Dopa dosage, supine and standing blood pressure, weight, and physical examination, the clinical assessments included the UPDRS (15), Hoehn and Yahr (H&Y) stage, and Activities of Daily Living (ADL) instruments, as well as the CAPIT (16). The patients also underwent a variety of timed tasks tests such as movement time, reaction time, and pegboard (10). Additional timed tests included a 25-foot timed walk (TW), five repeated chair sit-to-stand (CS) movements, and five repeated step-ups (SU) onto a 7.5-inch ledge (17). A variety of measures of gait and balance have been used to assess postural control in patients with PD, including Functional Reach (FR) and the Performance-Oriented Assessment (POA) (18–21). FR evaluates the individual's ability to reach forward without stepping and has been correlated with risk of falling in older adults (20). A significant negative correlation has been reported with the H&Y as well as the motor and ADL subscores of the UPDRS (22). During the performance of the FR test the subject stands behind a line and is asked to reach as far forward as possible while maintaining his or her balance. The distance of the forward reach is measured along a yardstick that is placed at the level of the subject's acromion and secured to a wall and is the distance from the startpoint to the endpoint of the reach. The POA is a screening tool that evaluates balance and gait components of mobility (21). It has been reported as a relevant predictor of individuals who suffer recurrent falls (23). The balance section (POAB) is comprised of nine items: sitting balance, standing balance with a progressively narrowed base of support, external perturbations, and turning in a 360-degree circle. The gait section (POAG) contains seven items, including hesitancy, step length, step symmetry, and step height. Significant negative correlations have been reported for both the POAB and POAG with the H&Y and the ADL subscore of the UPDRS (23). The mean Postural Instability Gait Difficulty (PIGD) score was calculated as the mean of the following five items on UPDRS: falling, freezing, walking difficulty by history, and gait and postural instability by examination (15).

Using the Vicon Motion Analysis System, a subset of patients underwent a quantitative assessment of arising from chair, gait, and turning (24). In this system, surface electromyography (EMG) electrodes were placed on the following muscles: quadriceps, hamstrings, tibialis anterior, and triceps surae. The EMG data, recorded during the various tasks at 2,000 samples per second, was integrated offline using a root-mean-square (RMS) algorithm analysis. In addition, a pair of footswitches was placed on the sole of the patient's shoes to identify heel-strikes and toe-offs during walking. A strip of conductive tape was attached to the patient's shorts to identify when the patient had risen from the chair and sat down in the chair. Two path beam sensors were used to identify when the patient crossed a particular point during a maneuver. During various paradigms the patients were instructed to rise from the chair, walk 3 meters to the square, turn 180 degrees inside the square, walk back 3 meters to the chair, turn 180 degrees inside the square in front of the chair, and sit down in the chair.

Sway or the limits of stability (LOS) were measured by posturography using the Smart Balance Master (Neurocom International, Portland, OR, U.S.A.) (25). Posturography was performed at quiet stance with the eyes open (EO), eyes closed (EC), and visual feedback. A target that represented the patient's center of gravity (COG) was presented on the screen for the visual feedback condition as a center target (CT) and the patients were asked to keep their COG within this target for 20 seconds. The limits of stability (LOS) test was performed with the presentation of an ellipse of eight targets arrayed around a center target on a computer screen. These targets were arranged at 75% of the theoretical LOS as determined by each individual's height. The subjects were asked to shift their COG toward the cued target while keeping their feet in place on a force plate.

Finally, an extensive battery of neuropsychological tests was performed. All patients had an MRI scan of the brain preoperatively and at 2 days after PVP; most patients also underwent another scan at 6 months to identify the precise location of their lesion. Assessments of motor function were made at 3 months (short-term), 12 months (long-term), and at the final evaluation (extended).

Statistical Analysis

Descriptive statistics (means, standard deviations, and sample sizes) were calculated. The change between preoperative and postoperative results in the ordinal level data was tested using the Wilcoxon signed ranks test. A one factor (four levels of time—presurgery and postsurgery at 3, 6, and 12 months) repeated measures analysis of variance (ANOVA) with a multivariate approach was used for all of the tests except for the nonparametric POAB, POAG, and TM. These variables were analyzed using the Friedman's two-way ANOVA. The 0.05 level of significance with a Bonferroni adjustment was used for the different variable construct categories in both the "on" and "off" state.

RESULTS

Our results of PVP and its effects on bradykinesia, dyskinesia, and other PD symptoms have been reported elsewhere. Here we describe our findings related to changes in gait and balance following PVP. There were 101 patients enrolled into the study, 89 with unilateral and 12 with bilateral PVP (total of 114 procedures). The mean age of patients at the time of surgery was 61.9 years (range, 36.6 to 76.6), at onset was 47.2 years (range, 19 to 68) and the mean duration of symptoms was 13.9 years (range, 2 to 26.5) (Table 28.1). L-Dopa equivalents showed no significant change in daily dosage from baseline to last follow-up (954.7 ± 683.7 versus 932.2 ± 581.3 mg). Fifteen patients who underwent PVP in our center did not return for their 3-month follow-up. Nine patients cited travel expenses for not returning (four of them eventually returned for their 6-month evaluation and medication adjustment), four continued to benefit from their procedure and, therefore, did not feel compelled to return. Two patients were too ill to

TABLE 28.1. *Baseline characteristics of the patients*

Characteristic	Unilateral PVP N = 89	Bilateral PVP N = 12
Sex (no. of patients)		
Male	46	6
Female	43	6
Side of surgery		
Right	39	6
Left	50	6
Age (yr)		
Mean SD	62.0 ± 9.4	61.2 ± 8.5
Range	36.6–76.6	47.1–72.3
Duration of symptoms (yr)		
Mean SD	13.7 ± 5.8	15.8 ± 7.5
Range	2.0–25.0	3.5–26.5
Duration of follow-up (yr)		
Mean SD	1.4 ± 0.9	1.0 ± 0.8
Range	0.2–3.4	0.2–2.2

TABLE 28.2. *Clinical outcome after unilateral pallidotomy*

	Off-period scores			
	Pre-PVP[1] N = 89	Short-term[2] N = 88	Long-term[3] N = 62	Extended[4] N = 41
Hoehn and Yahr	4.02 ± 0.70	3.08 ± 0.80[a]	3.08 ± 0.79[b]	3.28 ± 0.65[d]
Schwab and England	42.81 ± 14.83	60.45 ± 14.11[a]	59.76 ± 14.33[b]	56.22 ± 11.66[d]
UPDRS ADL	30.84 ± 5.72	20.58 ± 6.56[a]	19.60 ± 5.70[b]	20.88 ± 5.45[d]
UPDRS motor	57.17 ± 13.02	36.85 ± 12.60[a]	34.40 ± 10.61[b]	32.90 ± 15.82[d]
Walking	3.07 ± 0.78	2.14 ± 0.87[a]	2.31 ± 0.82[b]	2.37 ± 0.92[d]
Freezing	2.72 ± 0.97	1.67 ± 0.89[a]	1.52 ± 0.80[b]	1.90 ± 0.83[d]
Fall	1.48 ± 1.16	0.57 ± 0.91[a]	0.53 ± 0.72[b]	0.88 ± 0.95[e]
Postural stability	2.67 ± 0.86	1.80 ± 0.86[a]	1.71 ± 0.91[b]	1.94 ± 0.95[d]
Gait	2.94 ± 0.84	2.09 ± 0.94[a]	2.10 ± 1.04[b]	2.41 ± 0.96[e]
Total PIGD	12.92 ± 3.54	8.29 ± 3.47[a]	8.16 ± 3.32[b]	9.35 ± 3.26[d]
	On-period scores			
	Pre-PVP[1] N = 89	Short-term[2] N = 88	Long-term[3] N = 62	Extended[4] N = 41
Hoehn and Yahr	2.78 ± 0.73	2.07 ± 0.89[a]	1.96 ± 0.92[b]	2.11 ± 0.67[d]
Schwab and England	72.53 ± 13.25	85.00 ± 10.53[a]	85.32 ± 11.27[b]	84.02 ± 8.16[d]
UPDRS ADL	17.02 ± 4.80	10.53 ± 5.51[a]	9.26 ± 4.29[b]	10.12 ± 4.79[d]
UPDRS motor	31.53 ± 9.87	19.30 ± 10.22[a]	17.48 ± 9.49[b]	20.10 ± 7.86[d]
Walking	1.89 ± 0.70	1.14 ± 0.75[a]	1.18 ± 0.67[b]	1.39 ± 0.92[e]
Freezing	1.37 ± 0.80	0.77 ± 0.78[a]	0.63 ± 0.61[b]	0.93 ± 0.79
Fall	0.81 ± 0.96	0.40 ± 0.75[a]	0.29 ± 0.52[c]	0.44 ± 0.71
Postural stability	1.63 ± 0.87	1.01 ± 0.89[a]	0.94 ± 0.92[b]	0.95 ± 0.80[d]
Gait	1.80 ± 0.77	1.28 ± 0.89[a]	1.18 ± 0.95[b]	1.32 ± 0.79[e]
Total PIGD	7.49 ± 2.92	4.58 ± 3.14[a]	4.21 ± 2.71[b]	5.02 ± 3.01[d]

Mean (± SD) "off" and "on" scores.
Lower scores indicate better function except for the Schwab and England score.
P-values calculated from the signed rank test for paired values.
[a]1 versus 2. $P < 0.001$.
[b]1 versus 3. $P < 0.001$.
[c]1 versus 3. $P = 0.002$.
[d]1 versus 4. $P < 0.001$.
[e]1 versus 4. $P = 0.002$.

return. One of them was hospitalized at the time of his 3-month visit for evacuation of a subdural hematoma sustained in a fall. He recovered without deficits and completed his subsequent scheduled visits.

United Parkinson's Disease Rating Scale Gait and Balance Assessments

In this chapter, we analyze those items in UPDRS that are considered relevant measures of gait and balance (Table 28.2). The preoperative UPDRS score for walking was 3.07 ± 0.78 during the "off" period, which indicated a severe disturbance of walking (requiring assistance); the score was 1.89 ± 0.70 during the "on" period (moderate difficulty walking requiring little or no assistance). In addition, the patients exhibited freezing, as indicated by their preoperative "off" and "on" scores, 2.72 ± 0.97 and 1.37 ± 0.80, respectively. They were able to compensate quite well for their gait abnormalities and reported falling only occasionally or rarely: 1.48 ± 1.16 and 0.81 ± 0.96, respectively. Postural stability (2.67 ± 0.86 versus 1.63 ± 0.87) and gait (2.94 ± 0.84 versus 1.80 ± 0.77) were clearly impaired on neurologic examination. The PIGD score, a composite UPDRS score for walking, freezing, and falling (by history), and postural stability and gait (by examination), improved during "off" period from mean of 12.92 ± 3.54 at baseline to 8.29 ± 3.47 at 3 months ($P < 0.001$) and was still substantially lower at 9.35 ± 3.26 at the last follow-up ($P < 0.001$) (1). The respective scores during "on" period were: 7.49 ± 2.92,

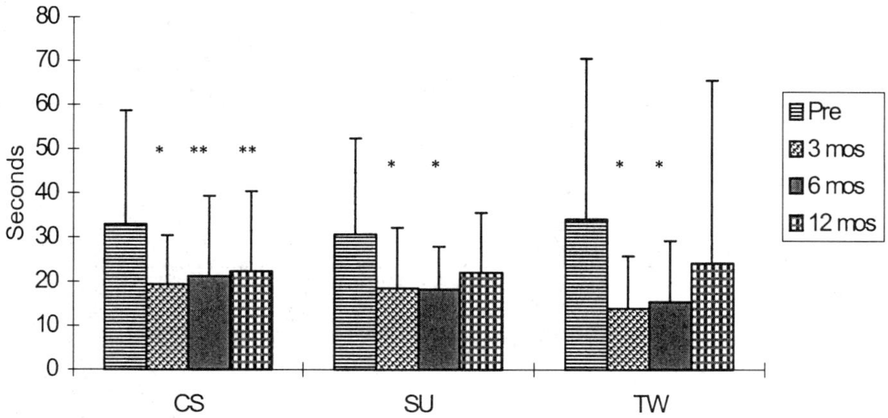

FIG. 28.1. Means and standard deviations for chair stands (*CS*), step-ups (*SU*), and timed walk (*TW*) in seconds when patients are "off" parkinsonian medications at presurgical baseline and 3, 6, and 12 months post-posteroventral pallidotomy. *P ≤ 0.010, **P ≤ 0.05.

4.58 ± 3.14 (P < 0.005) and 5.02 ± 3.01 (P < 0.001). In summary, all the UPDRS measures improved significantly at 3 months after PVP, and this improvement was maintained during the duration of follow-up (mean 2.6 ± 0.6 years).

In the 12 patients who underwent bilateral PVP, the "off" UPDRS gait scores improved from 2.5 to 1.6 at 3 months postoperatively, but increased again to 2.0 at 12 months and at last follow-up during the "off' state. There was no significant change during the "on" state. The sum of UPDRS trunk and lower extremity scores decreased from 18.6 to 12.7 at 3 months but increased again to 14.0 at last follow-up during "off" state; the respective scores for the "on" state were 11.1, 7.1, and 7.7.

Postural Control

Postural control testing, including assessments of strength and relevant components of gait, was performed by 27 patients (16 men and 11 women) at baseline and 12 months post-PVP. Mean age of this subset at baseline was 60.4 ± 9.4 years and the mean symptom duration was 14.7 ± 5.6 years. Their mean Hoehn and Yahr stage was 2.6 during "on" and 4.1 during "off." Means and standard deviations for the postural control

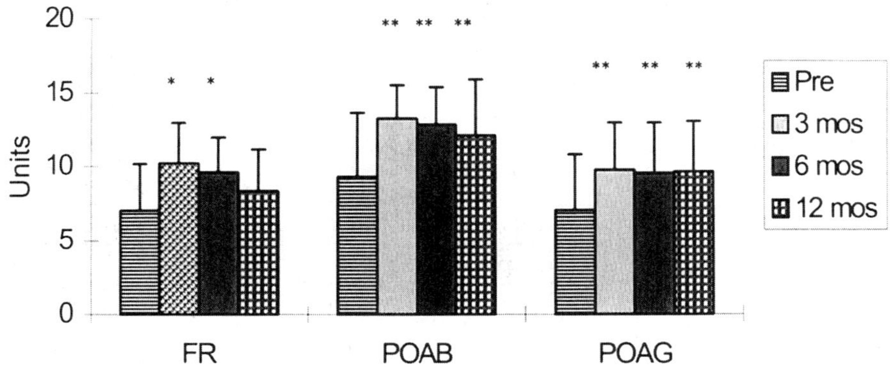

FIG. 28.2. Means for functional reach (*FR*) in inches and performance-oriented assessment of balance (*POAB*) and gait (*POAG*) in ordinal units (higher score is the better score) when patients are "off" parkinsonian medications at presurgical baseline and 3, 6, and 12 months post-posteroventral pallidotomy. *P ≤ 0.001, **P ≤ 0.025.

TABLE 28.3. *Scores for posturography "off" parkinsonian medications presurgery and postsurgery*

	Presurgery		3 Months		6 Months		12 Months	
Variable	Mean	SD	Mean	SD	Mean	SD	Mean	SD
APL	199.37	39.94	185.44	44.22	175.89	37.56	180.38	50.29
ATM	6.60	1.26	5.73	1.42	5.56	1.54	5.85	1.39
TM	0.49	0.34	0.28	0.33	0.27	0.31	0.30	0.34
EPE	437.77	91.60	487.78	74.82	492.39	74.61	474.70	86.21
MXE	524.16	96.73	569.30	64.62	563.81	65.92	545.86	82.29
MV	12.55	4.94	15.02	5.38	15.35	5.81	13.93	5.26

APL, average path length (expressed in % LOS [limits of stability]); ATM, average time (measured in seconds. Maximum time to reach target is 8 seconds); TM, targets missed (percentage of targets missed); EPE, endpoint excursion; MXE, maximum endpoint excursion (expressed in combined units in % LOS for all eight targets); MV, movement velocity (measured in degrees/sec).

variables are seen in Figures 28.1 and 28.2. After unilateral pallidotomy, SU improved by 24% (P = 0.001) and CS by 25% (P = 0.009) at 3 months when compared to baseline during "off" state and a significant improvement persisted for CS during the 12-month follow-up. These variables designed to assess strength, functional balance, and gait showed no significant change in performance after unilateral pallidotomy during "on" time. The maximum distance obtained in the FR test during "off" increased by 33% (P < 0.0005) in 3 months; however the improvement diminished by 12 months, although the mean score was still higher than baseline. The balance scores of the POA (POAB) improved by 37% during "off" at 3 months (P = 0.0002) when compared to baseline and the improvement was still present at 12 months (P = 0.0167). Turning both directions in a 360-degree circle did not demonstrate a significant change post-PVP either during "off" or "on" states. Four patients, however, were unable to turn in either direction before surgery and were able to turn post-PVP. During "off" period, the amount of time needed to complete a 25-foot walk decreased by 42% (P = 0.007) when measured at 3 months after surgery; however, at 12 months the mean speed slowed from the 3-month assessment, although it still remained above baseline. One patient was unable to walk at baseline while "off" but was able to walk the 25-foot distance throughout the post-PVP follow-up. The POAG "off" gait scores improved by 45% (P < 0.0005) at 3 months and were still better at 12 months as compared to baseline (P = 0.025).

Motion Analysis

Using the motion analysis system in five patients during their "off" state, the mean time to perform rise-step decreased at 3 months after PVP compared to baseline from 5.7 to 2.9 seconds, the walk-stop-walk from 22.4 to 7.1 seconds, turning from 16 to 3.2 seconds and walk without stopping from 25.8 to 7.1 seconds. There was a similar but less robust reduction during "on" state.

Posturography

Means and standard deviations for the posturography variables during "off" and "on" states are shown in Tables 28.3 and 28.4, respectively. The difference in LOS tracings is illustrated for

TABLE 28.4. *Scores for posturography "on" parkinsonian medications*

	Presurgery		3 Months		6 Months		12 Months	
Variable	Mean	SD	Mean	SD	Mean	SD	Mean	SD
APL	335.04	254.70	198.95	32.84	188.02	42.26	223.16	84.05
ATM	5.87	1.37	5.12	1.39	5.03	1.39	5.18	1.43
TM	0.35	0.33	0.19	0.25	0.16	0.21	0.20	0.27

APL, average path length (expressed in % LOS [limits of stability]); ATM, average time (expressed in seconds. Maximum time to reach target is 8 seconds); TM, targets missed (percentage of targets missed).

two patients at baseline and 12 months post-PVP during the "off" and "on" states in Figures 28.3 and 28.4, respectively. Average improvement for path deviation during "off" time improved 9% with peak path efficiency being seen at 6 months. The time to reach a target (ATM) and the number of targets missed (TM) improved by 13% and 43%, respectively during "off" time and by 13% and 47%, respectively during "on" time. Improvement for both of these variables remained significant at 12 months post-PVP. There was a significant improvement in movement velocity (MV), endpoint excursion (EPE), and maximum endpoint excursion (MXE) after surgery during "off" state, but not during "on" state. During the "on" state path length deviation decreased significantly. This improvement in path trajectory efficiency was probably owing to decreased postural dyskinesias. There was no change in sway after pallidotomy while the patients were tested during quiet stance either in "off" or "on" state.

DISCUSSION

Abnormalities of gait and balance are among the most disabling symptoms of PD, and these "axial" symptoms often do not respond to dopaminergic or other pharmacologic therapy. Surgical series using thalamotomy, pallidotomy, pallidal or subthalamic deep brain stimulation, and brain grafts have shown benefits in tremor, rigidity, bradykinesia, and L-Dopa-induced dyskinesias, but the effects on gait and balance have been less well documented (3–12,26–38). In our series of 101 patients who underwent a total of 114 pallidotomies we sought to specifically assess the effects of the procedure on measures of gait and balance during short-term and long- term follow-up. Measures related to gait and balance (UPDRS items 27 to 30, score range 0 to 16)

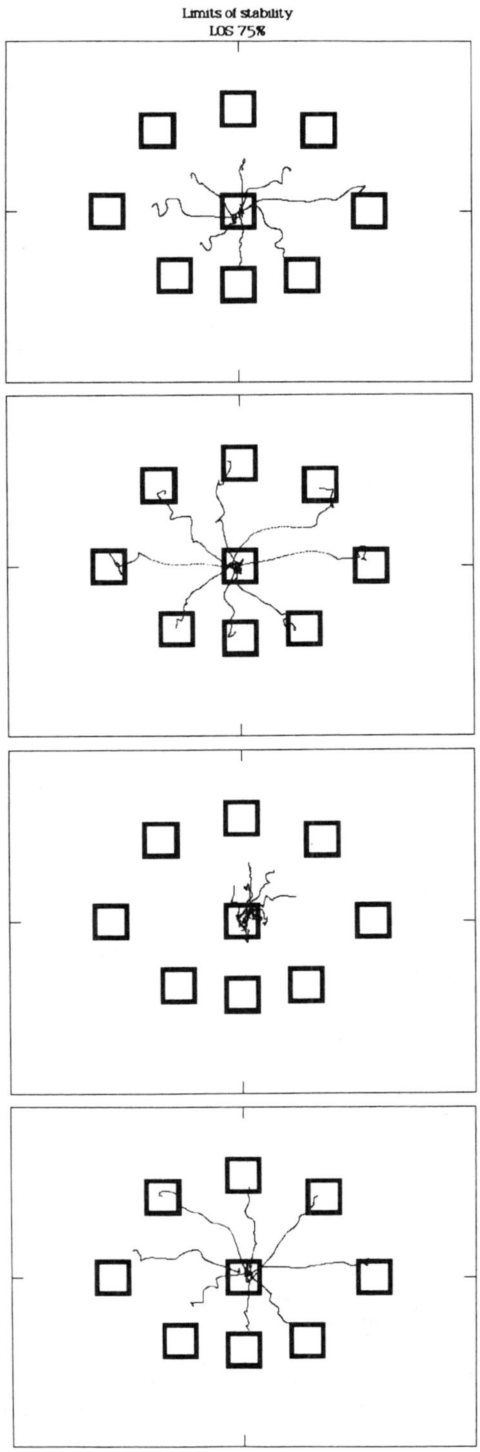

A B C D

FIG. 28.3. LOS path tracings of two patients' performance during the "off" state. The lines indicate the path trajectory of the individuals' attempt to shift their weight towards the cued target. Baseline tracings are represented for patients 1 (A) and 2 (C). Twelve-month follow-up tracings are represented for patients 1 (B) and 2 (D). The range of excursion is very restricted pre-posteroventral pallidotomy. The maintenance of increased range is evident at the 12-month follow-up.

showed a significant improvement from before PVP in both the "off" (33.2% reduction, $P < 0.0001$) and "on" (12.2% reduction, $P < 0.0001$) states at 3 months. The PIGD "off" scores improved 36% at 3 months and 28% at last follow-up; the "on" scores improved 39% and 33%, respectively. After bilateral PVP, the sum of UPDRS trunk and lower extremity "off" scores decreased by 32% at 3 months and by 25% at last; the percent reduction in these scores for the "on" state was 36% and 31%, respectively. Significant improvements were sustained through 12 months and at last evaluation (2.6 ± 0.6 years following PVP). There was also a significant improvement in freezing, but the overall functional improvement was less robust because the benefit was mostly unilateral (contralateral to the PVP) in some patients. In fact, two of our patients who had unilateral improvement in their freezing noted increasing falling, presumably because of loss of balance as a consequence of propulsion with the improved (contralateral) foot while the ipsilateral foot remained stationary. Improvements in measures of postural stability were marked at 3 months but declined for some variables by the 12 months follow-up. Chair sit-to-stand, POA, and posturography variables (LOS) retained significant improvements at 12 months. We conclude that PVP improves axial symptoms of PD, such as gait disturbance and postural instability, in the "off" and "on" state. Generally, the maximum improvement is seen at 3 months, but meaningful benefits can be sustained for up to 3 years following PVP.

The re-emergence of surgical treatment of PD, particularly pallidotomy, has been fueled in part by improved understanding of the basal ganglia

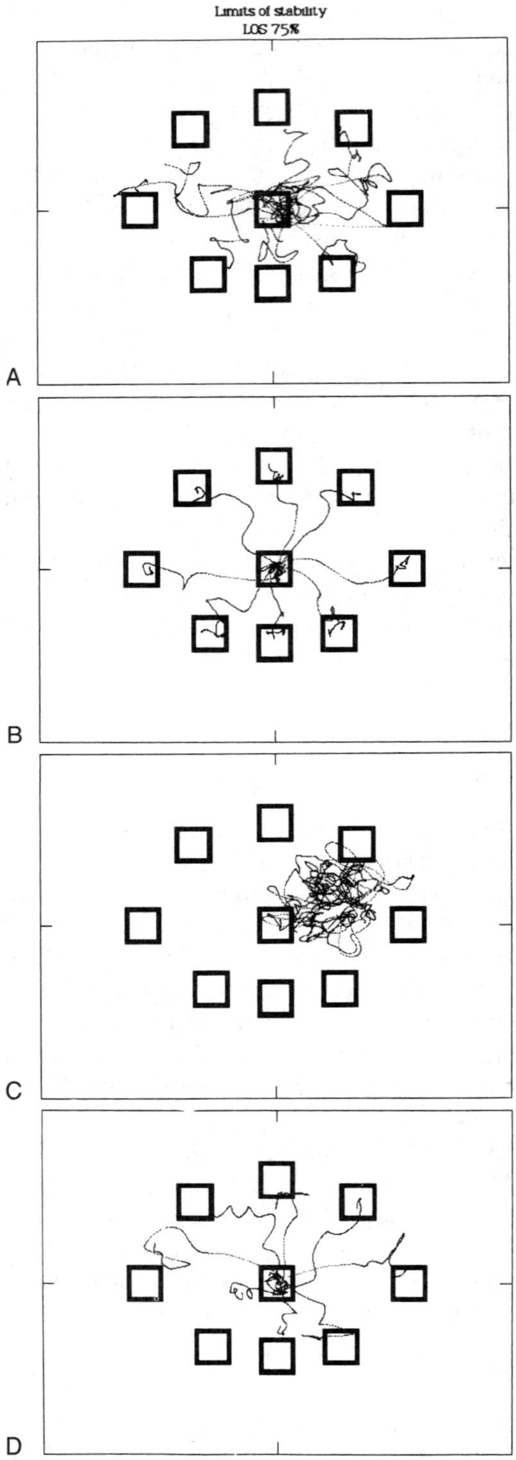

FIG. 28.4. Limits of stability path tracings of two patients' performance during the "on" state. The lines indicate the path trajectory of the individuals' attempt to shift their weight toward the cued target. Baseline tracings are represented for patients 1 (A) and 2 (C). Twelve-month follow-up tracings are represented for patients 1 (B) and 2 (D). Range of excursion is increased in the "on" state but is not controlled and restrictions in some directions are still evident pre-posteroventral pallidotomy (PVP). Maintenance of excursion toward all directions with more control is seen at the 12-month follow-up. Difficulty controlling the trajectory at the endpoint of the excursion is noticeable at 12 months post-PVP.

circuitry, including the recognition that the subthalamic nucleus (STN) and the GPi are overactive in experimental and human parkinsonism (39). Posteroventral pallidotomy improves motor performance in patients with PD, presumably by interrupting inhibitory pallidal projections to ventrolateral thalamus, which in turn projects to the cortex. Measurements by positron emission tomography (PET) of regional cerebral blood flow have shown that the activity of supplementary motor area (SMA) and premotor cortex (but not in primary motor cortex) is increased after PVP (40,41). Because SMA and premotor cortex have been thought to play an important role in gait, the increased activity of these areas after PVP may partly explain the observed improvement in gait following this procedure. What is the evidence that SMA is important in the execution of gait? Lesions in the SMA are associated with pronounced grasp in the contralateral hand (42). Freezing may be considered analogous to a grasp (involving the foot instead of the hand); therefore, restoration of SMA normal function by PVP may lead to an amelioration of freezing. Furthermore, Hanakawa et al. showed enhanced regional cerebral blood flow in the lateral premotor area during paradoxical gait, the well-known phenomenon during which a variety of visual, auditory, and tactile cues and other strategies are used to overcome freezing (43,44). The observed improvements in gait and balance, however, may be additionally mediated by the pallidal–brainstem connections, particularly to the pedunculopontine nucleus (PPN), which has been postulated to represent the mesencephalic locomotor center (45). Electrical stimulation of PPN can induce coordinated, rhythmic stepping movements on a treadmill in a cat or rat, even after intercollicular brainstem transection. Pathological changes have been documented in the PPN in various parkinsonian disorders and isolated lesions of this nucleus can cause gait disorders (45). Located in the caudal mesencephalic tegmentum, PPN receives direct inhibitory (GABA) projections from the striatum, pallidum, and substantia nigra reticulata (SNr) as well as glutamatergic input from the subthalamic nucleus. The pedunculopontine nucleus in turn projects via excitatory cholinergic and glutamatergic pathways to the SNr and to the striatum. In PD, increased activity of the GPi presumably leads to an abnormal inhibition of the PPN, which in turn results in impaired locomotion. It has been, therefore, postulated that the observed improvement in gait after PVP is owing to at least partial restoration of the normal activity of the PPN.

When a lesion is precisely localized to the GPi by neuroimaging or microelectrode recording techniques the benefits can be quite dramatic (3–9,12,13). The most robust effect of pallidotomy is on L-Dopa–induced dyskinesias, although most studies have also demonstrated improvement in contralateral rigidity, tremor, and bradykinesia. Although gait, balance, and freezing may also improve, these axial symptoms usually return within a few months after surgery. In our study the percent time the patients were "on" with dyskinesias decreased from 71.0 to 22.9 ($P < 0.0001$), the percent of patients with troublesome (moderate to violent) dyskinesia decreased from 86 prior to surgery to only 12 after surgery ($P < 0.0001$), and the daily "on" time increased by 52% ($P < 0.0001$) (11). In a blinded review of videotapes of patients during their true "off" time we showed a significant improvement in "off" UPDRS scores in patients undergoing pallidotomy, including a 21.9% improvement in gait score (6). Our longitudinal studies summarized here provide additional evidence that PVP can be helpful not only in PD-related cardinal signs and in L-Dopa–induced complications, but also in gait and postural control. An improvement in postural stability and falls was demonstrated in 9 of 16 (56%) patients who underwent unilateral PVP, the only other study that specifically examined the effects of PVP on postural control (46).

Although our data suggest that PVP improves gait and balance in some patients with PD, we do not recommend this procedure if ambulatory abnormalities are the most troublesome manifestations of the disease. Several studies have provided useful guidelines for inclusion–exclusion criteria but, unfortunately, there are no gait and balance rating scales that can be used to predict the response of these symptoms to PVP (47,48). We relied on clinical assessments based on relevant items of the UPDRS and additional quantitative assessments utilizing validated measures for gait and balance (20,21). There is a need for an easy-to-use, reliable assessment of ambulation and postural stability. A clinical instrument, the Gait And Balance Scale (GABS), is currently being validated and, hopefully, will be utilized in future studies of therapeutic interventions.

REFERENCES

1. Jankovic J, McDermott M, Carter J, et al. Variable expression of Parkinson's disease: a base-line analysis of the DATATOP cohort. *Neurology* 1990;40:1529–1534.
2. Lang AE, Lozano AM. Parkinson's disease. *N Engl J Med* 1998;339:1044–1053;1130–1143.
3. Baron MS, Vitek JL, Bakay RAE, et al. Treatment of advanced Parkinson's disease by posterior GPi pallidotomy: 1-year results of a pilot study. *Ann Neurol* 1996;40:355–366.
4. Fazzini E, Dogali M, Sterio D, et al. Stereotactic pallidotomy for Parkinson's disease: a long-term follow-up of unilateral pallidotomy. *Neurology* 1997;48:1273–1277.
5. Lang AE, Lozano A, Montgomery E, et al. Posteroventral-medial pallidotomy in advanced Parkinson's disease. *N Engl J Med* 1997;337:1036–1042.
6. Ondo W, Jankovic J, Lai E, et al. Assessment of motor function following stereotactic pallidotomy. *Neurology* 1998;50:266–270.
7. Samuel M, Caputo E, Brooks DJ, et al. A study of medial pallidotomy for Parkinson's disease: clinical outcome, MRI location and complications. *Brain* 1998;121:59–75.
8. Gross RE, Lombardi WJ, Lang AE, et al. Relationship of lesion location to clinical outcome following microelectrode-guided pallidotomy for Parkinson's disease. *Brain* 1999;122 405–416.
9. Samii A, Turnbull IM, Kishore A, et al. Reassessment of unilateral pallidotomy in Parkinson's disease. A 2-year follow-up study. *Brain* 1999;122:417–425.
10. Jankovic J, Ben-Arie L, Schwartz K, et al. Movement and reaction times and fine coordination tasks following pallidotomy. *Mov Disord* 1999;14:57–62.
11. Jankovic J, Lai E, Ben-Arie L, et al. Levodopa-induced dyskinesias treated by pallidotomy. *J Neurol Sci* 1999;167:62–67.
12. Krauss JK, Desaloms M, Lai EC, et al. Microelectrode-guided posteroventral pallidotomy for treatment of Parkinson's disease: postoperative magnetic resonance imaging analysis. *J Neurosurg* 1997;87:358–367.
13. Krauss JK, Grossman RG. Operative techniques for pallidal surgery. In: Krauss JK, Grossman RG, Jankovic J, eds. *Pallidal surgery for the treatment of Parkinson's disease and movement disorders*. Philadelphia: Lippincott–Raven, 1998:121–134
14. Desaloms JM, Krauss JK, Lai EC, et al. Posteroventral medial pallidotomy for Parkinson's disease: Preoperative magnetic resonance imaging features and clinical outcome. *J Neurosurg* 1998;89:194–199.
15. Fahn S, Elton RI, Members of the UPDRS Development Committee. Unified Parkinson's Disease Rating Scale. In: Fahn S, Marsden CD, Calne DB, et al, eds. *Recent developments in Parkinson's disease*, vol 2. Florham Park, NJ: Macmillan Health Care Information, 1987:153–164.
16. Langston JW, Widner H, Goetz CG, et al. Core Assessment Program for Intracerebral Transplantations (CAPIT). *Mov Disord* 1992;7:2–13.
17. Overby AS, Roberts-Warrior D, Jankovic J, et al. Does bradykinesia improve after pallidotomy? [abstract] *Ann Neurol* 1996;40:535.
18. Shumway-Cook A. Critical analysis of measurement of balance: a clinical approach. Eugene Michels Research Forum. *APTA* 1996:5–8.
19. Winter DA, Patla AE, Frank JS. Assessment of balance control in humans. *Med Prog Technol* 1990;16:31–51.
20. Duncan P, Weiner DK, Chandler JM, et al. Functional reach: a new clinical measure of balance. *J Gerontol* 1992;47:M93–M98.
21. Tinetti ME. Performance-oriented assessment of mobility problems in elderly patients. *JAGS* 1986;34:119–126.
22. Overby T, Roberts-Warrior D, Lai E. Changes in postural control after pallidotomy. In: Krauss JK, Grossman RG, Jankovic J, eds. *Pallidal surgery for the treatment of Parkinson's disease and movement disorders*. Philadelphia: Lippincott-Raven, 1998:191–210.
23. Tinetti ME, Williams TF, Mayewski R. Fall risk index for elderly patients based on number of chronic disabilities. *Am J Med* 1986;80:429–434.
24. Pollo FE. Clinical gait analysis in biomechanics. *IEEE Eng Med Biol Mag* 1998;17:32–33.
25. Nashner LM. Computerized dynamic posturography. In: Jacobson GP, Newman CW, Kartush JM, eds. *Handbook of balance function testing*. St. Louis: Mosby Year Book, 1993:280–307.
26. Cardoso F, Jankovic J, Grossman RG, et al. Outcome after stereotactic thalamotomy for dystonia and hemiballismus. *Neurosurgery* 1995;36:501–508.
27. Zirh A, Reich SG, Dougherty PM, et al. Stereotactic thalamotomy in the treatment of essential tremor of the upper extremity: reassessment including a blinded measure of outcome. *J Neurol Neurosurg Psychaitry* 1999;66:772–775.
28. Dalvi A, Winfield L, Yu Q, et al. Stereotactic posteroventral pallidotomy: clinical methods and results at 1-year follow up. *Mov Disord* 1999;14:256–261.
29. Schrag A, Samuel M, Caputo E, et al. Unilateral pallidotomy for Parkinson's disease: results after more than 1 year. *J Neurol Neurosurg Psychiatry* 1999;67:511–517.
30. Limousin P, Speelman JD, Gielen F, et al. Multicenter European study of thalamic stimulation in parkinsonian and essential tremor. *J Neurol Neurosurg Psychiatry* 1999;66:289–296.
31. Krack P, Pollak P, Limousin P, et al. Subthalamic nucleus or internal pallidal stimulation in young onset Parkinson's disease. *Brain* 1998;121:451–457.
32. Merello M, Nouzeilles MI, Kuzis G, et al. Unilateral radiofrequency lesion versus electrostimulation of posteroventral pallidum: a prospective randomized comparison. *Mov Disord* 1999;14:50–56.
33. Kumar R, Lozano AM, Sime E, et al. Comparative effects of unilateral and bilateral subthalamic nucleus deep brain stimulation. *Neurology* 1999;53:561–566.
34. Pollak P, Benabid AL, Krack P, et al. Deep brain stimulation. In: Jankovic J, Tolosa E, eds. *Parkinson's disease and movement disorders,* 3rd ed. Baltimore: Williams & Wilkins, 1998:1085–1102.
35. Starr PA, Vitek JL, Bakay RAE. Ablative surgery and deep brain stimulation for Parkinson's disease. *Neurosurgery* 1998;43:989–1015.

36. Wenning GK, Odin P, Morrish P, et al. Short- and long-term survival and function of unilateral intrastriatal dopaminergic grafts in Parkinson's disease. *Ann Neurol* 1997;42:95–107.
37. Lindvall O. Update on fetal transplantation: the Swedish experience. *Mov Disord* 1998;13:84–87.
38. Hauser RA, Freeman TB, Snow BJ, et al. Long term evaluation of bilateral fetal nigral transplantation in Parkinson disease. *Arch Neurol* 1999;56:179–187.
39. Bergman H, Wichmann T, DeLong MR. Reversal of experimental parkinsonism by lesions of the subthalamic nucleus. *Science* 1990;249:1436–1438.
40. Grafton ST, Waters C, Sutton J, et al. Pallidotomy increases activity of motor association cortex in Parkinson's disease: a positron emission tomographic study. *Ann Neurol* 1995;37:776–783.
41. Eidelberg D, Moeller JR, Ishikawa T, et al. Regional metabolic correlates of surgical outcome following unilateral pallidotomy for Parkinson's disease. *Ann Neurol* 1996;39:450–459.
42. Hashimoto R, Tanaka Y. Contribution of the supplementary motor area and anterior cingulate gyrus to pathological grasping phenomenon. *Eur Neurol* 1998;40:151–158.
43. Hanakawa T, Fukuyama H, Katsumi Y, et al. Enhanced lateral premotor activity during paradoxical gait in Parkinson's disease. *Ann Neurol* 1999;45:329–336.
44. Hanakawa T, Katsumi Y, Fukuyama H, et al. Mechanisms underlying gait disturbance in Parkinson's disease. A single photon emission computed tomography study. *Brain* 1999;122:1271–1282.
45. Masdeu JC, Alampur U, Cavaliere R, et al. Astasia and gait failure with damage of the pontomesencephalic locomotor region. *Ann Neurol* 1994;35:619–621.
46. Melnick ME, Dowling GA, Aminoff MJ, et al. Effect of pallidotomy on postural control and motor function in Parkinson's disease. *Arch Neurol* 1999;56:1361–1365.
47. Defer G-L, Widner H, Marié R-M, et al. Core assessment program for surgical interventional therapy in Parkinson's disease (CAPSIT-PD). *Mov Disord* 1999;14:572–584.
48. Tan EK, Jankovic J. Movement disorder surgery: patient selection and evaluation of surgical results. In: Lozano AM, ed. *Movement disorder surgery: progress and challenges, progress in neurological surgery*. Basel: Karger, 2000:78–90.

Gait Disorders. Advances in Neurology, Vol. 87,
edited by E. Růžička, M. Hallett, and J. Jankovic.
Lippincott Williams & Wilkins, Philadelphia © 2001.

29

The Role of the Pallidum in Parkinson's Disease Gait

Lessons from Pallidal Stimulation

*†Philippe Damier, ‡Jean-Luc Houeto, ||¶Boulos-Paul Bejjani, §Isabelle Arnulf, ‡Anne-Marie Bonnet, ‡Malika Miloudy, and ‡Yves Agid

**Department of Neurology, Faculty of Medicine, University Hospital of Nantes, Nantes F-44035, France; †Department of Neurology, Laennec Hospital, CHU Nantes, Nantes F-44093; ‡Federation of Neurology, Clinical Investigation Center, §Service of Functional Pneumological Explorations, Salpetriere Hospital, Paris 75013, France; ||Department of Neurology, Faculty of Medicine, University of Saint Joseph, Beruit, Lebanon; and ¶Parkinson & Movement Disorders Center, Notre Dame des Secours Hospital, Byblos-Jbeil, Lebanon*

Gait impairment is a complex symptom of Parkinson's disease (PD), varying in its presentation from one patient to another. It is typically manifested by slowness, ignition failure, freezing and postural instability. The pathophysiology of this disabling symptom is still poorly known and is probably linked to different mechanisms. Striatal dopamine deficiency, resulting from degeneration of the dopaminergic nigrostriatal pathway, clearly plays a role since in some patients gait impairment is improved by exogenous dopamine provided by L-Dopa or by direct activation of dopamine receptors with dopamine agonists. Most gait disturbances, however, are not improved or only partially improved by dopamine replacement, suggesting that nondopaminergic lesions are involved in this symptom (1). In particular, lesions of the noradrenergic locus ceruleus or the pedunculopontine nucleus have been suspected (2). Moreover, many other factors, such as side effects of the medical treatment (e.g., dyskinesias, orthostatic hypotension), posture abnormalities, fear of falls, likely account for the difficulties that patients experience in walking. Surgical treatment, recently proposed in patients with PD, acts downstream from the dopamine deficiency and might therefore act on the nondopaminergic factors responsible for gait impairment.

HIGH-FREQUENCY STIMULATION: AN ACTION DOWNSTREAM FROM DOPAMINE DEFICIENCY

From the classical model of the functioning of basal ganglia circuitry, dopamine deficiency in the striatum leads to a neural hyperactivity of the subthalamic nucleus (STN), the substantia nigra pars reticulata (SNr), and the internal part of the globus pallidus (GPi) (3). The resulting increased inhibitory outflow to the lateral thalamus and the pedunculopontine nucleus is considered to be responsible for most of the motor features observed in patients with PD. In contrast to the medical treatment, which aims to re-establish normal dopamine transmission in the striatum, the goal of surgical treatment is to act directly on the abnormal hyperactive nuclei in order to restore normal outflow to the output nuclei of the basal ganglia. A first approach is to lesion the

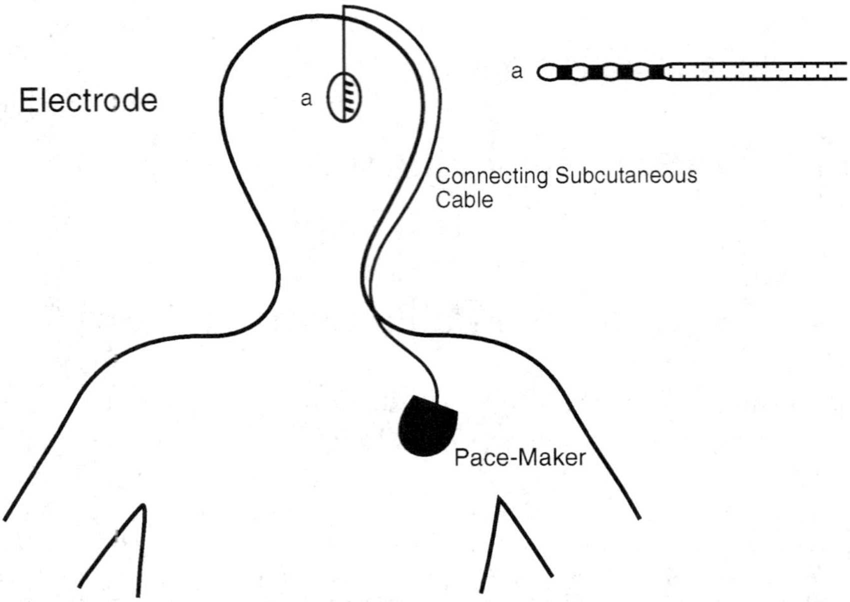

FIG. 29.1. High-frequency stimulation in the treatment of Parkinson's disease. A quadripolar electrode (3387, Medtronic, Minneapolis, MN, U.S.A.) is implanted in the target nucleus (subthalamic nucleus, globus pallidus) by stereotaxic surgery. Ventriculography and/or magnetic resonance imaging are used to visualize the target, and intraoperative microrecordings and clinical testing of the effects of stimulation in a patient under local anesthesia ensure that the optimal functional site is targeted. In most cases, surgery is performed bilaterally, with one electrode on each side of the brain. Each electrode is connected by a cable to a programmable pulse generator (ITREL II, Medtronic) implanted subcutaneously in the subclavicular area. The system allows continuous, 24-hour, high-frequency stimulation to be applied through the target nucleus. By telemetry, the pulse generator can be stopped or fine-tuned [voltage, frequency, pulse width, choice of one of the electrode's four stimulation contacts (*a*)] in order to obtain the maximal improvement of parkinsonian motor signs without inducing side effects. In contrast to a lesion, this technique has the advantage of reversibility of the effects and adaptability of the fine-tuning.

hyperactive nuclei. Lesioning of the GP (pallidotomy) in PD patients and of the STN in monkeys rendered parkinsonian through administration of 1-methyl-4-phenyl-1,2,3,6-tetrahydropyridine (MPTP), a selective toxic for dopamine-containing neurons, has been shown to significantly reduce parkinsonian motor disability (4,5). After having demonstrated that continuous high-frequency stimulation (Fig. 29.1) applied to the ventrolateral thalamus and the lesioning of this structure have a similar effect in reducing essential or PD tremor, Benabid et al. proposed applying the same technique to the hyperactive nuclei in order to treat patients with severe PD (6). This group and others have now clearly demonstrated that STN stimulation is highly effective in ameliorating most of the motor features of PD, with a marked reduction in patient disability and a decrease in the need for dopaminergic drug treatment (7). Results of pallidal stimulation, however, are more conflicting, with a dramatic suppression of drug-induced dyskinesias but a less consistent effect on PD motor signs (8–12).

From these considerations, a surgical approach to these abnormal nuclei can be expected to act mainly on the direct consequences of striatal dopamine deficiency, thus mimicking the effect of the drug treatment but with the advantage of a continuous action and the absence of the dopaminergic drug's side effects. These advantages might contribute to a more beneficial effect of surgical treatment compared to the drug treatment on PD motor features. Moreover, rather than being solely the consequence of dopamine deficiency, the abnormal hyperactivity of the STN, GP, and SNr might also result from neural dysfunction owing to nondopaminergic lesions. For example, direct connections between the STN and the pedunculopontine nucleus might account for the abnormal activity of the STN observed in PD (13). Therefore, treatment at the level of these abnormally hyperactive nuclei might also provide a beneficial effect on symptoms resulting from mechanisms other than the dopamine deficiency.

EFFECT OF PALLIDAL STIMULATION ON GAIT IMPAIRMENT

Five studies analyzed the effect of pallidal stimulation on gait impairment (Table 29.1). Gait was assessed before and after GP stimulation had been applied continuously for 3 months, the patients being deprived of dopaminergic treatment ("off" drug state). All but one of the studies found that pallidal stimulation significantly improved gait impairment. Volkmann and colleagues investigated in detail the effect of pallidal stimulation on PD gait using a computer-assisted analysis system (9). They found that the improvement of gait velocity was owing to both a significant increase in cadence and a significant decrease in step time, the latter being explained by a reduction in the double support time, whereas the duration of the swing phase was unchanged. These authors also found a clear improvement in the pattern of gait in seven of the nine subjects analyzed in this study. Hypokinetic gait disturbance with propulsion and tiptoeing as well as severe freezing was found to be dramatically improved with the restoration of an almost normal gait pattern in some patients under pallidal stimulation. In these four studies, most of the patients received bilateral GP stimulation. From our own experience, although unilateral pallidal stimulation can have a beneficial effect on gait impairment, the beneficial effect is stronger with bilateral GP stimulation.

These studies demonstrated an unequivocal improvement of parkinsonian gait when high-frequency stimulation was applied to the GP in patients deprived of striatal dopamine ("off" drug state). On the other hand, several studies have already reported the efficacy of L-Dopa or dopamine agonists in the treatment of some of the gait disorders observed in PD (14). This raises the question of whether or not pallidal stimulation and dopamine restoration treatment have similar effects on PD gait impairment. The significant improvement in gait after 3 months of pallidal stimulation in comparison to gait before surgery while patients are under the effect of dopaminergic treatment ("on" drug state) reported by

TABLE 29.1. *Effects of pallidal stimulation on gait impairment in Parkinson's disease*

Studies (reference)	Number of patients[a]	Assessment	Percentage of improvement (significance)
Pahwa et al., 1997 (8)	5 (3)	Walking time test (15 feet from a standing start, turn around and return)	27 (NS)
Volkmann et al., 1998 (9)	9 (9)	Gait velocity (computer-assisted analysis system)	32 ($P < 0.05$)
Krack et al., 1998 (10)	5 (5)	Gait score (UPDRS)	41 ($P < 0.05$)
Kumar et al., 1998 (11)	8 (4)	Gait + postural stability (UPDRS)	55 ($P < 0.01$)
Author's series	5 (5)	Gait score (UPDRS)	37 ($P < 0.05$)

Assessed 3 months after surgery in patients deprived of antiparkinson medication ("off" drug state).
NS, not significant, UPDRS, Unified Parkinson's Disease Rating Scale.
[a] The number of patients with bilateral implantation is indicated in parentheses.

Pahwa and colleagues, might suggest that pallidal stimulation provides an additional improvement in PD gait to that linked to the medical treatment (8). In this study, however, the patients' gait was also significantly improved 3 months after surgery when medical treatment was withdrawn and stimulation turned off for 1 hour ("off" drug, "off" stimulation state) compared to before surgery in the "off" drug condition. One possible explanation is a long-term effect of pallidal stimulation, still exerting a beneficial action on gait after the stimulator has been turned off for 1 hour. An alternative explanation is that gait improvement was not owing to a direct effect of pallidal stimulation but was related to several nonspecific factors improved by continuous pallidal stimulation, such as the reduction in motor fluctuations and drug-induced dyskinesias. For example, the reduction of disabling, drug-induced dyskinesias may lead to an improvement in abnormal posture, helping the patient to walk more easily, and may also make the patient more confident and less afraid of falling. To date, only one study has assessed the effect of pallidal stimulation on PD gait with a detailed comparison of the effect of drug treatment and GP stimulation (15). In this study, gait was assessed with a computer-assisted analysis system before surgery in the "off" and "on" drug states and, in the same drug conditions, while patients were being treated by continuous pallidal stimulation. In line with other studies, they found that the improvement in most gait parameters was owing solely to pallidal stimulation by comparing gait before and after surgery in patients deprived of drug treatment. The study also found a better effect of the combined treatment ("on" stimulation, "on" drug) compared to the effect of L-Dopa alone before surgery or pallidal stimulation alone after surgery. The additional improvement provided by the combined treatment was, however, mild and a significant interaction between L-Dopa treatment and stimulation was noted only for the single and double support time. These preliminary data might suggest that pallidal stimulation also corrects some factors responsible for gait disorders that are not directly linked to dopamine deficiency. Further studies are, however, still required to clearly differentiate between the respective effects of drugs and GP stimulation on PD gait. From a practical point of view, although encouraging, these data and the mildness of the additional effect of stimulation on the effect of the drug lead us not to recommend at this stage the use of pallidal stimulation in PD patients with severe L-Dopa–unresponsive gait disorders.

CONTRASTING EFFECT OF INTERNAL AND EXTERNAL PALLIDAL STIMULATION ON GAIT IMPAIRMENT

In contrast to the STN, a small nucleus in which the application of high frequency stimulation improves all cardinal motor features of PD, the GP is a large nucleus in which the effect of stimulation varies from one part to another (16,17). Stimulation applied to the dorsal part of the GP (GPe) improved all PD motor signs (i.e., rigidity, gait, and tremor) and could induce dyskinesias at voltages higher that 4 volts in patients in the "off" drug state. Stimulation applied to the ventral part of the GP (GPi) improved only rigidity but worsened akinesia. When the patient was in the "on" drug state and experienced dyskinesias, stimulation applied to the GPi dramatically reduced them, whereas stimulation applied to the GPe had no significant effect. As observed in the case of akinesia, GPe stimulation improved gait impairment, whereas GPi stimulation worsened it (Fig. 29.2). A great deal of uncertainty remains as to the pathophysiologic explanation for these clinical observations. In particular, they are difficult to reconcile with the model of functioning of the basal ganglia circuitry and the generally accepted postulate that the global mechanism of high frequency acts through neuroinactivation (3,6). If it were indeed the case, according to the classic model of basal ganglia functioning one might have expected an improvement of all parkinsonian signs when stimulation was applied to the GPi and a worsening of such signs when stimulation was applied to the GPe. However, the results of our study on the effect of stimulation on gait and akinesia clearly showed the opposite. These discrepancies might suggest that in contrast to the STN or the lateral thalamus, high-frequency stimulation does not act through a simple neural inactivation in the GP. Overall,

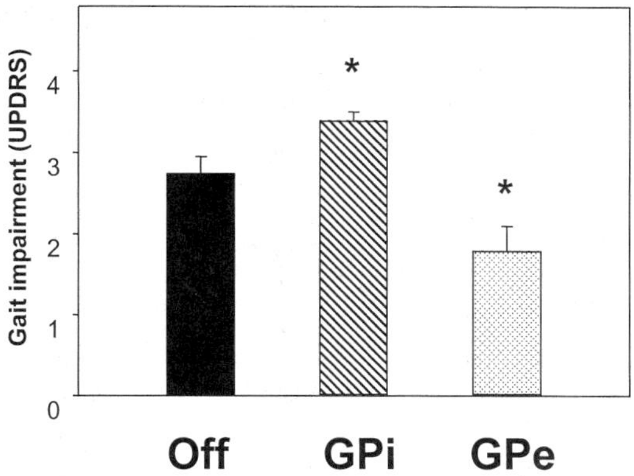

FIG. 29.2. Comparison of gait impairment (assessed by item 20 of the Unified Parkinson's Disease Rating Scale) before (*Off*) and during unilateral stimulation through the internal (*GPi*) and the external (*GPe*) globus pallidus in five patients deprived of drug treatment ("off" drug state). For each patient the voltage applied was that which had the maximal effect on parkinsonian symptoms without inducing side effects (range, 1 to 4.5 V). $^{*}P < 0.05$.

the beneficial effect of pallidal stimulation on gait impairment reported by several groups could indeed be owing to a combination of the antiakinetic effects of stimulation through the GPe and of the antidyskinetic effects through the GPi (Table 29.1). In our pathophysiologic study, however, these effects were observed after a unilateral stimulation had been applied for a few minutes in the different parts of the GP. The global effect of stimulation applied continuously and bilaterally in the chronic treatment of the patients might well be different. Further studies are needed to improve our understanding of the function of the basal circuitry and of the mechanisms of high-frequency stimulation.

LONG-TERM EFFECT OF PALLIDAL STIMULATION

There are no published data on the long-term effects of pallidal stimulation. Our own experience, however, is that most patients seem to lose the *initial* improvement in gait provided by pallidal stimulation after 1 year of treatment, as was noted after pallidotomy (Chapter 12) (18). A recent observation has led to the suggestion that pallidal stimulation might in fact also contribute to the development of motor side effects. A 66-year-old woman with a 19-year history of L-Dopa–responsive PD was implanted with stimulation electrodes bilaterally in the GP for high-frequency stimulation treatment. At the time of surgery she was severely disabled with motor fluctuations and L-Dopa–induced dyskinesias despite optimized medical treatment. Gait impairment with freezing was noticed during the "off" phase, but resolved totally in the "on" drug phase although intense dyskinesias often accompanied this state. The best therapeutic effect was obtained with stimulation applied chronically to the left GPi (2.4 V, 130 Hz, 60 μs pulse width) and the right GPe (2.8 V, 130 Hz, 60 μs pulse width). A few weeks after surgery, the patient greatly improved, with a significant reduction in L-Dopa–induced dyskinesias and motor fluctuations. The drug treatment was unchanged. One year after surgery, motor fluctuations progressively reappeared with intermittent gait freezing. Despite various changes in stimulation parameters and drug treatment, the patient's medical status worsened, with a more and more prolonged "off" phase and severe dyskinesias when an attempt was made to increase L-Dopa dosage. As her status worsened she also presented a progressive stooped posture, which gradually became fixed. The kyphoscoliotic posture resulted in dorsal pain and breathing difficulties. Prolonged inactivation of the stimulators was not feasible because of the severity of the resulting parkinsonian state. The medical status of the patient gave such cause for concern that we decided to remove her pallidal electrodes and implant bilateral STN electrodes. A few days after high-frequency stimulation had been applied to the STN, the patient significantly improved, with a reduction in the duration and intensity of the "off" phase and an almost total resolution of the stooped posture. Chronic pallidal stimulation might have been directly responsible for the kyphoscoliotic posture, possibly related to the putative "dyskinetic effect" of the GPe stimulation. The efficacy of STN stimulation in reducing PD motor signs without inducing dyskinesias allowed pallidal stimulation to be stopped and may thus have suppressed this stimulation-induced side effect. An alternative explanation could be that the abnormal posture and progressive worsening of the parkinsonian state was owing to the disease itself, but that STN stimulation constituted a more effective treatment than pallidal stimulation. This latter hypothesis is in accordance with reported comparative, albeit noncontrolled, evaluations suggesting that STN stimulation is more efficient than pallidal stimulation in the treatment of severe PD.

CONCLUSION

The role of the GP in PD-related gait impairment remains poorly understood. Unequivocally, this nucleus plays a role because high-frequency stimulation applied in the GP improves this disabling symptom. Whether this effect corresponds solely to the correction of pallidal dysfunctions induced by striatal dopamine deficiency or also results from an action on other neural dysfunctions owing to nondopaminergic mechanisms is still not known. However, the available data provide no indication that such treatment can have a strong effect on gait disturbances unresponsive to L-Dopa, which constitute one of the major problems in the practical management of patients.

REFERENCES

1. Marsden CD, Parkes JD. Success and problems of long-term levodopa therapy in Parkinson's disease. *Lancet* 1977;1:345–349.
2. Jellinger KA. Pathology of Parkinson's disease. Changes other than the nigrostriatal pathway. *Mol Chem Neuropathol* 1991;14:153–197.
3. DeLong MR. Primate model of movement disorders of basal ganglia origin. *Trends Neurosci* 1990;13:281–289.
4. Laitinen LV, Bergenheim AT, Hariz MI. Leksell's posteroventral pallidotomy in the treatment of Parkinson's disease. *J Neurosurg* 1992;76:53–61.
5. Bergman H, Wichmann T, DeLong MR. Reversal of experimental parkinsonism by lesions of the subthalamic nucleus. *Science* 1990;249:1436–1438.
6. Benabid AL, Pollak P, Gervason C, et al. Long-term suppression of tremor by chronic stimulation of the ventral intermediate thalamic nucleus. *Lancet* 1991;337:403–406.
7. Limousin P, Krack P, Pollak P, et al. Electrical stimulation of the subthalamic nucleus in advanced Parkinson's disease. *N Engl J Med* 1998;339:1105–1111.
8. Pahwa R, Wilkinson S, Smith D, et al. High-frequency stimulation of the globus pallidus for the treatment of Parkinson's disease. *Neurology* 1997;49:249–253.
9. Volkmann J, Sturm V, Weiss P, et al. Bilateral high-frequency stimulation of the internal globus pallidus in advanced Parkinson's disease. *Ann Neurol* 1998;44:953–961.
10. Krack P, Pollak P, Limousin P, et al. Subthalamic nucleus or internal pallidal stimulation in young onset Parkinson's disease. *Brain* 1998;121:451–457.
11. Kumar R, Lozano AM, Montgomery E, et al. Pallidotomy and deep brain stimulation of the pallidum and subthalamic nucleus in advanced Parkinson's disease. *Mov Disord* 1998;13:73–82.
12. Durif F, Lemaire JJ, Debilly B, et al. Acute and chronic effects of anteromedial globus pallidus stimulation in Parkinson's disease [In Process Citation]. *J Neurol Neurosurg Psychiatry* 1999;67:315–322.
13. Smith Y, Hazrati L-N, Parent A. Efferent projections of the subthalamic nucleus in the squirrel monkey as studied by the PHA-L anterograde tracing method. *J Comp Neurol* 1990;294:306–323.
14. O'Sullivan JD, Said CM, Dillon LC, et al. Gait analysis in patients with Parkinson's disease and motor fluctuations: influence of levodopa and comparison with other measures of motor function. *Mov Disord* 1998;13:900–906.
15. Krystkowiak P, Defebvre JL, Blatt JL, et al. Pallidal stimulation improves gait in Parkinson's disease: a study using the optoelectronic vicon system. *Parkinsonism Rel Disord* 1999;5:107A.
16. Bejjani B, Damier P, Arnulf I, et al. Pallidal stimulation for Parkinson's disease: two targets? *Neurology* 1997;49:1564–1569.
17. Krack P, Pollak P, Limousin P, et al. Opposite motor effects of pallidal stimulation in Parkinson's disease. *Ann Neurol* 1998;43:180–192.
18. Lang AE, Lozano AM, Montgomery E, et al. Posteroventral medial pallidotomy in advanced Parkinson's disease. *N Engl J Med* 1997;337:1036–1042.

Gait Disorders. Advances in Neurology, Vol. 87,
edited by E. Růžička, M. Hallett, and J. Jankovic.
Lippincott Williams & Wilkins, Philadelphia © 2001.

30

Bilateral Subthalamic Stimulation and Parkinsonian Gait

[†]Francesc Valldeoriola, [‡]José L. Molinuevo, and [*†]Josep Valls-Solé

[*]Department of Medicine, University of Barcelona; [†]Department of Neurology, Hospital Clinic Universitari 08036 Barcelona, Spain; and [‡]Department of Neurology, Hospital de Palamos, Palamos, 17230 Girona, Spain

Excessive neuronal driving onto the internal pallidum is one of the most important functional disturbances taking place in Parkinson's disease (PD) according to the currently accepted functional model of the basal ganglia circuitry (1). Despite several deficiencies, this model allows us to generate hypotheses to explain the functional changes taking place in the brain in patients with PD. In this model the striatum represents the main afferent structure of the basal ganglia and the most important striatal afferent is the dopaminergic nigrostriatal projection, whose lesion or degeneration results in parkinsonism. In addition, all cortical areas project to the striatum: The somatosensory and motor cortices project mainly to the putamen and the caudate nucleus receives projections from the prefrontal and other cortical areas. The striatum projects somatotopically to both the internal and external pallidal segments from different cell populations. There is a GABA-ergic pathway from the putamen to the internal pallidum (direct pathway) and another pathway from the putamen to the external pallidum (indirect pathway). The external pallidum inhibits the subthalamic nucleus (STN) and the subthalamus exerts a glutamate-mediated excitatory action over the internal pallidum and the substantia nigra pars reticulata (SNr). The internal segment of the pallidum (GPi) and the SNr are the main efferent nucleus of the basal ganglia, projecting to the motor thalamus and from the thalamus to the cortex, mainly the supplementary motor area. In the parkinsonian state, dopaminergic depletion causes a reduction of the activity of striatal neurons projecting directly to the GPi and an increase of the activity of the striatal neurons projecting to the external pallidum, leading to an increased activity of STN neurons. Such increased activity of STN excitatory neurons enhances the GPi and SNR output and leads in turn to an increased inhibition of the thalamus and thalamocortical circuits (2–4). This results in the inhibition of the cortical motor system, with the consequence of akinesia, rigidity, and tremor. The inhibitory descending projections of the GPi and SNr may contribute to abnormalities of gait and posture. In this setting, STN neuron blockade could induce a substantial amelioration of parkinsonian symptoms, which results in large part from excessive STN and pallidal activity. It has been shown in MPTP-treated primates that subthalamotomy and subthalamic stimulation can improve parkinsonian symptoms such as akinesia, tremor, and rigidity (5–11). In humans with PD, there is also recent evidence that chronic STN stimulation induces an important amelioration of parkinsonian symptoms (12–18). All these physiological and clinical data reinforce the important role of the STN in the control of the basal ganglia outflow.

MECHANISMS

The rationale for the observed improvement of gait and posture disturbances in PD after subthalamotomy or STN stimulation is largely based on the observation that such procedures restore pallidal outflow. The STN has been demonstrated to be the major excitatory input to the SNr (19,20). Therefore, inactivation of the STN not only reduces the efferent activity of the GPi, but also of the SNr. This effect may not be achieved with the blockade of either of the GPi or the motor thalamus because these structures do not exert direct influence over the SNr, and might explain the clinical and functional effect obtained by STN stimulation, which is probably greater than that obtained with pallidal stimulation (21).

Blockade of the STN can also exert influence at the level of the midbrain tegmentum, mainly the pedunculopontine nucleus (PPN). This nucleus is located in the caudal mesencephalic tegmentum extending from the caudal border of the red nucleus to the parabrachial nucleus. As an extension of this nucleus, the pedunculopontine area includes the cuneiform nucleus, the central tegmental field, the pontine-tegmental field, and a group of cholinergic neurons in the vicinity of the superior cerebellar peduncle (22,23). In the last decades evidence has accumulated in both primates and subprimates that this area receives direct bilateral descending and ascending projections from the STN, the dorsal and ventral striatum, the pallidum, and the SNr (24–29). GABA mediates descending projections from the pallidum and the SNR, and ascending projections from the PPN to the striatal output are mediated both by acetylcholine and glutamate; descending connections between the STN and the PPN are probably glutamatergic. Electrophysiologic studies in animals demonstrated that SNR inputs are inhibitory to the PPN (30), whereas reciprocal connections of the PPN cholinergic neurons with the SNR are excitatory (31). Consequently, the PPN is an additional source of excitatory inputs to the SNR, and the excitation of this structure results in feedback inhibitory regulation of PPN neurons. Although the functional role of these descending projections to PPN is not well known, they constitute one of the anatomic substrates by which the basal ganglia and related nuclei can influence the motor mechanisms of the brainstem and spinal cord. The PPN has been implicated as a major component of the mesencephalic motor region, a functional area in which electrical stimulation can induce coordinated locomotion on a treadmill in the cat and rat after intercollicular brainstem transection (32–34). The mesencephalic locomotor region is located within a large area centered on the posterior cuneiform nucleus, and its descending influences probably modulate the activity of putative locomotor pattern generators presumably present in the spinal cord (35). Acute stimulation of the PPN in the cat seems to produce stepping and other rhythmic events and blockade of neuronal activity in the area of the PPN leads to a reduction of locomotor activity. Furthermore, an injection of cholinergic agonists into the PPN appears to decrease locomotor activity; on the other hand, injection of GABA antagonists induces stepping (36). The activity of the PPN is abnormal in MPTP monkeys and distinct functional and pathologic alterations have been shown in the mesencephalic cholinergic nuclei in parkinsonian syndromes such as progressive supranuclear palsy (PSP) and multiple system atrophy (37–41). A loss of cholinergic neurons in the lateral part of the PPN has been confirmed in the brains of PD patients (42). This fact further supports the hypothesis that pathologic involvement of PPN neurons may contribute to some of the clinical features of PD such as abnormalities of posture and gait (43). This is largely based on the assumption that the PPN participates in rhythmic motor functions. This theory is supported by some clinical evidences showing isolated gait and balance disturbances owing to hemorrhagic or ischemic lesions at the region of the PPN or within its projections to the pontine tegmental nuclei (44–46).

In summary, there is at least theoretical evidence that STN blockade can improve gait and postural disturbances in PD secondary to the dopaminergic nigrostriatal breakdown. This effect is mainly achieved by resetting the excessive neuronal drive from the internal pallidum and the

SNR to the thalamocortical loop and toward the brainstem locomotor regions.

CLINICAL EXPERIENCE

There is, at the present moment, only limited clinical experience with the effects of STN ablation or stimulation on parkinsonian gait disturbances. In a study with MPTP-treated monkeys, gait was assessed before and after the lesion. In this study, subthalamotomy dramatically improved bilateral freezing, both during spontaneous behavior and while performing a task; however, complete recovery of a normal posture was not observed (9). In patients with PD, several clinical studies have pointed out that chronic high-frequency electrical stimulation of the STN is a safe and effective procedure that can be used to alleviate parkinsonian motor symptoms. Several authors have found an overall improvement of the motor scores and activities of daily living between 30% and 60% after surgery (12–18). In one study with 24 patients the score for axial symptoms (gait, arising from a chair and postural stability) in basal conditions, improved by 61%, 1 year after surgery (15). Separately, the score for gait improved by 65%. The Hoehn and Yahr staging system, based on the progression of the disease and the presence or absence of axial and postural disturbances, decreased from 4.6 ± 0.5 to 2.8 ± 0.6. In another survey involving nine patients, axial symptoms improved 67% 6 months after surgery, but gait was not analyzed independently (17). The authors, however, stated that patients unable to walk without medication before surgery were able to walk after bilateral STN stimulation. One study compared the efficacy of bilateral STN stimulation with that of bilateral pallidal stimulation in young onset patients with PD (16). Overall, improvement of parkinsonian symptoms was greater in STN-stimulated patients. Gait was analyzed by means of a "gait score" that included items of the Unified Parkinson's Disease Rating Scale (UPDRS), parts II and III. Although patients' scores were similar preoperatively, after surgery the "gait score" also showed a significant difference in favor of STN-stimulated patients. The differences were attributed to both the larger dimensions of the internal pallidum, which probably make more difficult a complete inhibition of the nucleus, and the lack of influence of pallidal stimulation on the SNr output.

We studied at our center the clinical outcome of 15 patients with PD, in whom bilateral electrodes for chronic deep brain stimulation were implanted in the STN with stereotactic neurosurgery techniques and intraoperative microrecording guidance following standardized methods (47,48). Patients were 10 men and five women, with a mean age of 60.9 years (± 6.8; range: 52 to 74 years), mean disease duration of 15.8 years (± 9.2; range: 7 to 38 years), and Hoehn and Yahr stage of 3.8 (± 0.8). Clinical assessments were done following the Core Assessment Program for Intracerebral Transplantation (CAPIT) (49) instructions 4 days before surgery and 6 months after surgery by means of the UPDRS (50), the Hoehn and Yahr staging system (51), and the Activities of Daily Living (ADL) Scale of Schwab and England (52). Motor assessments were carried out during the "off" drug periods following an overnight withdrawal of medication. The "on" drug condition was defined as the best motor state following a single dose of standard L-Dopa between 100% and 150% of the usual morning L-Dopa dose, depending on the predictability of the response. After surgery, assessments were performed using the UPDRS scale in "on" and "off" drug conditions and for each drug condition the stimulation device was switched on and off. One of the main objectives of the study was to compare the effects induced by L-Dopa with those produced by STN stimulation. Therefore, we aimed to maintain patients without dopaminergic drugs after surgery when it was possible and well tolerated. We evaluated some patients of the study several months after the complete withdrawal of antiparkinsonian drugs. Thus, we compared the motor status of patients before surgery in the previously defined "on" drug situation with the motor status after surgery in "off" drug/"on" stimulation condition without the artifacts possibly induced by the clinical long-term effect of L-Dopa and dopamine agonists. Coupled with drug tapering, electrical

TABLE 30.1. *Mean scores and standard deviation in 15 patients with Parkinson's disease before and after bilateral subthalamic nucleus stimulation*

	UPDRS-III	Axial	Akinesia	Rigidity	Tremor	ADL	H & Y
Maximum score	108	36	32	16	24	52	5
Before surgery							
Off medication	49.6 (14)	17.1 (6)	17.7 (6)	8.5 (3)	6.3 (6)	26.7 (9)	3.8 (0.7)
On medication	20.1 (8)	8.1 (3)	8.1 (4)	3.2 (2)	0.7 (1)	10.6 (8)	2.7 (0.6)
After surgery ("off" drug)							
Off stimulation	51.1 (17)	16.0 (7)	17.9 (5)	7.6 (3)	9.5 (7)	NA	3.6 (0.9)
On stimulation	16.9 (7)	5.9 (4)	7.0 (3)	2.9 (2)	1.2 (2)	7.5 (6)	1.9 (0.5)

UPDRS, Unified Parkinson's Disease Rating Scale; ADL, activities of daily living; H & Y, Hoehn and Yahr; NA, not aplicable.

parameters were adjusted at each visit. All patients were instructed to maintain stimulator on during all day and night.

Chronic bilateral STN stimulation significantly reduced parkinsonian motor symptoms 6 months postoperatively when comparing the preoperative "off" drug scores with the "off" drug/"on" stimulation scores after surgery (Table 30.1). No major adverse effects were seen as a consequence of the surgical procedure. Total UPDRS part III score decreased by 65.9% ($P < 0.0001$); bradykinesia, rigidity, and tremor improved by 60.4%, 66.1%, and 81.1%, respectively ($P < 0.0001$). "Off" period dystonia disappeared in all patients presenting with this complication. The Hoehn and Yahr stage changed from 3.8 ± 0.7 preoperatively to 1.9 ± 0.5 after surgery ($P < 0.0001$). Patients' ADL improved markedly as reflected by the change in the UPDRS-II and Schwab and England scale scores. UPDRS-II scores were reduced by 71.8% and Schwab and England scale scores improved by 45.3% when compared with preoperative "off" drug condition ($P < 0.0001$), and 28.9% (not significant) and 14.7% ($P < 0.001$), respectively, when compared with the "on" drug condition.

UPDRS motor scores of those symptoms whose clinical manifestation probably rely on the bilateral effect of stimulation, such as posture, gait, arising from a chair, postural stability, axial tremor, and axial rigidity were examined independently. The total score for axial symptoms in "off" drug condition significantly improved by 66.5%, from 17.1 ± 6.3 before surgery to 5.9 ± 3.66 months after surgery. The symptom "gait" (UPDRS part III, item no. 29) improved by 73.5%, from 2.8 ± 0.8 to 0.7 ± 0.6 after bilateral STN stimulation.

The daily L-Dopa equivalent dose was reduced by 76.3%, from 1,338 (±656) mg/day to 262 (±332) mg/day ($P < 0.0001$). Eight patients had stopped all dopaminergic medication at 12 months follow-up, without reappearance of parkinsonian symptoms and good tolerance. Two patients have completed an 18-month follow-up and two other patients a 1-year follow-up period and remain without medication. We did not find preoperative significant differences in age, disease duration, and disease severity among patients who were taking L-Dopa postoperatively and those who were not. The eight patients who were completely free of antiparkinsonian treatment, and three still taking small doses of L-Dopa, did not report daytime or nocturnal fluctuations. The other four patients recognized the existence of brief wearing-off periods characterized by the reappearance of mild parkinsonian symptoms. UPDRS-IV item no. 39, which measures the proportion of the day that the patient is in an "off" period, decreased from 2.6 (±1) before surgery to 0.3 (±0.5) after surgery (89.7% reduction, $P < 0.0001$). Nine of 15 patients were completely relieved from dyskinesias after surgery. The remaining six patients presented only mild choreiform dyskinesias. The severity of dyskinesias decreased by 80.6% after surgery ($P < 0.0001$) in the whole group and by 63.7% ($P < 0.0001$) in the patients still presenting dyskinesias.

Comparison between preoperative "on" drug motor scores and postoperative "on" stimulation scores in the eight patients who were completely

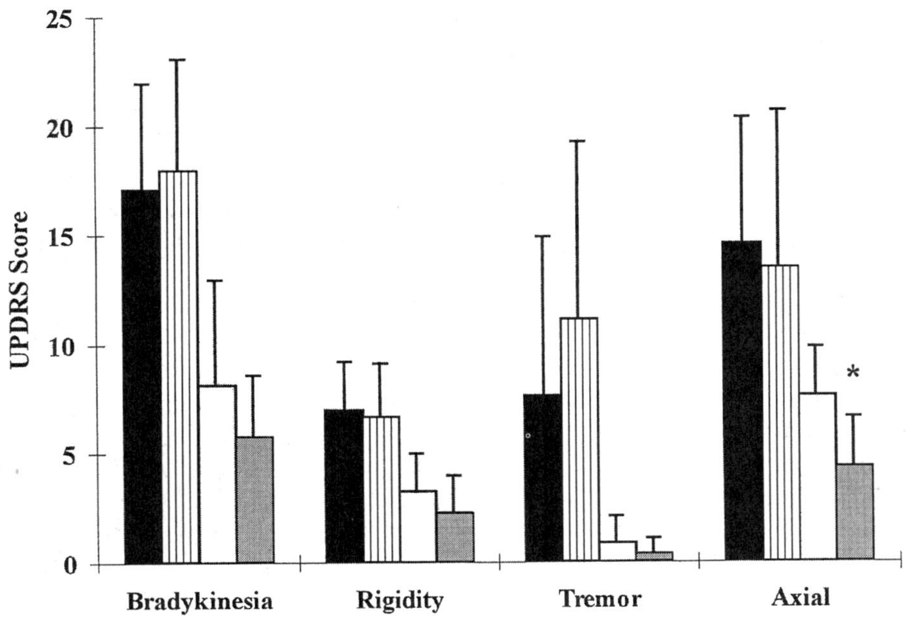

FIG. 30.1. Comparison of the antiparkinsonian action of L-Dopa before surgery with the effect obtained after chronic subthalamic nucleus stimulation 6 months after surgery measured by means of the Unified Parkinson's Disease Rating Scale (*UPDRS*) scores in eight patients free of L-Dopa for several months. Bars represent the mean score and standard deviation of the UPDRS scores in patients with Parkinson's disease. Before surgery while "off" drug (*black*) and "on" drug condition (*white*); after surgery, "off" drug/"off" stimulation (*stripes*) and "off" drug/"on" stimulation (*gray*) condition. *$P < 0.001$ in the comparison of "on" drug with "off" drug/on stimulation scores.

free of medication, showed no significant differences in general, except for the axial items of the UPDRS-III (Fig. 30.1). The ADL and the Hoehn and Yahr scales were also significantly better after surgery when compared with the preoperative "on" drug condition ($P < 0.001$).

These studies demonstrate that bilateral STN stimulation improves axial symptoms and gait. Such improvement is greater than 60% for axial symptoms and over 65% for gait when comparing the postoperative motor status with the "off" drug preoperative condition. In our study, the motor effect of bilateral STN stimulation on axial symptoms was significantly better than that obtained with L-Dopa before surgery. The standard rating scales, used to assess changes in axial symptoms, can be considered a valid clinical outcome measure because changes in these scales correlate well with modification of gait parameters in patients with PD and motor fluctuations (53). This effect could be caused by an action of STN stimulation beyond the effect of dopamine, improving some dopaminergic-resistant symptoms. The effect of STN stimulation resulted in improvement of dyskinesia scores, disappearance of the "off" period dystonia, and maintenance of a constant motor status during all the day. None of these improvements could be obtained with pharmacologic treatment. This continuous effect along with the improvement of dyskinesias and "off" period dystonia could explain the better results obtained in axial symptoms with STN stimulation when compared with those produced by L-Dopa. The procedure resulted in a greater degree of independence in patients, as measured by the Schwab and England scale, both when rated by patients and their relatives.

GAIT ANALYSIS

We studied gait parameters reflecting locomotor pattern (stride length, velocity, and cadence) in five patients (three men and two women) with advanced PD. These five patients were included in the study previously described in this chapter and were selected because of their ability to walk 7 meters several times in an overnight "off" drug condition without showing immediate fatigue, marked tendency to fall, or multiple freezing episodes that would have prevented the performance of the test. Their mean age was 63.6 years (range: 56 to 67), disease duration was 17.8 years (range: 7 to 38), mean weight was 74 kg (range: 68 to 85), and mean height was 167 cm (range: 157 to 181). We also analyzed gait parameters of ten healthy age- and height-matched control subjects.

We used a commercially available device to analyze gait designed by Bessou et al. (54). The apparatus permits an automatic recording of gait parameters and has previously been used for gait analysis in PD by other authors (55,56). Longitudinal locomotor displacements are transmitted to the recording equipment by means of threads attached with adhesive straps to each foot. The traction of the threads during gait leads to rotation of a pulley system, which is connected to an optical recording device. Signal output is transmitted to a computer. Appropriate software allows calculation of measures related to gait parameters.

Once the threads were attached to each foot, patients were requested to walk 7 meters in a corridor in a quiet ambiance. After several training trials, patients were instructed to walk at three self-selected different velocities (at the preferred velocity, as fast as possible, and at a leisurely pace) in order to analyze the adaptation of cadence and stride length to velocity changes. Patients were assessed preoperatively a few days before surgery while in "off" drug and "on" drug conditions, as described in the preceding. Postoperatively the test was performed in the "off" drug/"on" stimulation condition (two patients in overnight "off," and three patients several weeks after the complete withdrawal of L-Dopa and dopamine agonists). The "off" drug/"off" stimulation condition was not evaluated because

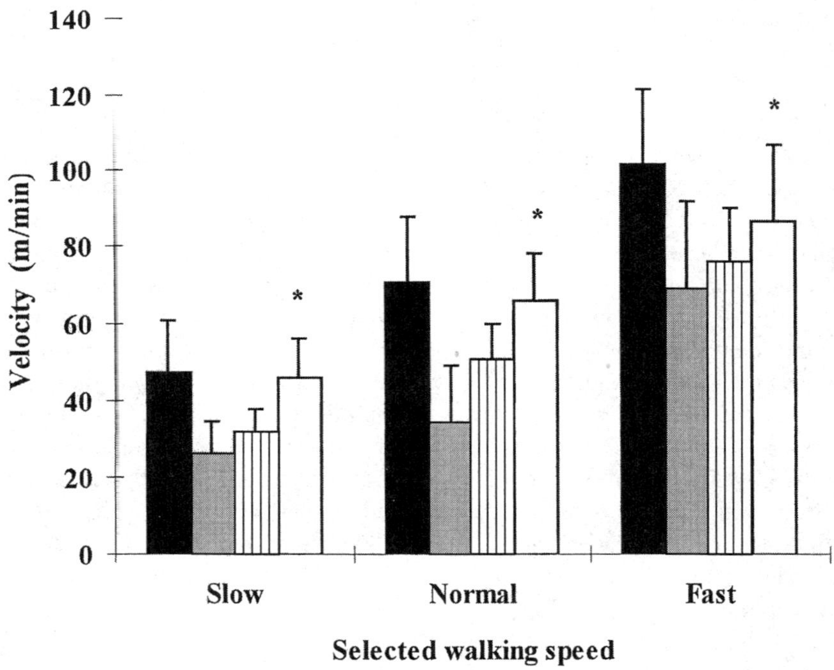

FIG. 30.2. Mean gait velocity, with the standard deviation within brackets, for selected walking speed (see text) in control patients (*black*), "off" drug PD patients before surgery (*gray*), "on" drug PD patients before surgery (*stripes*), and after subthalamic nucleus stimulation in "off" drug condition (*white*). *Statistically significant ($P < 0.05$) with respect to "off" drug condition.

gait and balance rapidly deteriorated after the stimulation device was switched off, and patients suffered such severe discomfort that it was impossible to test performance.

All patients showed significantly improved velocity and gait parameters compared with the preoperative "off" drug condition (Fig. 30.2). When walking at the preferred velocity, bilateral STN stimulation increased stride length from 60 ± 27 to 108 ± 37 cm, velocity from 34.1 ± 9 to 66.3 ± 12 m/min, and cadence from 116 ± 14 to 127 ± 17 steps/min (means ± standard deviation of the five patients). Slow ambulation also showed changes in stride length from 52 ± 16 to 90 ± 20 cm, velocity from 26.3 ± 6 to 46 ± 10 m/min, and cadence from 103 ± 17 to 112 ± 15 steps/min. Walking as fast as possible showed a change in the stride length from 69 ± 25 to 124 ± 30 cm and in velocity from 69.5 ± 14 to 86.4 ± 20 m/min; interestingly, cadence decreased from 145 ± 22 to 141 ± 20 steps/min.

Decreased stride length is the hallmark of PD, whereas cadence control is mostly preserved and can be modulated (57–59). Step rate is disproportionately increased in PD, whereas stride length increase is lower than in control subjects when the speed of walking is increased. Patients with PD, therefore, have a higher cadence rate than control subjects for any given velocity; it has been suggested that such increased cadence is a compensatory mechanism for reduced step size (59–61). Thus, temporal constrains allow identification of abnormalities of gait motor control that are not revealed when only the preferred velocity or cadence of walking is studied (57–59). Bilateral STN stimulation, although significantly increased the stride length in our patients with PD, did not completely correct the relationship between cadence and stride length at increasing velocities. This fact is evidenced in Figure 30.3, which illustrates that operated patients still present a higher cadence rate

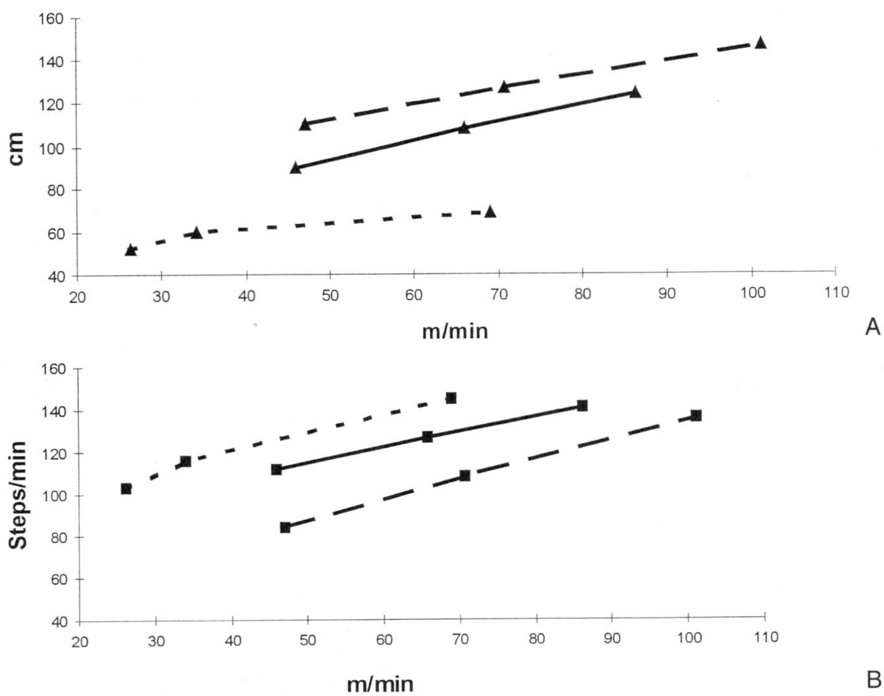

FIG. 30.3. Mean stride length (**A**) and cadence (**B**) as a function of velocity for patients with Parkinson's disease before surgery while "off" drug (*short-dashed lines*) and after surgery while stimulated (*solid line*) and age-matched controls (*long-dashed lines*).

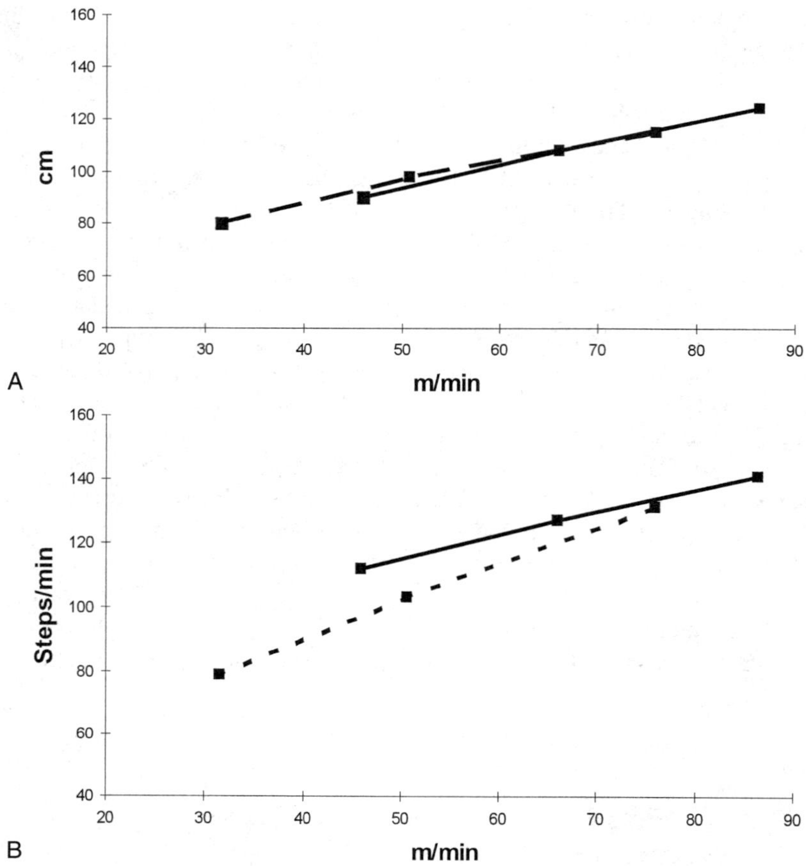

FIG. 30.4. Changes observed in the stride length (**A**) and cadence (**B**) with increasing walking velocities in patients with Parkinson's disease after bilateral subthalamic nucleus stimulation (*solid lines*) compared with those seen in the same patients before surgery while "on" drug (*dashed lines*).

and lower stride length than control subjects for any given velocity.

Comparison between gait parameters with STN stimulation in the "off" drug condition and those observed in the preoperatively "on" drug condition showed only scarce, insignificant differences. At the preferred velocity of walking, patients with STN stimulation presented a mean velocity of 66.3 ± 12 m/min, cadence of 127 ± 17 steps/min, and stride length of 108 ± 37 cm, whereas patients showed a slightly inferior velocity of 50.8 ± 15 m/min, cadence of 103.1 ± 20 steps/min, and stride length of 98 ± 33 cm when "on" drug. These results are in agreement with a single previous report showing gait analysis in patients with PD before and after bilateral STN stimulation in which a marked improvement in velocity and stride length after STN stimulation was also observed but with no further improvement beyond that given by medication (62). Abnormalities in stride length–cadence relation in PD, which probably express a defective scaling of stride size, are not completely mended by STN stimulation (63); however, we observed a lower tendency to increase in excess the cadence of walking to obtain faster velocities than that observed in patients before surgery in the "on" drug condition (Fig. 30.4). Although the beneficial effect of L-Dopa on gait is beyond doubt, some authors have suggested that complex disturbances of gait such as freezing and start hesitation sometimes do not consistently respond to L-Dopa and can even be aggravated by this treatment (64). According to our clinical findings, some aspects of gait disturbances associated with PD could be further improved by bilateral STN stimulation, beyond the benefits produced by L-Dopa.

Stride length and velocity showed only minor improvements after unilateral pallidotomy, in contrast to our results with bilateral STN stimulation (65). This finding is in keeping with other reports that showed small, waning, or transient effects on gait and postural disturbances after unilateral pallidotomy (66,67). In some studies, however, gait and balance items of the UPDRS improved after pallidotomy by about one-third, and this improvement, which was sustained for over 2 years follow-up, was even more robust after bilateral pallidotomy (Chapter 28). In our experience, axial symptoms after pallidotomy improved by 25% compared to the preoperative "off" drug condition at 3 months follow-up and only by 18% at the 1-year follow-up (68,69). These relatively poor results may result from the need of a bilateral intervention to succeed with such axial symptoms, although bilateral pallidal stimulation also seems to afford lesser clinical effects than bilateral STN stimulation (16). By contrast, a study did not find substantial differences in the antiparkinsonian effects achieved through these different brain targets (70) and a recent report revealed that bilateral pallidal stimulation made kinematic gait features closer to control subjects (71).

CONCLUSION

Bilateral STN stimulation should be considered a safe procedure, which improves all dopamine-sensitive parkinsonian symptoms (e.g., posture, balance, and gait); minimizes or eliminates motor fluctuations; and diminishes the need for dopaminergic drugs, thereby contributing to a marked amelioration of L-Dopa–induced dyskinesias. Complete dopaminergic drug withdrawal is possible if electrode placement into the sensorimotor subthalamus is accurate. The overall motor effect of STN stimulation is at least equal to or even better than that obtained with L-Dopa on axial symptoms, but avoids the inconvenience of pulsatile dopaminergic stimulation and non–motor drug-related adverse side effects. Abnormalities in the relationship between step-length and cadence in patients with PD are not completely corrected by STN stimulation, although they are significantly improved.

ACKNOWLEDGMENTS

This study was partially supported by a grant from "La Caixa" no. 97/072-00. The authors also thank Dr. Georg Ebersbach for technical support.

REFERENCES

1. Alexander GE, Crutcher MD. Functional architecture of basal ganglia circuits: neural substrates of parallel processing. *Trends Neurosci* 1990;13:266–271.
2. DeLong MR. Primate models of movement disorders of basal ganglia origin. *Trends Neurosci* 1990;13:281–285.
3. Miller WC, DeLong MR. Altered tonic activity of neurons in the globus pallidus and subthalamic nucleus in the primate MPTP model of parkinsonism. In: Carpenter MB, Jayaraman A, eds. *The basal ganglia II.* New York: Plenum Press, 1987:415–427.
4. Bergman H, Wichmann T, Karmon B, et al. The primate subthalamic nucleus II. Neuronal activity in the MPTP model of parkinsonism. *J Neurophysiol* 1994;72:507–520.
5. Bergman H, Wichman T, DeLong MR. Reversal of experimental parkinsonism by lesions of the subthalamic nucleus. *Science* 1990;249:1436–1438.
6. Aziz TZ, Peggs D, Sambrook MA, et al. Lesion of the subthalamic nucleus for the alleviation of 1-methyl-4-phenyl-1,2,3,6-tetrahydropiridine (MPTP)-induced parkinsonism in the primate. *Mov Disord* 1991;6:288–292.
7. Aziz TZ, Peggs D, Agarwal E, et al. Subthalamic nucleotomy alleviates parkinsonism in the 1-methyl-4-phenyl-1,2,3,6–tetrahydropiridine (MPTP)-exposed primate. *Br J Neurosurg* 1992;6:575–582.
8. Guridi J, Luquin R, Herrero Y, et al. The subthalamic nucleus: a possible target for stereotaxic surgery in Parkinson's disease. *Mov Disord* 1993;8:421–429.
9. Guridi J, Herrero MT, Luquin MR, et al. Subthalamotomy in parkinsonian monkeys. Behavioural and biochemical analysis. *Brain* 1996;119:1717–1727.
10. Benazzouz A, Gross C, Féger J, et al. Reversal of rigidity and improvement in motor performance by subthalamic high-frequency stimulation in MPTP-treated monkeys. *Eur J Neurosci* 1993;5:382–389.
11. Benazzouz A, Boraud T, Féger J, et al. Alleviation of experimental hemiparkinsonism by high-frequency stimulation of the subthalamic nucleus in primates: a comparison with l-dopa treatment. *Mov Disord* 1996;11:627–632.
12. Benabid AL, Pollack P, Gross C, et al. Acute and long term effects of subthalamic nucleus stimulation in Parkinson's disease. *Sterotact Funct Neurosurg* 1994;62:76–84.

13. Limousin P, Pollack P, Benazzouz A. Effect on parkinsonian signs and symptoms of bilateral subthalamic nucleus stimulation. *Lancet* 1995;345:91–95.
14. Limousin P, Pollak P, Hoffmann D, et al. Abnormal involuntary movements induced by subthalamic nucleus stimulation in parkinsonian patients. *Mov Disord* 1996;11:231–235.
15. Limousin P, Krack P, Pollack P, et al. Electrical stimulation of the subthalamic nucleus in advanced Parkinson's disease. *N Engl J Med* 1998;339:1105–1111.
16. Krack P, Pollak P, Limousin P, et al. Subthalamic nucleus or internal pallidal stimulation in young onset Parkinson's disease. *Brain* 1998;121:451–457.
17. Kumar R, Lozano AM, Kim YJ, et al. Double-blind evaluation of subthalamic nucleus deep brain stimulation in advanced Parkinson's disease. *Neurology* 1998;51:850–855.
18. Moro E, Scerrati M, Romito LMA, et al. Chronic subthalamic nucleus stimulation reduces medication requirements in Parkinson's disease. *Neurology* 1999;53:85–90.
19. Nakanishi H, Kita H, Kitai ST. Intracellular study of rat substantia nigra pars reticulata neurons in an in vivo slice preparation: electrical membrane properties and response characteristics of subthalamic stimulation. *Brain Res* 1987;437:45–55.
20. Van der Kooi, Hattori D. Single subthalamic neurones project to both the globus pallidus and substantia nigra in the rat. *J Comp Neurol* 1980;192:751–768.
21. Limousin P, Greene J, Pollak P, et al. Changes in cerebral activity pattern due to subthalamic nucleus or internal pallidum stimulation in Parkinson's disease. *Ann Neurol* 1997;42:283–291.
22. Armstrong DA, Saper CB, Levey AI, et al. Distribution of cholinergic neurons in the rat brain demonstrated by the immunohistochemical localization of choline-acetyltransferase. *J Comp Neurol* 1983;200:53–68.
23. Mesulam MM, Mufson EJ, Levey AI, et al. Atlas of cholinergic neurons in the forebrain and upper brainstem of the macaque based on monoclonal choline acetyltransferase immuno-histochemistry and acetylcholinesterase histochemistry. *Neuroscience* 1984;12:669–686.
24. Graybiel AM. Direct and indirect preoculomotor pathways of the brainstem: an autoradiographic study of the pontine reticular formation in cat. *J Comp Neurol* 1977;175:37–78.
25. Beckstead RM, Domesick VB, Nauta WJH. Efferent connections of the substantia nigra and ventral tegmental area in the rat. *Brain Res* 1979;412:169–174.
26. Jackson A, Crossman AR. Nucleus tegmenti pedunculopontinus: efferent connections with special reference to the basal ganglia, studied in the rat by anterograde and retrograde transport of horseradish peroxidase. *Neuroscience* 1981;10:725–765.
27. Hammond C, Rouzaire-Dubois B, Féger J, et al. Anatomical and electrophysiological studies on the reciprocal projections between the subthalamic nucleus and nucleus tegmenti pedunculopontinus in the rat. *Neuroscience* 1983;9:41–52.
28. Lavoie B, Parent A. Pedunculopontine nucleus in the squirrel monkey: Projections to the basal ganglia as revealed by anterograde tract-tracing methods. *J Comp Neurol* 1994;344:210–231.
29. Lavoie B, Parent A. Pedunculopontine nucleus in the squirrel monkey: cholinergic and glutamatergic projections to the substantia nigra. *J Comp Neurol* 1994;344:232–241.
30. Granata AR, Kitai ST. Inhibitory substantia nigra inputs to the pedunculopontine neurons. *Exp Brain Res* 1990;86:459–466.
31. Scarnati E, Proia A, Campana E, Pacitti C. A microiontophoretic of the putative neurotransmitter involved in the pedunculopontine-substantia nigra pars compacta excitatory pathway of the rat. *Exp Brain Res* 1986;62:470–478.
32. Shik ML, Severin FV, Orlovskii GN. Control of walking and running by means of electrical stimulation of the midbrain. *Biophysics* 1966;11:756–765.
33. Grillner S, Shik ML. On the descending control of the lumbosacral spinal cord from the "mesencephalic locomotor region." *Acta Physiol Scand* 1973;81:320–333.
34. Coles SK, Iles JF, Nicolopoulos-Stournaras S. The mesencephalic centre controlling locomotion in the rat. *Neuroscience* 1989;28:149–157.
35. García-Rill E, Skinner RD, Gilmore SA, et al. Connections of the mesencephalic motor region (MLR). II Afferents and efferents. *Brain Res Bull* 1983;10:57–62.
36. García Rill E. The pedunculopontine nucleus. *Prog Neurobiol* 1991;36:363–389.
37. Mitchell IJ, Clatke CE, Boyce S, et al. Neural mechanisms underlying parkinsonian symptoms based upon regional uptake of 2-deoxyglucose in monkeys exposed to 1-methyl-4-phenyl-1,2,3,6-tetrahydropiridine. *Neuroscience* 1989;32:213–226.
38. Juncos JL, Hirsch EC, Malessa S, et al. Mesencephalic cholinergic nuclei in progressive supranuclear palsy. *Neurology* 1991;44:2015–2019.
39. Fearnley JM, Lees AJ. Striatonigral degeneration. A clinicopathological study. *Brain* 1990;113:1823–1842.
40. Wenning GK, Tisson F, Ben Shlomo Y, et al. Multiple system atrophy: A review of 203 pathologically proven cases. *Mov Disord* 1997;12:133–147.
41. Zweig RM, Whitehouse PJ, Casanova MF, et al. Loss of pedunculopontine neurons in progressive supranuclear palsy. *Ann Neurol* 1987;22:18–25.
42. Zweig RM, Jankel WR, Hedreen JC, et al. The pedunculopontine nucleus in Parkinson's disease. *Ann Neurol* 1989;26:41–46.
43. Inglis W, Winn P. The pedunculopontine tegmental nucleus: where the striatum meets the reticular formation. *Prog Neurobiol* 1995;47:1–29.
44. Masdeu JC, Alampur U, Cavaliere R, et al. Astasia and gait failure with damage of the pontomesencephalic locomotor region. *Ann Neurol* 1994;35:619–621.
45. Caplan L, Goodwin J. Lateral tegmental brainstem hemorrhages. *Neurology* 1982;32:252–260.
46. Kwa VIH, Zaal LH, Verbeeten B, et al. Disequilibrium in patients with atherosclerosis. Relevance of pontine ischemic rarefaction. *Neurology* 1998;51:570–573.
47. Hutchison WD, Allan RJ, Opitz H, et al. Neurophysiological identification of the subthalamic nucleus in surgery for Parkinson's disease. *Ann Neurol* 1998;44:622–628.
48. Hutchison WD, Lozano AM, Tasjer RR, et al. Identification and characterization of neurons with tremor-frequency activity in human globus pallidus. *Exp Brain Res* 1997;113:557–563.
49. Langston JW, Widner H, Goetz CG, et al. Core assessment program for intracerebral transplantations (CAPIT) *Mov Disord* 1992;7:2–13.
50. Fahn S, Elton RL, members if the UPDRS Development Committee. Unified Parkinson's Disease Rating Scale.

In: Fahn S, Marsden CD, Calne DB, et al, eds. *Recent developments in Parkinson's disease,* vol 2. Florham Park, NJ: Macmillan Health Care Information, 1987:153–164.
51. Hoehn MM, Yahr MD. Parkinsonism: onset, progression and mortality. *Neurology* 1967;17:427–442.
52. Schwab RS, England RC. In: Gillingham FJ, Donaldson IML, eds. *Projection technique for evaluating surgery in Parkinson's disease.* Edinburgh: E and S Livingstone, 1969:152–157.
53. O'Sullivan JD, Said CM, Dillon LC, et al. Gait analysis in patients with Parkinson's disease and motor fluctuations: influence of levodopa and comparison with other measures of motor function. *Mov Disord* 1998;13:900–906.
54. Bessou P, Dupui P, Montoya R, et al. Simultaneous recording of longitudinal displacements of both feet during human walking. *J Physiol (Paris)* 1988;83:102–110.
55. Blin O, Ferrandez A-M, Serratrice G. Quantitative analysis of gait in Parkinson patients: increased variability of stride length. *J Neurol Sci* 1990;98:91–97.
56. Blin O, Ferrandez AM, Pailhous J, et al. Dopa-sensitive and Dopa-resistant gait parameters in Parkinson's disease. *J Neurol Sci* 1991:103:51–54.
57. McIntosh GC, Brown SH, Rice RR, et al. Rhythmic auditory-motor facilitation of gait patterns in patients with Parkinson's disease. *J Neurol Neurosurg Psychiatry* 1997;62;22–26.
58. Ebersbach G, Heijmemberg M, Kindermann L, et al. Interference of rhythmic constraint on gait in healthy subjects and patients with early Parkinson's disease: evidence for impaired locomotor pattern generation in early Parkinson's disease. *Mov Disord* 1999;14:619–625.
59. Morris ME, Iansek R, Matyas TA, et al. The pathogenesis of gait hypokinesia in Parkinson's disease. *Brain* 1994;117:1169–1181.
60. Morris ME, Iansek R, Matyas TA, et al. Ability to modulate walking cadence remains intact in Parkinson's disease. *J Neurol Neurosurg Psychiatry* 1994;57:1532–1534.
61. Morris ME, Iansek R, Matyas TA, et al. Stride length regulation in Parkinson's disease. Normalization strategies and underlying mechanisms. *Brain* 1996;119:551–568.
62. Xie J, Pollak P, Krack P, Benabid AL. Effect of bilateral subthalamic stimulation on parkinsonian gait. *Mov Disord* 1998;13:135.
63. Morris M, Iansek R, Matyas T, et al. Abnormalities in the stride length-cadence relation in parkinsonian gait. *Mov Disord* 1998;13:61–69.
64. Giladi N, McMahon D, Przedborski S, et al. Motor blocks in Parkinson's disease. *Neurology* 1992;42:333–339.
65. Valldeoriola F, Molinuevo JL, Valls-Solé J, et al. Gait analysis in parkinsonian patients after pallidotomy (abstract) at the International Symposium on Gait Disorders. Prague, Czech Republic, 1999.
66. Baron MS, Vitek JL, Bakay RAE, et al. Treatment of advanced Parkinson's disease by posterior Gpi pallidotomy: 1-year results of a pilot study. *Ann Neurol* 1996;40:355–366.
67. Lozano AM, Lang AE, Galvez-Jimenez N, et al. Effect of GPi pallidotomy on motor function in Parkinson's disease. *Lancet* 1995;346:1383–1387.
68. Molinuevo JL, Valldeoriola F, Rumià J, et al. Contribution of neurophysiological guidance to stereotactic posteroventral pallidotomy for Parkinson's disease. *Acta Neurochir (Wien)* 1999;141:1195–1201.
69. Molinuevo JL, Valldeoriola F, Rumià J, et al. Eficacia y seguridad de la palidotomía posteroventral en el tratamiento de la enfermedad de Parkinson. *Med Clin (Barc)* 2000;114:205–208.
70. Rodríguez MC and the Deep Brain Stimulation Parkinson's Disease Study Group. Estimulación del núcleo subtalámico y globo pálido interno en la enfermedad de Parkinson. Resultados del estudio multicéntrico al año de evolución. *Neurología* 1998;13:452.
71. Grasso R, Peppe A, Stratta F, et al. Basal ganglia and gait control: apomorphine administration and internal pallidum stimulation in Parkinson's disease. *Exp Brain Res* 1999;126:139–148.

Gait Disorders. Advances in Neurology, Vol. 87,
edited by E. Růžička, M. Hallett, and J. Jankovic.
Lippincott Williams & Wilkins, Philadelphia © 2001.

31

Evaluation of Gait in Normal Pressure Hydrocephalus Before and After Shunting

*Joachim K. Krauss, †Michael Faist, †‡Martin Schubert, §Jan J. Borremans, †Carl H. Lücking, and †Wiltrud Berger

**Department of Neurosurgery, University Hospital Mannheim, Ruprecht-Karls-University, 68167 Mannheim, Germany; Departments of †Neurology, ‡Neurophysiology, and §Neurosurgery, Albert-Ludwigs-University, 79106 Freiburg, Germany*

The diagnosis of idiopathic normal pressure hydrocephalus (NPH) of the elderly is raised in patients with widening of the supratentorial ventricular system on imaging studies who present with gait disturbance, cognitive impairment, and urinary urge or incontinence (1–4). Intensive research and effort have been exerted to elucidate the etiology, pathogenesis, and pathophysiology of this enigmatic disease of the elderly since its first description in 1965 (5–8). Numerous studies have shown the benefit of cerebrospinal fluid (CSF) shunting, which can be achieved with the careful preoperative selection of patients. There is little consensus, however, about which investigations are best suited to confirm the suspected diagnosis and which tests have the highest predictive value for outcome after shunting. The differential diagnosis between idiopathic NPH and vascular encephalopathy has been puzzling (8–11). This issue is further complicated by the fact that coexistence of both conditions occurs in many patients (12,13).

When Hakim and colleagues first described the clinical syndrome of symptomatic occult hydrocephalus with normal CSF pressure, they reported gait difficulties and impaired memory as the most evident symptoms (5,6). Later, attention shifted to idiopathic NPH as a cause of treatable dementia. Shunting has not led to gratifying results, however, in patients with marked dementia and little gait disturbance (14). The importance of gait disturbance for the diagnosis of idiopathic NPH and the outcome after CSF shunting has been shown by various investigators (15–17). Although it is commonly accepted nowadays that gait disturbance is the predominant clinical symptom of idiopathic NPH, few studies have analyzed its features and pathophysiologic mechanisms. This chapter focuses on various aspects of gait disturbance in idiopathic NPH.

IDIOPATHIC NORMAL PRESSURE HYDROCEPHALUS OF THE ELDERLY

Epidemiology of Idiopathic Normal Pressure Hydrocephalus

The frequency of idiopathic NPH in the elderly remains unclear. There are no systematic studies. Some have thought that it is a rather rare disease, with an estimated incidence of 1.3 to 2.2 per million per year (18). On the other hand, it has been demonstrated that hydrocephalus is present in a considerable number of elderly patients with otherwise unexplained gait disturbances. Sudarsky and Ronthal found hydrocephalus responsible for the clinical picture in two out of 50 patients (4%) with previously undiagnosed gait disorders (19). Fisher demonstrated hydrocephalic dilation of the ventricular system in 46 of 50 patients (92%) over the age of 60 with otherwise unexplained disturbance of gait, whereas hydrocephalus was seen in only 6.3% of a control group of similar age (20).

Most patients are in their seventh decade when they are diagnosed with idiopathic NPH. We have investigated several clinical aspects in a prospective series of 65 consecutive patients with idiopathic NPH of the elderly (4,21–25). The mean age of those 65 patients was 70.8 years (±7.4), with a range from 50 to 87 years. There were 35 women (54%) and 30 men (47%).

The Classic Triad and Other Clinical Symptoms

The frequency of clinical symptoms in patients with idiopathic NPH has varied considerably among different series. These differences are mainly owing to conceptual and methodological issues. The frequency and severity of the three cardinal symptoms of idiopathic NPH found in our cohort of 65 patients are shown in Table 31.1. We found gait disturbance in all instances. Gait disturbance was classified as mild (cautious gait or difficulty on tandem gait) in 12 of 65 patients (18%), marked (evident difficulty walking or considerable unstable gait) in 32 of 65 patients (49%), and severe (unaided gait not possible) in 21 of 65 patients (32%). In contrast, the distribution in the severity of cognitive deficits and urinary problems differed. Cognitive deficits were categorized as mild in 38%, marked in 40%, and severe in only 20%. It has been stressed by Fisher that disturbance of gait usually is the earliest symptom of idiopathic NPH, preceding mental changes by months to years (15). A variety of other symptoms may occur in addition to the classic triad (26). Parkinsonian movement disorders have been described repeatedly in patients with idiopathic NPH (27,28). We have identified other movement disorders apart from gait disturbance in 86% of our patients (25). After excluding other possible causes in this population of elderly patients, the idiosyncratic movement disorder of idiopathic NPH included hypomimia (55%), hypokinesia (42%), bradykinesia (55%), tremor at rest (6%), rigidity (8%), and dystonia (3%). The clinical picture was dominated in some patients by a parkinsonian appearance. These data, along with electrophysiologic observations on motor disturbances in the upper extremities, suggest that gait disturbance in patients with idiopathic NPH can be part of a more generalized motor function disorder (29,30). After CSF shunting, there is not only improvement of the gait disturbance but also of bradykinesia and other parkinsonian features (25).

TABLE 31.1. *Frequency and severity of gait disturbance, urinary symptoms, and cognitive deficits in 65 patients with idiopathic normal pressure hydrocephalus*

	Gait disturbance		Urinary problems		Cognitive deficits	
	N	%	N	%	N	%
Symptom absent	0	0	11	17	1	2
Symptom present	65	100	54	83	64	98
Severity: I	12	18	18	28	25	38
Severity: II	32	49	24	37	26	40
Severity: III	21	32	12	18	13	20

Severity of symptoms: mild impairment, I; marked impairment, II; severe impairment, III. Gait disturbance; I, cautious gait/difficulties on tandem gait; II, evident difficulties walking/considerable unstable gait; III, unaided gait not possible. Urinary symptoms: I, urge, rare incontinence; II, frequent incontinence; III, little or no control of micturition. Cognitive deficits: I, mild impairment of attention and recent memory; II, marked impairment, oriented within situative context; III, not fully oriented within situative context.

N, number of patients; %, related to total number of patients.

Idiopathic Normal Pressure Hydrocephalus, White Matter Lesions, and Vascular Risk Factors

Idiopathic NPH has been thought to be primarily a disorder of CSF absorption. There is increasing evidence, however, that changes in the cerebral parenchyma may initiate the pathomechanisms and that altered fluid dynamics seen in patients with idiopathic NPH are secondary (8,31,32). After the introduction of magnetic resonance imaging (MRI), correlates of subcortical vascular encephalopathy were found frequently in patients with idiopathic NPH (9,33). We evaluated the extent and severity of white matter lesions by MRI in 37 patients with idiopathic NPH, all of whom improved after shunting (23). In comparison to an age-matched control group, both periventricular and deep white matter lesions were significantly more frequent in patients with idiopathic NPH. Remarkably, a significant negative correlation was found between ventricular width and the severity of white matter lesions in the NPH group, whereas there was a positive correlation in the control group. This finding may be interpreted as evidence for a coexistence of idiopathic NPH and vascular encephalopathy in some patients but it does not support the assumption that vascular encephalopathy actually causes NPH. Deep white matter lesions in patients with NPH are secondary to ischemic demyelination, which may be true also for most periventricular lesions (34). The common link between the frequent coexistence of idiopathic NPH and white matter lesions might be an underlying condition such as arterial hypertension. Few studies in the past investigated the frequency of vascular risk factors in NPH patients (11,35–37). Graff-Radford and Godersky found arterial hypertension prevalent in 74% of their patients with NPH (35). Jacobs reported that diabetes was present in 52% of patients with NPH (36). The investigation of vascular risk factors in our collective yielded a prevalence of arterial hypertension (83%) and diabetes (49%) that was significantly higher than in a control group (24). Univariate analysis demonstrated a highly significant association between arterial hypertension and idiopathic NPH and a weaker association with diabetes. Multivariate analysis confirmed the strong association between arterial hypertension and NPH, whereas the adjusted odds ratio for diabetes was no longer significant. There were also significant associations between cardiac and arteriosclerotic diseases and idiopathic NPH.

Clinical Outcome After Cerebrospinal Fluid Shunting

The benefit of shunting depends primarily on the preoperative selection of patients. The selection process is based on multiple factors, including clinical, hydrodynamic, and morphologic and functional imaging variables. The importance of the presence of a gait disturbance cannot be overemphasized. Cerebrospinal fluid diversion was performed widely after the discovery that shunting can improve the clinical symptoms of idiopathic NPH. Subsequently, shunting also was performed in patients who were unlikely to have idiopathic NPH; some authors even regarded shunting as the definitive diagnostic test (18). Under these circumstances results of shunting for idiopathic NPH were highly variable in different series and were met by some with heavy skepticism. Most centers have applied more rigid criteria for selection of patients for shunting within the past 10 years. Postoperative improvement is seen in 70% to 100% of patients in most contemporary studies (4,26,38–45). In general, gait disorders tend to improve more than cognitive deficits.

Patients with idiopathic NPH and concomitant correlates of subcortical vascular encephalopathy may benefit from shunting, although the degree of improvement in general correlates with the extent and severity of the accompanying white matter changes (21). It may not always be appropriate to ask whether a patient with gait disturbance and hydrocephalus suffers from idiopathic NPH or subcortical vascular encephalopathy. There appears to be a broad overlap and some patients may actually have both conditions.

CLINICAL ASPECTS OF THE GAIT DISTURBANCE OF IDIOPATHIC NORMAL PRESSURE HYDROCEPHALUS

Phenomenology of Hydrocephalic Gait

The severity and clinical aspects of gait disturbance vary widely, depending on the progression of idiopathic NPH and the general condition of the patient (3,15,46). In the early phase of the disease, patients often describe themselves as being dizzy or feeling unstable, even though there is little objective evidence of a gait disorder. Patients with mild impairment of gait walk more carefully and they have considerable difficulty with tandem gait. The number of paces may be increased on turning. With further progression of the disease gait becomes evidently unstable, with a decrease of walking speed, stride length, stride frequency, step height, and foot-floor clearance. Then the gait can adopt a shuffling appearance somewhat resembling parkinsonian gait disorder. Patients may complain about leg weakness, but formal neurologic assessment usually does not detect motor deficit. Ultimately, hydrocephalic gait is characterized by marked slowness and many patients are barely able to walk without support. In late stages, the inability to walk can be embedded in a clinical picture of akinetic mutism.

The typical clinical picture of the gait disturbance of idiopathic NPH is most commonly seen during the second phase of clinical deterioration. Various terms have been used to describe the characteristic features of this gait disturbance. Patients were said "to walk as if they were glued to the floor" in the original description by Adams and colleagues (6). Magnetic gait is another expression that fairly well depicts the clinical appearance (7). There is little to justify use of the expressions apraxia or ataxia of gait, although they have been used most frequently. There is no evidence for ideokinetic apraxia of the lower limbs. Even those patients who are unable to stand may lift their legs when they are supine and perform cycling movements, for example. Usually, there are also no signs for cerebellar ataxia or for dysmetria on tests such as the heel-knee test.

The frequency of several other features of disturbed gait and postural stability have not been investigated extensively in patients with idiopathic NPH. According to our experience many patients with idiopathic NPH demonstrate propulsion or retropulsion on balance tests. In a group of 13 patients with NPH, 30% were described with gait ignition failure (47). Freezing was a common finding in another study, occurring in 56% of NPH patients (48). Dementia and incontinence were significantly associated with the presence of freezing. We have seen festination in single patients, but its frequency remains unknown.

The gait disorder seen in patients with idiopathic NPH, however, is neither pathognomonic nor unique. Similar gait disturbances are seen in patients with frontal lobe pathology. It has even been suggested that various gait disturbances in elderly people are similar to each other regardless of etiology. Elble and colleagues investigated quantitative gait kinematics by infrared computed stroboscopic photometry in a heterogeneous group of 10 patients with symmetrical neurological gait disturbance who were diagnosed with vascular dementia, Alzheimer's disease, peripheral neuropathy, and NPH (49). Although the patients' gait kinematics deviated markedly from control values, the characteristics of these gait disturbances were heavily veiled by nonspecific stride-dependent changes compromising the syndrome of senile gait.

Hydrocephalic Gait Disturbance and Vascular Disease

The severity of symptoms in idiopathic NPH, in general, is not associated with the width of the ventricular system. It is not known whether there is any relation between the severity of the gait disturbance and accompanying white matter lesions. We have analyzed possible relationships between clinical presentation and arterial hypertension and diabetes in our cohort of 65 patients with idiopathic NPH (24). A positive association was recognized between the presence of a marked or severe gait disturbance and arterial hypertension. A weaker association also was found for diabetes. No consistent associations were found when other vascular risk factors were examined, however. The association between arterial hypertension and more severe clinical symptoms allows several interpretations.

Although it is possible that these patients have a more severe coexistent vascular encephalopathy, it is also conceivable that arterial hypertension per se might have an impact on disease progression.

Impact of Gait Disturbance on Prediction of Outcome After Shunting

Graff-Radford and colleagues prospectively assessed different variables predicting surgical outcome in 30 elderly patients with NPH (50). The order of initial onset of either dementia or gait disturbance was highly significant in the prediction of outcome. None of the patients in whom dementia preceded the gait disturbance improved after shunting. In addition, duration of dementia but not gait disturbance was a negative predictor for outcome. In the series of Jacobs and colleagues, no patient who had good walking preoperatively showed improvement in cognitive deficits after shunting (16).

Probatory removal of 30 to 50 mL CSF by spinal tap is now frequently being used to select possible candidates for shunting (26,44,51). Improvement of the gait disturbance after probatory CSF removal has been described to be predictive of both amelioration of gait and general outcome. We investigated the predictive value of ventricular CSF removal on outcome in idiopathic NPH in a previous study (52). Eleven out of 13 patients who underwent subsequent shunting had good functional and symptomatic improvement at a mean follow-up of 12.5 months. Those six patients who showed marked amelioration of their gait disturbance after diagnostic CSF removal had both improvement of gait and functional disability. The predictive value of CSF removal was more variable, however, in those six patients who had only a moderate response.

BIOMECHANICAL EVALUATION OF GAIT BEFORE AND AFTER CEREBROSPINAL FLUID SHUNTING

Review of Biomechanical Studies of Gait in Normal Pressure Hydrocephalus

Knutsson and Lying-Tunell were the first to report their findings on gait recordings in 11 patients with NPH (53). Seven of these patients were thought to have idiopathic NPH of the elderly, and in four instances hydrocephalus was secondary to subarachnoid hemorrhage. Gait patterns were evaluated with intermittent light photography or with polarized light goniometry. In addition, muscle activation was investigated by integrated surface EMG from six muscles of one leg. The gait assessments were performed during free-speed walking along a walkway over a distance of 5 meters. Different phases of the gait cycle were indicated by foot switch signals for heel, foot, and toe contacts to the floor. Gait disturbance was characterized by slow and small angular displacements in the hip, knee, and ankle joints. In particular, foot-floor clearance in the swing phase of the leg was markedly low. Overall, walking speed was reduced and steps were short. Gait cycles were significantly longer in patients with NPH, with a mean cycle duration of 1.8 sec, as compared to 1.1 sec in healthy controls. Furthermore, the swing-to-stance ratio was reduced to 0.2 to 0.5. Continuous activity in antigravity muscles acting on the hip and knee joints was recorded in patients with severe gait disturbance, whereas activity in the triceps surae was low.

Movement and muscle activation patterns could be assessed after lumbar spinal CSF removal in three patients, and after CSF shunting in two. The pathologic EMG pattern shifted toward normal including greater innervation of the triceps surae after lumbar CSF tap in two patients. There was an increase of angular displacement, stride length, and walking speed after CSF shunting. It was thought that the abnormal activation of antigravity muscles was secondary to a release of proprioceptive supporting reactions. This is also supported by the clinical observation that proprioceptive stimuli elicit grasping responses and marked Gegenhalten or paratonic rigidity in patients with idiopathic NPH (25,46). In particular, disturbed supraspinal control of spinal mechanisms for the coordination of gait has been suggested by these authors with regard to the abnormal EMG activation patterns.

Sudarsky and Simon investigated gait disturbances in six elderly patients with hydrocephalus

(54). Diminished cadence, reduction of step height, and decreased counterrotation of the shoulders relative to the pelvis characterized hydrocephalic gait when compared to other groups. Electromyographic studies demonstrated cocontraction in antagonist leg muscles.

Soelberg Sorensen and colleagues performed a prospective study in 16 patients with NPH (30). Postural stability was investigated with a computer-assisted force plate to determine sway of the patient. Gait was evaluated by measuring ground reaction forces during treadmill walking. The vertical, transverse, and sagittal forces of each foot were measured separately to evaluate gait unsteadiness. Postural instability measured on the force plate was more pronounced when the patients had their eyes closed. The mean sway was significantly increased in NPH patients as compared to controls. There were significant differences in speed and stride length; however, these authors did not find differences in various temporal factors in comparison to the control group. Calculations of the external work expressed in joules per kilogram of body weight per meter of gait demonstrated much more energy consumption in NPH patients. Three to six months after CSF shunting, postural instability was similar to those of controls, stride length and speed were increased, and the parameters of unsteadiness were normalized. Interestingly, several patients were unable to walk as slowly as before the operation.

Biomechanical Evaluation of Gait in Normal Pressure Hydrocephalus

Recently we performed a quantitative prospective study to clarify the characteristics of gait disturbance in idiopathic NPH and to investigate its changes after CSF shunting (55). Eleven out of 20 consecutive patients with a diagnosis of idiopathic NPH were able to complete the study protocol. Treadmill walking with freely chosen walking speed was investigated before and at 11 weeks after CSF shunting. Patients were instructed to walk at their maximal comfortable speed. The self-driven treadmill was equipped with separate belts for the right and left foot. Each belt was connected to a force-measuring system. A closed-loop control system was used to adjust the treadmill velocity to the subject's chosen walking velocity. The speed of the treadmill was continuously monitored. The findings were compared to those of a group of 10 age-matched healthy subjects and a group of 10 patients with idiopathic Parkinson's disease (IPD). Gait disorder and general disability were improved in 10 of the 11 patients with idiopathic NPH after CSF shunting.

Several biomechanical parameters of gait were found to be abnormal in patients with idiopathic NPH in the preoperative assessment. Mean values of the quantitative gait assessment preoperatively and at 11 weeks postoperatively are shown in Table 31.2. Walking speed increased significantly after shunting, from 0.39 to

TABLE 31.2. *Biomechanical evaluation of gait before and after cerebrospinal fluid shunting in 11 patients with idiopathic normal pressure hydrocephalus*

Treadmill walking		Walking velocity in m/s	Stride length in m	Stride frequency	Swing phase in % of stride	Stance phase in % of stride	Double supp. in % of stride	Knee joint angle range	Ankle joint angle range	Swing in % of stance phase
Before shunt operation	Mean	0.39	0.43	0.92	32.66	68.98	38.77	35.3	18.0	50.80
	SD	0.26	0.28	0.15	10.80	11.95	12.17	13.3	7.4	23.70
11 weeks after operation	Mean	0.57	0.65	0.88	37.54	63.22	31.48	47.0	25.0	59.81
	SD	0.24	0.27	0.16	2.83	4.24	9.83	13.2	6.7	7.99
P value		0.007	0.005	0.19	0.17	0.21	0.08	0.004	0.049	0.28

Mean values of N = 11 subjects.
SD, standard deviation.

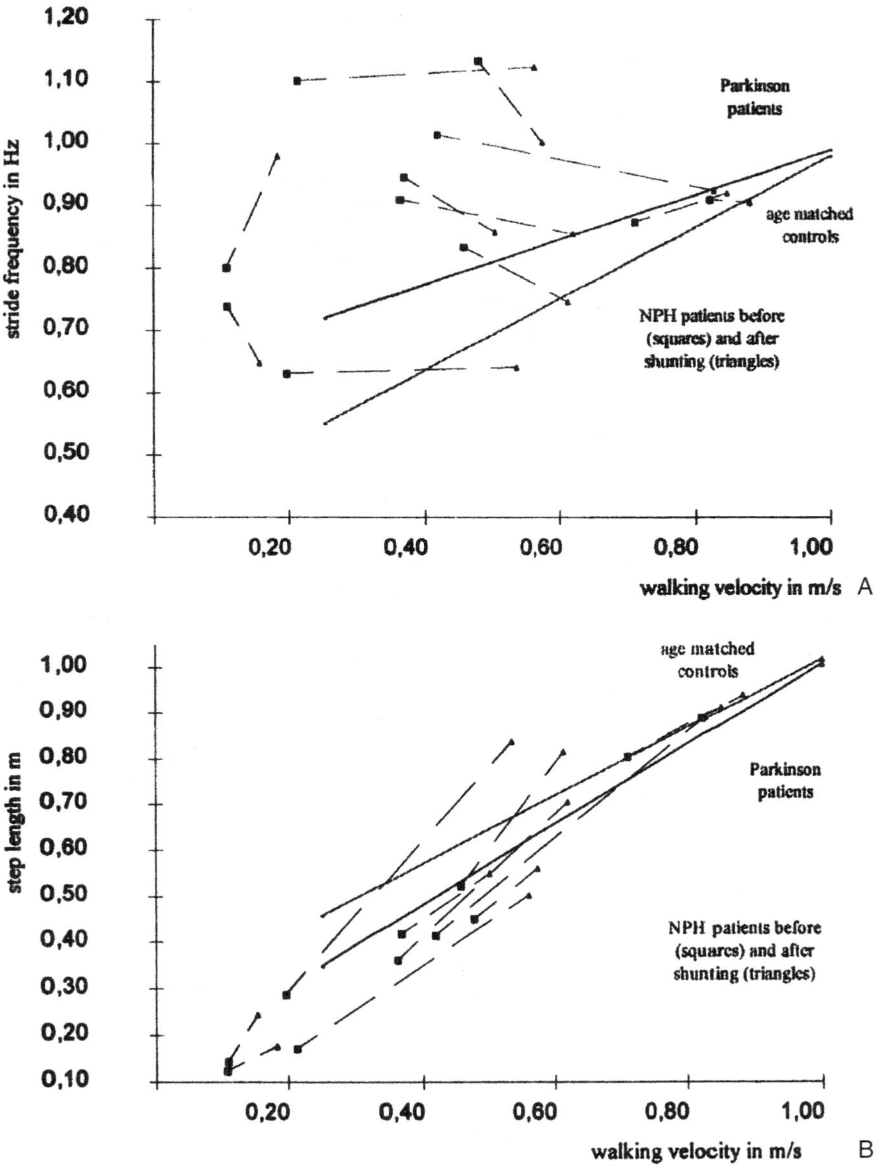

FIG. 31.1. Walking velocity plotted against stride frequency (**A**) and step length (**B**) before and after shunting. The long lines present the regression lines of age-matched controls and patients with Parkinson's disease (PD). Measurements in individual patients with idiopathic normal pressure hydrocephalus (*NPH*) before (*square*) and after (*triangle*) shunting are connected by shorter lines. Preoperative step length in patients with NPH is similar or shorter than in patients with PD. Increased walking velocities after shunting are achieved by increasing step length, not stride frequency.

0.57 cm/sec ($P < 0.01$), and stride length increased from 0.43 to 0.65 m ($P < 0.01$); however, there was no significant change in stride frequency, which was determined at 0.92 Hz preoperatively and 0.88 Hz postoperatively. Joint angle displacements increased from 35 degrees preoperatively to 47 degrees postoperatively in the knee joint ($P < 0.01$), and from 18 to 25 degrees in the ankle ($P < 0.05$), which was close to the range of normal subjects. The similarities between hydrocephalic gait and parkinsonian gait are evident when the walking velocity is plotted against the stride frequency or the step length comparing NPH patients with age-matched controls and patients with PD (Fig. 31.1). The postoperative change in walking velocity by an increase in step length but at constant stride frequency probably reflects both a shift from a parkinsonian-like gait pattern toward normalcy and a disturbed ability of frequency modulation in NPH patients before and after shunting. This finding may indicate that the integrative process of gait is still disturbed at least at an intermediate follow-up despite marked clinical improvement.

CONSIDERATIONS ON THE PATHOPHYSIOLOGY OF HYDROCEPHALIC GAIT

Gait disturbance in patients with idiopathic NPH may have features of both a middle-level and highest-level gait disorder with regard to its clinical presentation and biomechanical evaluations (56). It is best categorized as a frontal gait disorder in the majority of patients, and as such shares several features with the gait disorder of subcortical vascular encephalopathy, or lower-body parkinsonism (57,58). According to the classification proposed by Nutt and colleagues, it may evolve from cautious gait to typical frontal gait disorder to frontal disequilibrium (56). Involvement of the subcortical white matter also is compatible with the presence of other frontal release signs, accompanying cognitive deficits, and urinary control problems. The presence of parkinsonism in several patients in addition suggests a varying degree of functional disturbance of the basal ganglia circuitry and its connections.

How hydrocephalic ventricular enlargement induces gait disturbance and other motor symptoms in NPH is not fully understood. It has been assumed that this is caused by distention of fibers of the corticospinal tract along their course around the enlarged ventricles. Simple mechanical stretching of motor fibers appears to be unlikely given the fact that gait disturbance improves after shunting despite little or no change of the ventriculomegaly seen in postoperative imaging studies in some patients. Furthermore, motor evoked potentials do not indicate dysfunction of the central motor pathways in NPH (59). It is more likely that gait disturbance in patients with idiopathic NPH is associated with disturbed neural control mechanisms of gait secondary to compromised autoregulation and blood flow in the periventricular and deep white matter. This is in accordance with positron emission tomography (PET) and single photon emission computed tomography (SPECT) studies that have shown disturbed hemodynamics predominantly in the frontal and temporal subcortical white matter in patients with idiopathic NPH (60–64). Both functional disturbances and structural lesions most likely contribute to the development of clinical symptoms. Clinical improvement after CSF removal or shunting may be attributed to several factors, including increased periventricular blood flow along with improvement of metabolism subsequent to reduction of intracranial pressure, decrease of CSF pulse pressure, and normalization of compliance. The parallel existence of morphologic white matter damage, on the other hand, may explain why and to what extent recovery of clinical symptoms is incomplete in most of these elderly patients.

REFERENCES

1. Black PM, Ojemann RG, Tzouras A. CSF shunts for dementia, incontinence, and gait disturbance. *Clin Neurosurg* 1985;32:632–651.
2. Pickard JD. Adult communicating hydrocephalus. *Br J Hosp Med* 1982;27:35–44.
3. Symon L, Hinzpeter T. The enigma of normal pressure hydrocephalus: tests to select patients for surgery and to predict shunt function. *Clin Neurosurg* 1977;24:285–315.
4. Krauss JK, Droste DW, Mergner T. [Idiopathic normal pressure hydrocephalus]. *Deutsches Aerzteblatt* 1997; 94:A589–595.
5. Hakim S, Adams RD. The special clinical problem of symptomatic hydrocephalus with normal cerebrospinal fluid pressure. *J Neurol Sci* 1965;2:307–327.
6. Adams RD, Fisher CM, Hakim S, et al. Symptomatic occult hydrocephalus with "normal" cerebrospinal fluid pressure. A treatable syndrome. *N Engl J Med* 1965;273:117–126.
7. Bret P, Chazal J. L'hydrocéphalie chronique de l'adulte. *Neurochirurgie* 1990;36:1–159.
8. Vanneste J. Three decades of normal pressure hydrocephalus: are we wiser now? *J Neurol Neurosurg Psychiatry* 1994;57:1021–1025.
9. Bradley WG, Whittemore AR, Watanabe AS, et al. Association of deep white matter infarction with chronic

communicating hydrocephalus: implications regarding the possible origin of normal-pressure hydrocephalus. *AJNR* 1991;12:31–39.
10. George AE. Chronic communicating hydrocephalus and periventricular white matter disease: a debate with regard to cause and effect. *AJNR* 1991;12:42–44.
11. Casmiro M, d'Allesandro R, Cacciatore FM, et al. Risk factors for the syndrome of ventricular enlargement with gait apraxia (idiopathic normal pressure hydrocephalus): a case-control study. *J Neurol Neurosurg Psychiatry* 1989;52:847–852.
12. Koto A, Rosenberg G, Zingesser LH, et al. Syndrome of normal pressure hydrocephalus: possible relation to hypertensive and arteriosclerotic vasculopathy. *J Neurol Neurosurg Psychiatry* 1977;40:73–79.
13. Earnest MP, Fahn S, Karp JH, et al. Normal pressure hydrocephalus and hypertensive cerebrovascular disease. *Arch Neurol* 1974;31:262–266.
14. Avant DS, Toole JF. Diagnostic guidelines in hydrocephalic dementia. *NC Med J* 1972;33:120–125.
15. Fisher CM. The clinical picture in occult hydrocephalus. *Clin Neurosurg* 1977;24:270–284.
16. Jacobs L, Conti D, Kinkel WR, et al. "Normal-pressure" hydrocephalus. Relationship of clinical and radiographic findings to improvement following shunt surgery. *JAMA* 1976;235:510–512.
17. Graff-Radford NR, Godersky JC. Normal pressure hydrocephalus: onset of gait abnormality before dementia predicts a good surgical outcome. *Arch Neurol* 1986; 43:940–942.
18. Vanneste J, Augustijn P, Dirven C, et al. Shunting normal-pressure hydrocephalus: do the benefits outweigh the risks? *Neurology* 1992;42:54–59.
19. Sudarsky L, Ronthal M. Gait disorders among elderly patients. A survey study of 50 patients. *Arch Neurol* 1983;40:740–743.
20. Fisher CM. Hydrocephalus as a cause of disturbances of gait in the elderly. *Neurology* 1982;32:1358–1363.
21. Krauss JK, Droste DW, Vach W, et al. Cerebrospinal fluid shunting in idiopathic normal-pressure hydrocephalus of the elderly: effect of periventricular and deep white matter lesions. *Neurosurgery* 1996;39:292–300.
22. Krauss JK, Regel JP, Vach W, et al. Flow void of cerebrospinal fluid in idiopathic normal pressure hydrocephalus of the elderly: can it predict outcome after shunting? *Neurosurgery* 1997;40:67–74.
23. Krauss JK, Regel JP, Vach W, et al. White matter lesions in patients with idiopathic normal pressure hydrocephalus and in an age-matched control group: a comparative study. *Neurosurgery* 1997;40:491–496.
24. Krauss JK, Regel JP, Vach W, et al. Vascular risk factors and arteriosclerotic disease in idiopathic normal pressure hydrocephalus of the elderly. *Stroke* 1996;27:24–29.
25. Krauss JK, Regel JP, Droste DW, et al. Movement disorders in adult hydrocephalus. *Mov Disord* 1997;12: 53–60.
26. Larsson A, Wikkelsö C, Bilting M, et al. Clinical parameters in 74 consecutive patients shunt operated for normal pressure hydrocephalus. *Acta Neurol Scand* 1991;84:475–482.
27. Curran T, Lang AE. Parkinsonian syndromes associated with hydrocephalus: case reports, a review of the literature, and pathophysiological hypotheses. *Mov Disord* 1994;9:508–520.
28. Jacobs L, Kinkel W. Computerized axial transverse tomography in normal pressure hydrocephalus. *Neurology* 1976;26:501–507.
29. Blomsterwall E, Bilting M, Stephensen H, et al. Gait abnormality is not the only motor disturbance in normal pressure hydrocephalus. *Scand J Rehabil Med* 1995;27:205–209.
30. Soelberg Sorensen P, Jansen EC, Gjerris F. Motor disturbances in normal-pressure hydrocephalus. Special reference to stance and gait. *Arch Neurol* 1986;431: 34–38.
31. Krauss JK. Idiopathic normal pressure hydrocephalus: primary disorder of CSF absorption or parenchymal cerebral disease? The relevance of vascular risk factors and cerebral white matter lesions. In: Reid A, Marchbanks R, Ernst A, eds. *Intracranial and inner ear physiology and pathophysiology.* London: Whurr Publishers, 1998: 67–78.
32. Bech RA, Juhler M, Waldemar G, et al. Frontal brain and leptomeningeal biopsy specimens correlated with cerebrospinal fluid outflow resistance and B-wave activity in patients suspected of normal-pressure hydrocephalus. *Neurosurgery* 1997;40:497–502.
33. Jack CR, Mokri B, Laws ER, et al. MR findings in normal-pressure hydrocephalus: significance and comparison with other forms of dementia. *J Comput Assist Tomogr* 1987;11:923–931.
34. Munoz DG, Hastak SM, Harper B, et al. Pathologic correlates of increased signals of the centrum ovale on magnetic resonance imaging. *Arch Neurol* 1993;50:492–497.
35. Graff-Radford NR, Godersky JC. Idiopathic normal pressure hydrocephalus and systemic hypertension. *Neurology* 1987;37:868–871.
36. Jacobs L. Diabetes mellitus in normal pressure hydrocephalus. *J Neurol Neurosurg Psychiatry* 1977;40:331–335.
37. Tanaka K, Yonekawa Y, Miyake H, et al. [Idiopathic normal pressure hydrocephalus in elderly patients: its pathophysiology and diagnosis.] *Neurol Surg* 1993; 21:403–409 (Jap).
38. Benzel EC, Pelletier AL, Levy PG. Communicating hydrocephalus in adults: prediction of outcome after ventricular shunting procedures. *Neurosurgery* 1990;26:655–660.
39. Boon AJ, Tans JT, Delwel EJ, et al. Dutch normal-pressure hydrocephalus study: prediction of outcome after shunting by resistance to outflow of cerebrospinal fluid. *J Neurosurg* 1997;87:687–693.
40. Cardoso ER, Piatek D, Del Bigio MR, et al. Quantification of abnormal intracranial pressure waves and isotope cisternography for diagnosis of occult communicating hydrocephalus. *Surg Neurol* 1989;31:20–27.
41. Kristensen B, Malm J, Rabben T. Effects of transient and persistent cerebrospinal fluid drainage on sleep disordered breathing in patients with idiopathic adult hydrocephalus syndrome. *J Neurol Neurosurg Psychiatry* 1998;65:497–501.
42. Raftopoulos C, Deleval J, Chaskis C, et al. Cognitive recovery in idiopathic normal pressure hydrocephalus: a prospective study. *Neurosurgery* 1994;35:397–405.
43. Raftopoulos C, Massager N, Baleriaux D, et al. Prospective analysis by computed tomography and long-term outcome of 23 adult patients with chronic idiopathic hydrocephalus. *Neurosurgery* 1996;38:51–59.
44. Malm J, Kristensen B, Karlsson T, et al. The predictive value of cerebrospinal fluid dynamic tests in patients

with the idiopathic adult hydrocephalus syndrome. *Arch Neurol* 1995;52:783–789.

45. Sahuquillo J, Rubio E, Codina A, et al. Reappraisal of the intracranial pressure and cerebrospinal fluid dynamics in patients with the so-called "normal pressure hydrocephalus" syndrome. *Acta Neurochir* 1991;112: 50–61.
46. Estanol BV. Gait apraxia in communicating hydrocephalus. *J Neurol Neurosurg Psychiatry* 1981;44:305–308.
47. Petzinger G, Perez E, Fahn S. Motor features of normal pressure hydrocephalus [abstract]. *Mov Disord* 1994;9:126.
48. Giladi N, Kao R, Fahn S. Freezing phenomenon in patients with parkinsonian syndromes. *Mov Disord* 1997;12:302–305.
49. Elble RJ, Hughes L, Higgins C. The syndrome of senile gait. *J Neurol* 1992;239:71–75.
50. Graff-Radford NR, Godersky JC, Jones MP. Variables predicting surgical outcome in symptomatic hydrocephalus in the elderly. *Neurology* 1989;39:1601–1604.
51. Wikkelsö C, Andersson H, Blomstrand C, et al. Normal pressure hydrocephalus: predictive value of the cerebrospinal fluid tap-test. *Acta Neurol Scand* 1986;73: 566–573.
52. Krauss JK, Regel JP. The predictive value of ventricular CSF removal in normal pressure hydrocephalus. *Neurol Res* 1997;19:357–360.
53. Knutsson E, Lying-Tunell U. Gait apraxia in normal-pressure hydrocephalus: patterns of movement and muscle activation. *Neurology* 1985;35:155–160.
54. Sudarsky L, Simon S. Gait disorder in late-life hydrocephalus. *Arch Neurol* 1987;44:263–267.
55. Krauss JK, Faist M, Schubert M, et al. Biomechanical evaluation of gait in normal pressure hydrocephalus (NPH) of the elderly before and after shunting [abstract]. *Mov Disord* 1998;13:77.
56. Nutt JG, Marsden CD, Thompson PD. Human walking and higher-level gait disorders, particularly in the elderly. *Neurology* 1983;43:268–279.
57. Fisher CM. Binswanger's encephalopathy: a review. *J Neurol* 1989;236:65–79.
58. FitzGerald PM, Jankovic J. Lower body parkinsonism: evidence for vascular etiology. *Mov Disord* 1989;4:249–260.
59. Zaaroor M, Bleich N, Chistyakov A, et al. Motor evoked potentials in the preoperative and postoperative assessment of normal pressure hydrocephalus. *J Neurol Neurosurg Psychiatry* 1997;62:517–521.
60. Meyer JS, Tachibana H, Hardenberg JP, et al. Normal pressure hydrocephalus: influences on cerebral hemodynamic and cerebrospinal fluid pressure—chemical autoregulation. *Surg Neurol* 1984;21:195–203.
61. Tanaka A, Kimura M, Nakayama Y, et al. Cerebral blood flow and autoregulation in normal pressure hydrocephalus. *Neurosurgery* 1997;40:1161–1167.
62. Waldemar G, Schmidt JF, Delecluse F, et al. High resolution SPECT with [^{99m}Tc]-d,l-HMPAO in normal pressure hydrocephalus before and after shunt operation. *J Neurol Neurosurg Psychiatry* 1993;56:655–664.
63. Tedeschi E, Hasselbalch SG, Waldemar G, et al. Heterogeneous cerebral glucose metabolism in normal pressure hydrocephalus. *J Neurol Neurosurg Psychiatry* 1995;59:608–615.
64. Kristensen B, Malm J, Fagerlund M, et al. Regional cerebral blood flow, white matter abnormalities, and cerebrospinal fluid hydrodynamics in patients with idiopathic adult hydrocephalus syndrome. *J Neurol Neurosurg Psychiatry* 1996;60:282–288.

Gait Disorders. Advances in Neurology, Vol. 87,
edited by E. Růžička, M. Hallett, and J. Jankovic.
Lippincott Williams & Wilkins, Philadelphia © 2001.

32

Patterns of Upper Motoneuron Dysfunction in the Lower Limb

*†Nathaniel H. Mayer, ‡§Alberto Esquenazi, and ||¶Mary Ann E. Keenan

**Department of Rehabilitation Medicine, Temple University, Philadelphia, Pennsylvania 19140; †Motor Control Analysis Laboratory and ‡Gait and Motion Laboratory, MossRehab, Philadelphia, Pennsylvania 19141; Departments of §Physical Medicine and Rehabilitation and ||Orthopaedic Surgery, Thomas Jefferson University School of Medicine, Philadelphia, Pennsylvania 19107; and ¶Neuro-Orthopaedic Surgery Program, Department of Orthopaedic Surgery, Albert Einstein Medical Center, Philadelphia, Pennsylvania 19141*

In the 1930s, Nikolai A. Bernstein suggested that a basic problem of motor control relates to overcoming redundant degrees of freedom in our multijointed skeletal system (1). Because we live in a three-dimensional world but we have more than three degrees of freedom in our multijointed limb segments, the issue for Bernstein and many others in his tradition was to discover the coordinative rules or priorities used by the brain to constrain redundant degrees of freedom when performing motor tasks. Latash has pointed out that the "Bernstein problem" can occur even at the level of single-joint, single degree of freedom movements where there is seemingly no room for peripheral redundancy (2). Commonly, there are multiple "agonists" and "antagonists" for virtually any movement direction. In order to match a required joint torque even across a single joint, the question regarding which muscles should be activated and at what levels of activity is likely to have a very variable answer without a unique solution. For a given patient, however, there may be a unique solution in that equinovarus deformity may be solely attributable to an overactive tibialis anterior in one patient, whereas in another it may be an overactive tibialis posterior or some other muscle. This concept, namely, identifying which muscles contribute dynamically and statically to upper motoneuron gait dysfunction, serves as a conceptual basis for this chapter and Chapters 33 and 34. Simply put, identifying muscles that produce deforming maladaptive joint movements and postures statically and dynamically is an important endeavor in aiding clinical interpretation of gait dysfunction and in rationalizing subsequent treatment interventions (3).

PRIORITIES, FEATURES, AND FUNCTIONAL PRODUCTS

Core motor control priorities of gait include translation of the body's center of gravity (COG) from place to place and stability of the upright body during that translation (4). Stability during translation is both a swing phase and a stance phase priority and implies no falling in stance and no tripping in swing (i.e., adequate clearance of obstacles in a cluttered environment). Translation of the COG is enabled by mechanisms that control swing and stance phase advancement within a range of stable parameters. Stability of the COG is enabled by control of a range of ground reaction forces generated by the stance limb and control of a range of clearances generated by the swing limb.

As viewed by a clinician, operational features of gait include swing phase advancement, clearance stability, loading and unloading (i.e., transferring weight from one limb to another), stability of single-limb support and stance phase advancement (i.e., advancement of the COG over the stance limb). It is well recognized that the COG progresses continuously throughout the gait cycle. Pathologies that affect the swing limb and the stance limb will have an impact on translation of the COG; therefore, operational features of swing limb advancement and stance limb advancement (i.e., mechanisms that affect swing phase and stance phase advancement) are intimately linked to the gait priority of COG translation. On the other hand, antigravity support of the COG is linked to the operational features of swing phase clearance, stance phase loading, and stability of single-limb support.

Core motor control priorities and their operational features give rise to the functional products of locomotion. Some of the functional products of locomotion include the production of a range of the following:

1. Step and stride lengths
2. Velocities
3. Base widths
4. Cadences
5. Single-limb support postures
6. Changes in directionality
7. Elevations and descents
8. Articulations with uneven surfaces
9. Clearances

Functional products of locomotion are practical clinical parameters of gait that may be used by clinicians, at least in part, to evaluate gait dysfunction and to measure changes as a result of clinical interventions. Functional products of gait are commonly impaired in patients with an upper motoneuron syndrome because patterns of upper motoneuron dysfunction in the lower limb commonly influence core priorities of gait, operational features of gait, and functional products of gait (5,6).

PATTERNS OF UPPER MOTONEURON DYSFUNCTION

Patterns of upper motoneuron dysfunction in the lower limb that have been selected for presentation in this chapter include:

1. Equinovarus foot
2. Equinovalgus foot
3. Hyperextended great toe
4. Flexed knee
5. Stiff knee
6. Adducted (scissoring) thighs
7. Flexed hip (Table 32.1) (7)

The first four patterns are considered to be deviant throughout the gait cycle. "Stiff knee" and adducted thigh are predominantly deviations of swing phase. The flexed hip is considered a stance phase deviation. All patterns potentially influence translation or stability of the COG in some way.

EQUINOVARUS

Equinovarus foot is the most common upper motoneuron (UMN) posture seen in the lower

TABLE 32.1. *Impact of upper motoneuron dysfunction patterns on functional products of gait*

Functional products	Equinovarus	Equinovalgus	Hyperextended great toe	Flexed knee	Stiff knee	Adducted thigh	Flexed hip
Step and stride lengths	R	R	R	R		R	R
Velocities	R	R	R	R	R	R	R
Base widths	R	R		R		R	
Single limb support postures	R	R	R	R	R	R	R
Uneven surfaces	R	R	R	R	R	R	R
Clearances	R	R			R	R	
Elevations and descents	R	R	R	R	R	R	R
Changes in direction	R	R		R		R	R

Normal gait exhibits a range of capabilities and values for the functional products of gait. As identified in the table, persons with upper motoneuron dysfunction frequently demonstrate a restricted (R) range.

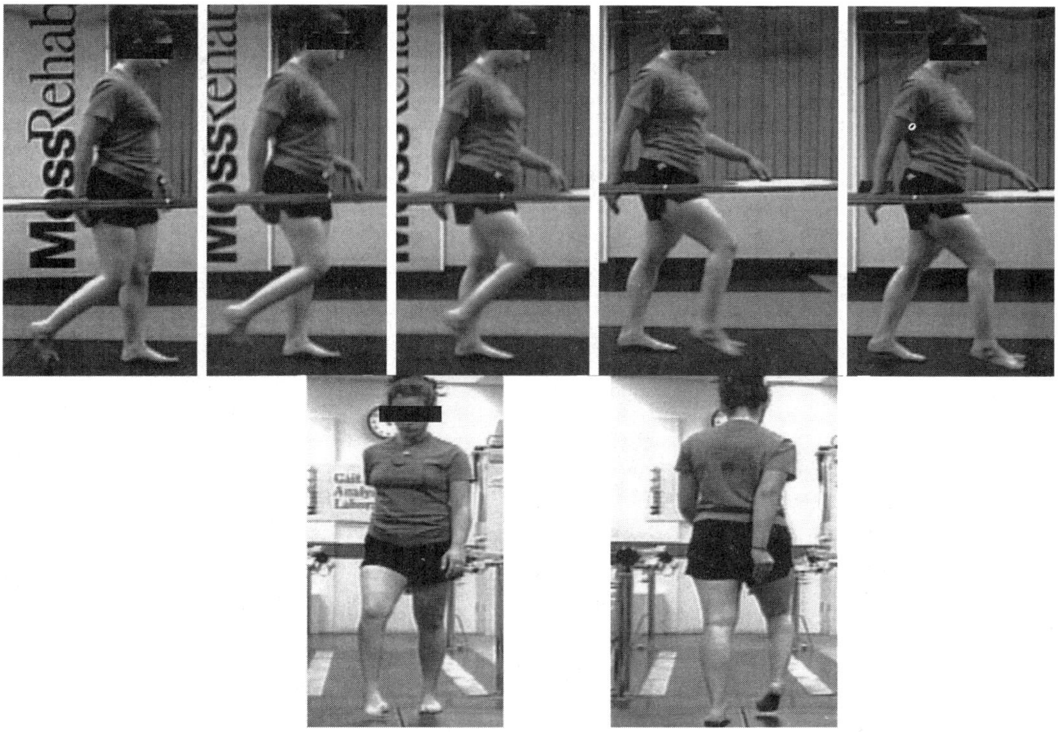

FIG. 32.1. Gait dysfunction illustrating equinovarus.

extremity. The foot and ankle are turned down and in (Fig. 32.1). Toe curling or toe clawing may coexist. The lateral border of the foot, particularly the fifth metatarsal head, is typically compressed against the floor or against the footrest of a wheelchair. Skin breakdown over the metatarsal head may develop from unrelieved pressure. During stance phase of gait, the forefoot makes contact with the ground first, weight is borne primarily on the lateral border of the foot, and toe flexion typically is present. During weight bearing, the patient often complains of pain over the lateral border and callus and skin breakdown can be seen. Equinovarus limits dorsiflexion motion during single-limb support when the foot is stationary. The tibia ordinarily progresses forward by means of ankle dorsiflexion but the lack of available dorsiflexion in the equinovarus foot results in hyperextension thrust of the knee and restrained forward translation of the body's COG. Walking on uneven ground is difficult and overall balance is compromised. During early swing phase, toe drag associated with equinovarus may make floor clearance and limb advancement difficult. Equinovarus affects the priority of COG translation during stance limb advancement. It affects the priority of COG stability during swing phase clearance and during stance phase loading and single-limb support. Functional products of gait affected by equinovarus include a reduced range of: step and stride lengths, velocities, base widths, single-limb postures, elevations and descents, articulation with uneven surfaces, and clearance stability. A patient's ability to change direction is more difficult as well.

A number of muscles may generate unbalanced forces with respect to the equinovarus pattern (8). Deforming muscles may include tibialis anterior, tibialis posterior, gastrocnemius, soleus, long toe flexors, and extensor hallucis longus (EHL). Weak muscles may include peroneus longus and peroneus brevis in stance phase and the long toe extensors in swing phase.

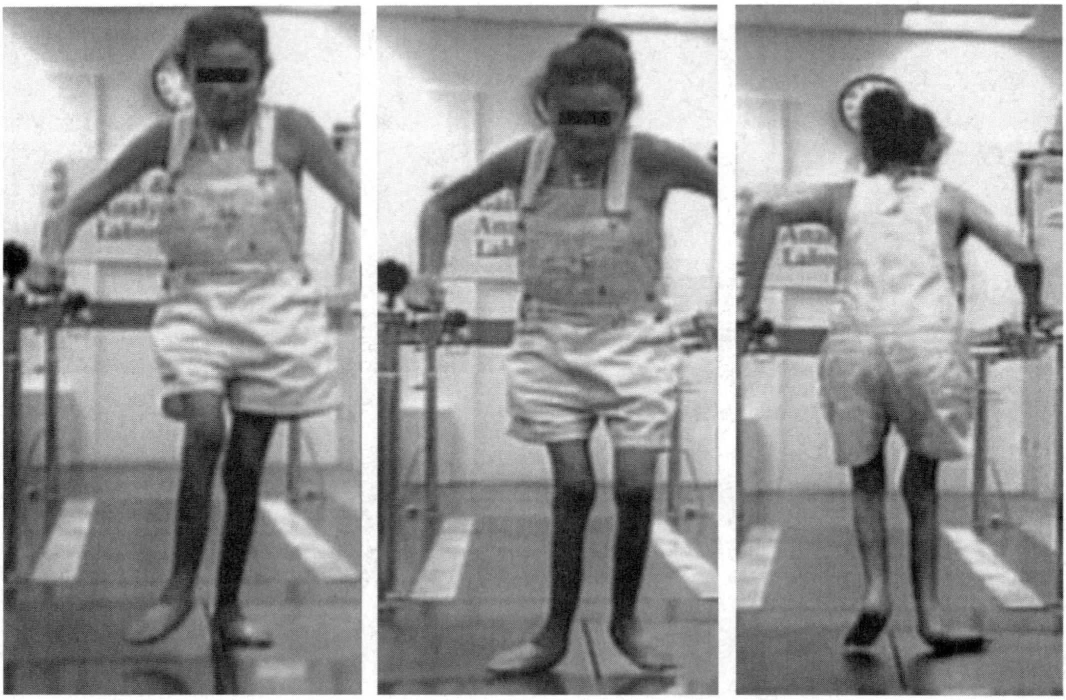

FIG. 32.2. Gait dysfunction illustrating equinovalgus pattern. Note weight bearing on medial aspect of the foot.

EQUINOVALGUS

In the equinovalgus foot deformity, the foot and ankle are turned down and out. Toe curling or clawing may be present. The medial border of the foot, particularly the first metatarsal head, is often compressed against the floor or the footrest of a wheelchair (Fig. 32.2). Skin breakdown may develop and contact of the forefoot with the ground may produce pain as weight is borne on the medial aspect of the foot. Equinovalgus has an impact on COG translation during stance limb advancement. Equinovalgus has an impact on COG stability during swing phase clearance and during stance phase loading and single-limb support. Functional products of gait affected by equinovalgus include a reduced range of the following: step and stride lengths, velocities, base widths, single-limb postures, elevations and descents, articulation with uneven surfaces, clearances, and changes in direction.

A number of muscles may generate unbalanced forces in stance phase with respect to equinovalgus pattern. Deforming muscles may include peroneus longus, peroneus brevis, gastrocnemius, soleus, and the long toe flexors. Weak muscles may include tibialis anterior and EHL in both phases of the gait cycle and tibialis posterior in stance phase.

HYPEREXTENDED GREAT TOE

Hyperextended great toe is a deformity that is characterized by toe extension throughout the gait cycle. Ankle equinus and varus may accompany this abnormal foot posture. When wearing shoes, the patient complains of pain at the tip of the toe and under the first metatarsal head during stance. During gait, toe extension during early and mid-stance complicates weight bearing. The patient will shorten stance time of the affected limb and there is interference with push off and forward propulsion in terminal stance and preswing. There may be sustained hallux extension during swing phase. Thus, hyperextended great toe has an impact on COG translation during stance limb advancement. It also has an impact on COG stability during stance phase loading and single-limb support. Functional products affected by hyperextended great toe include a reduced range of the following: step and stride lengths, velocities, single-limb postures, elevations and descents, and articulation with uneven surfaces. A number of muscles may generate unbalanced forces with respect to the hyperextended great toe pattern. EHL provides a deforming force causing great toe hyperextension. A weak flexor hallucis longus may not be able to compensate and offset the hyperextension force of EHL. When equinovarus is present, analysis of the contributions of tibialis anterior, tibialis posterior, gastrocnemius, soleus, and the long toe flexors are taken into account as well.

FLEXED KNEE

In the flexed knee deformity, the knee remains flexed throughout swing and stance. A flexed knee during stance phase requires compensatory hip flexion on the same side and increased hip and knee flexion during swing contralaterally. Bilateral knee flexion deformity results in a crouch pattern (Fig. 32.3). The impact of a flexed knee on translation of the COG may be seen in the operational feature of swing limb advancement. Lack of full knee extension in terminal swing limits limb advancement and results in a short step length. The flexed knee also has an impact on stance phase advancement because knee extension from mid- to terminal stance is absent. Center of gravity stability is affected by a flexed knee deformity during the operational features of limb loading and single-limb support. The impact of flexed knee on the functional products of gait includes a reduction in the range of step and stride lengths, velocities, base widths, single-limb postures, elevations and descents, articulation with uneven surfaces, and changes in direction.

Muscles that may generate deforming forces with respect to the flexed knee pattern include medial and lateral hamstrings in both phases of the gait cycle, gastrocnemius in stance phase, and iliopsoas in swing. A weak quadriceps may be unable to counterbalance the hamstrings. In addition, a weak gastrocnemius and soleus group may lead to a "drop off" pattern of gait in terminal stance (i.e., sudden and simultaneous ankle dorsiflexion and knee flexion).

STIFF KNEE

The stiff knee is a swing phase deformity by definition. The term "stiff knee" is often placed in quotation marks to signify that it refers to a

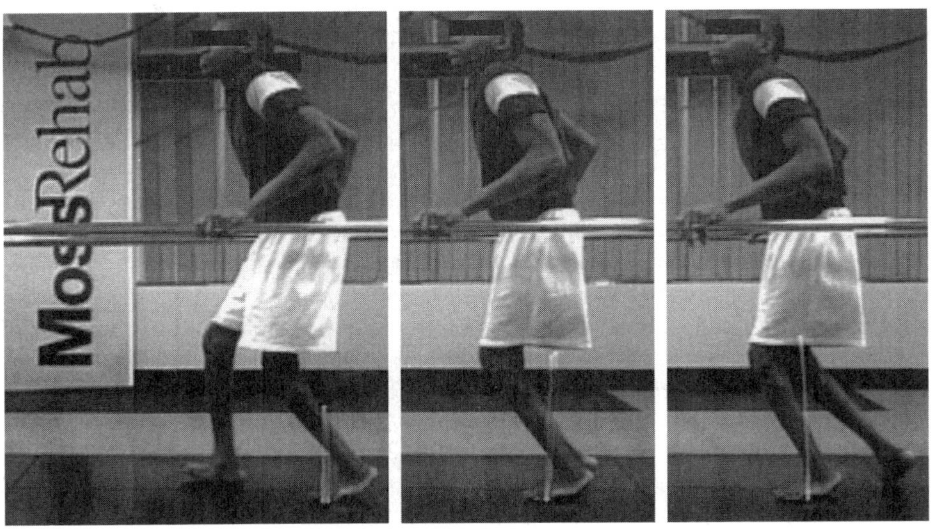

FIG. 32.3. Gait dysfunction with bilateral flexed knee in swing and stance.

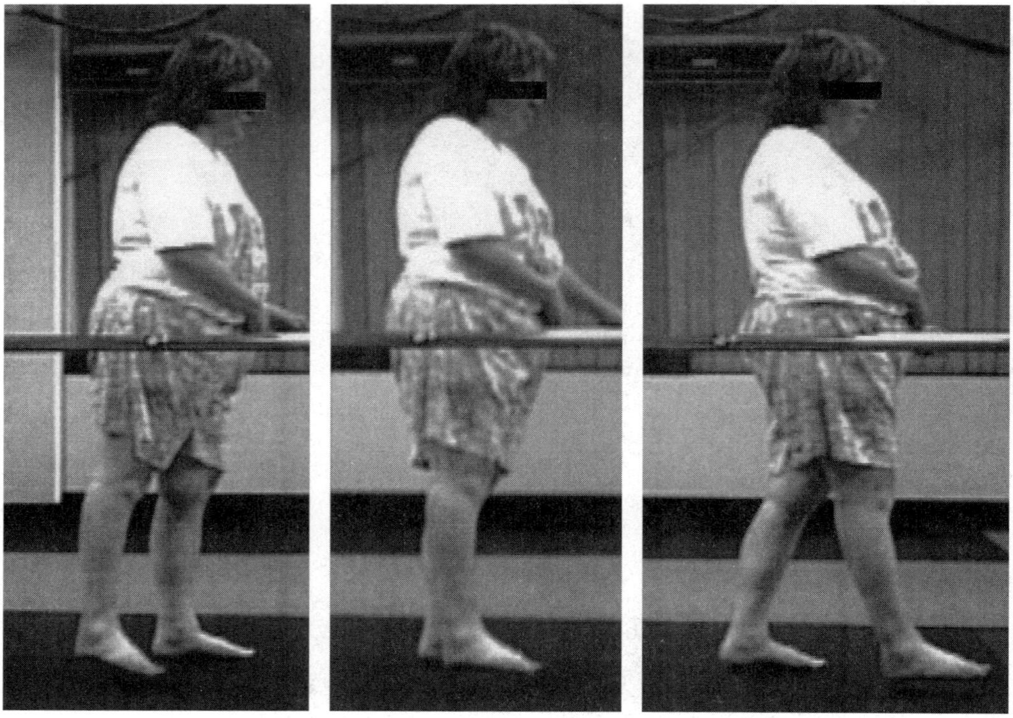

FIG. 32.4. Gait dysfunction with stiff knee pattern during swing phase.

dynamic deformity created by muscle contraction rather than an intrinsic structural deformity of the knee causing loss of passive motion. In stiff knee gait, the knee typically remains extended during swing phase and frequently in stance phase as well (Fig. 32.4). A stiff knee lengthens the limb and poses problems, particularly during the preswing and swing phases of gait. Toe drag and early swing may cause tripping and falling if there is an associated equinovarus. The limb appears to be functionally longer because it remains extended throughout the swing phase. In order to achieve clearance of the floor during swing phase, the patient may attempt to compensate for this relative leg length discrepancy by ipsilateral limb circumduction, by hiking the pelvis or by contralateral vaulting that consumes increased energy. The impact of stiff knee includes an increase in the inertial load of the swinging limb (by virtue of its longer moment arm when the knee is extended compared with a flexed knee), thereby potentially influencing COG translation during swing-limb advancement. An extended knee may become problematic during swing phase clearance and its associated effect on COG stability. The impact of stiff knee on functional products of gait includes a reduced range of velocities, single-limb postures, elevations and descents, articulation with uneven surfaces, and clearance of a cluttered environment.

Muscles that may generate deforming forces with respect to the stiff knee pattern include rectus femoris, vastus lateralis, intermedius and medialis, gluteus maximus, and the gastrocsoleus group. An overactive gluteus maximus in swing phase may act to restrain hip flexion and swing limb advancement, resulting in a nonswinging extended knee. An overactive calf muscle group, especially if contractured in equinus, promotes compensatory hip flexion in stance phase. Ankle equinus causes the knee to hyperextend by preventing forward progression of the tibia during stance phase and the hip flexes to bring body mass forward and compensate for the posterior oblique angling of the tibia. Knee hyperextension of stance phase typically carries over into the subphase of preswing and often into the other subphases of swing as well. When iliopsoas is weak in swing phase, weak hip motion is accompanied by weak knee flexion as well.

ADDUCTED (SCISSORING) THIGH

The patient with adductor spasticity sits with scissoring thighs or walks with a scissoring pattern characterized by both lower limbs exhibiting medial thigh contact throughout the gait cycle. Nevertheless, as a deviant pattern of gait, the scissoring thigh pattern is largely considered to originate in swing phase. Scissoring thighs may interfere with hygiene, dressing, sexual intimacy, sitting, transfers, standing, and walking. During swing phase, severe hip adduction interferes with limb advancement (Fig. 32.5). The adducted posturing at the end of swing phase generates a narrow base of support during stance, ultimately making upright balance precarious. When adductor spasticity is complicated by hip flexor spasticity, toileting functions and perineal access are markedly hampered and frequent repositioning of the patient sitting in a chair is required and usually does not work well. The impact of scissoring thighs on translation of the COG may be seen during swing limb advancement and stance limb advancement. Stability of the COG may be challenged by scissoring thighs, which can pose a problem of clearance in swing phase. The adducted position of the lower limb at the end of terminal swing has an impact on subsequent loading and single support in stance. Functional products affected by scissoring thighs include a reduced range of the following: step and stride lengths, velocities, base widths, single-limb postures, elevations and descents, articulation with uneven surfaces, and changes in direction.

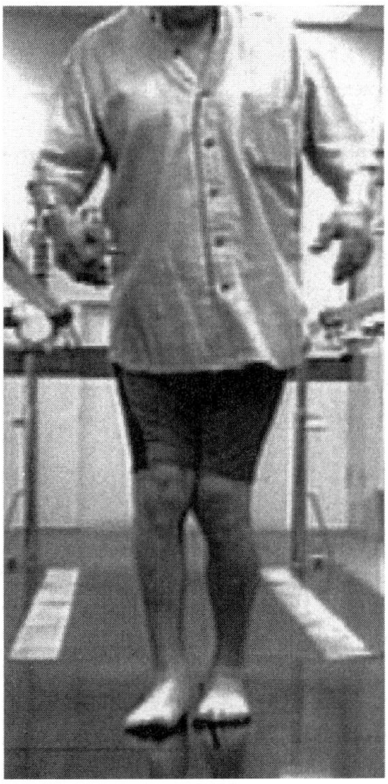

FIG. 32.5. Gait dysfunction with adducted thighs. Note narrow base width and "kissing" thighs that hinder limb advancement.

A number of muscles may generate unbalanced forces in swing phase with respect to the adducted (scissoring) thigh pattern. Muscles that may contribute deforming forces include adductor longus, brevis, and magnus, gracilis, and pectineus muscles that may generate unbalanced forces. Weak muscles may include iliopsoas and sartorius. The patient may adduct the thigh in swing phase by using adductors to compensate for these weak hip flexors. The patient may develop stance phase difficulties after an adduction deviation in swing phase because of the subsequently narrow base width. Control of stance phase stability with a narrow base width of support requires strong hip abductors. If gluteus medius and tensor fascia lata are weak, stance phase stability may be impaired.

FLEXED HIP

The patient with excessive hip flexion experiences difficulty when standing up from a seated position during both phases of the gait cycle and potentially during positioning efforts for perineal care and sexual intimacy. In normal gait, the hip is flexed at initial contact but thereafter extends throughout stance phase. The UMN pattern of hip flexion is defined as persistent hip flexion throughout stance (Fig. 32.6). Severe hip flexion deformity may promote development of

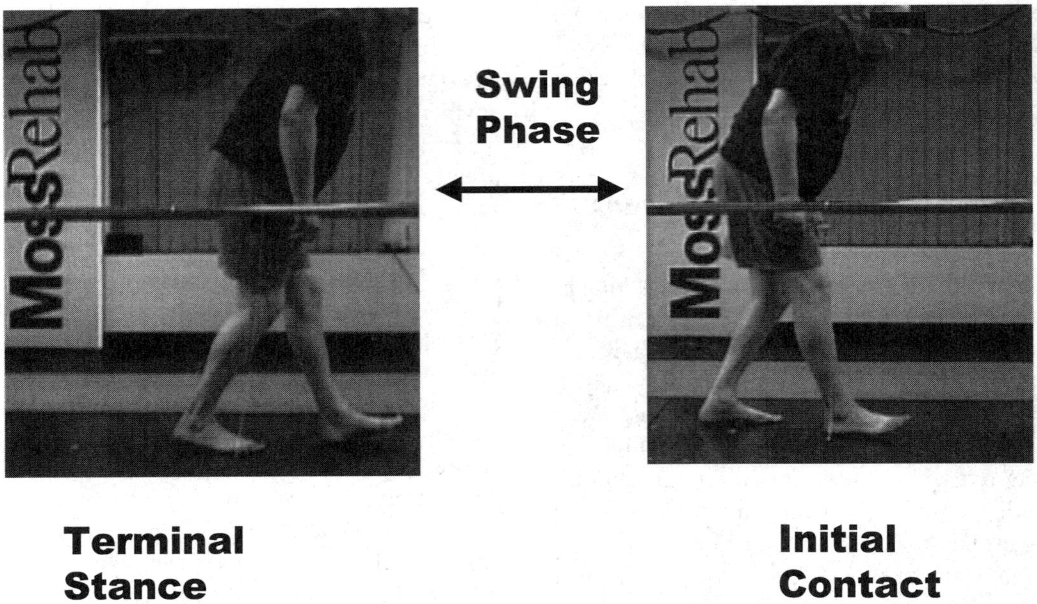

FIG. 32.6. Gait dysfunction with flexed hip. The hip remained flexed throughout stance phase from initial contact through terminal stance. Note short step length secondary to inadequate hip extension in terminal stance.

a knee flexion deformity. When the limb with excessive hip flexion is in stance phase, forward advancement of the body over this limb is markedly restricted. The result is a shortened contralateral step. Excessive hip flexion also affects stability of the COG by influencing single-limb support during stance. Excessive hip flexion has an impact on the functional products of gait including a reduced range of step and stride lengths, velocities, single-limb postures, elevations and descents, articulation with uneven surfaces, and changes in direction. A number of muscles may generate unbalanced forces in stance phase with respect to the flexed hip pattern. Excessive activity in iliopsoas, pectineus, and rectus femoris may generate dynamically deforming hip flexor forces in stance phase. A weak gluteus maximus may not be strong enough to counterbalance flexor forces.

CONCLUSION

Patterns of lower limb dysfunction in the upper motoneuron syndrome have an impact on the core priorities, operational features, and functional products of gait. A number of muscles typically cross major joints of the lower extremity; identifying the *actual* muscles that contribute dynamically and statically to a UMN deformity is an important key to clinical management of the resulting gait dysfunctions (9). Clinical evaluation contributes to the analysis of gait dysfunction but gait laboratory evaluation using dynamic electromyography (EMG) is often necessary to identify the particular contributions of offending muscles with confidence. The correct selection of target muscles that contribute to any one pattern of dysfunction may serve as a rational basis for interventions that focus on specific muscles including chemodenervation with botulinum toxin, neurolysis with phenol and surgical lengthenings, and transfers and releases of individual muscles (10). In a sense, the Bernstein "degrees of freedom problem" for any given patient is "solved" through clinical hypothesis development based on the combined findings of the clinical examination and gait laboratory data. Treatment interventions, whether conservative or surgical, may be considered as empirical tests of these clinically formulated hypotheses.

REFERENCES

1. Rosenbaum DA. *Human motor control.* San Diego, CA: Academic Press, 1991.
2. Latash ML, Anson JG. What are "normal movements" in atypical populations? *Behavioral and Brain Sciences.* 1996;19:55–106.
3. Mayer NH, Esquenazi A, Wannstedt G. Surgical planning for upper motoneuron dysfunction: the role of motor control evaluation. *J Head Trauma Rehabil* 1996;11: 37–56.
4. Esquenazi A, Keenan MA. Gait analysis. In: Delisa JA, ed. *Rehabilitation medicine: principles and practice,* 2nd ed. Philadelphia: J.B. Lippincott, 1991.
5. Lance JW. Symposium synopsis. In: Feldman RG, Young RR, Koella WP, eds. *Spasticity: disordered motor control.* Chicago: Yearbook, 1980.
6. Mayer NH. Clinical physiologic concepts of spasticity and motor dysfunction in adults with an upper motoneuron lesion. *Muscle Nerve* 1997;6:S1–S13.
7. Mayer NH, Esquenazi A, Childers MK. Common patterns of clinical motor dysfunction. *Muscle Nerve* 1997; 6:S21–S35.
8. Keenan MA, Mayer NH, Esquenazi A, et al. A neuro-orthopaedic approach to the management of common patterns of upper motoneuron dysfunction after brain injury. *Neuro Rehabilitation* 1999;12:119–143.
9. Mayer NH, Esquenazi A, Keenan MA. Analysis and management of spasticity contracture and impaired motor control after brain injury. In: Horn LJ, Zasler ND, eds. *Medical rehabilitation of traumatic brain injury.* Philadelphia: Hanley & Belfus, 1996.
10. Keenan MA. Surgical decision-making for residual limb deformities following traumatic brain injury. *Orthop Rev* 1988;27:1185–1192.

Gait Disorders. Advances in Neurology, Vol. 87,
edited by E. Růžička, M. Hallett, and J. Jankovic.
Lippincott Williams & Wilkins, Philadelphia © 2001.

33

Dynamic Polyelectromyography, Neurolysis, and Chemodenervation with Botulinum Toxin A for Assessment and Treatment of Gait Dysfunction

*‡Alberto Esquenazi, †¶Nathaniel H. Mayer, and §‖Mary Ann E. Keenan

**Gait and Motion Analysis Laboratory and †Motor Control Analysis Laboratory, MossRehab, Philadelphia, Pennsylvania 19141; Departments of ‡Physical Medicine and Rehabilitation and §Orthopaedic Surgery, Thomas Jefferson University School of Medicine, Philadelphia, Pennsylvania 19107; ‖Neuro-Orthopaedic Program, Department of Orthopaedic Surgery, Albert Einstein Medical Center, Philadelphia, Pennsylvania 19141; and ¶Department of Rehabilitation Medicine, Temple University, Philadelphia, Pennsylvania 19140*

Problems of movement control and limb deformities are common consequences of the upper motoneuron syndrome (UMN) (1). The genesis of limb deformity is based, in large part, on the concept that UMN features such as paresis, spasticity, and impaired motor control generate an imbalance of muscular forces affecting joint position statically and joint movement dynamically.

Typical patterns of UMN deformities are diagnostically evaluated to identify which muscles contribute dynamically and statically to the observed deformity and impaired motor control. Dynamic electromyography (EMG), gait, motion analysis, and diagnostic nerve blocks frequently provide the necessary detailed information about specific muscle groups that guide decision making for treatment. Techniques to improve passive and active motion can be carried out based on such information. These techniques frequently include the use of motor point blocks with phenol, nerve blocks (primarily motor nerves) with phenol, and chemodenervation with botulinum toxin A (Botox A) (Allergan, Inc., Irvine, CA, U.S.A.). These interventions can be followed by rehabilitation techniques such as muscle strengthening, stretching, retraining, EMG biofeedback, serial casting, and bracing. Frequently, surgery is necessary to achieve a more permanent correction of deforming forces.

Prior to selecting interventions, the clinical team and the patient should explicitly develop functional goals. Functional goals may be classified as passive or active in nature (2). Passive function refers to the passive manipulation of limbs to achieve functional ends, typically performed by caregivers, although patients may also manipulate their limbs passively with noninvolved limbs. Active functions, on the other hand, refer to patient's direct use of the limb to carry out a functional activity. Identifying muscles with volitional capacity is important to the achievement of this goal. Another requirement is behavioral compliance and the ability to incorporate the newly gained increases in motion into the daily routine.

In broad terms, clinical evaluation focuses on the identification of three factors:

1. The clinical pattern of motor dysfunction (Chapter 32) (3)
2. The patient's ability to control muscles involved in the pattern of dysfunction

3. The role of rheologic properties of muscles, including contracture, as they relate to the functional problem (4)

The treatment interventions suggested in this chapter are usually muscle-specific, and the outcome of a detailed evaluation using dynamic EMG and other techniques available in the gait laboratory is to identify muscle-specific motor behaviors that are linked to specific interventions. This implies that the unit level of evaluation is typically a joint and individual muscles affecting this joint.

Clinical examination is the mainstay of evaluation and seeks information about the following questions: (a) Is there selective voluntary control of a given muscle? (b) Is the muscle activated dyssynergically (i.e., as an antagonist in movement)? (c) Is the muscle resistive to passive stretch? (d) Does the muscle have fixed shortening (contracture)? The clinical examination alone may not be sufficient to answer these questions and laboratory assessment, including dynamic polyelectromyography (polyEMG), kinetic and kinematic studies, as well as nerve blocks, may be helpful. In the gait laboratory, dynamic EMG is acquired and examined in reference to simultaneous measurements of joint motion (kinematics) and ground reaction forces (kinetics) obtained from force platforms. Kinetic, kinematic, and dynamic EMG data augment the clinician's ability to interpret whether voluntary function is present in a given muscle and whether that muscle behavior is also out of phase (dyssynergic). In addition, evaluation before and after temporary diagnostic nerve or motor point blocks can help the clinician distinguish between obligatory and compensatory gait patterns and postures.

Combined with clinical information, the laboratory measurements of muscle function often provide the degree of detail and confidence necessary to optimize the rehabilitation interventions.

The three main functional goals of human ambulation are to move from one place to another, to move safely, and to move efficiently. These three goals are frequently compromised in the patient with residual effects of acquired or congenital brain injury. The great majority of patients are able to perform limited ambulation, but they often have problems because of inefficient movement strategies, the presence of pain caused by abnormal limb postures, and decreased safety. Often, the compensatory movements necessary for ambulation produce exaggerated displacements of the center of gravity (COG), which result in increased energy expenditure. Impaired balance, sensation, and problems with limb clearance can contribute to the anxiety of ambulation and may increase the frequency of loss of balance and falls (5).

Some generalizations can be made about the gait of a patient with residual effects of acquired or congenital brain injury. These include a decrease in walking velocity with a reduction in the duration of stance phase, impairment of weight bearing in the affected limb with an increase in the duration of stance time of the less affected limb. Ochi et al. reported on differences in temporospatial parameters of locomotion among patients with residual stroke and traumatic brain injury (6). Gait deficiencies can be categorized with respect to the gait cycle from a functional perspective. In the stance phase, an abnormal base of support can be caused by equinovarus, toe flexion, or ankle valgus. Limb instability can occur because of knee buckling (sudden flexion) or hyperextension, which may result in knee joint pain. This may make walking unsafe, energy-inefficient, and painful.

Inadequate limb clearance (e.g., caused by a stiff knee) and inadequate limb advancement (e.g., caused by limited hip flexion or knee extension) may interfere with the safety and energy efficiency of walking during the swing phase.

Formal gait analysis in a laboratory may be required to focus more appropriately on the essence of multifactorial gait dysfunction. Combining clinical evaluation with laboratory measurements increases the degree of information resolution needed to understand the common patterns of gait dysfunction in the UMN.

EQUINOVARUS

Equinovarus deformity is the most common pathologic posture seen in the lower limb after central nervous system injuries. The foot and ankle are in a toe-down and turned in position. Toe curling may coexist. The patient frequently develops a painful bursa in the lateral aspect of the foot, particularly in the area of the base of the fifth metatarsal. During ambulation, initial contact of the foot with the ground occurs at the forefoot and weight is borne primarily on the lateral border. Toe flexion is typically present. Equinovarus is frequently maintained throughout stance phase and inversion may increase, causing ankle instability as weight bearing is applied. Limited dorsiflexion during early and mid-stance prevents the appropriate forward advancement of the tibia over the stationary foot, which frequently promotes knee hyperextension. Impairment in dorsiflexion range of motion in the late stance and preswing phases interferes with push-off and forward propulsion, resulting in significant reduction in joint power generation. During swing phase, equinus posture of the foot may result in a limb clearance problem, whereas the lack of adequate posture of the foot in stance phase may result in instability of the body as a whole. Under these circumstances, correction of this problem is essential even for limited ambulation.

Muscles that can potentially contribute to the equinovarus deformity include the tibiales anterior, tibiales posterior, long toe flexors, gastrocnemius, soleus, extensor hallucis longus and the peroneus longus. The dynamic polyelectromyographic (polyEMG) recordings of the mentioned muscles in combination with the clinical examination provide a more detailed understanding of the genesis of this deformity (7). Dynamic polyEMG recordings often demonstrate prolonged activation of the gastrocnemius and soleus complex as well as the long toe flexors as the most common cause of plantar flexion (Fig. 33.1). Occasionally, the gastrocnemius and soleus may activate differentially and treatment interventions must take this into consideration. Inversion is the result of the overactivation of the tibiales posterior and anterior in combination with the gastrocnemius and soleus and, at times, the extensor hallucis longus. If the tibiales posterior and anterior are both contributing to the varus deformity, a decision has to be made about which one of the two muscles is the main contributor. Two approaches are possible. The first one is to use the joint powers obtained as part of the kinematic data in routine gait analysis. The second consideration is a diagnostic tibial nerve block with lidocaine. One has to be mindful that reducing the activation of the gastrocnemius soleus complex tend to increase dorsiflexion and that tightness of the toe flexors usually becomes more apparent as a result of toe flexor tenodesis brought on by the increased dorsiflexion. Plantar fasciitis may also become evident after interventions to reduce ankle plantar flexor spasticity are carried out and the patient increases his or her walking.

Based on dynamic polyEMG correlated with clinical findings, the treatment of choice is injection of botulinum toxin into the tibiales posterior, gastrocnemius, soleus, and long toe flexors. When a contracture is evident, surgical intervention needs to be considered.

VALGUS FOOT

The foot and ankle are turned outwards and the patient walks on the medial aspect of the foot. The patient may develop callus over the navicular and may complain of pain over the medial border of the foot. During walking, weight bearing occurs primarily on the medial aspect of the foot. If present, limitation in ankle dorsiflexion prevents the forward progression of the tibia over the stationary foot and increase the valgus posture. This frequently is seen in young individuals who sustain neurologic injuries when skeletal maturation has not been reached. Muscles that can potentially contribute to this deformity include peroneus longus, peroneus brevis, gastrocnemius, soleus, the long toe flexors, and reduced activation or weakness of the tibiales anterior and tibiales posterior. Dynamic polyEMG recordings obtained from the mentioned muscles in combination with clinical examination should provide detailed information to formulate a hypothesis about the underlying deforming forces. Electromyographic recordings may demonstrate prolonged activation of the peroneus longus and/or brevis, abnormal activation of the gastrocnemius, and soleus. In some cases, lack of activation of the tibiales anterior or posterior may also be encountered.

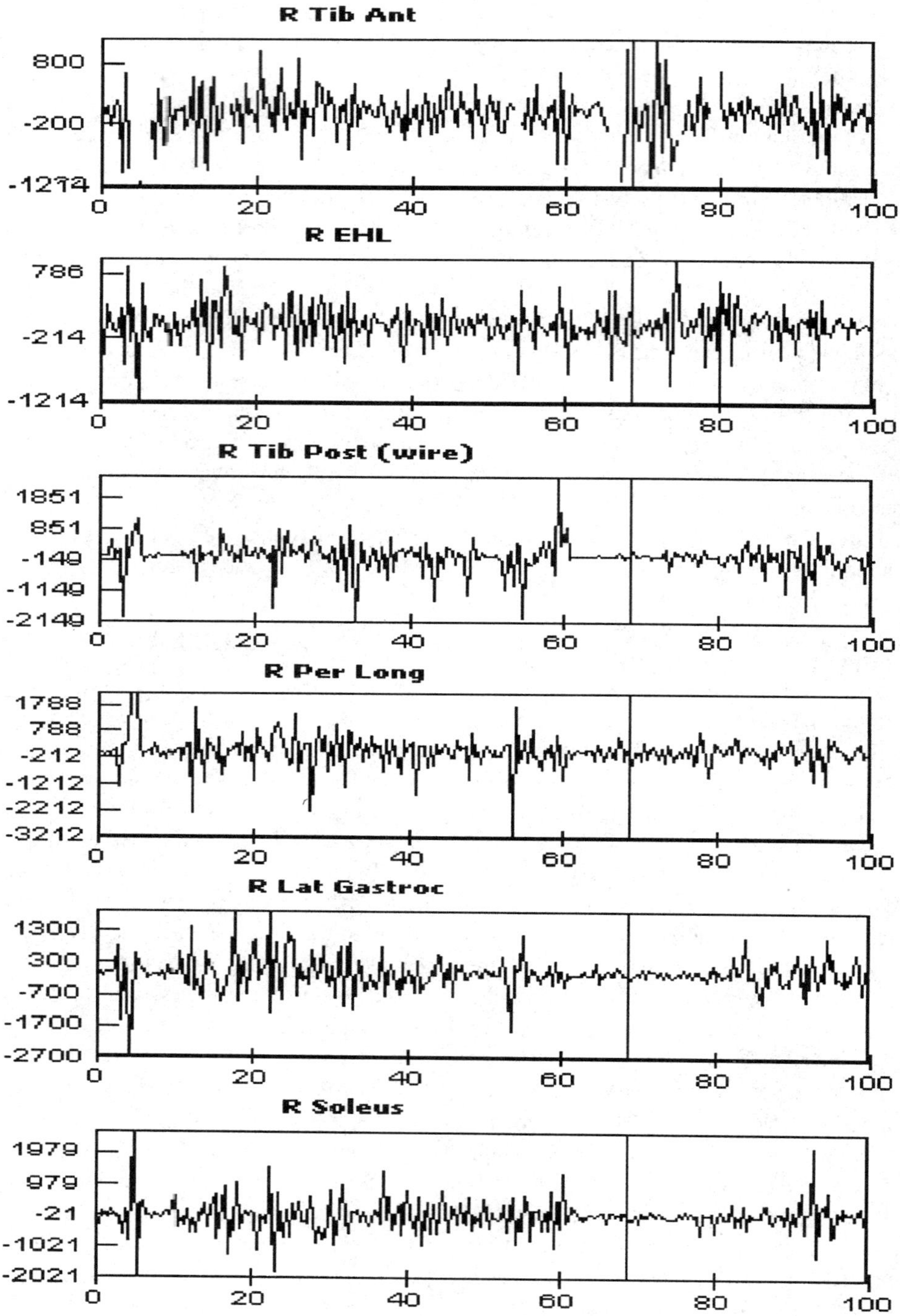

FIG. 33.1. Equinovarus. One cycle of gait in a patient with an upper motoneuron syndrome who clinically demonstrated ankle inversion during swing phase. Dynamic polyEMG obtained during swing phase reveals activity in tibialis posterior and anterior combined with gastrocnemius, soleus, and the extensor hallucis longus. Stance phase is on the left side of the record as demarcated from 0% to approximately 65% of the gait cycle; swing phase is on the right side of the record from 65% to 100%. *R Tib Ant,* right tibialis anterior; *R EHL,* right extensor hallucis longus; *R Tib Post,* right tibialis posterior; *R Per Long,* right peroneus longus; *R Lat Gastroc;* right lateral gastrocnemius; *R Soleus;* right soleus.

Occasionally, it is difficult to differentiate the contribution of peroneus longus from peroneus brevis in the deformity. In those few instances, a lidocaine diagnostic motor point block to one of the muscles can be used to ascertain the respective contributions.

Botox injected into the peroneus longus and/or brevis followed by aggressive strengthening of the ankle invertors and stretching of the ankle evertors is pursued. The use of motor point blocks with phenol to the peroneus brevis is possible. Motor point block of the peroneus longus with phenol is not advisable because the motor points are close to the peroneal nerve, a mixed sensorimotor nerve, and phenol may produce dysesthesia if it leaks onto nearby sensory nerve fibers.

HYPEREXTENDED GREAT TOE

Sometimes referred to as striated toe or hitchhiker's toe, the great toe is held in extension throughout the gait cycle. Ankle equinus and varus may accompany this foot posture. At times, lesser toe flexion is also noted. Dynamic polyEMG can elucidate the contribution of overactive gastrocsoleus group or underactive tibiales anterior to this deformity as the extensor hallucis longus (EHL) may be overactive in an effort to compensate for lack of dorsiflexion in swing phase (Fig. 33.2). A motor point block of the EHL with phenol or chemodenervation with Botox following the recommended dose can easily be achieved. Stretching of the EHL into flexion and strengthening of the tibiales anterior should follow this intervention.

STIFF KNEE

The knee is kept extended during preswing and initial swing, resulting in a reduction of the arc of motion with its peak below 40 degrees (normal reference approximately 60 degrees). In addition, there may be delay in the timing of flexion and a concomitant reduction in hip flexion. Knee flexion during walking is generated by hip flexion. Reduced hip flexion moment may result in decreased knee flexion in swing phase. This deviation may cause foot drag, for which the patient attempts to compensate by circumduction, hip hiking, or contralateral vaulting (early heel rise). Frequently, a reduction is noted in the activation of iliopsoas along with excessive activation of the rectus femoris, vastus intermedius, vastus medialis, vastus lateralis and, at times, excessive activation of the gluteus maximus. If an ankle equinus deformity is also present, a reduction in joint power generation and plantarflexion moment may result in further reduction of knee flexion.

Based on clinical laboratory findings, phenolization of the motor branch of the femoral nerve innervating the quadriceps mechanism or chemodenervation with botulinum toxin to individual heads of the quadriceps may be considered. Aggressive stretching of the rectus femoris using the modified Ely technique should follow this. This technique requires that the patient lie prone on a hard surface and that the knee be flexed as the hip is maintained in full extension producing a stretch on the rectus femoris. Marching exercises and walking in water are also beneficial in promoting hip flexor strength.

FLEXED KNEE

In this deviation, the knee is kept flexed in stance and swing. The patient does not achieve full knee extension after the loading response in stance nor in terminal swing. This deviation requires the patient to utilize compensatory mechanisms during stance phase, particularly in the period of double support. The flexed knee deviation results in a limitation of step length because of the patient's inability to extend the knee joint fully in the terminal part of swing phase.

Dynamic polyEMG recordings obtained from medial and lateral hamstrings, quadriceps, gastrocnemius, and soleus should clarify the contribution of each of these muscles to the deformity. Electromyographic recordings frequently demonstrate overactivation of the hamstrings, medial more than lateral. Excessive activity in the gastrocnemius may also be present, particularly during swing phase. Kinematic data demonstrate limited knee extension and, frequently, accompanying hip flexion.

Interventions that may be considered to reduce spasticity of the hamstrings include phenol

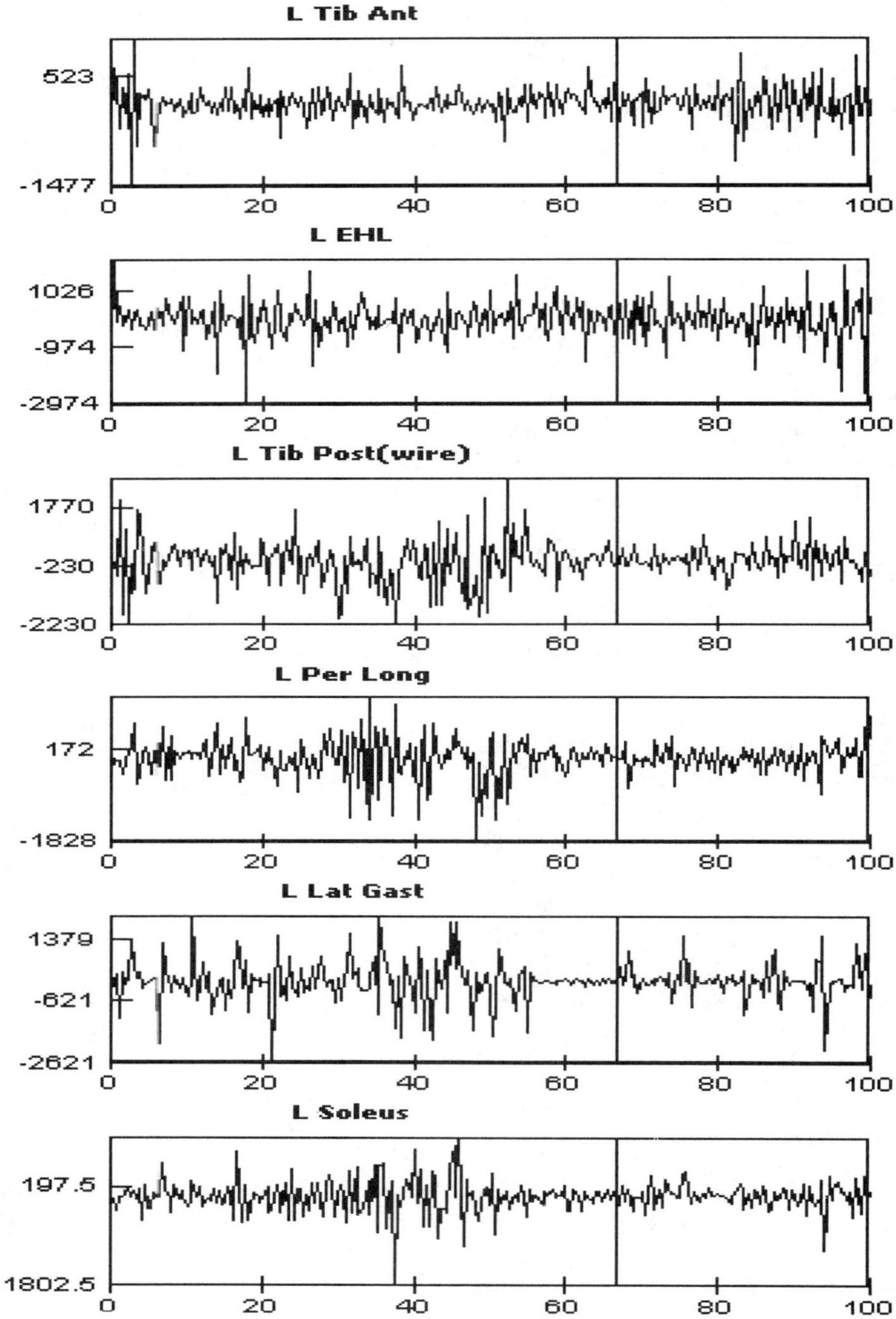

FIG. 33.2. EHL hyperextension. One cycle of gait in a patient with an upper motoneuron syndrome who clinically demonstrated a hyperextended great toe during swing and stance. Dynamic polyEMG obtained during swing and stance phases reveals persistent activity in extensor hallucis longus. The patient also had equinovarus posturing. Stance phase is on the left side of the record as demarcated by a vertical line at approximately 65% of the gait cycle; swing phase is on the right side of the record. *L Tib Ant,* left tibialis anterior; *L EHL,* left extensor hallucis longus; *L Tib Post,* left tibialis posterior; *L Per Long,* left peroneus longus; *L Lat Gast,* left lateral gastrocnemius; *L Soleus,* left soleus.

neurolysis to the motor branches of the sciatic nerve, motor point blocks to the hamstrings, or chemodenervation with Botox. Patients who have large muscle mass and severe spasticity will require large doses of Botox and phenol may be more appropriate in these patients. Gastrocnemius motor point blocks or chemodenervation with Botox can be achieved easily.

ADDUCTED (SCISSORING) THIGH

This deformity is characterized by adduction of the hip during the swing phase of locomotion. Adducted thigh results in a narrow base of support in stance phase with potential impairment of balance. It also can interfere with limb clearance and advancement because the adducting swing phase limb may collide with the stance limb.

Dynamic polyEMG recordings demonstrate overactivation of the hip adductors, medial hamstrings, and pectineus (Fig. 33.3). Weakness of the hip abductors and the iliopsoas may also contribute to this deformity because the patient may attempt to use the hip adductors compensatorily to advance the limb forward in swing phase.

It is essential to ascertain if the deformity is obligatory (the result of adductor spasticity) or compensatory (the result of weak hip flexors) because treatment will differ for each. Percutaneous temporary diagnostic obturator nerve block can

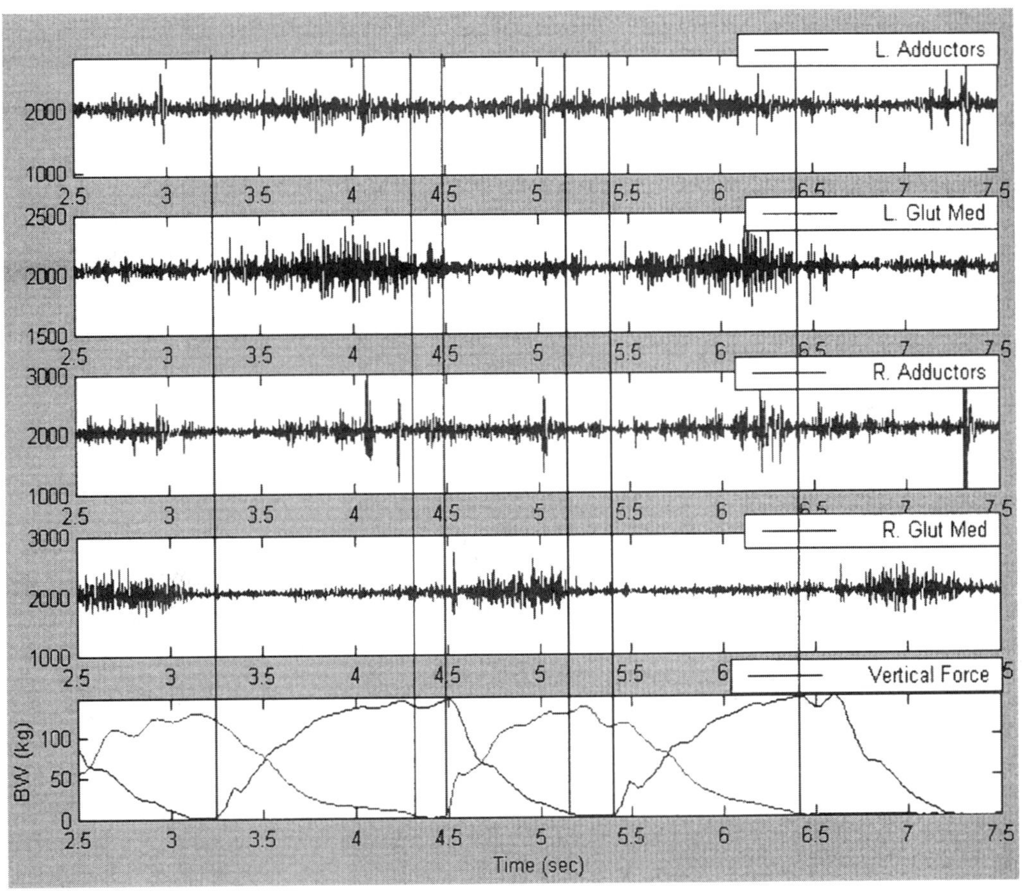

FIG. 33.3. Hip adduction. Multiple cycles of gait in a patient with an upper motoneuron syndrome who clinically demonstrated bilateral scissoring of the thighs. Dynamic polyEMG obtained during swing phase (*narrow parallel lines* in the figure at about 4.4 and 5.2 seconds, respectively) reveals adductor activity. Right gluteus medius activity in stance phase is reduced. *BW*, body weight; *L.*, left; *R.*, right; *Glut Med,* gluteus.

be used to differentiate the role of hip adduction if the clinician is uncertain. Longer-term interventions, such as percutaneous phenol nerve block, are easily carried out. After the intervention, aggressive stretching of the hip adductors, strengthening of the hip flexors, and abductors is pursued. Electrical stimulation to the hip abductors may be beneficial for this purpose.

FLEXED HIP

This gait deviation is characterized by sustained hip flexion during the stance phase of locomotion. This is particularly evident in mid- to late stance when the hip is extending. A shortening of contralateral step length is noted when this condition is unilateral.

Dynamic polyEMG recordings of iliopsoas, pectineus, gluteus maximus, rectus femoris, and lumbar paraspinals should help in determining the contribution of the different muscles in the gait cycle. Overactive iliopsoas, rectus femoris, hip adductors, or weakness of the hip extensors and paraspinals may be evident. Interventions to reduce spasticity of the hip flexors (iliopsoas and rectus femoris), particularly chemodenervation with Botox to the iliopsoas and chemodenervation with Botox to the rectus femoris or the use of phenol motor branch block to the rectus can be performed easily. This should be followed by aggressive stretching of the hip flexors with the patient positioned in the modified Thomas test for the hip flexors and the Ely test position for the rectus femoris. The Thomas test requires that the patient be in the supine position on a hard surface. Both legs are flexed up toward the chest, stabilizing the pelvis and preventing lumbar lordosis. One leg is allowed to extend and brought down to the examination table, resulting in stretching of the hip flexors. Strengthening of the hip extensors and paraspinals should also be encouraged.

Gait dysfunction resulting from spasticity, contracture, and impaired motor control after upper motor neuron injury can be quite complex. Kinematic, kinetic, and dynamic polyEMG analysis along with diagnostic selective temporary blocks can help optimize rehabilitation planning and treatment interventions. It is important to clearly identify the muscles involved by a combination of focused clinical examination supplemented by evaluation in the Gait and Motion Analysis Laboratory. The imbalance of muscles can be improved by rehabilitation interventions aided by the use of motor point and motor nerve blocks with phenol and chemodenervation with Botox.

BOTULINUM TOXIN A

Botox has strong neuromuscular blocking properties that inhibit the release of acetylcholine causing a flaccid paralysis (8). The clinical effect of the toxin is primarily owing to its action at the neuromuscular junction by inhibiting the release of acetylcholine. Three steps are involved in the toxin mediated paralysis: (a) internalization, (b) disulfide reduction and translocation, and (c) inhibition of neurotransmitter release. The toxin must enter the nerve ending to exert its effect. The United States Food and Drug Administration currently approves Botox injection for the treatment of blepharospasm, facial spasm, strabismus, and torticolis. In Europe it is also approved for the management of spasticity secondary to cerebral palsy and stroke (9).

The purpose of Botox block is to reduce force produced by a contracting spastic muscle or muscle group. A reduction in spastic tension can lead to improvement in passive and active range of motion and allows for more successful stretching of tight musculature. More subtly, and more importantly, a patient's improved control over movement and posture may allow for compensatory behaviors during functional activities (unmasking). A reduction in spastic activity in one muscle or muscle group may have consequences for tone in other muscle groups of the limb through a reduction in the overall effort required to perform movement and/or through changes in sensory information going to the central nervous system from that limb. Finally, the application of external devices such as braces, splints, casts, even shoes, can be facilitated by chemodenervation.

Botox is injected directly into an offending muscle. The major advantages in its use are the ease of application that permits its injection without anesthesia and its predictable effect. The most

TABLE 33.1. *Suggested botox dosing for adults*

Clinical pattern	Potential muscles involved	Botox dose units/visit	# of injection sites
Flexed hip	Iliacus	50–150	2
	Psoas	50–200	2
	Rectus femoris	100–200	3
Flexed knee	Medial hamstrings	50–150	3
	Lateral hamstrings	50–150	3
	Gastrocnemius (knee flexors)	100–200	4
Adducted thighs	Adductor brevis-longus-magnus	200–400	4–6
Stiff knee	Quadriceps	100–300	6–8
	Gluteus maximus	200–300	4
Equinovarus foot	Gastrocnemius	100–300	4
	Soleus	100–300	2
	Tibiales posterior	50–100	1
	Tibiales anterior	50–100	2
	Flexor dig. longus	20–75	1
	Extensor hallucis longus	30–100	2
Valgus foot	Peroneus longus	50–150	2
	Peroneus brevis	50–100	1
Hyperextended (hitchhiker's) great toe	Extensor hallucis longus	50–150	2

common adverse effect is excessive weakness of injected muscles; however, nausea, headache, and fatigue have also been reported. No effect on the sensory system is evident with Botox. Strength gradually returns even when the patient may have a strong response to the paralytic effect of the toxin with overweakening. No anaphylactic response has ever been reported because of Botox injection.

Therapeutic doses have ranged between 10 and 300 units, depending on the size of the muscle being injected (Table 33.1). Extrapolation from animal studies would place the lethal dose to a 70-kg human at an estimated dose of 3,200 U. An antitoxin is available in cases of accidental poisoning. Because of the potential risk of migration out of the muscle and the possibility of antibody formation, usually no more than 400 U are administered in a single treatment session. This may be sufficient, however, to treat a number of muscles in that one session. Development of resistance to Botox A therapy is an important clinical issue. To minimize the risk of immunoresistance use the smallest possible effective dose, extend the interval between treatments for at least 3 months or longer if possible, and avoid the use of booster injections between treatments. Careful documentation of muscle selection, dose, and effects is encouraged so in the next treatment cycle one may adjust the dose as necessary. In our practice we limit dose per treatment to no more than 400 U of Botox A, we try to concentrate the available dose to a few muscles if multiple large muscles are to be injected, and we consider using other interventions (e.g., phenol) to other muscles or motor nerves to achieve a complete treatment strategy. With the currently available information we recommend not injecting Botox in patients who are pregnant or lactating.

The physician should be knowledgeable about the diagnosis and medical management of the condition producing spasticity before using Botox A in the clinical management of spasticity and he or she should be proficient in the relevant anatomy and kinesiology. The physician should have a clear understanding of the potential benefits of unmasking function and of the limitations of this therapeutic intervention. A patient may require several sessions to optimize the dose that seems to be necessary for optimal treatment because there is a several day delay between injection of toxin and onset of action. Unlike the dystonias, where voluntary capacity is not an issue, spastic muscles may very well have voluntary capacity, which the clinician would like to preserve, and, therefore, titration of the paralytic effect of the toxin becomes a much more critical factor in its administration because unmasking of function may occur. The duration of toxin effectiveness is usually 10 weeks to 4 months, but injections should be spread at intervals of more than 3 months because of the risk of developing antibodies. In our experience, patients received 300 to 400 U at 3-month intervals for more than 3 years without evident loss of effectiveness of the medication. It would seem that the toxin might be most effective as a temporizing management agent in spasticity, particularly in the period of expected neurologic recovery in which spasticity is changing as motor recovery occurs or as an effective tool to "simulate" the effects of surgery, to the benefit of the surgeon and patient alike.

The strategy of performing a Botox injection is as follows: Botulinum toxin A is available worldwide under the tradename Botox (Allergan) and in Europe Dysport (Speywood, U.K.). Botox is available in 100-U vials that arrive frozen as a white powder. To prepare 100 U, reconstitute it with 1 to 3 cc of normal saline solution *without* preservative based on the desired dilution. Gentle agitation of the vial is performed and the toxin is loaded into a syringe. The skin is prepared by cleaning it with alcohol prior to insertion of the Teflon-coated, 22-gauge stimulating injecting needle. The electrically conductive inner core of the tip of the needle is used to pass current to the tissues. After injection, muscle activation should be encouraged to increase the uptake and internalization of the toxin. As the paralytic effect appears evident aggressive stretching, muscle reeducation, and functional training are performed.

Phenol

This drug, a derivative of benzene, is also known as carbolic acid, it denatures the protein membrane of peripheral nerves in aqueous concentrations of 5% or more. When phenol is injected in or near a nerve bundle, phenol's neurolytic action on the myelin sheath or the cell membrane of axons with which it makes contact serves to reduce neural traffic along the nerve and its usefulness in treating spasticity. The onset of the destructive process with higher concentrations of phenol may begin to show effects several days after injection, but phenol also has a local anesthetic feature that allows a clinician and the patient to see "partial results" shortly after the phenol block is performed. The denaturing process induced by phenol extends biologically on the order of weeks, perhaps months, but eventually regeneration occurs, so that a phenol block clinically is used as a temporizing measure rather than a permanent intervention. In our clinical experience and the experience of others, the effect of a phenol block typically lasts 3 to 5 months. Histologically, it has been shown that phenol destroys axons of all sizes, probably is a patchy distribution but more so on the outer aspect of the nerve bundle, onto which phenol is dripped. In such a model, interior axons within a nerve bundle theoretically are more spared than their sibling axons located more peripherally in a nerve bundle where phenol has access to them. When phenol is injected percutaneously, it is extremely likely that the nerve block will be incomplete. This is especially useful in situations where a spastic muscle also has volitional capacity because under these circumstances it is desirable to reduce spasticity while still preserving the volitional capacity of that muscle.

The technique of phenol injection is based on electrical stimulation. Except in few circumstances we generally inject motor branches close to the offending muscle or muscle group (motor point). Several tests are available that identify muscles and their motor points. A surface stimulator is briefly used to approximate the percutaneous stimulation site in advance. The skin is prepared with alcohol and a local anesthetic can be injected or rubbed on to the skin. The purpose is to eliminate cutaneomotor reflexes that may cause the limb to jump when the blocking needle is subsequently inserted. A 25-gauge Teflon-coated hypodermic needle (which is the same needle used for Botox injections) is advanced toward the motor nerve. Depth of penetration and directional orientation of the needle tip require a steady hand, a competent knowledge of anatomy and a good assistant. Electrical stimulation is adjusted by noting whether muscle contraction of the desired muscle takes place. As one gets closer to the motor nerve, less current intensity is required to produce a contractile response. The motor nerve is injected when minimal current produces a visible or palpable contraction. We use a duo stim electrical stimulator with pulse frequencies of 1 per second, we typically inject when the milliampere reading on the unit reads less than 0.4 mA. We generally inject 3 to 7 cc of 5% or 7% aqueous solution of phenol. For longer effects, larger concentrations, larger volumes, and longer distances between the site of injection and the distance to the neuromuscular junction of the muscle are used. The literature does report that phenol applied to sensory nerves may produce a disesthesia that is troublesome. For this reason we do not recommend injection of mixed peripheral nerves except in a patient who is vegetative and indifferent to any sensory consequences. (Actually, sensory blockade may help reduce spasticity by reducing afferent input to a hyperexcitable motor system.) After the block, we recommend that ice be applied to the injection site for 10 to 15 minutes every 2 hours in order to reduce any local irritation or swelling. Because a certain amount of needling is required to find the best place for injecting the motor nerve, we prefer not to use phenol in patients who are anticoagulated. The technique for botulinum toxin injection (see the preceding) may be preferable in this circumstance. As with any injection, care needs to be taken not to inject into a blood vessel and this is done by aspirating prior to the injection. We use the help of an assistant to perform the injection while the physician holds the needle still. In contrast, a physician alone generally performs injection with botulinum toxin. The literature has reported a range of injections between 1 and 10 mL of phenol in various concentrations, usually not exceeding 7%. The lethal range of phenol that gets into the central nervous system is approximately 8.5 g. Ten milliliters of a 7% solution of phenol contains 0.7 g of phenol (a tenfold factor of safety). We generally do not inject more than 15 mL of 7% phenol in one session. If a phenol block seems ineffective after several weeks, it may be repeated. With repeated phenol injections, an increase in fibrous tissue at the site of injection may occur and this may make repeat injections more difficult. Overall, phenol is a very useful technique when pursuing the focal strategy of spasticity management during the period of motor recovery after brain injury. In clinically effective concentrations (5% to 7%), phenol causes peripheral nerve injury that reverses itself over the course of months approximately proportional to the recovery rate of a motor nerve whose injury extends from the site of phenol installation to the neuromuscular junction of that nerve, taking into account an additional 3 to 4 weeks of Wallerian degeneration as well. Phenol injections are a good temporizing measure during the period of motor recovery, and it facilitates serial casting, range of motion exercises, passive activities of daily living, active movements, and function. Phenol is very inexpensive and its injection may be repeated fairly soon after it becomes clear that the desired effect has not been obtained. In this sense it is a titratable drug.

REFERENCES

1. Griffith ER, Mayer NH. Hypertonicity in movement disorders. In: Rosenthal M, Griffith ER, Bond MR, et al., eds. *Rehabilitation of the adult and child with traumatic brain injury,* 2nd ed. Philadelphia: F.A. Davis, 1990.
2. Lance JW. Symposium synopsis. In: Feldman RG, Young RR, Koelia WP, eds. *Spasticity: disorder motor control.* Chicago: Yearbook, 1980.
3. Mayer NH, Esquenazi A, Childress MK. Common patterns of clinical motor dysfunction. *Muscle Nerve* 1997;56:S21–35.
4. Keenan MA, Mayer NH, Esquenazi A, et al. A neuroorthopedic approach to the management of common patterns of upper motor neuron dysfunction after brain injury. *Neurol Rehabil* 1999;12:119–143.
5. Esquenazi A, Keenan MA. Gait analysis. In: DeLisa JA, Gans BM, eds. *Rehabilitation medicine: principles and practice,* 2nd ed. Philadelphia: J.B. Lippincott, 1993:122–130.
6. Ochi F, Esquenazi A, Hirai B, et al. Temporal-spatial features of gait after traumatic brain injury. *J Head Trauma Rehabil* 1999;14:105–115.
7. Esquenazi A, Talaty M. Gait analysis, technology and clinical applications. In: Braddom R, ed. *Physical medicine and rehabilitation,* 2nd ed. Philadelphia: W.B. Saunders, 2000:93–108.
8. Clinical use of botulinum toxin. A National Institutes of Health consensus development statement. *Arch Neurol* 1991;48:1294–1297.
9. Jankovic J, Hallett M, eds. *Therapy with botulinum toxin.* New York: Marcel Dekker, 1994.

Gait Disorders. Advances in Neurology, Vol. 87,
edited by E. Růžička, M. Hallett, and J. Jankovic.
Lippincott Williams & Wilkins, Philadelphia © 2001.

34

Surgical Treatment of Common Patterns of Lower Limb Deformities Resulting from Upper Motoneuron Syndrome

*‡Mary Ann Keenan, †§Alberto Esquenazi, and ||¶Nathaniel H. Mayer

*Departments of *Orthopaedic Surgery and †Physical Medicine and Rehabilitation, Thomas Jefferson University School of Medicine, Philadelphia, Pennyslvania 19107; ‡Neuro-Orthopedics Program, Department of Orthopaedic Surgery, Albert Einstein Medical Center; §Gait and Motion Laboratory and ||Motor Control Analysis Laboratory, MossRehab Hospital, Philadelphia, Pennsylvania 19141; and ¶Department of Rehabilitation Medicine, Temple University, Philadelphia, Pennsylvania 19140*

Neuro-orthopedics is the field of orthopedic surgery that treats limb deformities resulting from neurologic disease or injury. Upper motoneuron dysfunction (UMN) commonly follows injuries to the brain from stroke, traumatic brain injury, anoxia, infections of the brain, and perinatal trauma. The surgical management of limb dysfunction follows the same principles regardless of etiology. A number of common patterns of lower extremity movement dysfunction are seen in patients with UMN (Table 34.1) (1–3). These patterns typically develop against a background of weakness, impaired voluntary and postural motor control, spasticity, and contracture that come with the territory of UMN. All of these abnormal movement patterns have a direct adverse effect on gait.

Many complications result from spasticity (Table 34.2) (4–10). The most common are extremity contractures. Limb contracture leads to skin maceration, difficulty with hygiene, and decubitus ulcers. Uncontrolled spasticity can lead to fracture malunions in brain-injured patients with fractures. Extremes of limb position often result in peripheral nerve lesions (9,11). Sciatic neuropathy can be caused by the pronounced inflammation associated with heterotopic bone formation posterior to the hip joint. The bone can encase the sciatic nerve in some cases. Joint subluxation or dislocation can happen with severe spasticity. Hip dislocation occurs with severe longstanding adductor spasticity. Posterior subluxation of the knee can occur in the presence of hamstring spasticity. Iatrogenic fractures can happen in the presence of spasticity and contracture. Heterotopic ossification is thought to be stimulated in part by the mechanical tension caused by the spasticity (8).

In the past, UMN patterns have been attributed to increased muscle tone in specific groups of muscles that were reflexly excited. Muscle tone, however, is not a simple construct. It depends on complex mechanisms, of which hyperexcitable reflexes are just one part. The biomechanics of joint motion, the active contractile and passive properties of soft tissues all contribute to the resistance the examiner perceives as increased tone. They also contribute to the resistance that the patient must overcome when trying to generate a voluntary movement. For clinicians, the manifestations of spasticity, muscle stiffness, and contracture become intertwined with the issue of how much motor control has been spared and how much will recover.

Although neurologic damage after acquired brain injury is obviously central in nature,

TABLE 34.1. *Common extremity deformities in upper motoneuron syndrome*

Clinical problem	Possible deforming muscle forces
Equinovarus foot	Gastrocnemius, soleus, tibialis, anterior, tibialis posterior, EHL, FDL, FHL
Equinovalgus foot	Gastrocnemius, soleus, peroneus longus, peroneus brevis
Hyperextended great toe	Extensor hallucis longus
Stiff knee gait	Rectus femoris, vastus intermedius, v. lateralis, v. medialis
Flexed knee	Gracilis, semimembranosus, semitendinosis, biceps femoris
Adducted (scissoring) thighs	Adductor longus, adductor brevis, gracilis
Flexed hip	Iliopsoas, pectineus, sartorius, rectus femoris

EHL, extensor hallucis longus; FDL, flexor digitorum longus; FHL, flexor hallucis longus.

neuro-orthopedic interventions are based on the principle that central damage generates altered and unbalanced forces in peripheral actuators and that the latter may be manipulated orthopedically. Centrally mediated UMN features such as paresis, spasticity, and impaired motor control ultimately alter the ability of peripheral actuators to generate movement. Using a variety of techniques that aim at components of peripheral actuators such as tendons, nerves, bones, and joints, neuro-orthopedic interventions aim to rebalance deforming forces, thereby enabling some degree of functional restoration that, for all intents and purposes, is not dependent on central neurologic recovery.

EXPECTATIONS AND TIMING OF NEURO-ORTHOPEDIC SURGERY

When evaluating patients with UMN, questions arise regarding the indications for surgery, the cost, what outcome to expect, and the practicality of this approach. These issues should be considered on an individual basis for each patient. General principles have been delineated that can serve as decision-making guidelines.

Operate early, before deformities are severe and fixed. Neuro-orthopedic surgery is a powerful rehabilitation tool. Surgery often is the only treatment that will correct a limb deformity or improve function. Surgery should not be considered a treatment of last resort when conservative measures have failed. Physical and occupational therapy cannot effect a permanent change in motor control. Drug therapy for increased muscle tone has generalized effects and cannot be targeted to specific offending muscles. Phenol blocks and botulinum toxin injections provide only temporary modulation of muscle tone. Surgery should be considered when a permanent treatment is needed to decrease muscle tone or redirect muscle force. The results of surgical intervention are improved when deformities are corrected early. Less muscle lengthening is needed when deformities are mild and there is little or no fixed contracture to overcome. Early surgery preserves maximum muscle strength, joint capsule and ligament flexibility, and articular cartilage integrity. In general, the patient will also be in better physiologic condition to undergo surgery if there has not been a period of several years of immobility.

Better underlying motor control means better function for the extremity. Neuro-orthopedic surgery cannot impart control to a muscle. Lengthening a spastic muscle can improve its function by diminishing the overactive stretch response and uncovering the volitional control that was present. Successful surgery depends on a careful preoperative evaluation to determine the amount of volitional control present in each individual muscle that is effecting limb posture and movement.

Motor performance is a continuous scale, with the disabled at the lower end and the elite athlete at the upper end. Infinitesimal improvements in the performance of elite athletes distinguish between the winner and loser. Incremental changes in limb function also result in performance improvements for the disabled individual. Surgery should not be reserved for patients with severe

TABLE 34.2. *Complications of spasticity*

Contractures
Decubitus ulcers
Hygiene difficulties
Fracture malunion
Joint subluxation or dislocation
Heterotopic ossification
Peripheral neuropathy

impairment and deformity. Individuals with milder degrees of impairment can benefit greatly from relatively simple procedures. The amount of improvement correlates best with the degree of underlying motor control and not the severity of the deformity.

Distinguish between the function of the extremity and the function of the individual. We commonly speak of "functional" and "nonfunctional" surgical procedures. These terms refer to the expected outcomes for a limb but do not indicate the outcome for the person as a whole. Surgical releases of a leg contracted in a flexed and adducted position in a nonambulatory, quadriplegic patient often allows the person to sit comfortably in a wheelchair to become interactive with others.

Consider the cost of not correcting limb deformities. The cost of motor control evaluation using dynamic electromyography (EMG) is relatively modest for the benefits it provides. Dynamic EMG is a one-time expense. The cost of performing an incorrect surgical procedure that fails to correct or worsens a limb deformity is much greater. The cost of performing a surgical procedure likewise is limited when compared to a lifetime of attendant care, spasticity medications, repeated blocks, orthotics to control limb position, complications such as skin ulceration and infection, and lost productivity for the patient and caretakers.

PREOPERATIVE EVALUATION OF LOWER LIMB DEFORMITIES

Assessment of Cognition and Communication

The goals of surgery must be practical and clearly understood by all. The patient must be capable of following simple commands and should also be able to cooperate with a postoperative therapy program. Adequate memory is needed to retain what is taught during the postoperative therapy (1).

Sensory Evaluation

The ability to maintain balance and ambulate is dependent on adequate sensation in the foot and ankle. The basic modalities of light touch and pain sensation are essential. Proprioception must be present at the level of the ankle joint for good balance reactions. If proprioception is impaired at the ankle, an ankle foot orthosis may be needed during ambulation to prevent a compensatory knee extension thrust (12).

Clinical Evaluation of Motor Control

It is difficult to distinguish between the many potential causes of limited joint motion in a neurologically impaired patient. The possibilities include increased muscle tone, a myostatic contracture, the presence of periarticular heterotopic ossification (HO), an undetected fracture or dislocation, joint subluxation, pain, or the lack of patient cooperation secondary to diminished cognition. Bony deformities may not exhibit an obvious clinical deformity but can be detected by radiography.

Evaluation of UMN focuses on identification of three factors: (a) the clinical pattern of motor dysfunction, (b) the patient's ability to control muscles involved in the clinical pattern, and (c) the role of muscle stiffness and contracture in relation to the functional problem (1,3,13–21). For purposes of convenience, we identify the seven clinical patterns of lower extremity motor dysfunction that are most commonly seen (Table 34.1). Other variations of motor dysfunction occur but are less common. Numerous muscles may contribute to motor dysfunction across joints and limb segments in these clinical patterns. Evaluation focuses on the following characteristics of the involved muscles: (a) voluntary or selective control, (b) spastic reactivity, (c) rheologic stiffness, and (d) contracture.

Passive range of motion of each joint should be established first. Anesthetic nerve blocks are extremely useful in differentiating between the relative contributions of pain, increased muscle tone, and contracture to a limb deformity. The strength and control of the antagonistic muscle group can also be evaluated. Unmasking of primitive patterning reflexes further contributes to the motor impairment. Spasticity (hyperactive response to quick stretch), rigidity (resistance to slow movement), or movement dystonias may be present. The degree of spasticity within selected muscles can be graded clinically in response to a quick

TABLE 34.3. *Clinical scale of motor control*

Grade	Type	Description
Grade 1	Flaccid posture	Hypotonic, no active motion
Grade 2	Rigid posture	Hypertonic, no active motion
Grade 3	Reflexive mass pattern	Mass flexion or extension synergies in response to examiner stimulation
Grade 4	Volitional mass pattern	Patient is able to initiate mass flexion or extension pattern volitionally
Grade 5	Selective with pattern overlay	Slow volitional movement of specific joints Physiologic stress results in mass action and obligatory movement of other joints
Grade 6	Selective control	Volitional control of individual joints without simultaneous obligatory movement of other joints

stretch. Another method of quantifying muscle tone is to measure the amount of intramuscular pressure generated by a passive quick stretch or during functional use of the limb. Intramuscular pressure can be measured using a wick or slit catheter technique. The pressure generated within the muscle is proportional to the force of contraction.

Motor control can be graded in the extremity using a clinical scale (Table 34.3) (22). The clinical questions of interest regarding a given muscle include the following: (a) Does the patient have selective voluntary control over the given muscle? (b) Is the muscle activated dyssynergically (i.e., in antagonism to movement) when the patient attempts to move the relevant joint? (c) Is the muscle resistive to passive stretch (i.e., spastic)? (d) Does the given muscle have fixed shortening (i.e., contracture)? These questions are best addressed with dynamic poly-EMG.

Laboratory-Assisted Assessment of Gait and Motor Control

Clinical examination supported by gait analysis and dynamic polyelectromyography (poly-EMG) is the mainstay of evaluation (1,3, 13–16,19,21,23–33). Laboratory gait analysis is performed preoperatively on all patients. This consists of bidirectional video recordings. Ground reaction forces are recorded and displayed using a laser vector superimposed on the video. Vertical load, horizontal shear force, and the mediolateral direction are measured. Temporospatial parameters obtained include walking velocity, cadence, stride time, and measurements of symmetry of gait. Dynamic multichannel EMG is acquired with simultaneous measurements of joint motion (kinematics) in the lower extremity while walking. Joint motion is recorded using electrogoniometers. Surface electrodes are used for the superficial lower limb muscles and wire electrodes for the deep muscles such as tibialis posterior and long toe flexors.

SURGICAL TREATMENT OF COMMON LOWER LIMB DEFORMITIES

The Equinovarus Foot Deformity

Equinus

Equinus is the most common deformity and results from the increased or premature activity of the gastrocnemius and soleus muscles (17,20,21,32,34–36). Surgical lengthening of the Achilles tendon is indicated when the patient foot and ankle position is not adequately controlled by an orthosis or when attempting to make the patient brace-free. Adequate lengthening of the Achilles tendon can be performed using the Hoke triple hemisection technique (Fig. 34.1) (37). Postoperative management requires 6 weeks of rigid immobilization. After this the patient uses an ankle foot orthosis for an additional 6 weeks.

Claw Toes

Toe clawing or curling is a common accompaniment of overactivity of the gastrocnemius muscles. Toe curling is caused by overactivity of the flexor hallucis longus and flexor digitorum muscle as well as the short toe flexor and intrinsic muscles of the foot (37,38). A longitudinal incision is made on the plantar surface of each

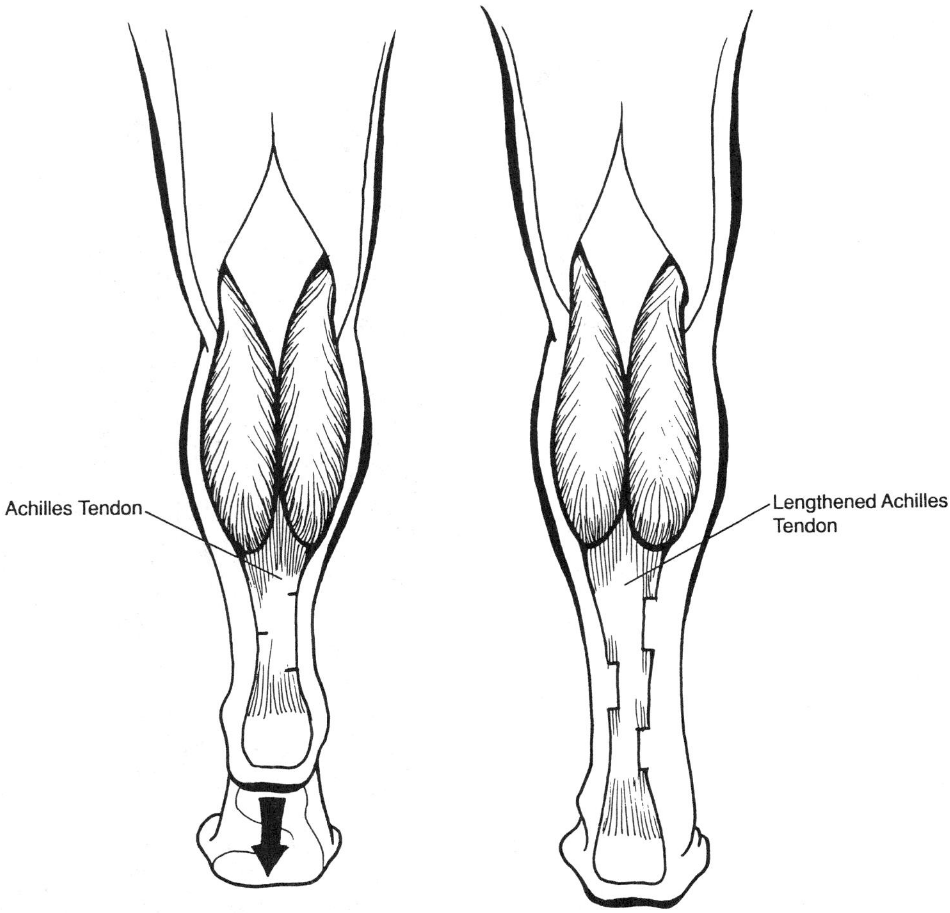

FIG. 34.1. Technique of percutaneous Achilles tendon lengthening. (From Keenan MA, Kozin SH, Berlet AC. *Manual of orthopedic surgery for spasticity.* New York: Raven Press, 1993, with permission.)

toe at the metatarsal phalangeal joint level. The flexor tendons are identified and released under direct vision (Fig. 34.2). This procedure is commonly done in combination with an Achilles tendon lengthening because bringing the foot into a plantigrade position will worsen the toe curling.

Ankle Plantarflexor Muscle Paresis

Muscle paresis (weakness) is an integral part of upper motoneuron syndrome. Lengthening the Achilles tendon to correct an equinus deformity weakens the gastrocnemius-soleus muscle group, which was already weak as a consequence of the underlying upper motor neuron syndrome. This calf paresis generally results in the need of an ankle foot orthosis (AFO) during ambulation. Thus transfer of the digitorum longus muscle can be done in order to augment calf strength. More patients eventually achieve brace-free ambulation with this transfer (31). In prior studies of treatment of a spastic equinovarus foot deformity, 30% of patients were able to walk safely without an AFO. When transfer of the flexor digitorum longus (FDL) to the os calcis augments the gastroc-soleus strength, 70% of patients achieve brace-free ambulation.

Postoperatively the patient is placed in a short leg-walking cast at surgery holding the foot in a neutral position. Gait training can be started on the first postoperative day, allowing the patient to bear full weight on the foot as tolerated. The cast is kept on the foot for 6 weeks. Six weeks after surgery the patient begins using a nonarticulated,

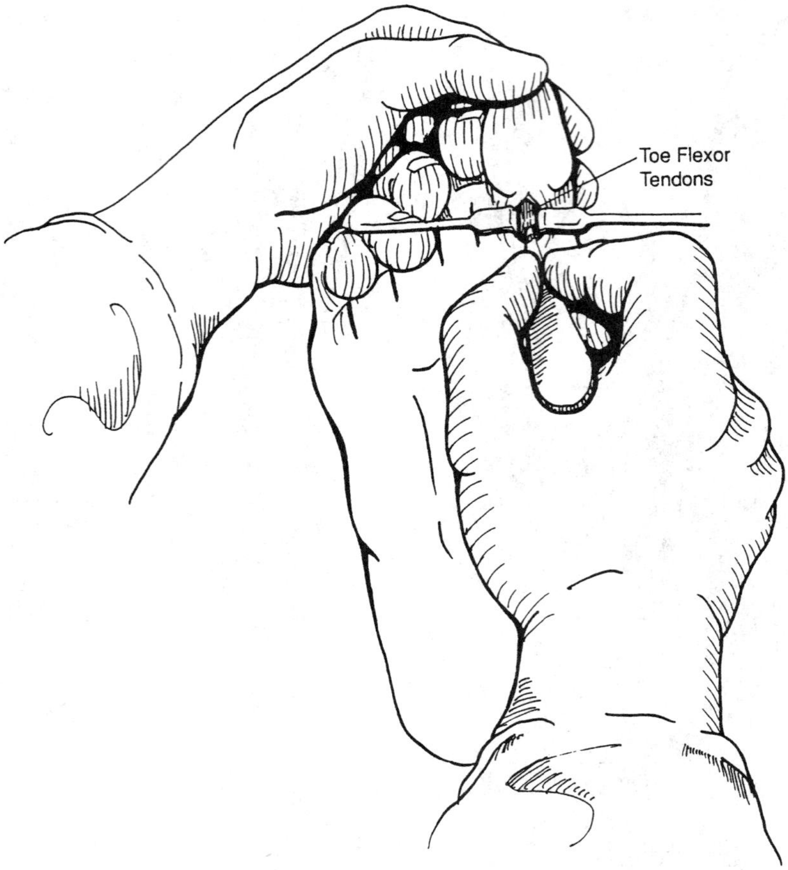

FIG. 34.2. Release of the toe flexor tendons to correct clawing. (From Keenan MA, Kozin SH, Berlet AC. *Manual of orthopedic surgery for spasticity.* New York: Raven Press, 1993, with permission.)

rigid ankle foot orthosis for an additional 6 weeks. The patient must sleep wearing AFO during this time to protect the foot from an inadvertent stretch. The brace can be removed for sleeping and gait training at 3 months after surgery. The AFO can be discontinued if and when the patient has established sufficient strength in the calf.

Varus

Split Anterior Tibial Tendon Transfer

Varus deformities most commonly occur as the result of increased and inappropriate activity of the tibialis anterior muscle. When dynamic EMG has documented the tibialis anterior to be the cause of varus, a split anterior tibial tendon transfer (SPLATT) corrects the deformity (14,17,20,21,27,29,31–36,38–47). The SPLATT maintains the half of the tendon on the medial aspect of the foot and transfers the other half of the tibialis anterior tendon to the lateral side of the foot (Fig. 34.3). A lengthening of the Achilles tendon should be performed first and the toe flexor tendons divided because equinus and toe curling usually accompany the varus deformity. An incision is made over the distal insertion of the tibialis anterior tendon on the medial aspect of the foot (37). The lateral half of the tendon is sharply divided from its insertion. A second incision is made approximately 10 cm proximal to the ankle joint just lateral to the crest of the tibia over the tibialis anterior muscle. The free end of the tendon is pulled into the proximal wound,

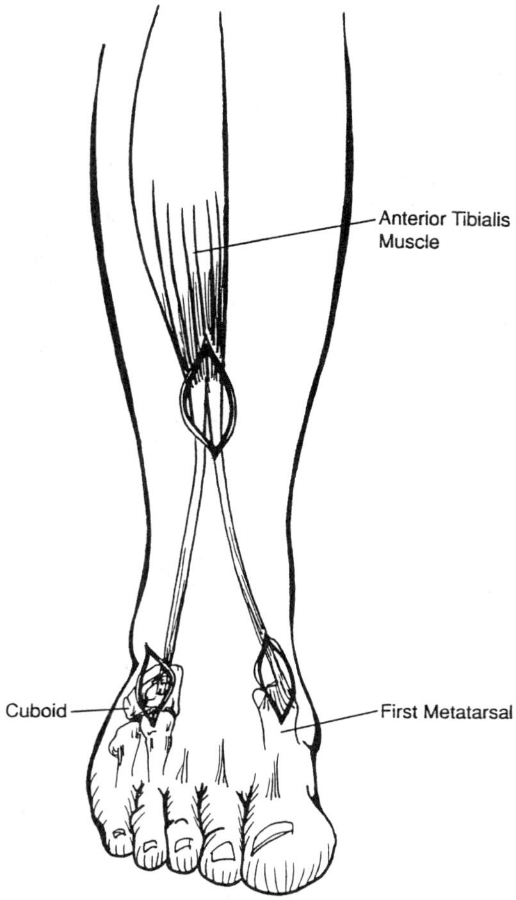

FIG. 34.3. The split anterior tibialis tendon transfer (SPLATT) to correct spastic varus. (From Keenan MA, Kozin SH, Berlet AC. *Manual of orthopedic surgery for spasticity.* New York: Raven Press, 1993, with permission.)

thereby splitting the tibialis anterior tendon. A third incision is then made on the lateral aspect of the foot and the lateral face of the cuboid is subperiosteally exposed. A drill is used to make a tunnel through the cuboid for anchoring of the lateral portion of the tendon. A subcutaneous tunnel is created from the proximal wound to the lateral incision using a long forceps. The lateral arm of the tibialis tendon is passed through this subcutaneous passage to protrude from the lateral incision. The tibialis anterior tendon is secured on the lateral side of the foot through the tunnel in the cuboid bone and sutured to itself to hold the foot in a neutral position.

The patient is placed in a short leg-walking cast for 6 weeks postoperatively. Then the patient begins using a nonarticulated, rigid ankle foot orthosis for an additional 6 weeks. The patient must sleep wearing AFO during this time to protect the foot from an inadvertent stretch. The brace can be removed for sleeping and gait training at 3 months postoperatively. The AFO can be discontinued if and when the patient has established sufficient strength in the calf muscles to permit safe walking.

Tibialis Anterior Lengthening

Occasionally a mild varus deformity is seen during walking that is owing to a moderate increase in tibialis anterior activity. A myotendinous lengthening is sufficient to control the varus deformity in this situation. An incision is made over the tibialis anterior muscle approximately 10 cm proximal to the ankle joint. The fascial sheath of the tibialis anterior is opened and the tendon is transected over the muscle belly of the tibialis anterior, thereby allowing the muscle to lengthen fractionally. No immobilization is needed after surgery if this is the only procedure performed.

Tibialis Posterior Lengthening

In approximately 10% of stroke and brain-injured patients the tibialis posterior muscle is also spastic and contributes to the varus deformity. Clinically, this is evidenced by the increased heel varus in addition to the forefoot varus caused by the tibialis anterior muscle. A myotendinous lengthening of the tendon is performed posterior and slightly proximal to the medial malleolus when spasticity of the tibialis posterior muscle is present. Complete release of the tibialis posterior tendon is not recommended because a planovalgus deformity may occur secondarily.

The Equinovalgus Foot Deformity

Peroneal Lengthening

Spastic valgus foot deformities are less common in the stroke and brain-injury population.

The deformity can result from overactivity of the peroneus longus, peroneus brevis, or both. Dynamic EMG is used to determine which muscles are causing the deformity (33). A myotendinous lengthening can be considered if the deformity is not severe. An incision is made over the lateral leg approximately 10 cm above the ankle joint. The fascia of the lateral compartment is opened and the offending peroneal muscles are fractionally lengthened. If no other procedures are performed simultaneously, no immobilization is needed after surgery and unrestricted ambulation is allowed.

Peroneus Longus Transfer

A spastic valgus deformity may be seen from overactivity of the peroneus longus muscle. This can occur as an isolated deformity but more commonly occurs in combination with spastic equinovarus. In the "spastic combination foot" deformity, equinovarus is observed during swing phase from premature and prolonged firing of the tibialis anterior and gastroc-soleus muscles. The planovalgus deformity occurs during stance from the inappropriate activity of the peroneus longus muscle. The pronation deformity may be accentuated by a premorbid tendency to flat foot or by the presence of an equinus contracture.

When a severe spastic valgus occurs, the peroneus longus tendon is transferred through the interosseous membrane to the tarsal navicular bone to support the longitudinal arch of the foot during stance (Fig. 34.4) (37). When a combined deformity is present, a SPLATT is performed along with a tendo-Achilles lengthening (TAL) and toe flexor release (TFR) to correct the swing

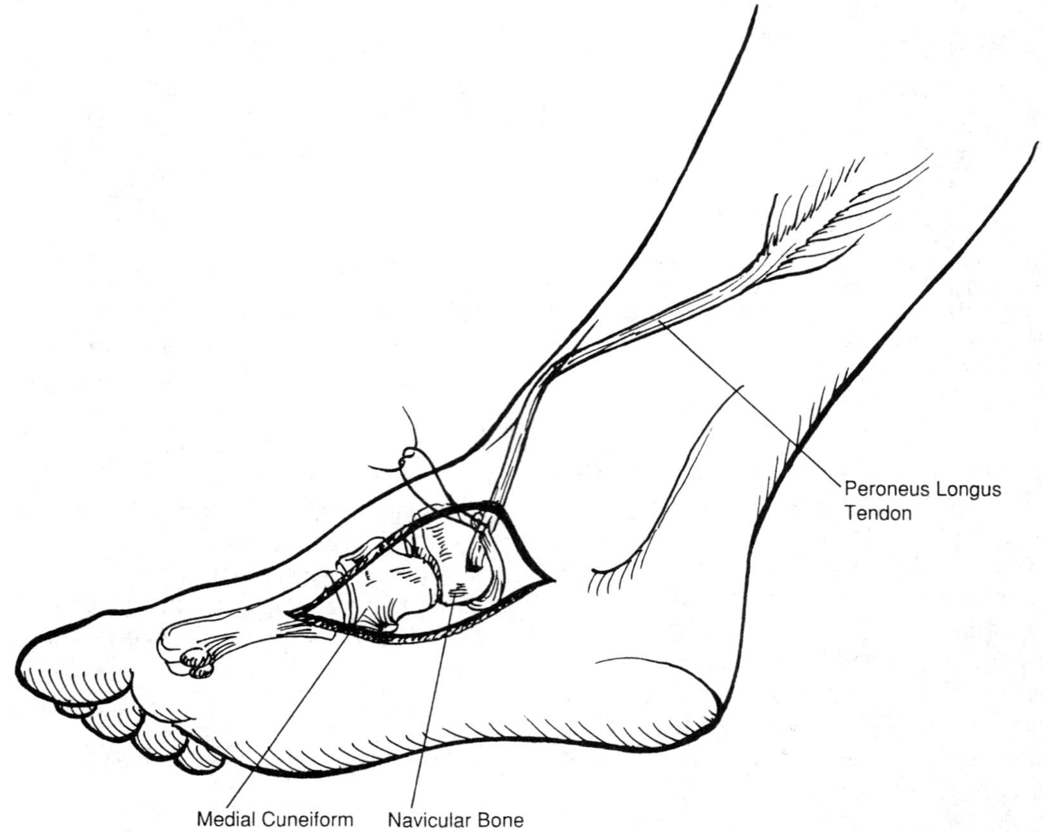

FIG. 34.4. Transfer of the peroneus longus tendon to the tarsal navicular to correct a spastic valgus deformity. (From Keenan MA, Kozin SH, Berlet AC. *Manual of orthopedic surgery for spasticity.* New York: Raven Press, 1993, with permission.)

phase abnormalities (33). The postoperative management is the same as for the SPLATT.

The Hyperextended Great Toe Deformity

Extensor Hallucis Lengthening

With the equinovarus deformity the patient may also have a hyperextended great toe secondary to spasticity of the extensor hallucis longus (EHL) tendon (3,13,16,28,48). The EHL also contributes to the varus deformity of the forefoot. Transecting the tendon as it overlies the muscle belly fractionally lengthens the EHL muscle.

The Stiff Knee Gait Deformity

Rectus Femoris to Gracilis Transfer for Dynamic Stiff Knee Gait

Patients with a stiff knee gait are unable to flex the knee during the swing phase of gait (24,25,49–58). The deformity is a dynamic one, meaning that it only occurs during walking. Usually the knee is maintained in extension throughout the gait cycle. Toe drag, which is likely in the early swing phase, may cause the patient to trip. The limb appears to be functionally longer. Circumduction of the involved limb, hiking of the pelvis, and/or contralateral limb vaulting may occur as compensatory maneuvers.

A gait study with dynamic EMG should be performed preoperatively to document the activity of the individual muscles of the quadriceps. Dyssynergic activity is commonly seen in the rectus femoris from preswing through terminal swing throughout the gait cycle. Abnormal activity is also common in the rectus intermedius. The patient should be able to ambulate with a reasonable velocity in order to benefit from surgery because the amount of knee flexion during swing is directly related to the speed of walking. Hip flexion strength is also needed for a good result because it is the forward momentum of the leg that normally provides the inertial force to

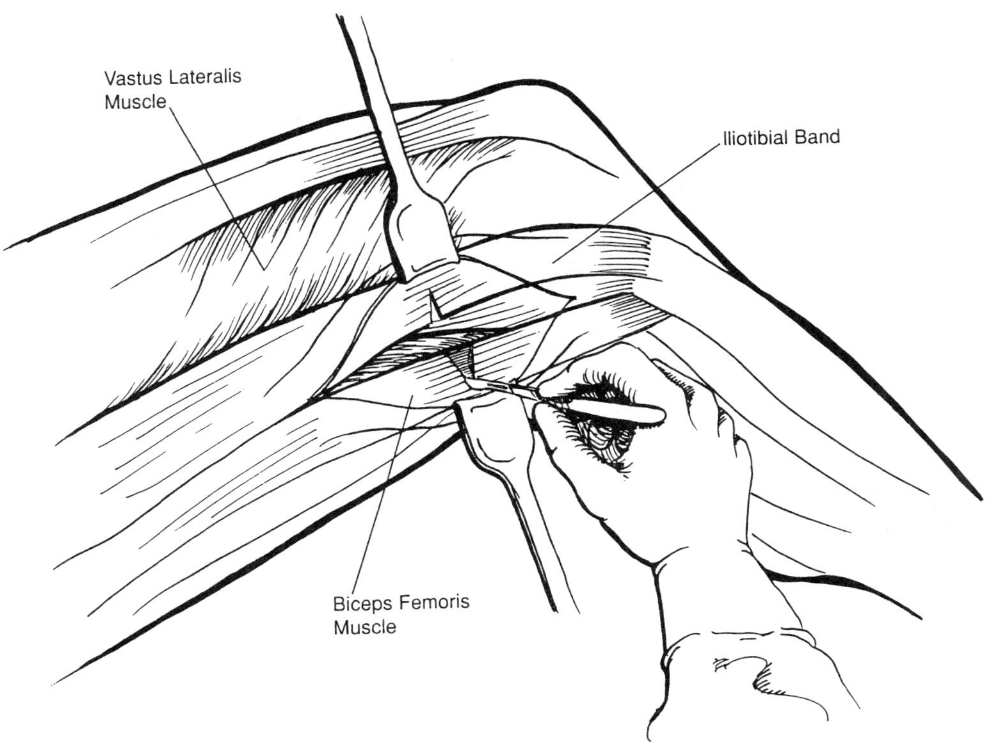

FIG. 34.5. Lengthening of the hamstring muscles distally to correct spastic knee flexion. (From Keenan MA, Kozin SH, Berlet AC. *Manual of orthopedic surgery for spasticity.* New York: Raven Press, 1993, with permission.)

flex the knee. Transfer of the rectus femoris to the gracilis hamstring tendon not only removes it as a deforming muscle force; it also converts the rectus into a corrective (flexion) force. If significant spasticity was seen in the vasti muscle on the dynamic EMG study, they are fractionally lengthened. The patient is placed in a knee immobilizer splint for 1 week after surgery to prevent a knee flexion deformity from occurring secondary to the tension and discomfort of the transfer. A marching gait pattern is stressed during therapy to facilitate knee flexion during swing.

Quadriceps Lengthening

Extensor spasticity can cause a knee extension contracture after a brainstem injury. This usually is seen in combination with a hip extension contracture. Both deformities result in problems with sitting. The knee extension deformity can be corrected by lengthening the quadriceps. Quadriceps weakness is not a problem in these patients because they are not ambulatory. In the past a V-Y lengthening of the quadriceps tendon was done routinely. More recently, we have performed a fractional lengthening of the individual muscles of the quadriceps. This procedure is more easily performed and has less morbidity than V-Y lengthening. It also does not cause a patella baja deformity. Even severe hyperextension knee deformities can be corrected with this procedure.

The Flexed Knee Deformity

Distal Hamstring Lengthening

A knee flexion deformity is caused by overactivity of the hamstring muscles (14,19,20,56,59–61). When the knee flexion deformity is less than 60 degrees and the patient has documented volitional activity in the hamstring muscles, then a lengthening procedure is done (Fig. 34.5). This will correct the flexion deformity while

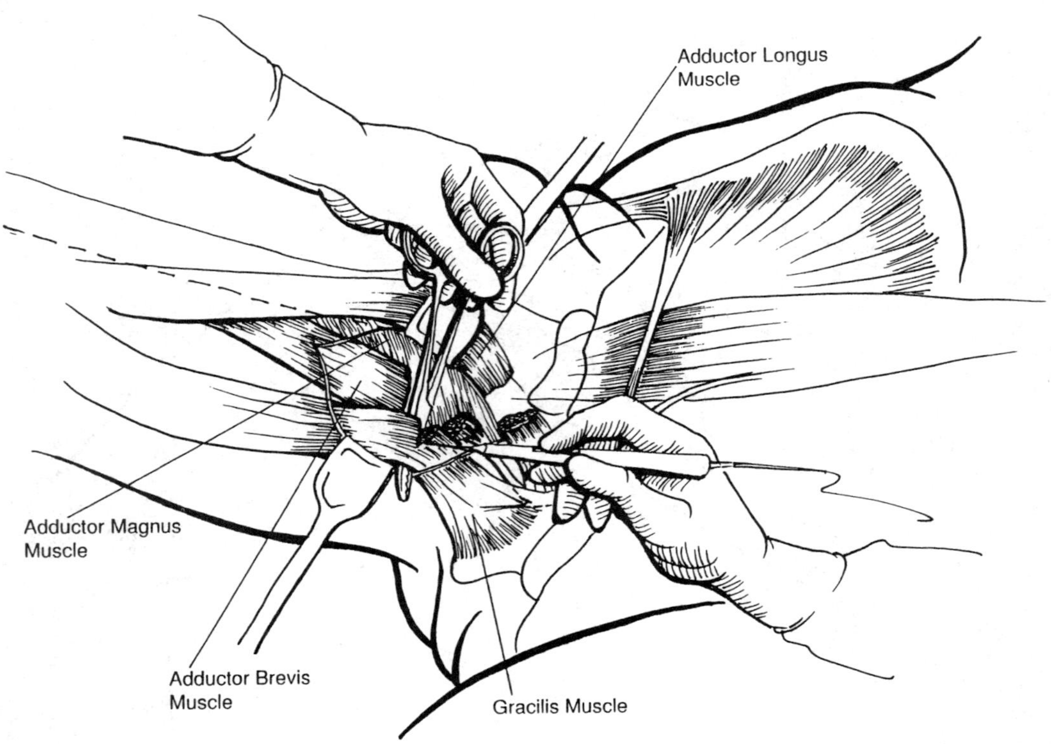

FIG. 34.6. Release of the hip adductor muscles to correct scissoring of the thighs. (From Keenan MA, Kozin SH, Berlet AC. *Manual of orthopedic surgery for spasticity.* New York: Raven Press, 1993, with permission.)

preserving the function of the hamstrings. The extremity is immobilized in a long leg cast after surgery. The cast is changed weekly until full knee extension has been obtained.

Distal Hamstring Release

In a patient with severe spasticity of the hamstring muscles or a knee flexion contracture of greater than 60 degrees is present, attempts to correct the knee position with casting or bracing may result in posterior subluxation of the tibia. Lengthening of the hamstring muscles is not sufficient to correct the knee deformity so a distal release is performed (14,20,37,61–63). Distal release of the hamstring tendons does not prevent a patient from becoming ambulatory. A recurrent knee flexion contracture is likely to develop that is very resistant to surgical correction if the hip flexion contracture or spasticity is not corrected at the same time as the hamstring release. In severe contractures, release of the sartorius muscle is also performed. The posterior joint capsule may need to be released in longstanding contractures. The extremity is immobilized in a long leg cast after surgery.

The Adducted (Scissoring) Thighs Deformity

Obturator Neurectomy

Scissoring of the legs in an ambulatory patient gives the patient a narrow base of support while standing and results in poor balance (3,13,16,28,37,62,64–68). When no fixed adduction contracture is present, transection of the anterior branches of the obturator nerve will denervate the adductors and allow the patient a broader base of support (37). Gait training is instituted in the postoperative period.

Hip Adductor Tenotomy

A hip adduction contracture that interferes with nursing care and hygiene in a nonambulatory patient or excessive limb scissoring during attempted transfers and ambulation in a patient with active function are indications for surgical release (Fig. 34.6).

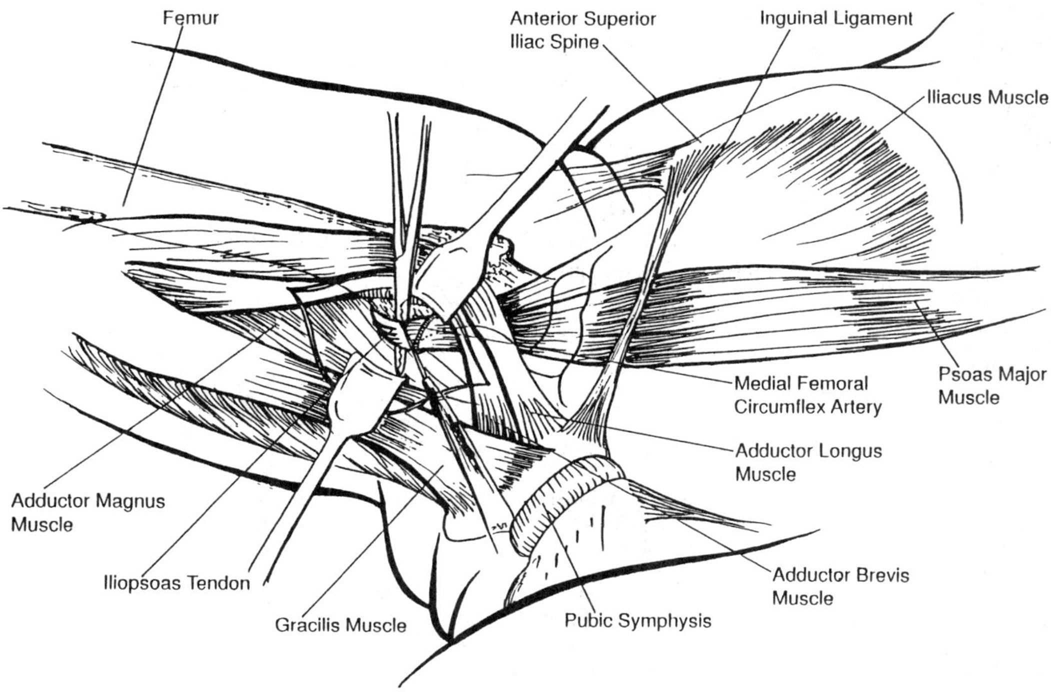

FIG. 34.7. Release of the iliopsoas tendon from the lesser trochanter of the femur to correct a hip flexion deformity. (From Keenan MA, Kozin SH, Berlet AC. *Manual of orthopedic surgery for spasticity.* New York: Raven Press, 1993, with permission.)

Daily wound care is essential to prevent infection in this potentially contaminated area. The hips should be kept in abduction for 4 weeks using casts or an abduction pillow splint to prevent recurrence of the deformity during wound healing.

Flexed Hip

Functional Release: Pectineus Release with Iliopsoas Recession

Spasticity of the hip flexors can result in a crouched gait with compensatory knee flexion to maintain balance (1,6,19,30,37,62,64,66,69). This is a very costly deformity because it requires constant use of the quadriceps, hip extensor, and calf muscles to maintain upright posture. The energy requirement for the continuous firing of these muscles is extremely high. Few patients are able to remain ambulatory with this deformity.

The hip flexor muscles are needed to advance the limb during gait. Complete release of the hip flexors should be avoided in any patient with the potential to ambulate. Release of the iliopsoas tendon from the lesser trochanter of the femur does not provide a complete release because the iliopsoas has capsular insertions. Release of the tendon from the lesser trochanter permits the iliopsoas to recess proximally, thereby diminishing its pull but retaining its function (Fig. 34.7) (37).

Postoperatively, the patient begins range of motion exercises and full weight-bearing gait training as tolerated. Prone lying and electrical stimulation of the gluteus maximus muscle are helpful to correct any residual hip flexion deformity.

REFERENCES

1. Keenan MAE, Waters RL. Surgical treatment of the lower extremity after stroke. In: Chapman MS, ed. *Operative orthopaedics*. Philadelphia: J.B. Lippincott, 1993:3449–3466.
2. Kolessar D, Keenan MAE. Surgical management of upper extremity deformities following traumatic brain injury. In: Stone LR, ed. *Neurologic and orthopedic sequelae of TBI*. Philadelphia: Hanley & Belfus, 1993: 623–636.
3. Mayer NH, Esquenazi A, Keenan MAE. Analysis and management of spasticity, contracture, and impaired motor control. In: Horn LJ, Zasler ND, eds. *Medical rehabilitation of traumatic brain injury*. Philadelphia: Hanley & Belfus, 1996:411–458.
4. Botte MJ, Nickel VL, Akeson WH. Spasticity and contracture. *Clin Orthop* 1988;233:7–18.
5. Garland DE, Keenan MA. Orthopedic strategies in the management of the adult head-injured patient. *Phys Ther* 1983;63:2004–2009.
6. Perry J. Contractures. A historical perspective. *Clin Orthop* 1987:8–14.
7. Keenan MA, Kauffman DL, Garland DE, et al. Late ulnar neuropathy in the brain-injured adult. *J Hand Surg* 1988;13:120–124.
8. Keenan MA, Haider T. The formation of heterotopic ossification after traumatic brain injury: a biopsy study with ultrastructural analysis. *J Head Trauma Rehabil* 1996;11:8–22.
9. Stone L, Keenan MA. Peripheral nerve injuries in the adult with traumatic brain injury. *Clin Orthop* 1988:136–144.
10. Young S, Keenan MAE. Extremity fractures in the brain-injured patient. In: Nickel VL, Botte MJ, eds. *Orthopedic rehabilitation*. New York: Churchill Livingstone, 1992:401–410.
11. Orcutt SA, Kramer WG, Howard MW, et al. Carpal tunnel syndrome secondary to wrist and finger flexor spasticity. *J Hand Surg* 1990;15:940–944.
12. Keenan MA, Perry J, Jordan C. Factors affecting balance and ambulation following stroke. *Clin Orthop* 1984:165–171.
13. Esquenazi A, Keenan MA. Gait analysis. In: DeLisa JA, ed. *Rehabilitation medicine: principles and practice*. Philadelphia: J.B. Lippincott, 1993:122–130.
14. Keenan MA. Surgical decision making for residual limb deformities following traumatic brain injury. *Orthop Rev* 1988;17:1185–1192.
15. Kerrigan DC, Annaswamy TM. The functional significance of spasticity as assessed by gait analysis. *J Head Trauma Rehabil* 1997;12:29–39.
16. Mayer N, Esquenazi A, Wannstedt G. Surgical planning for upper motoneuron dysfunction: the role of motor control evaluation. *J Head Trauma Rehabil* 1996;11: 37–56.
17. Perry J, Waters RL, Perrin T. Electromyographic analysis of equinovarus following stroke. *Clin Orthop* 1978:47–53.
18. Perry J, Giovan P, Harris LJ, et al. The determinants of muscle action in the hemiparetic lower extremity. *Clin Orthop* 1978;131:71–89.
19. Perry J. Determinants of muscle function in the spastic lower extremity. *Clin Orthop* 1993;288:10–26.
20. Waters RL, Perry J, Garland D. Surgical correction of gait abnormalities following stroke. *Clin Orthop* 1978:54–63.
21. Waters RL, Frazier J, Garland DE, et al. Electromyographic gait analysis before and after operative treatment for hemiplegic equinus and equinovarus deformity. *J Bone Joint Surg* 1982;64:284–288.
22. Keenan MA, Haider TT, Stone LR. Dynamic electromyography to assess elbow spasticity. *J Hand Surg* 1990;15:607–614.
23. Etnyre B, Chambers CS, Scarborough NH, et al. Preoperative and postoperative assessment of surgical intervention for equinus gait in children with cerebral palsy. *J Pediatr Orthop* 1993;13:24–31.

24. Miller F, Cardoso Dias R, Lipton GE, et al. The effect of rectus EMG patterns on the outcome of rectus femoris transfers. *J Pediatr Orthop* 1997;17:603–607.
25. Sutherland DH, Santi M, Abel MF. Treatment of stiff-knee gait in cerebral palsy: a comparison by gait analysis of distal rectus femoris transfer versus proximal rectus release. *J Pediatr Orthop* 1990;10:433–441.
26. O'Byrne JM, Jenkinson A, O'Brien TM. Quantitative analysis and classification of gait patterns in cerebral palsy using a three-dimensional motion analyzer. *J Child Neurol* 1998;13:101–108.
27. Synder M, Kumar SJ, Stecyk MD. Split tibialis posterior tendon transfer and tendo-Achilles lengthening for spastic equinovarus feet. *J Pediatr Orthop* 1993;13: 20–23.
28. Anmuth C, Esquenazi A, Keenan MAE. Lower extremity surgery for the spastic patient. In: Katz R, ed. *Spasticity*. Philadelphia: Hanley & Belfus, 1994:547–564.
29. Keenan MA, Creighton J, Garland DE, et al. Surgical correction of spastic equinovarus deformity in the adult head trauma patient. *Foot Ankle* 1984;5:35–41.
30. Keenan MAE. Rehabilitation of the neurologically disabled patient. In: Wilkens R, ed. *Neurosurgery*. New York: McGraw–Hill 1996:445–457.
31. Keenan MAE, Lee GA, Tuckman A, et al. Improving calf muscle strength in patients with spastic equinovarus deformity by transfer of the long toe flexors to the os calcis. *J Head Trauma Rehabil* 1999;14:163–175.
32. Piccioni L, Keenan MA. Surgical management of the spastic equinovarus foot deformity. *Op Tech Orthop* 1992;2:146–150.
33. Young S, Keenan MA, Stone LR. The treatment of spastic planovalgus foot deformity in the neurologically impaired adult. *Foot Ankle* 1990;10:317–324.
34. Edwards P, Hsu J. SPLATT combined with tendo Achilles lengthening for spastic equinovarus in adults: results and predictors of surgical outcome. *Foot Ankle* 1993;14:335–338.
35. Lawrence SJ, Botte MJ. Management of the adult, spastic, equinovarus foot deformity. *Foot Ankle Int* 1994;15:340–346.
36. O'Byrne JM, Kennedy A, Jenkinson A, et al. Split tibialis posterior tendon transfer in the treatment of spastic equinovarus foot. *J Pediatr Orthop* 1997;17:481–485.
37. Keenan MAE, Kozin SH, Berlet AC. *Manual of orthopedic surgery for spasticity*. New York: Raven Press, 1993.
38. Keenan MA, Gorai AP, Smith CW, et al. Intrinsic toe flexion deformity following correction of spastic equinovarus deformity in adults. *Foot Ankle* 1987;7:333–337.
39. Lawrence SJ, Botte MJ. Current topic review: management of the adult spastic equinovarus foot deformity. *Foot Ankle Int* 1994;15:340–346.
40. Morita S, Yamamoto H, Furuya K. Anterior transfer of the toe flexors for equinovarus deformity due to hemiplegia. *J Bone Joint Surg* 1994;76-B:447– 449.
41. Roper BA, Williams A, King JB. The surgical treatment of equinovarus deformity in adults with spasticity. *J Bone Joint Surg* 1978;60-B:533–535.
42. Waters RL, Frazier J, Garland D, et al. Electromyographic gait analysis before and after treatment for hemiplegic equinus and equinovarus deformity. *J Bone Joint Surg* 1982;64-A:284–288.
43. Reiter F, Danni M, Lagalla G, et al. Low-dose botulinum toxin with ankle taping for the treatment of spastic equinovarus foot after stroke. *Arch Phys Med Rehabil* 1998;79:532–535.
44. Vogt JC. Split anterior tibial transfer for spastic equinovarus foot deformity: retrospective study of 73 operated feet. *J Foot Ankle Surg* 1998;37:2–7; discussion 78.
45. Hoffer MM, Barakat G, Koffman M. 10-year follow-up of split anterior tibial tendon transfer in cerebral palsied patients with spastic equinovarus deformity. *J Pediatr Orthop* 1985;5:432–434.
46. Ireland ML, Hoffer M. Triple arthrodesis for children with spastic cerebral palsy. *Dev Med Child Neurol* 1985;27:623–627.
47. Pinzur MS, Sherman R, DiMonte-Levine P, et al. Adult-onset hemiplegia: changes in gait after muscle-balancing procedures to correct the equinus deformity. *J Bone Joint Surg* 1986;68:1249–1257.
48. Esquenazi A, Keenan MA, Mayer N. *Evaluacion y manejo de espasticidad, contracturas y disfuncion del control motor. Kinesiologia* 1995;42:60–65.
49. Ounpuu MS, Muik E, Davis III RB, et al. Rectus femoris surgery in children with cerebral palsy. Part II: a comparison between the effect of transfer and release of the distal rectus femoris on knee motion. *J Pediatr Orthop* 1993;13:331–335.
50. Chambers H, Lauer A, Kaufman K, et al. Prediction of outcome after rectus femoris surgery in cerebral palsy: the role of co-contraction of the rectus femoris and vastus lateralis. *J Pediatr Orthop* 1998;18:703–711.
51. Riley PO, Kerrigan DC. Torque action of two-joint muscles in the swing period of stiff-legged gait: a forward dynamic model analysis. *J Biomech* 1998;31: 835–840.
52. Piazza SJ, Delp SL. The influence of muscles on knee flexion during the swing phase of gait. *J Biomech* 1996;29:723–733.
53. Damron TA, Breed AL, Cook T. Diminished knee flexion after hamstring surgery in cerebral palsy patients: prevalence and severity. *J Pediatr Orthop* 1993;13:188–191.
54. Sutherland DH, Davids JR. Common gait abnormalities of the knee in cerebral palsy. *Clin Orthop* 1993:139–147.
55. Ounpuu MS, Muik E, Davis III RB, et al. Rectus femoris surgery in children with cerebral palsy. Part I: the effect of rectus femoris transfer location of knee motion. *J Pediatr Orthop* 1993;13:325–330.
56. Gage JR. Surgical treatment of knee dysfunction in cerebral palsy. *Clin Orthop* 1990: 45–54.
57. Perry J. Distal rectus femoris transfer. *Dev Med Child Neurol* 1987;29:153–158.
58. Waters RL, Garland DE, Perry J, et al. Stiff-legged gait in hemiplegia: surgical correction. *J Bone Joint Surg* 1979;61:927–933.
59. Waters RL, Perry J, McDaniels JM, et al. The relative strength of the hamstrings during hip extension. *J Bone Joint Surg* 1974;56:1592–1597.
60. Bauman JU, Ruetsch H, Schurman K. Distal hamstring lengthening in cerebral palsy. *Int Orthop* 1980;3:305–309.
61. Keenan MA, Ure K, Smith CW, et al. Hamstring release for knee flexion contracture in spastic adults. *Clin Orthop* 1988:221–226.
62. Botte MJ, Waters RL, Keenan MAE, et al. Orthopedic management of the stroke patient. Part II: treating deformities of the upper and lower extremities. *Orthop Rev* 1988;27:891–910.

63. Keenan MA, Waters RL. Surgical treatment of the upper extremity after stroke or brain injury. In: Chapman MS, ed. *Operative orthopaedics*. Philadelphia: J.B. Lippincott, 1993:1529–1544.
64. Botte MJ, Waters RL, Keenan MAE, et al. Orthopedic management of the stroke patient. Part I: pathophysiology, limb deformity, and patient evaluation. *Orthop Rev* 1988;27:637–646.
65. Perry J, Keenan MAE. Rehabilitation of the neurologically disabled patient. In: Aminoff MJ, ed. *Neurology and general medicine*. New York: Churchill Livingstone, 1989:747–778.
66. Pinzur MS. Surgical correction of lower extremity problems in patients with brain injury. *J Head Trauma Rehabil* 1996;44:69–77.
67. Smith CW, Levanthal L. Surgical management of lower extremity deformities in adult head injured patients. *J Head Trauma Rehabil* 1987;2:53–61.
68. Waters RL, Clifford B, Jordan C. Surgical correction of spastic lower extremity deformities. *Acta Orthop Belg* 1984;50:172–179.
69. Jordan C. Current status of functional lower extremity surgery in adult spastic patients. *Clin Orthop* 1988:102–109.

Gait Disorders. Advances in Neurology, Vol. 87,
edited by E. Růžička, M. Hallett, and J. Jankovic.
Lippincott Williams & Wilkins, Philadelphia © 2001.

35

Gait Disorders and Gait Rehabilitation in Parkinson's Disease

*Meg E. Morris, †Frances E. Huxham, †Jennifer McGinley, and ‡§Robert Iansek

**School of Physiotherapy, La Trobe University, Bundoora, 3086, Australia; †Geriatric Research Unit, and ‡Department of Geriatric Neurology, Kingston Centre, Southern Health, Cheltenham, Victoria 3192, Australia; and §Department of Medicine, Monash University, Clayton, 3168 Victoria, Australia*

Gait disorders are common in idiopathic Parkinson's disease (PD), affecting the vast majority of people with this chronic progressive condition. The most common gait disorders in PD are hypokinesia, start hesitation, and freezing, although dyskinesia also can be troublesome in people who have advanced disease and have been on L-Dopa medication for many years. Gait disorders are accentuated when people with PD attempt to perform secondary motor or cognitive tasks at the same time as walking (1,2). Hypokinesia and freezing are further exacerbated when the person attempts to turn or negotiate environmental obstacles during ambulatory tasks. In the advanced stages of the disease, postural instability can further compromise gait, with more than 38% of people with PD falling every year and 18% suffering fractures as a result of falls (3). In this chapter we review the pathogenesis of gait disorders in PD and discuss current findings on the biomechanics and motor control of gait derived as a basis for structuring rehabilitation.

GAIT HYPOKINESIA

Approximately 80% of people with PD experience gait hypokinesia at some stage in the course of the disease. The word "hypokinesia" means reduced movement amplitude (size) and speed. Hypokinesia is accentuated in the performance of long or repetitive movement sequences, particularly when movements are performed as part of well-learned, complex motor skills (4).

The majority of studies on gait hypokinesia in PD have investigated abnormalities in the spatial and distance parameters of the footstep pattern, such as stride length, cadence (stepping rate), gait speed, and the proportion of the walking cycle spent in double-limb support, which affords maximum stability (4–13). Our early studies on gait hypokinesia demonstrated that the short-stepped, shuffling gait pattern in PD was characterized by a deficit in stride length regulation (4,10). Despite the difficulty in controlling the size of footsteps within complex gait sequences, patients with mild to moderately severe disease had mean cadence rates that were within the normal range (4,10,11,13). The overall speed of walking was markedly reduced because the size of footsteps substantially decreased for each 10-m walk, even though the mean rate of footsteps was not different from age-matched control subjects. The portion of the gait cycle in double-limb stance was close to average, suggesting that balance disturbance was not a major factor limiting gait in these patients.

Although the mean stepping rate for a standard 10-m gait sequence in PD subjects is within the normal range (100 to 120 steps/min), there is new evidence that locomotor pattern generation is impaired in the early stages of the disease (7). Whereas our earlier studies had used a clinical stride analyzer to gather data on *mean* values for each of the footstep parameters for a 10-m walk (15 to 20 seconds duration), new technology used by Ebersbach et al. and Hausdorff et al. permitted quantification of variations in the footstep pattern from *one stride to the next* in long walking sequences (7,14). These studies revealed that, under certain conditions, stride length and stride duration variability were two to three times that observed in unimpaired subjects. These conditions were when subjects had to walk 10 m in time to a metronome with the auditory cue set at a rate 20% lower than self-selected cadence (7) or when subjects were instructed to walk for 5 minutes along a 77-m long hallway (14).

For the metronome entrainment task, Ebersbach and colleagues found that slowing cadence down to around 80 steps/min produced significantly more interstride variability of stride length and stride *time* in PD subjects than in controls, even though the mean stepping rate was close to 80 steps/min (7). The finding that the coefficient of variance (COV) for stride *length* was markedly increased in patients with PD is not surprising, given the accumulation of evidence that footstep size diminishes during the execution of gait sequences owing to a disorder in amplitude regulation (5,6,13). However, the finding that the COV for stride *time* was large for the metronome entrainment task implies that subjects with PD had added difficulty in maintaining rhythmical footstep timing. Ebersbach's data show that subjects with PD were both overshooting and undershooting their temporal targets (7). This would suggest a disorder in the central time-keeping mechanism thought to provide periodic signals enabling accurate timing subcomponents within motor sequences (15).

For the gait endurance task (5-minute walk) measured by Hausdorff et al., the COV for stride time in subjects with PD was nearly twice that of control subjects (14). Walking up and down a long corridor for 5 minutes without stopping can be quite difficult for people with PD, who appear to rely heavily on attentional mechanisms to maintain walking speed. Over this long period of time attention to the task of walking could wane, allowing the full extent of disturbances in rhythmical stepping and amplitude to be revealed. Subjects who performed 10 walks at their preferred speed for our earlier experiments (4,10,11,13) and those in the preferred walking condition (without the metronome) in Ebersbach's study (7) might have been able to compensate for a central timing disorder by focusing their attention on maintaining rhythmicity. In contrast, those in Hausdorff's experiment might have found it difficult to compensate for timing difficulties over the longer time period, thereby yielding more variable cadence than their age-matched counterparts. Hausdorffs' results again suggest that the underlying motor control mechanisms controlling footstep timing are abnormal in PD, leading to considerable stride-to-stride variability in footstep timing despite the fact that the mean cadence values for each 10-m walk are within the normal range.

A number of upper limb studies have previously shown that movement timing is impaired in PD (16–19). For example, Pastor et al. showed that subjects with PD could not maintain synchrony with a rhythmical finger-tapping task, even though they had no difficulty in either hearing or perceiving the auditory signal (16). Soliveri et al. also found that subjects with PD could not accurately maintain a rhythmical tapping sequence of the feet or fingers and Nakamura et al. identified a hastening phenomenon, whereby finger tapping movements became faster and faster during the execution of long motor sequences (18,19). In addition, Ho et al. found disordered timing in articulatory movements subserving speech in subjects with PD (20). Together, these results suggest that neurotransmitter imbalance in PD leads to a generalized disorder in the control of both movement timing and movement amplitude.

Notwithstanding, the stride-length amplitude regulation disorder remains the most prominent and troublesome problem in PD gait. This is evidenced by experiments that have employed a dual-task paradigm to elucidate the pathogenesis of gait disturbance in hypokinesia. In one example, Bond and Morris evaluated the effects of secondary motor task performance on the spatial and temporal parameters of gait in PD subjects compared with elderly control subjects (1). Participants performed a series of trials walking freely, carrying a tray, and carrying a tray with glasses.

For all of the conditions subjects with PD walked more slowly than controls owing to their shorter steps, even though mean cadence rates were comparable for the two groups. Although there was little change in the footstep pattern when a tray was carried while walking, subjects in the PD group showed more marked reductions than controls in stride length and walking velocity when instructed to carry a tray with glasses at the same time. When opportunities for compensation using attentional mechanisms and visual guidance were minimized (the tray obscured view of the feet, preventing visual guidance of step length), the deficit in stride length regulation was accentuated in subjects in PD. Both groups slowed their cadence rate during this difficult dual task, although the rate of reduction in cadence was comparable for the two groups. In agreement with these results, O'Shea et al. showed that both secondary motor and cognitive tasks led to significant reductions in stride length and speed that were much greater in subjects with PD than controls (2). In O'Shea's experiment, the secondary motor task involved transferring coins from one hip pocket to another, whereas the secondary cognitive task was the digits backward test. Although the cadence rate decreased during secondary task conditions in the PD group, the magnitude of decline was less than for stride length.

The disorder in stride length regulation in PD is in agreement with the results of upper limb studies. Berardelli et al. showed that sequential wrist movements in PD subjects were reduced in size because of underscaling of the first burst of activity in muscle agonists (21). Under certain circumstances, subjects with PD could produce large bursts of muscle activity; however, force generation did not always match the size of movement required. Nonhuman primate studies provide some insight into the nature of the amplitude regulation problem. The basal ganglia project to the motor cortex via the supplementary motor area (SMA) and premotor cortex. Animal models of parkinsonism have shown that set-related activity in the SMA is defective, leading to inadequate preparation of the primary motor cortex for forthcoming movements (22). As a result, movements are underscaled in size and therefore performed more slowly than usual because more catch-up bursts of muscle activity are required to complete a task (23). In relation to stride length regulation, it could be speculated that defective set-related activity of the SMA owing to abnormal output from the internal globus pallidus to the SMA could compromise neural recruitment in the primary motor cortex, resulting in diminution of step size. Because nonhuman primates do not typically generate bipedal gait in upright stance, this hypothesis has not yet been confirmed with neurophysiologic investigations.

To date, little has been reported on the kinematics and kinetics of gait hypokinesia in PD. Early descriptive studies using cinematography provided two-dimensional kinematic analysis of people with PD of varied etiology (24–26). Movement size (amplitude) was reduced in the lower limb joints, with decreased hip and knee flexion in swing phase. Foot contact was also abnormal in many subjects and plantarflexion in late stance was reduced. As these early studies used a single camera only for two-dimensional analysis, it seems likely that measurement error owing to out-of-plane movements (such as foot rotation) may have confounded the results.

More recently our team has used three-dimensional analysis to quantify the kinematics of gait hypokinesia. In one experiment we described the effect of L-Dopa and visual cues on the kinematics and kinetics of gait in a single subject with idiopathic PD (27). Movement excursion (amplitude) was markedly reduced in all lower limb joints at end-of-dose in the medication cycle, with kinematic profiles shifted toward flexion (27). With the introduction of L-Dopa and visual cues (white strips of cardboard placed on the floor at the correct step length for that person's age and height), movement amplitude increased toward normal range, with improved extension noted at the hip and knee. Although kinetics also altered with L-Dopa and visual cues, abnormalities in both joint moments and powers persisted. The patient continued to exhibit irregular, underscaled, multiple bursts of muscle power in achieving a normal-looking pattern of movement with treatment. Most noticeably, power generation at the calf was markedly underscaled at pushoff. The knee power profile showed a burst of absorption at terminal stance, rather than a slight amount of power generation that is normally the case. Maintaining walking with such abnormal kinetics is very energy consuming, and from that point of view inefficient (27). If walking with normal kinematic patterns comes at such a high energy cost, it is not surprising that people with PD find it difficult to maintain normal movement patterns after training with visual or auditory cues, as has been demonstrated previously (4,8,10). The attentional and cognitive energy cost may provide one reason why patients tend to stop performing optimally after brief gait training sessions.

Figure 35.1 illustrates a typical example of the kinematics of gait disturbance in PD hypokinesia, as well as an individual patient's response to L-Dopa medication. The figure illustrates pelvic, hip, knee, and ankle kinematics in the sagittal plane as measured by a four-camera Vicon 140 three-dimensional motion analysis system (Oxford Metrics, Oxford, U.K.) and Kistler force platform (Kistler, Winterthur, Switzerland). This subject (Mr. A) was a 68-year-old man (height 162 cm, weight 65 kg) with a 16-year history of idiopathic PD. Despite motor fluctuations he was an independent community ambulator, and was on a liquid form of L-Dopa. Gait was measured at the end-of-dose and at peak-dose, using a protocol described elsewhere (27). Disability and impairment were measured using the Unified Parkinson's Disease Rating Scale (UPDRS); scores on this scale were 65 and 37 in the end-of-dose and peak-dose condition, respectively. Mr. A was assessed to be at stage 4 on the Hoehn and Yahr scale (29). At the end-of-dose, reduced amplitude of movement was seen at the hip, knee, and ankle, with compression (underscaling of amplitude) of each of these profiles. In addition, the hip, knee, and ankle profiles were shifted upward into

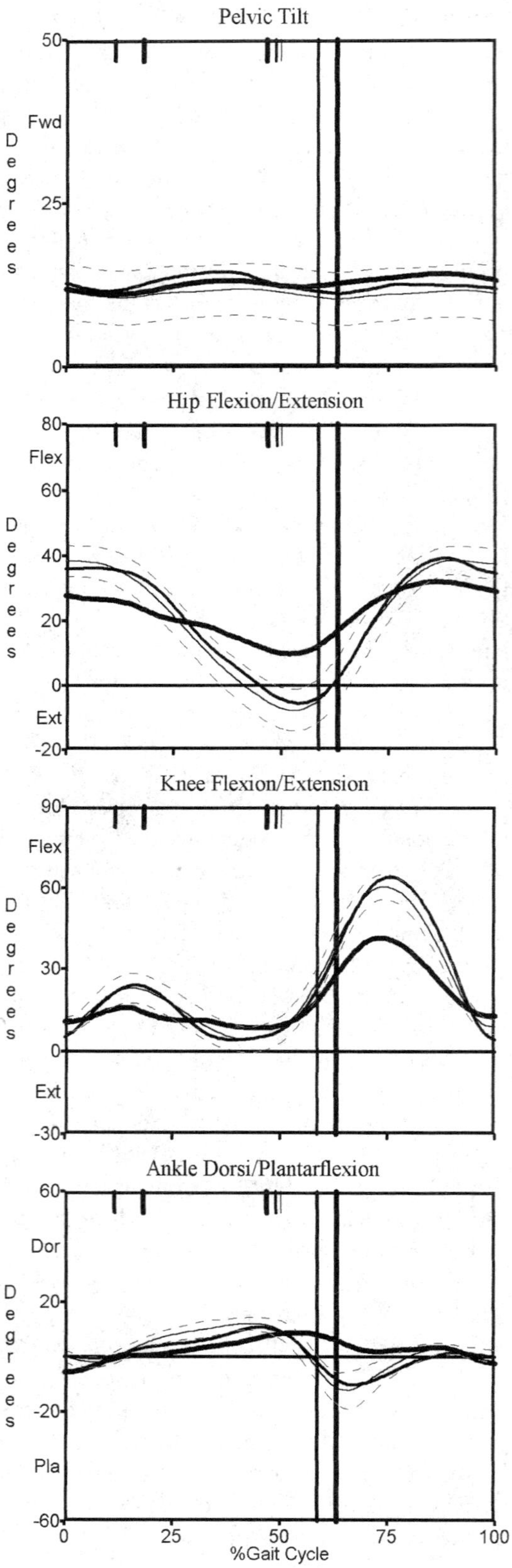

FIG. 35.1. Kinematics at the pelvis, hip, knee, and ankle for Mr. A with gait hypokinesia. *Thick black lines* represent end-of-dose performance, *lines of medium thickness* represent peak-dose performance, and *thin lines* together with *dashed lines* represent mean and one standard deviation for age-matched control subjects (N = 10).

TABLE 35.1. *Spatial and temporal parameters of gait for Mr. A with gait hypokinesia at end-of-dose, peak-dose, and compared with control subject data*

Variable	End-of-dose	Peak-dose	Matched controls (N = 10)
Speed (m/sec)	0.5	1.26	1.5
Cadence (steps/min)	122	117	122
Stride length (m)	0.49	1.28	1.45
Step time (sec)	0.52	0.52	0.48
Single support (% cycle)	28.6	37.3	39.0
Double support (% cycle)	34.7	21.6	19.5
Opposite foot off (% cycle)	18.4	11.8	11.3
Foot off (% cycle)	63.3	58.3	58.5
Opposite foot contact (% cycle)	47.0	49.0	50.3

flexion, consistent with the observed flexed posture of this subject throughout the stance phase (Fig. 35.1). Power generation was markedly reduced with very low peaks, reflecting the slow velocity and short steps of this typical PD gait (Table 35.1). In the peak-dose condition, a marked increase in movement amplitude was noted at the hip, knee, and ankle joints, for both flexion and extension ranges. In mid-stance, Mr. A was decidedly straighter, with all joints extending into normal range (Fig. 35.1). Power profiles revealed more typically shaped curves with larger peaks of both power generation and absorption across all joints. Thus, L-Dopa medication led to considerable improvement in gait kinematics and kinetics, although normal values were not always achieved.

Inspection of the temporal-distance data for Mr. A showed typical medication response changes consistent with our previous reported data (Table 35.1) (13). In the end-of-dose condition, gait was slow and short-stepped, with a stride length of only 0.49 m and speed of 0.5 m/sec. With medication, a marked change was evident at peak-dose, with a stride length of 1.28 m and speed of 1.26 m/sec. Normal values are around 1.5 and 1.5 m/sec, respectively. Cadence remained essentially unchanged across conditions. Thus, in this subject L-Dopa medication enhanced the spatiotemporal parameters of gait, although a normal footstep pattern was not obtained.

The data from this gait analysis illustrate some of the classic features of gait hypokinesia in PD. First, the patient's movements were reduced in size, across all gait parameters. Second, the underlying patterns of force generation were abnormal, being jerky and underscaled. Moreover, these gait parameters showed only partial amelioration with L-Dopa medication. Although the medication improved the walking pattern, there was a limited response and some abnormalities in kinetics persisted despite the best attempts to optimize the dosage and scheduling of medication. This supports previous investigations that have demonstrated that gait hypokinesia is only partially responsive to pharmacotherapy (6,8,9,13,28,30).

AKINESIA: START HESITATION AND FREEZING

Around 20% of people with PD experience start hesitancy (also called akinesia) and freezing. Very little is known about the pathogenesis of akinesia or the short-term and longer-lasting effects of treatment on these movement disorders. Clinical reports by Giladi, Stern, Fahn, Gantchev, and Nutt et al. noted that akinesia manifests in two ways (31–35). Most commonly, there is a difficulty with initiating movement, known as start hesitancy or "ignition disorder," so that the person finds it extremely difficult to initiate the first step in the locomotor sequence. Start hesitancy is accentuated when a long or complex gait sequence needs to be performed, and when L-Dopa levels are very low. In these circumstances patients typically report that they feel their feet are "glued to the floor" and cannot lift the leg despite considerable effort (32). This is not related to weakness, disorders of muscle tone, or musculoskeletal disorders; rather, it appears to be a neurologic disorder of basal ganglia origin (33). Of interest, start hesitancy varies in severity according to the context in which a task is being performed. For example, at some times people find it exceedingly difficult to take the first step forward, yet when they use certain "tricks" or "strategies" such as saying "go," rocking from side-to-side, or visualizing stepping over a log they can move more normally (32–34). Clinically, it appears that the ability to initiate the walking sequence is not lost; rather, there is an activation problem.

With "freezing," people experience sudden and uncontrollable cessation of movement *during* the execution of the locomotor sequence. These freezing episodes may be triggered by environmental constraints, such as walking through a narrow doorway, negotiating obstacles such as a low tree branch or cobblestones, or the need to make a transition when walking from carpet to floorboards (36). Freezing can also be triggered by altered emotional states (36) and can occur when a person's attention is directed to a second task such as talking when walking. In other people, the footsteps become progressively shorter for no apparent reason just prior to the block. A major problem for people with freezing is the high falls rate, ranging from 38% to 65% (3).

Cortically generated movement-related potentials provide a window of opportunity for understanding the neural correlates of start hesitation and freezing. The movement-related potential (MRP) represents a build-up of negative electrical activity in the cortex of the brain. It is measured from the scalp, above the SMA and cingulate motor areas. This electrical activity precedes voluntary self-initiated movements. Movement-related potentials have been divided into two components, localized from different cortical areas. The early component is known as the Bereitschafts potential (BP) and slowly builds up over the SMA 1 to 2 seconds prior to movement. The late component is a rapidly increasing negative potential that begins at around 500 ms before movement onset. It is maximal over the contralateral primary motor cortex. As demonstrated by Cunnington et al., the movement-related potential has larger amplitude for noncued (internally regulated) voluntary movements than for externally cued movements (37). Vidailhet et al. examined cortical movement-related potentials preceding gait initiation in patients with mild to moderate PD (off their medication) compared with control subjects (38). Subjects were required to perform simple repetitive stepping movements of the foot in sitting, followed by gait initiation. Whereas control subjects demonstrated larger BPs for gait initiation than stepping, PD subjects showed no change. Their failure to change premovement activity according to task demands resulted in a disorder in movement preparation for gait initiation. No attempt was made to compare brain potentials for steps in which gait ignition failure occurred against steps in which gait was successfully ignited. In addition, the researchers did not simultaneously measure anticipatory postural adjustments or the kinematics of gait. Therefore, the severity of BP abnormality could not be correlated with the severity of gait and balance disturbance.

A more recent study by Burleigh-Jacobs et al. investigated anticipatory postural adjustments during gait initiation using force platform measures of the trajectories of center of mass (COM) and center of pressure (COP) (39). The COM is the point equivalent of the center of a person's body mass in three-dimensional space, whereas the COP is the point within the foot where the base of the vertical ground reaction force vector lies. They found that subjects with PD had moderately reduced lateral and posterior COP excursions as well as reduced vertical force production prior to push off. However, this experiment did not differentiate PD subjects with akinesia from those with hypokinesia. Even when L-Dopa medication was withheld for 12 hours only two of the six subjects with PD tested were unable to self-generate steps. This means that only two subjects in the sample actually had ignition disturbance, thereby limiting the generalizability of findings to the population of patients with akinesia. To date there has not been any attempt to measure the kinematics of gait (pattern of movement at the hips, knees, and ankles) at the same time as measuring the COM, COP, and premovement potentials in people with akinesia. Correlating kinematic disturbances with force platform and premovement potentials would provide clinicians with information on the underlying biomechanical and neural bases of ignition disturbance.

The pathogenesis of start hesitation and freezing episodes midway through walking has not been the topic of systematic evaluation despite the seminal clinical descriptions by investigators such as Nutt et al., Giladi et al., and Vidailhet et al. (35,36,38). Notwithstanding, a number of theories have been proposed to account for akinesia in PD. According to one theory the basal ganglia are involved in running motor skills automatically, once the skill has been selected and initiated by the motor cortical regions (40). Iansek argued that the basal ganglia regulate movement automaticity by: (a) providing the appropriate amount of set-related activity to the motor cortical regions to maintain cortically selected movement plans in a state of readiness until the movement has been completed; (b) providing internal cues to string submovements of motor plans together with the correct timing and sequence (41). Set-related activity is hypothesized to regulate movement gain, and is represented at a neuronal level as sustained premovement discharge (41). Cues are proposed to be represented at a neuronal level as phasic bursts of activity that are generated in the internal globus pallidus of the basal ganglia during or at the end of submovements (41).

Using this model, we hypothesize that two motor control problems may lead to start hesitancy and freezing. First, there may be disruption to the role of the basal ganglia in regulating the gain of complex motor sequences. This would result in a scaling down or miniaturization of movement. Scaling down of movement size to zero would prevent the person from initiating the first step in the sequence. Partial scaling down would presumably impair the person's ability to regulate the excursion of the COP and COM trajectories to initiate gait. Normally, when people initiate gait they move the COP backward and toward the foot that is about to swing (23). This causes the COM trajectory to accelerate forward and toward the stance limb, allowing the swing limb to unload in preparation for pushoff (23). If the COP were underscaled then insufficient weight would be transferred on to the stance limb, preventing the swing limb from leaving the ground (42).

Disorders in the internal "cue" role of the basal ganglia could also lead to a sequence effect in the cortex-basal ganglia-cortex motor feedback loop (41). As submovements in the locomotor sequence were processed by the faulty feedback loop, they would presumably become progressively smaller, resulting in "festination" (also known as the sequence effect) and eventual freezing. It is also possible that environmental stimuli such as doorways and mats as well as dual-task performance predispose patients toward freezing episodes as these factors distract attention away from compensating for the gait disturbance. By preventing the compensation, the full extent of the underlying akinesia emerges. These empirical observations need to be confirmed with controlled clinical trials.

GAIT DYSKINESIAS, INCLUDING DYSTONIA

Although it is agreed in clinical circles that dyskinesia is a major movement disorder compromising walking in people with PD, there has not yet been a study documenting the characteristic features of dyskinetic gait in PD or quantifying the effects of different treatment regimens on this problem. The term "dyskinesia" refers to extra, involuntary movements of the limbs, trunk, head, and neck, which can occur after patients have been on L-Dopa medication for many years. Whether dyskinesia is owing to prolonged medication use or the natural history of the disease is currently not known. Although usually choreiform in type, dyskinesia can also take the form of tics, athetosis, and dystonia (43). Dystonia refers to involuntary excessive contraction of a particular muscle group, such as the plantarflexors of the foot or lateral trunk flexors and leads to temporary abnormalities in postural alignment of that part. The patient may, for example, walk with their trunk excessively laterally flexed to one side, or with their foot plantarflexed during the swing phase of gait. In the latter case this would increase the risk of tripping the foot on an obstacle and falling.

TABLE 35.2. *Spatial and temporal parameters of gait for Mr. B with at end-of-dose, peak-dose, and compared with control subject data*

Variable	End-of-dose	Peak-dose	Matched controls (N = 10)
Speed (m/sec)	0.69	1.24	1.5
Stride length (m)	0.77	1.39	1.45
Cadence (steps/min)	106	106	122
Step time (sec)	0.58	0.56	0.48
Single support (% cycle)	28.6	35.7	39.0
Double support (% cycle)	35.7	23.2	19.5
Opposite foot off (% cycle)	19.6	14.3	11.3
Foot off (% cycle)	64.3	58.9	58.5
Opposite foot contact (% cycle)	48.2	50.0	50.3

Figure 35.2 shows an example of the kinematics of gait in a person with PD dystonia. Mr. B was a 55-year-old man (height 181 cm, weight 85 kg) with an 18-year history of PD. He was community ambulant, and also managed on liquid form of L-Dopa. At end-of-dose and peak-dose, UPDRS scores were 57 and 45, respectively (Hoehn and Yahr stage 4). Mr. B experienced severe motor fluctuations with marked dystonia. As with the previous patient, he demonstrated a slow short-stepped gait in the end-of-dose condition, with a stride length of 0.77 m and speed of 0.69 m/sec (Table 35.2). In contrast, stride length at peak-dose increased to 1.39 m and speed to 1.24 m/sec. Cadence remained unchanged across conditions. In terms of kinematic profiles, Mr. B showed characteristic movement amplitude increases at the hip, knee, and ankle consistent with a moderately strong medication response to gait hypokinesia. In addition, the influence of dystonia was apparent, varying across both body segment location and medication phase. For the end-of-dose condition, this subject reported a painful trunk extensor dystonia. This was reflected in the marked anterior (forward) tilt of the pelvis (Fig. 35.2). At peak dose, this dystonia was no longer present, with more normal pelvic tilt apparent. However, observation of gait at peak dose revealed dystonia present in the left foot, with the foot pulling into an inverted and plantarflexed position at the end of swing, just prior to foot contact. The ankle kinematic profile reflects this, with plantarflexion of about 17 degrees present prior to contact, and a flattened slope of ankle dorsiflexion during early stance (Fig. 35.2). Accordingly, marked abnormality of the peak-dose ankle power profile was present, with a large absorption peak in early stance, correlating with flexion at the knee and ankle joints.

This case history illustrates the marked effect dystonia can have on a person's walking pattern. It can affect not only the pattern of movement at the trunk, hips, knees, and ankles, but also the underlying powers and moments of force. Dystonia can, however, be difficult to treat as it is transient in nature and varies according to the locus of the PD medication cycle.

DISORDERS OF TURNING IN PARKINSONIAN GAIT

Much of the research into mobility in PD has been based on studies of walking in a straight line (10,42,44). However, difficulties with turning, whether to change direction or to sit down in a chair, are frequently reported by patients. The importance of such difficulties should not be under-rated for two reasons. One is that turning is a time of increased risk of falling, both in the elderly population (45,46) and those with PD (3). Further, it seems probable that many falls during turning would occur laterally, a position associated with increased risk of hip fracture (47). The other reason that turning difficulties are clinically important in any population is the frequency of the action, particularly within the home where most falls occur (48). Sedgman showed that people make as many as five turns every 10 m while performing common daily tasks, such as making a cup of tea, house cleaning, and walking to the toilet (49). Some existing standardized

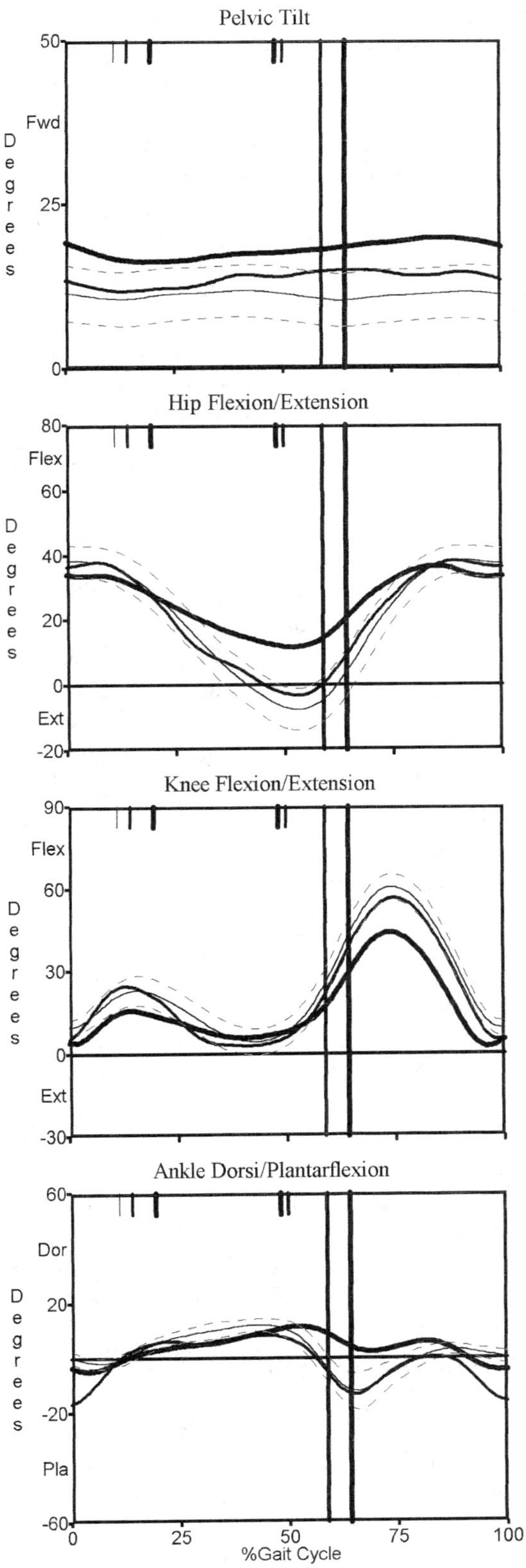

turn tests include a stationary 360-degree turn (e.g., Berg Balance Scale; Performance-Oriented Balance Assessment) (45,50). However, the external validity of these tests may be questioned given that Sedgman et al. found that nearly half of all turns during walking were between 76 and 120 degrees and none was greater than 225 degrees (49). Other tests utilize a 180-degree turn performed while walking (e.g., Timed Up and Go and Performance-Oriented Mobility Assessment) (45,51). However, Sedgman's study of turning in healthy elderly people noted that 180-degree turns were almost only used to sit down and that such turns were performed differently from a walking 180-degree turn.

The accurate assessment of turns in people with PD is further complicated by the lack of normative information and quantitative data against which to compare patient groups. Normally turns are performed smoothly, steadily, and independently (45,50,52). However, in people with PD where akinesia and dyskinesia are quite common, this is not always the case. In those with akinesia, there can be great difficulty initiating the turn and a person can cease moving midway through its execution. In people with dyskinesia, turning movements are usually made with excessively large amplitudes and the variability in footstep patterns is pronounced. Classification of turns used by those with PD has therefore resulted in six types, which Ashburn and Stack described as: festinating, forward, backward, twisting, wheeling, and sideways (53). Ashburn and Stack's study did not include a control group, so it is unclear which if any of these turn types represented "normal" patterns of turning. It is possible that some of the variation seen may occur in unimpaired subjects; however, no kinematic study of normal turning has been performed to date.

FIG. 35.2. Kinematics at the pelvis, hip, knee, and ankle for Mr. B with gait dystonia. *Thick black lines* represent end-of-dose performance, *gray lines* represent peak-dose performance, and *thin lines* together with *dashed lines* represent mean and one standard deviation for age-matched control subjects (N = 10).

One aspect of turning that has been investigated in unimpaired subjects is the time necessary to turn suddenly when walking at preferred speed. In one study, the success rate of sudden 90-degree turns was found to be directly related to the available response time (ART) to move (54). Cao et al. noted that unimpaired older subjects (mean 73.8 years) required an additional 112 ms ART to achieve the same success rate as younger subjects (mean 21.75 years). Another investigation found young healthy subjects were unable to make sudden 60 or even 30-degree turns when the stimulus occurred in the same step cycle (55). In examining the kinetics and strategies used to make these turns, the authors noted that control of the center of mass laterally is a major consideration in turning, whereas walking in a straight line requires the COM to be controlled only in the anteroposterior plane. As yet, neither of these paradigms has been investigated in PD. Nevertheless, it could be predicted that people with the disease would require longer ART because both reaction and movement time are increased (56). This could put them at risk when a turn must be made suddenly, such as to avoid an oncoming pedestrian or bicycle. Further, it appears from research performed in standing that control of COM, a critical factor in turning, is more difficult for people with PD because of altered postural reflexes (38,57,58). Altered sequencing of postural responses, reduced ability to control the COM and therefore reduced limits of stability, and underscaling of the forces that govern the position of COM could all be expected to make the important task of lateral and rotational control of COM during turning more problematic in people with PD (38,57,58).

As well as altered postural responses, people with PD frequently have difficulty with shifting motor set. The inflexibility of postural responses seen in response to support surface perturbations given with different supports (e.g., sitting, standing, and supported standing) demonstrates this difficulty and is likely to impact on turns during walking (57,59). Clinically, turning in people with PD frequently results in reduced step size, with or without motor blocks. These problems may occur in a subject for whom walking in a straight line is relatively trouble free. Turning can be seen not only to be an integral part of much goal-directed behavior but an activity that is adversely impacted on by many of the symptoms of PD, such as akinesia, set-shifting difficulties, and problems with dual-task performance. It also places greater demand on the balance control system because it requires greater control of the COM.

EFFECTS OF BALANCE DISTURBANCE ON GAIT IN PARKINSON'S DISEASE

Disturbances in balance and postural control may also compromise the ability to walk in people with PD, particularly in the latter stages of the disease. Even during unperturbed walking the control of balance and upright stance is biomechanically challenging because of the need to balance the large inertial mass of the head, arms, and trunk high above a narrow and constantly shifting base of support (60). Additional demands are placed on the balance control system by the need to use the upper limbs for manipulation and also by environmental constraints such as rough terrain and obstacles. The maintenance of balance during walking is normally achieved by a combination of proactive and reactive mechanisms (55,61,62). The visual system plays a vital role in proactive balance control by combining with experience to evaluate potential threats to stability (55). As a result, we may choose to steer away from or to step over obstacles, to slow our gait if the ground is slippery, or to run from an approaching car. In people with PD, vision is not compromised; however, several factors may make proactive use of visual information less effective and therefore impact on their balance control. One factor relates to the difficulty those with PD may have in shifting cognitive set (63). For example, although a person with PD may see a patch of water or ice on the ground, he or she may be slow to recognize it as a threat to balance and to modify the gait pattern appropriately. Even if the risk is recognized, the difficulty in shifting motor set may impede subjects' ability to alter the walking path or pattern appropriately. Another factor involves the ability to implement a correctly chosen strategy. In general, threats to stability may be managed by internal modification such as slowing down, shortening one's steps, and minimizing pushoff power to lessen the shear forces that occur at the foot–ground interface (55). Alternative proactive strategies to reduce balance demand include avoiding the threat altogether, either by steering away from it or by stepping over or bending under it (55).

In many people with advanced PD, such strategies are not adequately implemented. Slower response and movement times would be expected to increase the ART needed for suddenly occurring obstacles. A study of step initiation found slowed anticipatory postural adjustments with decreased force production and speed of movement (39). This may suggest that people with PD may have decreased pushoff power to accelerate away from a moving obstacle. In addition, while examining automatic postural reactions in response to support surface perturbation, Bloem and colleagues noted a medication-resistant delay in control of COM (64). This implies potential trouble in controlling COM if sudden stops or turns are needed. Akinetic blocks are also more likely to occur when an obstacle lies in the path than when the pathway is clear. All of these factors may affect implementation of proactive balance strategies in people with PD.

A third factor in the consideration of proactive balance control in PD is that most people with the condition are elderly. Much of proactive balance control is based on vision; therefore, it may be affected by concurrent age-related problems with visual acuity, contrast sensitivity, and slowed central processing. Age-associated changes in muscles, joints, and neural networks may also limit the second, nonvisual component of proactive balance control.

Proactive balance control not only acts to minimize balance threats from outside the body, but also to predict and control the forces that threaten to destabilize from within the body. Predictive balance control refers to the ability to keep the body's center of mass within manageable limits and to provide intersegmental stability during movement (61). For unimpaired people, these goals are achieved mainly by predicting what destabilization would arise from any movement or change of position and acting to prevent it before it occurs. Anticipatory postural adjustments (APAs) are patterns of muscle actions that commence before self-generated movements to adjust the COM position where necessary and to provide intersegmental stability. Anticipatory postural adjustments are supplemented during and after movement by accompanying and compensatory postural adjustments. To date, APAs during walking have not been studied in either unimpaired or patient groups. However, in standing, people with PD have been shown to correctly activate APAs less often than control subjects, although this may relate in part to slower focal movements, which may not elicit APAs in normal subjects (65,66). As discussed, the normal APAs in step initiation are seen to be slower in PD, with decreased force production and reduced speed of movement (39).

Predictive control of balance includes maintaining the COM within manageable limits of the base of support. The limits of stability for people with PD in standing are smaller than for healthy elderly people, and decrease further as the disease progresses (58). This may result in part from an altered relationship of the COM to the support surface, with the COM projection tending to be excessively anterior in the early stages and posterior later. Although this has not been investigated during walking, such alterations suggest impaired predictive control of gravitational forces. Another factor that is likely to impact on the provision of appropriate postural adjustments is the impaired modulation of both tonic stretch and phasic stretch reflexes in the soleus muscles of people with PD, demonstrated by Hayashi et al. (67). This impairment may be expected to impact on postural control in both standing and walking.

By accurate prediction of the forces acting on the body, the normal balance control system allows locomotion to proceed smoothly and with minimum intrasubject variability. In PD, however, variability is increased. Greater stride-to-stride variability of step length is seen to increase as the disease progresses (44) and has been associated with increased falls risk in older people without PD (68). A second measure, stride width, is more closely associated with balance during walking (69). People with PD demonstrate greater intraindividual variability of stride width than control subjects (70). The increase in variability suggests that predictive control of balance during walking is reduced in PD, which in turn contributes to postural instability and falls risk.

If a fall is threatened, owing to a failure of the proactive and predictive components of balance to maintain control or to perturbation by an unexpected external force, the reactive component of balance control is activated. A number of studies have examined how people with PD respond to perturbation, mainly to support surface movement in standing. The latencies of postural responses have been found to be normal (56,71). However, the patterns of muscle response may be abnormal with excessive antagonist activity and sometimes sequencing difficulties (57). Increased postural sway to displacement is seen with delayed correction (64,72). This reduced control of the COM is not improved with medication (64). Further, PD subjects do not modify their postural responses to reflect changes in the support conditions, showing similar patterns of response whether they are standing independently, with support, or sitting on a stool (57,59). Postural adjustments are delayed and inflexible with increased posterior sway in response to toe-up perturbation (73). In addition, the response to external perturbations to the center of mass is compromised in people with PD. For example, the Shoulder Tug test has been shown to differentiate between subjects with and without PD, and also between PD subjects who have and have not fallen (3,74).

In summary, people with PD may be impaired by their disease in several aspects of balance control during walking and their functional balance may be further compromised by concurrent aging and secondary disuse-related problems. The most dangerous components of their balance losses relate to the marked inability to execute effective reactive responses to perturbation as well as failure of their proactive balance mechanisms.

GAIT REHABILITATION

Gait rehabilitation in people with PD is reliant on clinicians having a clear understanding of whether gait dysfunction is owing to hypokinesia, akinesia, freezing, dyskinesia, balance impairment, secondary effects of aging or disuse, or a combination of these factors (43,75). If gait hypokinesia is the primary problem, then visual cues and attentional strategies can be beneficial (4). Visual cues may be markers placed on the floor for the person to step over, markers on the wall to direct the person to extend their thoracic spine or neck more, or written instructions detailing the strategy on a cue card. Attentional strategies include breaking gait tasks down into component parts and performing each part separately (76), mentally rehearsing the gait task before it is performed (75), avoiding secondary motor or cognitive tasks while walking (1,4), and focusing attention on walking with long strides (4,75). If freezing and difficulty initiating gait are troublesome, the person can again try visual cues, although they may find rhythmical auditory stimuli from music, clapping, or the voice more beneficial (8,9). "Tricking" the brain by visualizing stepping over a log or by actually stepping over an upturned walking stick also can be helpful (43,75). Choreiform dyskinesia and dystonia of lower limb muscles during gait appear less amenable to gait rehabilitation (75). Although it has been suggested that prolonged stretch can help to reduce dystonia, and compression, weight-bearing and resistance can assist in reducing choreiform movements, the effects of these interventions appear to be only transient and have not been confirmed with controlled trials (75). Balance disturbance is one of the most disabling sequelae of advanced PD, although there are no data on the effects of balance training on gait in people with PD. It could be speculated that teaching people with PD to deliberately prepare in advance for potential threats to their balance during walking, as well as how to consciously generate appropriate stepping responses on perturbation, might be beneficial. However, these strategies have not been validated with research.

Only two randomized controlled clinical trials have been conducted on the effects of physical therapy for PD. Comella et al. measured responses on the UPDRS of 16 people with PD randomly allocated to 4 weeks of physiotherapy or a 4-week control phase (77). The physiotherapy comprised exercises to enhance range of movement, endurance, balance, walking, and hand dexterity. Although the majority of people showed favorable improvements on the motor section of the UPDRS with training, the effects were short-lived, with performance returning to baseline within 6 months. Schenkman et al. randomly allocated 46 people with PD either to a group that received a 10-week, 30-session, individualized exercise program administered by a physiotherapist, or to a waiting list for therapy (78). Physiotherapy comprised exercises to "enhance participation of appropriate synergistic muscles, utilize relaxation to increase range of motion, and promote efficient movement of the axial skeleton" (78). Although Schenkman et al. found an increase in spinal flexibility, speed in moving from supine to sitting and the functional reach test, the underlying movement disorders such as hypokinesia, akinesia, and dyskinesia were not taken into account, and external cues and attentional strategies appear not to have been utilized (78). Randomized controlled clinical trials are now needed to measure the effects of external cues and attentional strategies on movement disorders in PD.

CONCLUSION

When structuring gait rehabilitation programs for people with PD, clinicians need to take into consideration the effects of hypokinesia, start hesitancy, freezing, dyskinesia, turning disturbance, and balance disturbance on walking capacity. There is clear evidence that people with PD have a disorder in the motor control mechanisms that regulate the size of consecutive footsteps in long or complex locomotor sequences. In agreement with these findings, kinematic analyses show that the amplitude of angular displacements at the hips, knees, and ankles is scaled-down in people with gait hypokinesia. Reduced movement amplitude correlates with reduced power generation, particularly in the ankle plantarflexors at the end of stance phase. In addition there are new data indicating that people with PD hypokinesia have a deficit in the internal timing regulation mechanisms that control the variability of walking cadence. In contrast, the pathogenesis of start hesitancy, freezing, and gait dyskinesia is poorly understood and is an area requiring concentrated research effort. Furthermore, people with late-stage disease commonly have balance disturbance that is exacerbated by age related changes in postural stability. Together these findings illustrate that gait disability can arise from a variety of underlying causes. By supplementing clinical gait analysis with data from three-dimensional motion analysis, clinicians can be in a much better position to diagnose the pathogenesis of locomotor disturbance and evaluate the patient's response to different forms of treatment. From the assessment findings gait rehabilitation programs can be tailored to individual needs.

ACKNOWLEDGMENT

Preparation of this manuscript was supported by grant number 971268 from the National Health and Medical Research Council of Australia.

REFERENCES

1. Bond J, Morris ME. Goal-directed secondary motor tasks: their effects on gait in subjects with Parkinson disease. *Arch Phys Med Rehabil* 2000;1:110–116.
2. O'Shea S, Morris ME, Iansek R. The effect of secondary cognitive and motor tasks on gait in Parkinson's disease. Proceedings International Symposium on Gait Disorders, Prague, Czech Republic, September 1999.
3. Smithson F, Morris ME, Iansek R. Predisposing factors for falls in Parkinson's disease. Preceedings in: *Older people in our society: a kaleidoscope.* Australian Association Gerontology, Perth, Australia, 1994.
4. Morris ME, Iansek R, Matyas TA, et al. Stride length regulation in Parkinson's disease: normalization strategies and underlying mechanisms. *Brain* 1996;119:551–568.
5. Behrman A, Teitelbaum P, Cauraugh JH. Verbal instructional sets to normalize the temporal and spatial gait variables in Parkinson's disease. *J Neurol Neurosurg Psychiatry* 1998;65:580–582.
6. Blin O, Ferrandez A-M, Pailhous J, et al. Dopa-sensitive and dopa-resistant gait parameters in Parkinson's disease. *J Neurol Sci* 1991;103:51–54.
7. Ebersbach G, Heijmenberg M, Kinderman L, et al. Interference of rhythmic constraint on gait in healthy subjects and patients with early Parkinson's disease: evidence for impaired locomotor pattern generation in early Parkinson's disease. *Mov Disord* 1999;14:619–625.

8. Thaut MH, McIntosh GC, Rice RR, et al. Rhythmic auditory stimulation in gait training for Parkinson's disease patients. *Mov Disord* 1996;11:193–200.
9. McIntosh GC, Brown SH, Rice RR, et al. Rhythmic auditory-motor facilitation of gait patterns in patients with Parkinson's disease. *J Neurol Neurosurg Psychiatry* 1998;62:22–26.
10. Morris ME, Iansek R, Matyas TA, et al. The pathogenesis of gait hypokinesia in Parkinson's disease. *Brain* 1994;117:1161–1182.
11. Morris ME, Iansek R, Matyas TA, et al. Ability to modulate walking cadence remains intact in Parkinson's disease. *J Neurol Neurosurg Psychiatry* 1994;57:1532–1534.
12. Morris ME, Matyas TA, Iansek R, et al. Temporal stability of gait in Parkinson's disease. *Phys Ther* 1996; 76:763–777.
13. Morris ME, Iansek R, Matyas TA, et al. Abnormalities in the stride length-cadence relationship in Parkinson's disease. *Mov Disord* 1998;13:61–69.
14. Hausdorff JM, Cudkowicz ME, Firtion R, et al. Gait variability and basal ganglia disorders: stride-to-stride variability of gait cycle timing in Parkinson's disease and Huntington's disease. *Mov Disord* 1998;13:428–437.
15. Rao SM, Harrington DL, Haaland KY, et al. Distributed neural systems underlying the timing of movements. *J Neurosci* 1997;14:5528–5535.
16. Pastor MA, Artieda J, Jahanshahi M, et al. Time estimation and reproduction is abnormal in Parkinson's disease. *Brain* 1992;115:211–225.
17. Artieda J, Pastor MA, Lacruz F, et al. Temporal discrimination is abnormal in Parkinson's disease. *Brain* 1992;115:199–210.
18. Soliveri P, Brown RG, Jahanshahi M, et al. Learning manual pursuit tracking skills in patients with Parkinson's disease. *Brain* 1997;120:1325–1337.
19. Nakamura R, Nagasaki H, Narabayashi H. Disturbances of rhythm formation in patients with Parkinson's disease: characteristics of tapping responses to the periodic signals. *Percept Motor Skills* 1978;46:63–75.
20. Ho AK, Bradshaw JL, Cunnington R, et al. Sequence heterogeneity in Parkinsonian speech. *Brain Language* 1998;64:122–145.
21. Berardelli A, Dick JPR, Rothwell JC, et al. Scaling of the size of the first agonist EMG burst during rapid wrist movements in patients with Parkinson's disease. *J Neurol Neurosurg Psychiatry* 1986;49:1273–1279.
22. Brotchie P, Iansek R, Horne MK. Motor function of the monkey globus pallidus: 1. Neuronal discharge and parameters of movement. *Brain* 1991;114:1667–1683.
23. Hallett M, Khashbin S. A physiological mechanism of bradykinesia. *Brain* 1980;103:301–314.
24. Murray MP, Sepic SB, Gardner GM, et al. Walking patterns of men with Parkinsonism. *Am J Phys Med* 1978;57:278–294.
25. Knuttson E. An analysis of parkinsonian gait. *Brain* 1972;95:475–486.
26. Knuttson E, Martensson A. Quantitative effects of L-dopa on different types of movements and muscle tone in parkinsonian patients. *Scand J Rehabil Med* 1971;3: 121–130.
27. Morris ME, McGinley J, Huxham F, et al. Constraints on the kinetic, kinematic and spatiotemporal parameters of gait in Parkinson's disease. *Hum Mov Sci* 1999;18: 461–483.
28. Leeman AL, O'Neill CJA, Nicholson PW, et al. Parkinson's disease in the elderly: response to and optimal spacing of night time dosing with levodopa. *Br J Clin Pharmacol* 1987;24:637–643.
29. Hoehn MM, Yahr MD. Parkinsonism: onset, progression and mortality. *Neurology* 1967;17:427–442.
30. Bowes SG, Clark PG, Leeman AL, et al. Determinants of gait in the elderly parkinsonian on maintenance levodopa/carbidopa therapy. *Br J Clin Pharmacol* 1990;30:13–24.
31. Giladi N, Kao R, Fahn S. Freezing phenomenon in patients with Parkinsonian syndromes. *Mov Disord* 1997;12:302–305.
32. Stern GM, Lander CM, Lees AJ. Akinetic freezing and trick movements in Parkinson's disease. *J Neural Transm* 1983;16:137–141.
33. Fahn S. The freezing phenomenon in Parkinsonism. In: Fahn S, Hallett M, Lüders HO, et al., eds. *Negative motor phenomena.* Philadelphia: Lippincott–Raven, 1995:53–63.
34. Gantchev N, Viallet F, Aurenty R, et al. Impairment of posturo-kinetic co-ordination during initiation of forward oriented stepping movement in Parkinsonian patients. *Electroencephalog Clin Neurophysiol* 1996;101:110–120.
35. Nutt JG, Marsden CD, Thompson PD. Human walking and higher-level gait disorders, particularly in the elderly. *Neurology* 1993;43:268–279.
36. Giladi N, McDermott M, Fahn S, et al. Freezing of gait in Parkinson's disease. *Neurology* 1996;46:A377.
37. Cunnington R, Iansek R, Bradshaw JL, et al. Movement-related potentials in Parkinson's disease: presence and predicability of temporal and spatial cues. *Brain* 1995;118:935–950.
38. Vidailhet M, Stocchi F, Rothwell JC, et al. The Bereitschafts potential preceding simple foot movement and initiation of gait in Parkinson's disease. *Neurology* 1993;43:1784–1788.
39. Burleigh-Jacobs A, Horak FB, Nutt JG, et al. Step initiation in Parkinson's disease: influence of levodopa and external sensory triggers. *Mov Disord* 1997;2:206–215.
40. Marsden CD. Slowness of movement in Parkinson's disease. *Mov Disord* 1989;4:S26–S37.
41. Iansek R, Bradshaw J, Phillips J, et al. Basal ganglia function and Parkinson's disease. In: Morris ME, Iansek R, eds. *Parkinson's disease: a team approach.* Blackburn, Australia: Buscombe Vicprint, 1997:173–188.
42. Elble RJ. Gait and freezing in Parkinson's disease. Proceedings Seminar 4.2, 5th International Congress of Parkinson's Disease and Movement Disorders, 1998: 1–33.
43. Morris ME, Iansek R. Gait disorders in Parkinson's disease: a framework for physical therapy practice. *Neurol Rept* 1997;21:125–131.
44. Blin O, Ferrandez A, Serratrice G. Quantitative analysis of gait in Parkinson patients: increased variability of stride length. *J Neurol Sci* 1991;98:91–97.
45. Tinetti ME. Performance-oriented assessment of mobility problems in elderly patients. *J Am Ger Soc* 1986; 34:119–126.
46. Tinetti ME. Risk factors for falls among elderly persons living in the community. *N Engl J Med* 1988;319:1701–1707.
47. Nevitt M, Cummings SR, Kidd S, et al. Risk factors for recurrent nonsyncopal falls. *JAMA* 1989;261:2663–2668.

48. Fildes B. *Injuries among older people: falls at home and pedestrian accidents*. North Blackburn, Australia: Collins Dove, 1994.
49. Sedgman R, Goldie P, Iansek R. Development of a measure of turning during walking. Paper presented at the Advancing Rehabilitation: Inaugural conference of Faculty of Health Sciences, La Trobe University, Melbourne, Australia, 1994.
50. Berg K, Wood-Dauphinee S, Williams JI, et al. Measuring balance in the elderly: preliminary development of an instrument. *Physiother Can* 1989;41:304–311.
51. Podsiadlo D, Richardson S. The timed "Up & Go": a test of basic functional mobility for frail elderly persons. *JAGS* 1991;39:142–148.
52. Topper, AK, Maki BE, Holliday PJ. Are activity-based assessments of balance and gait in the elderly predictive of risk of falling and/or type of fall? *JAGS* 1993;41:479–487.
53. Ashburn A, Stack E. Patterns of turning used by people with Parkinson's disease. Paper presented at the 13th International Congress of WCPT 1999, Yokohama, Japan.
54. Cao C, Ashton-Miller JA, Schultz AB, et al. Abilities to turn suddenly while walking: effects of age, gender and available response time. *J Gerontol Med Sci* 1997;52A:M88–M93.
55. Patla AE. Understanding the roles of vision in the control of human locomotion. *Gait Posture* 1997;5:54–69.
56. Jahanshahi M, Brown RG, Marsden CD. The effect of withdrawal of dopaminergic medication on simple and choice reaction time and the use of advance information in Parkinson's disease. *J Neurol Neurosurg Psychiatry* 1992;55:1168–1176.
57. Horak FB, Nutt JG, Nashner LM. Postural inflexibility in parkinsonian subjects. *J Neurol Sci* 1992;111:46–58.
58. Schiappati M, Hugon M, Grasso M, et al. The limits of equilibrium in young and elderly normal subjects and in parkinsonism. *Electroencephalograph Clin Neurophysiol* 1994;93:286–298.
59. Chong RK, Jones CL, Horak FB. Postural set for balance control is normal in Alzheimer's but not in Parkinson's disease. *J Gerontol Med Sci* 1999;54:M129–135.
60. Winter DA. *The biomechanics and motor control of human gait: normal, elderly and pathological.* 2nd edition. Ontario: University of Waterloo Press, 1991.
61. Patla A, Frank J, Winter D. Assessment of balance control in the elderly: major issues. *Physiother Can* 1990;42:89–97.
62. Patla AE. Neurobiomechanical bases for the control of human locomotion. In: Bronstein TBA, Woollacott M, eds. *Clinical disorders of balance, posture and gait*. London: Arnold, 1996:19–40.
63. Levin BE, Katzen HL. *Early cognitive changes and nondementing behavioural abnormalities in Parkinson's disease*. New York: Raven Press, 1995.
64. Bloem BR, Beckley DJ, van Dijk JG, et al. Influence of dopaminergic medication on automatic postural responses and balance impairment in Parkinson's disease. *Mov Disord* 1996;11:509–521.
65. Latash ML, Aruin AS, Neyman I, et al. Anticipatory postural adjustments during self-inflicted and predictable perturbations in Parkinson's disease. *J Neurol Neurosurg Psychiatry* 1995;58:326–334.
66. Horak FB, Esselmann P, Anderson ME, et al. The effects of movement velocity, mass displaced and task certainty on associated postural adjustments made by normal and hemiplegic individuals. *J Neurol Neurosurg Psychiatry* 1984;47:1020–1028.
67. Hayashi R, Tokuda T, Tako K, et al. Impaired modulation of tonic muscle activities and H-reflexes in the soleus muscle during standing in patients with Parkinson's disease. *J Neurol Sci* 1997;153:61–67.
68. Maki BE. Gait changes in older adults: predictors of falls or indicators of fear? *J Am Geriatr Soc* 1997;45:313–320.
69. Gabell A, Nayak USL. The effect of age on variability of gait. *J Gerontol* 1984;39:662–666.
70. Charlett A, Weller C, Purkiss AG, et al. Breadth of base whilst walking: effect of ageing and parkinsonism. *Age Ageing* 1998;27:49–54.
71. Bloem BR. Postural instability in Parkinson's disease. *Clin Neurol Neurosurg* 1992;94:S41–S45.
72. Beckley DJ, Bloem BR, van Dijk JG, et al. Electrophysiological correlates of postural instability in Parkinson's disease. *Electroencephalogr Clin Neurophysiol* 1991; 81:263–268.
73. Bloem BR, Beckley DJ, Remler MP, et al. Postural reflexes in Parkinson's disease during 'resist' and 'yield' tasks. *J Neurol Sci* 1995;129:109–119.
74. Pastor M, Day B, Marsden C. Vestibular induced postural responses in Parkinson's disease. *Brain* 1993;116:1177–1182.
75. Morris M. Movement disorders in Parkinson's disease: a model of physical therapy. *Phys Ther* 2000;80:578–597.
76. Yekutiel MP, Pinhasov A, Shahar G, et al. A clinical trial of the re-education of movement in patients with Parkinson's disease. *Clin Rehabil* 1991;5:207–214.
77. Comella CL, Stebbins GT, Brown-Toms N, et al. Physical therapy and Parkinson's disease: a controlled clinical trial. *Neurology* 1994;44:376–378.
78. Schenkman M, Cutson TM, Kuchibhatla M, et al. Exercise to improve spinal flexibility and function for people with Parkinson's disease: a randomized controlled trial. *J Am Geriatr Soc* 1998;46:1207–1216.

Gait Disorders. Advances in Neurology, Vol. 87,
edited by E. Růžička, M. Hallett, and J. Jankovic.
Lippincott Williams & Wilkins, Philadelphia © 2001.

36

Frontal Gait Apraxia

Pathophysiological Mechanisms and Rehabilitation

*¶Robert Iansek, §Noor H. Ismail, †Margaret Bruce, ‡Frances E. Huxham, and ||Meg E. Morris

**Department of Geriatric Neurology, †Movement Disorders Program, and ‡Geriatric Research Unit Kingston Centre, Southern Health, Cheltenham, Victoria, 3192 Australia; §Department of Geriatric Medicine, Tan Tock Seng Hospital, 308433 Singapore; ||School of Physiotherapy, La Trobe University, Bundoora, 3086 Australia; and ¶Department of Medicine, Monash University, Clayton, Victoria, 3168 Australia*

Gait and balance disturbances are common causes of morbidity in elderly people and can result in falls, fractures, loss of independence, and reduced quality of life. Among the numerous conditions affecting gait and balance in this population the most common are Parkinson's disease (PD), multiple lacunar infarcts, frontal gait apraxia (FGA), and senile gait disorder (1). Clinical descriptions of the latter three conditions suggest they may share similar pathophysiological mechanisms. However, underlying pathology cannot be easily identified in all clinical groups. The clinical manifestations of FGA encompass a number of pathological entities; thus, FGA represents the second most common neurologic cause of gait and balance disturbance in older adults after PD (2).

Considerable controversy exists as to the manifestations and etiology of FGA; some reports cover clinical manifestations, some examine the extent of subcortical ischemic load, and others consider the pathological mechanisms (3–6). It has been suggested that FGA is probably owing to loss of subcortical frontal projection fiber bundles caused by small vessel disease in the subcortical white matter or from normal pressure hydrocephalus (7).

The distribution and load of ischemia varies from patient to patient. Clinical symptoms also vary, but may include upper motor neuron, cerebellar, bulbar, and cognitive dysfunction as well as gait disturbance (6). The gait apraxia is characterized by a flexed posture, diminished stride length, and widened base of support with hesitation and difficulty in gait initiation; however, patients have no difficulty in performing isolated cycling or stepping movements (7). Amplitude of arm swing is retained, as are normal facial expression and social movements. Postural instability is commonly present. The capacity to produce protective motor responses to postural perturbations is impaired, especially in the anterior-posterior direction. The absence of upper body hypokinesia and tremor separates this clinical entity from PD, resulting in the terms lower half parkinsonism or vascular parkinsonism (7).

The possibility of a vascular etiology is strengthened by the presence of FGA in Binswanger's disease and subcortical progressive vascular encephalopathy (5,6). Microscopic vascular changes in the subcortical white matter have been documented at postmortem in patients with clinical FGA despite few changes on imaging studies (6).

Although a number of studies have attempted to correlate the clinical symptoms of FGA with neuroimaging and pathological findings at postmortem or to describe clinical presentations, we found no reports in the literature that systematically addressed the issue of treatment, and, in particular, movement rehabilitation for FGA (4–9). Fitzgerald and Jankovic briefly mentioned that one subject used a white upturned walking stick to overcome gait initiation difficulties (8). The absence of rehabilitation in this condition reflects the lack of knowledge of pathophysiological mechanisms that underlie the clinical gait disturbance. Thompson and Marsden suggested that the symptoms were owing to disruption of the pallidal projection fibers to the SMA with selective involvement of the legs explained by the more superficial location of the leg projection fibers to the periventricular region of the frontal horns compared with those from the arm (7). They drew attention to the similar gait disturbance in normal pressure hydrocephalus, frontal tumors, and senile gait disturbance. In all these conditions, the same fiber bundles would be subject to disruption and thus could produce the same clinical syndrome.

This study reports the effects of utilizing rehabilitation attentional strategies on FGA. After addressing the fear of falling, the strategies to normalize stride length and balance were taught in an intensive 3-week inpatient program. This approach produced dramatic improvement in gait and to a lesser degree in balance, although continued reinforcement of these strategies, generally on an outpatient basis, was required to ensure retention of training.

METHOD

The results of this study will be presented in three sections. The first provides a detailed analysis of the relationship between balance disturbance and gait disturbance in 10 subjects with FGA compared to 10 age-, height-, and sex-matched control subjects. The second details a retrospective analysis of 12 subjects who underwent the rehabilitative program on an inpatient basis over a 3-week period. The third section describes a prospective single case analysis with repeated measures of balance and gait parameters undertaken over a 3-week rehabilitation program.

Analysis of Frontal Gait Apraxia

A case-control study compared the temporal-spatial parameters of gait and postural stability of people with FGA compared with control subjects. All subjects were tested with and without a wheeled walking frame to determine the possible influence of the frame itself on improvement in the gait parameters.

Subjects

Community-dwelling subjects diagnosed with FGA who attended the Movement Disorders Program at Kingston Centre were recruited if they were willing and able to give informed consent. Subjects were excluded if they had concurrent pathology impacting on walking or balance. Control subjects were age-, height-, and sex-matched volunteers recruited from neighboring elderly citizens' clubs.

Apparatus

Gait parameters were measured over the central 10 m of a 14-m gait walkway, using a commercially available Clinical Stride Analyzer (CSA) (B&L Engineering, Sante Fe Springs, CA). This system enabled the collection of the temporal and spatial characteristics of the gait pattern using electronic footswitches placed in the subject's shoes. Information was downloaded from a data-logger worn around the subject's waist to a computer, using application software (Stride Analyzer, Version 3.1). All participants were assessed with this equipment, first walking freely and then using an adjustable walking frame with four wheels.

Procedure

Subject data on age, height, medical history, medication, smoking habits, and falls history were collected. Participants then completed three brief questionnaires. The Falls Efficacy Scale and the Modified Falls Efficacy Scale evaluated the effect of fear of falling on level of activity (10,11). The Mini Mental State Examination (MMSE) investigated cognitive status (12).

The CSA footswitches were then inserted into the subject's usual walking shoes. Participants were asked to walk the length of the walkway "at a comfortable speed" and footswitch data were collected over the central 10 m of each walk. After three trials, all participants were given a wheeled frame and again instructed to walk along the walkway at a comfortable speed for a further three trials. Stride width was measured by taping colored marker pens to the subjects' heels and asking them to walk along a 10 × 800-mm strip of paper stuck to the floor. Subjects walked at a comfortable speed, first independently then with the frame. Finally, the subjects' postural responses to an external perturbation were assessed by the shoulder tug test (13). This test examines the postural response to an external perturbation in the form of a backward tug on the shoulders.

Measurement

The following data were collected from the CSA: gait velocity (vel), cadence (cad), stride length (sl), and percent of the gait cycle spent in double-limb support (dls). Stride width was measured as follows: the midpoint of each step length was found and all points joined to provide the approximate center of the gait path. The distance from each heel contact to the path center was then measured and doubled to provide stride width. The shoulder tug test uses a 5-point scale scored as follows:

0 = Remains upright with no step
1 = Takes one step but steady
2 = Takes more than one step yet safe
3 = Takes several steps and must be caught
4 = Falls backward without taking a step

Retrospective Review of Inpatient Rehabilitation

The medical records of all FGA patients referred through the Movement Disorders Program at Kingston Centre were reviewed and the records of patients who had undergone inpatient rehabilitation were examined in detail. Data collected included demographics, morbidity, cognitive status, and functional level, as well as gait and balance parameters.

Demographic data included age, sex, duration of disease, and smoking history. Morbidity data considered comorbid medical illnesses of relevance to etiology and pathology. Functional level, including activities of daily living, was measured with the Barthel Index at admission and on discharge (14). Cognitive function was assessed with the MMSE (12). Gait and balance data included gait parameters measured by clinical timed tests of walking or with a commercially available stride analyzer. This provided measures of stride length, velocity, cadence, and double-limb support, prior and subsequent to intervention. Balance was assessed using differing clinical tests with a number of patients tested by the shoulder tug test (13).

Rehabilitation Protocol

Subjects were admitted to a ward with staff trained in the management of movement disorders. Length of stay ranged from 2 to 3 weeks, depending on the rate of progress made by the individual patient. Physiotherapy sessions were provided daily for 2 to 3 hours during the inpatient stay. The ward staff outside the therapy sessions reinforced strategies by use of the attentional techniques described in Table 36.1. In general terms, the rehabilitation approach utilized attentional motor control mechanisms to improve postural reflex mechanisms as well as stride length.

The program was structured to retrain balance responses and ambulation in a graduated manner, starting with simple movements and extending to more difficult reaching and stretching activities that further challenged balance in activities of daily living. External supports such as rails, frames, or therapist supervision were provided as necessary to ensure safety, with each advancing step in training minimizing external support so that activities of daily living were eventually safely performed independently. The protocol consisted of three separate categories that included balance, gait, and functional multilimb activities (Table 36.1). A separate outpatient category consisted of maintenance exercises.

Tests of statistical significance for comparison of numerical data prior to, and after intervention,

TABLE 36.1. *Protocol for frontal gait apraxia rehabilitation*

Activities	External supports
Balance	
Feet apart	Rails
Feet together	Wall
One foot	Frame
Step forward	Supervision
Step side	
Step backward	
Foam	
Balance board	
Self-generated perturbation responses	
External perturbation responses	
Gait	
Stepping	Rails
Treadmill	Wall
Large bicycle movements	Frame
Ramps	Supervision
Kerbs	
Slopes	
Functional ADLs	
Shelf reach	No external supports
Picking up objects from floor	
Hang clothes on line	
Bowling	
Sweeping floor	
Putting golf ball	
Cleaning large window	
Carrying objects	
Home examples	

Increasing level of difficulty (↓) — Decreasing level of external support (↓)

ADL, activities of daily living.

utilized a Wilcoxon Rank test. The alpha level was set at 0.05.

Single Case Study of Rehabilitation: A Time Series Analysis

Case Report

A 76-year-old man presented in August 1997 with walking difficulty and poor balance. Subjectively, he felt unsteady when walking as if he might fall. He described the frequent occurrence of falling backward onto the bed whenever he tried to put on his pajamas in the standing position. He denied difficulty with bed mobility or manipulative tasks. He had a past history of hypertension and cigarette smoking. He had no history of diabetes. His medication was comprised of Temazepam and Amlodipine. Examination revealed a blood pressure of 170/100. He had no precordial bruits. His facial expression and social movements were normal. He stood cautiously and slowly. He had a wide based stance and walked with a wide-based, small stepping gait with good arm swing. His postural reflexes were absent when tugged suddenly backward. His reflexes were brisker on the right side. He fell slowly backward while seated on the bed with his arms outstretched and eyes closed. Magnetic resonance imaging (MRI) of the brain showed periventricular lucencies with white matter changes consistent with chronic small vessel disease.

The patient was admitted to the movement disorder ward and underwent rehabilitation according to the protocol described in the "Methods" section of this chapter. Stride analysis was undertaken with a CSA.

Strategy for Statistical Analysis

Three walking trials were obtained from the patient for each condition (frame, no frame) and

TABLE 36.2A. *Mean values and standard deviation for subjects with frontal gait apraxia and controls*

Parameter	FGA mean	FGA SD	Control mean	Control SD	Significance
Age	78.8	6.05	79.4	5.93	NS
Height	167.55	6.25	168.3	9.42	NS
MMSE	26.4	3.03	29.1	1.29	$P < 0.004$
FES	75.15	22.12	97.5	5.68	$P < 0.021$
MFES	1.9	1.4	3.7	3.6	$P < 0.01$

FGA, frontal gait apraxia, SD, standard deviation; MMSE, Mini Mental State examination, FES, Fall Efficacy Scale; MFES, Modified Falls Efficacy Scale.

on each testing occasion (baseline and days 5, 8, 12, and 22 after physical therapy treatment commenced). Visual inspection of the box-plots for each of the trials with and without the walking frame indicated that the data for all of the dependent variables were skewed. We therefore calculated the median values for velocity, stride length, cadence, and double-limb support duration on each testing occasion. Before plotting these results, the median values were smoothed using the "moving median" technique. This reduces random variability owing to measurement error, allowing the underlying trend to be clearly seen.

RESULTS

The diagnosis of FGA in all three components of the project was based on the clinical signs, which included a wide-based stance and gait, reduced stride length, and good arm swing with a tendency to block and festinate, particularly on turning or on initiation of gait. In addition a positive perturbation test was necessary for diagnosis (13). Absence of PD signs such as facial masking, diminished or absent social movements, tremor, rigidity, reduced fine finger movements, and repetitive hand movements was mandatory.

Analysis of Frontal Gait Apraxia

Subjects with FGA were not significantly different in age, sex, and height to control subjects. The findings of the comparison are summarized in Tables 36.2 A, B, and C. Subjects with FGA were more cognitively impaired than control subjects, with a mean MMSE score of 26.4 compared to 29.1 in the control group. Both falls efficacy scales were significantly different in the FGA group from the control group, implying not only a greater fear of falling but also a significant consequence in daily activities owing to fear. The response to external perturbation (shoulder tug) was significantly more abnormal in the FGA group, with a score of 2.6 compared to a score of 0.9 for controls. Stride width was significantly greater in the FGA group (18.9 compared to 10 cm), and the use of a frame did not achieve significant reduction. Stride length and gait velocity were also significantly reduced in the FGA

TABLE 36.2B. *Mean and standard deviation for gait and balance parameters for patients with frontal gait apraxia and control subjects*

Parameter	FGA mean	FGA SD	Control mean	Control SD	Significance
Shoulder tug	2.8	1.3	1.7	0.6	$P < 0.002$
Speed	32.7	12.4	69.6	10.5	$P < 0.001$
Stride length	0.7	0.2	1.3	0.2	$P < 0.003$
Stride width	8.15	0.8	5.7	1.1	$P < 0.009$
%DLS	45.3	10.1	34.4	8.6	$P < 0.013$
Cadence	103.6	14.6	107.0	6.1	NS

FGA, frontal gait apraxia; SD, Standard deviation; NS, not significant; %DLS, percentage of gait cycle spent in double limb supports.

TABLE 36.2C. *Comparison of effect of walking aid as compared to no aid in subjects with frontal gait apraxia*

Parameter	No aid mean	No aid SD	Aid mean	Aid SD	Significance
Velocity	32.7	12.4	37.8	10.7	NS
Stride length	0.67	0.19	0.64	0.25	NS
Stride width	8.15	0.76	7.3	0.67	NS
%DLS	45.3	10.1	40.59	8.8	$P < 0.006$
Cadence	103.2	14.5	100.6	12.0	NS

SD, standard deviation; NS, not significant; %DLS, percentage of gait cycle spent in double limb support.

group compared to control subjects; again, the use of a frame failed to improve either parameter. A significant difference in double-limb support in the FGA group compared with controls was the only parameter significantly reduced by use of a frame.

Retrospective Review

Forty-five people with FGA were seen over 3 years. Of these, 12 more severe patients were admitted for inpatient rehabilitation (Table 36.3). Mean age was 81 years (range, 65 to 97), with a male to female ratio of approximately 2 to 1. Six patients had a past history of hypertension, two had diabetes, and two had experienced previous strokes. The majority of patients (nine of 12) had risk factors for atherosclerotic disease, with one of the others an exsmoker and the remaining two having normal pressure hydrocephalus. Three patients had computed tomography (CT) scans suggestive of normal pressure hydrocephalus; one patient had had a ventricular–peritoneal shunt inserted 6 months prior to his assessment in our clinic without any improvement in his gait. The other two patients had refused surgery. Six of the patients had a previous history of smoking; however, we were unable to quantify the duration of and time since cessation of smoking. One patient had dysphasia and was unable to do the MMSE; the average MMSE was 25 (range, 19 to 30). None of the patients had previously been diagnosed with Alzheimer's disease. The duration of the target complaint varied from 3 months to 6 years at time of first presentation.

Barthel Index Scores

The Barthel Index uses a 5-point scale to measure each of 10 categories of daily function, such as personal hygiene, bladder control, dressing, and ambulation. The mean total Barthel score (BI) of the 12 patients on admission was 78 out of a maximum of 100 (SD = 17) and 93 (SD = 5) on discharge. Significant change also occurred in the BI subscore for the activities of daily living component [mean on admission 49 (SD = 5); on discharge 52 (SD = 3)].

TABLE 36.3. *Summary means and standard deviations for gait and balance parameters for 12 patients who underwent inpatient rehabilitation demonstrating comparison between pre- and post-rehabilitation*

Parameter	Admission mean	Admission SD	Discharge mean	Discharge SD	Significance
Speed	44.2	26.0	66.03	26.8	$P < 0.004$
Stride length	0.54	0.31	0.80	0.24	$P < 0.008$
Shoulder tug 0 = best 4 = worst	3.5	0.55	2.0	1.25	$P < 0.007$
BI total	80.25	14.2	92.75	15.24	$P < 0.005$
BI ADL	48.67	4.81	51.92	9.74	$P < 0.02$
BI mobility	31.58	10.87	40.83	14.06	$P < 0.006$

SD, standard deviation; BI, Barthel Index; ADL, activities of daily living.

Gait Parameters

The average stride length was 0.54 m (SD = 0.31) on admission, improving to 0.80 m (SD = 0.24) on discharge. This difference was statistically significant. There were also significant gains in gait speed after rehabilitation, from 44.2 m/min on admission to 66.0 m/min on discharge, with cadence unchanged at 105 (SD = 17) steps/min on admission and 106 (SD = 16) steps/min on discharge.

Postural Reflexes

Postural response results were difficult to analyze because inconsistent measures had been used in the early patients who underwent rehabilitation. Of the six patients who were assessed using the shoulder tug test, five demonstrated improved scores. Prerehabilitation scores ranged from 3 to 4 and postrehabilitation scores ranged from 1 to 3. One patient's score did not improve following rehabilitation. These data are summarized in Table 36.3.

Neuroimaging

Computed tomography scans were available for 11 patients. Four patients demonstrated changes of subcortical white matter ischemia and three showed changes consistent with normal pressure hydrocephalus. Three other patients had evidence of cerebral atrophy and one had scarring from removal of frontal lobe tumor. One patient had had both MRI and cerebral perfusion positron emission tomography (PET) scan performed. His MRI showed subcortical white matter ischemia with the PET scan, demonstrating bilateral decrease in blood flow in both frontal and parietal regions.

Follow-up

Patients were discharged to a community rehabilitation center, which they attended 1 day a week for 3 months to maintain the level of improvement achieved in the inpatient setting. Maintenance of gains varied. One patient continued rehabilitation in the community for 9 months and then required a further period of inpatient rehabilitation following a 3-month break from community rehabilitation. Three other patients continued to improve while in community rehabilitation. Of these, one deteriorated after a 2-month therapy break and required further inpatient rehabilitation. Another patient was unable to follow through with rehabilitation following discharge from hospital because of cognitive impairment. This patient had normal pressure hydrocephalus on CT scan, refused surgery, and continued to have falls. Another patient with normal pressure hydrocephalus did not continue with rehabilitation on discharge and also refused surgery. One patient continued with outpatient rehabilitation for 6 months but 5 months later the gait pattern had deteriorated to baseline levels. One patient deteriorated within 2 months without follow-up rehabilitation in a Day Hospital. A final patient had significant comorbid illness that limited improvements in rehabilitation. Although there were some improvements in the early stages for this patient these were not sustained owing to repeated acute illnesses.

Single Case Study for Rehabilitation: A Time Series Analysis

The results of the rehabilitation program over time are illustrated in Table 36.4 and Figures 36.1 to 36.4. It can be seen that the patient discussed in the case study showed an improvement in walking speed, stride length, cadence, and double-limb support over the course of physical therapy treatment. The improvement was most rapid during the first 5 days of treatment. After that time, recovery was more gradual to the point where there was little change between days 8 and 22.

When walking independently without a frame, the patient's median baseline walking speed was very slow, at only 52.3 m/min (Fig. 36.1). After 5 days of physical therapy treatment, this had increased to 59.5 m/min, and following 8 days of treatment it had reached 69.3 m/min, which was normal for his age and height (15). Thereafter the walking speed reached a plateau at values between 70 and 72 m/min. Similar improvement trends with physical therapy were

TABLE 36.4. *Summary of gait and balance parameters for prospective single case study performed over 3-week period*

Condition	Day 1	Day 5	Day 8	Day 12	Day 22
Velocity No aid	52.3	59.5	69.3	70.2	71.7
Aid	45.7	65.1	66.0	69.8	69.8
Stride length No Aid	1.08	1.16	1.24	1.29	1.30
Aid	0.94	1.2	1.3	1.3	1.26
%DLS No Aid	42.5	34.2	34.2	34.2	32.2
Aid	43.8	31.9	31.9	31.3	31.2
Cadence No aid	97.0	102.3	107.8	108.6	109.5
Aid	97.7	106.9	106.9	107.0	109.4
Shoulder tug 0 = best 4 = worst	4	0	0	0	0

%DLS, percentage of time and gait cycle spent in double limb support.

observed for stride length (Fig. 36.2). The median stride length before therapy was only 1.08 m, rather than 1.3 to 1.5 m, which is more usual for healthy older men (15). This steadily improved over the course of treatment, reaching 1.29 m after 12 days of physical therapy and a maximum value of 1.3 m after 22 days of treatment. The percentage of the gait cycle spent in double-limb support showed rapid improvement from 42.5% GC at baseline to 34.2% by day 5, reaching the usual value for healthy elderly men of 32.3% after 22 days of physical therapy treatment

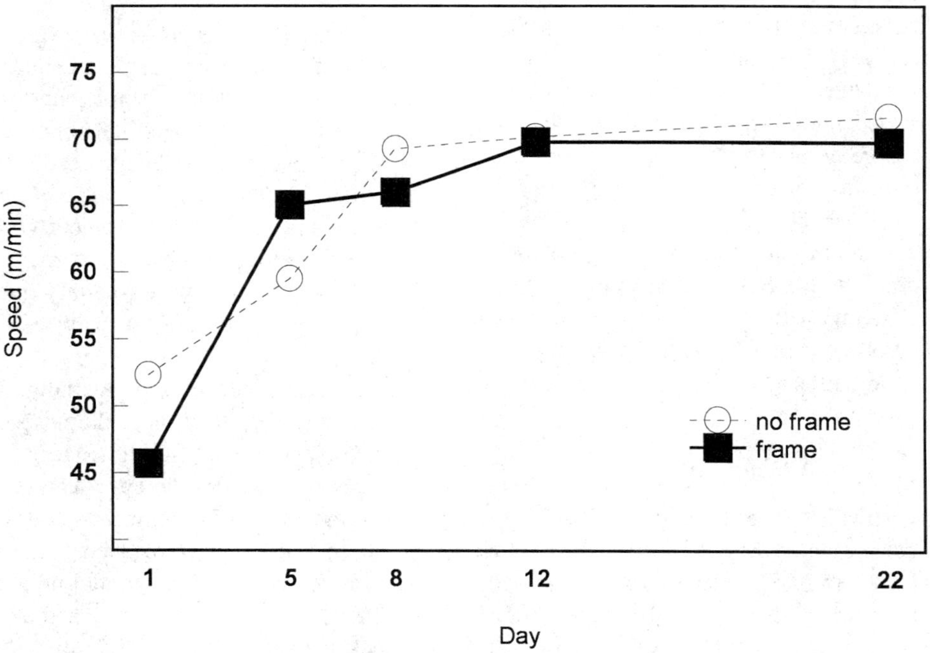

FIG. 36.1. Change in gait speed over time.

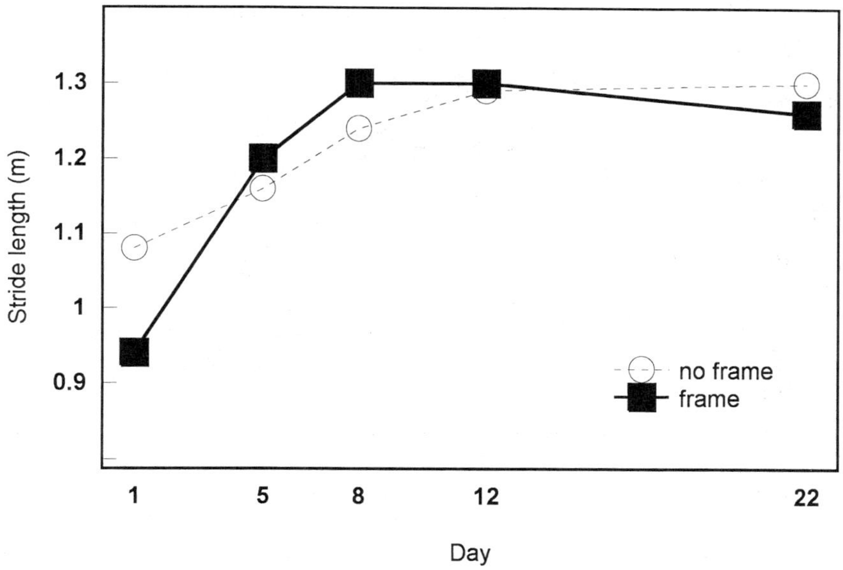

FIG. 36.2. Change in stride length over time.

(Fig. 36.3). Walking cadence was only 97.7 steps/minute before physical therapy (Fig. 36.4). It improved to a more usual value of 107 after only 8 days of treatment and remained normal thereafter.

Overall, the provision of a walking frame had little impact on the pattern or rate of recovery in walking speed, stride length, cadence, or the percentage of the gait cycle spent in double-limb support. Initially, when the frame was provided during baseline testing, the walking speed dropped from 52.3 m/min to 45.7 m/min (Fig. 36.1). Similarly, the median stride length reduced from 1.08 to 0.94 m, even though the

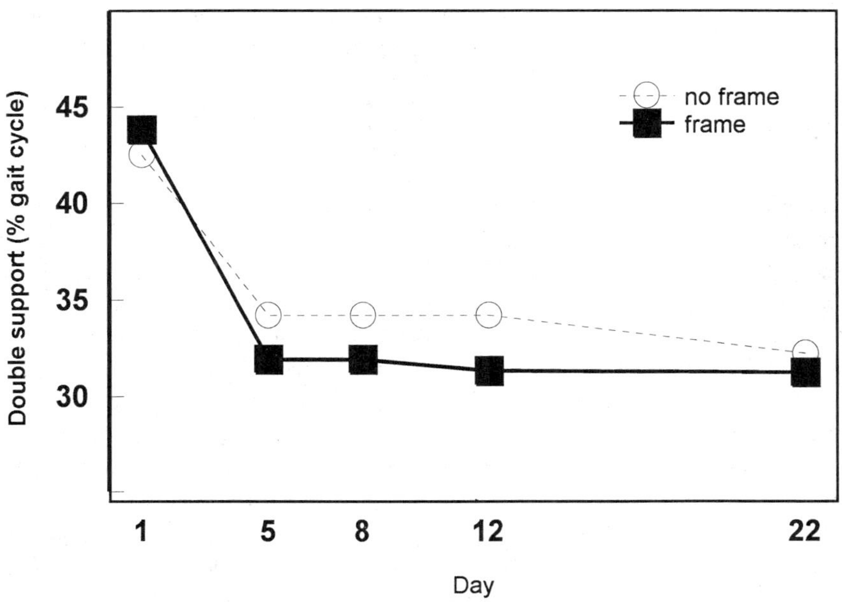

FIG. 36.3. Change in percentage of gait cycle spent in double-limb support over time.

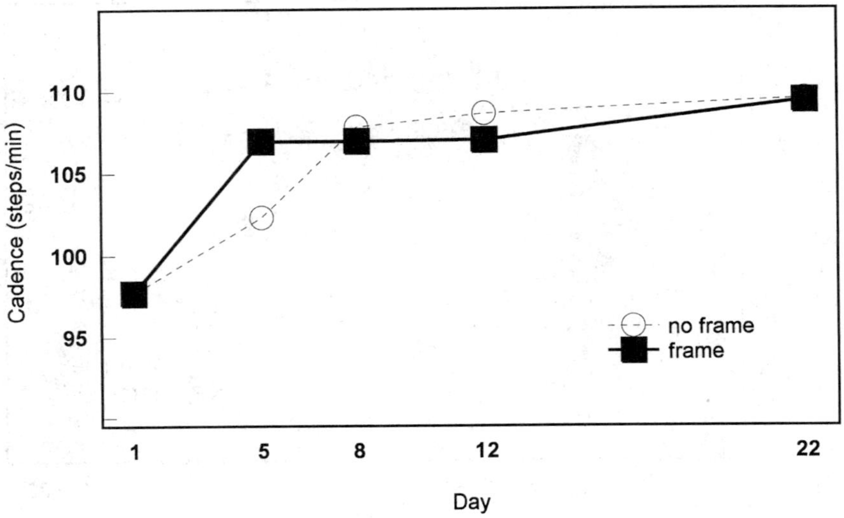

FIG. 36.4. Change in cadence over time.

stepping rate and severity of shuffling [as indicated by DS (%GC)] were similar with and without the frame (Figs. 36.2 and 36.3). During the course of physical therapy training the pattern of improvement was similar with the frame to that seen without the frame. After 22 days of treatment there were negligible differences in the walking pattern when the subject walked freely compared to walking with the frame. Thus the use of the frame did not appear to enhance his recovery.

DISCUSSION

Overall, the results of these studies confirmed clinical findings that subjects with FGA demonstrate a widened base of support, walk with reduced stride length and velocity, and spend more time in double-limb support than normal elderly subjects. They also confirmed that these patients have more cognitive impairment than control subjects, together with a greater fear of falling, which impacts on their daily activities. Another finding was that the use of a frame failed to improve any of the gait deviations, other than double-limb support time. The characteristics of the subject groups were consistent with the published literature, both in relation to the clinical manifestations of the condition and the imaging studies that confirmed a high incidence of subcortical white matter ischemia or normal pressure hydrocephalus.

The results suggested that the use of a frame in the FGA group did not significantly alter the clinical manifestations. Over the duration of the rehabilitation program, improvement did not differ between the use or nonuse of a frame. Instead, the benefit demonstrated in the retrospective review and in the single case study appeared to be owing to movement training rather than the use of walking frames.

An additional finding is apparent from the single case study. The results showed that this patient with gait apraxia was able to walk with a normal footstep pattern after a small number of physical therapy training sessions. Although he initially walked very slowly with short, slow, shuffling steps and low cadence after around 3 weeks of physical therapy he was confidently walking with a normal footstep pattern in a variety of contexts. Therefore, the ability to walk normally is not lost in patients with FGA. Rather, patients with FGA appear to lose the flexibility of adjusting their footstep parameters to the needs of the environment. For example, walking on a smooth but nonslip surface usually results in longer steps than walking on compliant surfaces such as grass. In turning to sit down, the leg on the outer side of the turn makes a bigger step than the inner foot. Such adaptability appears to be lost in people with FGA who tend to use the same, short-stepped, wide-based steps for all locomotor activities.

Postural responses appear to be similarly affected by the same process. In the descriptive part of this report, postural responses were significantly impaired compared to the control group. Similarly, in the retrospective review, patients who underwent the rehabilitative program, postural responses were abnormal and improved significantly following the rehabilitation program. This was further confirmed in the prospective single case study.

The rehabilitative approach utilized in this report depended on the use of attentional motor control mechanisms. Patients slowly progressed through a decreasing external support system as they utilized attentional mechanisms to improve stride length and postural responses. Eventually, when more proficient at these tasks, patients were taken through a series of activities that stressed both balance and stride length. These activities usually involved community type tasks, such as inclines, steps, rough ground, reaching, and bending. Finally, exercises were given to each subject to perform outside therapy sessions to maintain the attentional aspect of the program.

We have used such an approach quite successfully in the rehabilitation of people with PD (16). The basis of benefit in PD is the intact motor cortical function and the ability of cortical control mechanisms to bypass the defective basal ganglia and restore function to normal. The success of a similar approach in FGA suggests that a disconnection between the normal basal ganglia and the motor cortical regions exists in FGA. The disconnection is not in the basal ganglia but probably via its connections with the motor cortical regions. Thompson and Marsden have suggested that this disconnection occurs in the subcortical white matter and that the leg projection fibers are most commonly affected because their location is adjacent to the lateral ventricle (7). Certainly the findings of this report support this hypothesis, because the motor control areas were capable of activation and able to produce improved motor performance.

CONCLUSION

In summary, this report has demonstrated that FGA responds to a rehabilitation program that utilizes attentional motor control mechanisms. This suggests that investment of time and resources into gait and balance retraining in patients with FGA can reduce disability by teaching them how to compensate for this disabling movement disorder. The findings also support the hypothesis that the clinical manifestations arise from disconnection of the basal ganglia from the motor cortical region and also that gait and posture are more prone to involvement than face and upper limbs owing to the intimate location of the lower limbs basal ganglia projection fibers to the lateral ventricles.

ACKNOWLEDGMENT

The authors thank Robyn Tapp for advice on the time-series analysis.

REFERENCES

1. Sudarsky L, Ronthal M. Gait disorders among elderly patients. A survey study of 50 patients. *Arch Neurol* 1983;40:740–743.
2. Glatt SL, Koller WC. Gait apraxia. In: Spivack BS, ed. *Evaluation and management of gait disorders.* New York: Marcel Dekker, 1998:157–165.
3. Alexander NB. Gait disorders in older adults. *Progr Geriatr* 1996;44:434–451.
4. Nutt JG, Marsden CD, Thompson PD. Human walking and higher level gait disorders, particularly in the elderly. *Neurology* 1993;43:268–279.
5. Loizou LA, Kendall BE, Marshall J. Subcortical arterioscleroticencephalopathy: a clinical and radiological investigation. *J Neurol Neurosurg Psychiatry* 1981;44:294–304.
6. Babikian V, Ropper AK. Binswanger's disease: a review. *Stroke* 1987;18:2–11.
7. Thompson PD, Marsden CD. Gait disorder of subcortical arteriosclerotic encephalopathy: Binswanger's disease. *Mov Disord* 1987;2:1–8.
8. Fitzgerald PM, Jankovic J. Lower body Parkinsonism: evidence for vascular etiology. *Mov Disord* 1989; 4:249–260.
9. Thajeb P. Gait disorders of multi-infarct dementia. *Acta Neurol Scand* 1993;87:239–242.
10. Tinetti ME, Richman D, Powell L. Falls efficacy as a measure of fear of falling. *J Gerontol* 1990;45:239–243.
11. Hill K. Fear of falling revisited. *Arch Phys Med Rehabil* 1996;77:1025–1029.
12. Folstein MF, Folstein SE, McHugh PR. Mini-mental state: a practical method for grading the cognitive state of

patients for the clinician. *J Psychiatr Res* 1975;12:189–198.
13. Pastor MA, Day BL, Marsden CD. Vestibular induced postural responses in Parkinson's disease. *Brain* 1993; 116:1177–1190.
14. Collin C, Wade DT, Davis S. The Barthel ADL index; a reliability study. *Int Dis Stud* 1988;10:61–63.
15. Winter DA. *The biomechanics and motor control of human gait: normal, elderly and pathological,* 2nd ed. Ontario: University of Waterloo Press, 1991.
16. Iansek R. Interdisciplinary rehabilitation in Parkinson's disease. In: Stern GM, ed. *Parkinson's disease.* Philadelphia: Lippincott Williams & Wilkins, 1999:555–559.

Gait Disorders. Advances in Neurology, Vol. 87,
edited by E. Růžička, M. Hallett, and J. Jankovic.
Lippincott Williams & Wilkins, Philadelphia © 2001.

37

Gait Dysfunction in Huntington's Disease: Parkinsonism and a Disorder of Timing

Implications for Movement Rehabilitation

*¶Andrew J. Churchyard, ‡Meg E. Morris, §Nellie Georgiou, ||Edmond Chiu, ‡Randall Cooper, and †¶Robert Iansek

**Movement Disorders Unit and †Department of Geriatric Neurology, Kingston Centre, Cheltenham, Victoria, 3192, Australia; ‡School of Physiotherapy, La Trobe University, Bundoora, Victoria, 3086, Australia; Departments of §Psychology and ¶Medicine, Monash University, Clayton, Victoria, 3168, Australia; and ||Academic Unit of Psychiatry of Old Age and Huntington's Disease Clinic, University of Melbourne, St. George's Health Service, Kew, Victoria, 3101, Australia*

Huntington's disease (HD) is an autosomal dominant degenerative disease caused by 37 or more CAG triplet repeats of a gene located at sub-band 4p16.3 of the short arm of chromosome 4 (1). Huntington's disease is manifest primarily as a combination of involuntary movements (chorea), parkinsonism (rigidity and akinesia and bradykinesia, slowness in initiating and executing movement, respectively), and predominantly "frontostriatal" cognitive impairment that may ultimately result in dementia (2). Rare cases of HD characterized by cerebellar ataxia occur (2). Hypokinesia of the limbs appears to be invariable, even in the absence of marked parkinsonism (3,4). As with Parkinson's disease (PD), reaction (RT), and movement (MT) times in a variety of tasks are slowed in HD (3,5–8). Moreover, patients with HD are more impaired than controls in changing cognitive set and in holding and shifting attention (9,10). Whether or not upper limb MT and RT correlate with lower limb gait parameters is unknown.

The studies described in this chapter sought to quantify gait patterns in patients with HD and control subjects using spatiotemporal variables obtained from stride analysis, with the goal of providing an intellectual basis from which to develop rehabilitative strategies to compensate for abnormalities in walking. In addition, we tested the hypothesis that basal ganglia destruction is the major cause of gait dysfunction and abnormal postural control in patients with HD by examining the relationship between gait dysfunction and overall disease severity as measured by the Unified Huntington's Disease Rating Scale (UHDRS), which is assumed to be an index of striatal and pallidal damage. A further aim was to examine whether abnormalities in gait correlated with deficits in cognition so as to quantify the impact of cognitive impairment on difficulties in walking.

METHODS

Symptomatic community-dwelling HD patients (more than 37 triplet repeats) were recruited by EC and by advertisement in the Huntington's Disease Association of Victoria newsletter. Control subjects were cognitively intact (MMSE greater than 26), had no history of neurological, psychiatric, or rheumatologic disease and were matched to the patients for age and height.

Patients were examined by AC for severity of HD with the UHDRS. Upper limb motor parkinsonism was assessed objectively with RT and MT time tasks. MT was quantified by serially pressing buttons at choice points along a designated sequential pathway in response to visual stimuli (7). Varying the stimulus allowed the reliance on advance visual information to be examined (7). RT was measured as the difference in the time of onset of the overall response to relevant and irrelevant stimuli (Simon effect) (7). Cognitive function was determined with the Mini Mental State Examination (MMSE), Stroop test, Trails A and B, Controlled Oral Word Association, and Montgomery–Asberg Depression Scale (11–15). Scores obtained by patients and controls with each of the RT, MT, Trails, Controlled Word Association Test, MMSE, Stroop, and Montgomery–Asberg scales were compared with t-tests. An Interference score was calculated for the Stroop test and Trails B was subtracted from Trails A so as to obtain a switching score for each patient and control.

The spatial (distance) and temporal (time) parameters of gait were quantified by RC, MM and RG using a Clinical Stride Analyzer (CSA; B&L Engineering, Santa Fe Springs, CA, U.S.A.), which comprised four pressure-sensitive switches worn as inner soles in the subject's shoes connected to a 0.5-kg microcomputer suspended from a belt (16–19). Data from each of the footswitches were sampled every 2 ms and stored prior to being analyzed (PCSA software, Version 6, B&L Engineering). Recording was activated and terminated by a hand-held trigger that was activated by the examiner at the beginning and end of the walkway. Five 10-m walking trials for free (preferred), slow, and fast walking were conducted; the order of the conditions were counterbalanced to control for series effects. The variables measured were gait velocity (m/min), stride length (m), cadence (steps/min), and duration of the double-support phase (expressed as a percent of the gait cycle). To determine if patients could utilize external cues to normalize gait, walking in time to a metronome (80 bpm) was also examined. In order to deterine if attentional mechanisms have an impact on gait in HD, walking was examined while counting digits backward (distraction task).

For each subject, the mean of trials 2 and 3 from a series of five successive trials for each gait condition were entered into an SPSS (Version 6) data file. Distributions of each of the variables for each condition were inspected and the descriptive statistics obtained. Normalcy of distribution of velocity, stride length, cadence and duration of double stance in free walking was confirmed with the Kolmogorov-Smirnov and Shapiro-Wilks statistics. Velocity, stride length, cadence, and duration of double stance in the HD and control groups were compared using univariate analyses of variance and t-tests.

Objective parameters of gait (velocity, stride length, cadence, and duration of double stance) were related to the UHDRS motor score, RT, and MT, all measures of cognitive function, and the duration of symptoms with Pearson's correlation. The relationship between gait dysfunction and disease severity was explored to test the hypothesis that basal ganglia destruction is a major contributing factor to gait disorders in HD by relating the UHDRS motor score to gait velocity, stride length, cadence, and duration of double stance, RT, and MT.

RESULTS

Data from 20 patients with symptomatic HD (chorea with 37 triplet repeats) were compared to 16 age-matched controls (Table 37.1). The initial presentation of HD was with chorea in 15, psychiatric disease in three, and cognitive impairment in two. Inheritance was maternal in 13, paternal in four, and unknown in three. Six patients received neuroleptics for suppression of chorea and seven were taking antidepressants. The mean duration of symptomatic disease was 9.9 years (range, 1 to 27). The mean UHDRS motor score was 44.1. The UHDRS motor score and duration of symptomatic illness correlated ($r = 0.67$, $P < 0.05$).

Preferred Gait (Free Walking)

The preferred velocity of free walking for HD subjects was slower than for control subjects. Whereas control subjects walked on average at 84.5 m/min, those with HD had an average

TABLE 37.1. *Demographic characteristics of Huntington's disease and control subjects (mean [SD])*

	Gender	Age	Disease duration (yr)	UHDRS	MMSE
Huntington's disease	16M 4F	58.2 (12.9)	9.9 (6.6)	44.1 (25.5)	24.6 (3.8)
Controls	13M 3F	55.4 (10.5)	NA —	NA —	29.4 (0.7)

HD subjects and controls were matched for age. The mean duration of symptomatic disease was 9.9 years and the mean United Huntington's Disease Rating Scale (UHDRS) motor score was 44.1.

SD, standard deviation; MMSE, Minimental State Examination; NA, not applicable.

velocity of only 59.7 m/min [$F(1,35) = 19.3$, $P < 0.005$] (Table 37.2). Velocity is the product of stride length × cadence × 1/2. Double stance is the time when both feet are on the ground at the beginning and end of the gait cycle. For preferred (self-selected) speed of walking, the mean stride length in HD of 1.16 m was significantly less than the controls (1.51 m) [$F(1,35) = 17.5, P < 0.005$] (Fig. 37.1; Table 37.1). That is, parkinsonism of gait (reduced velocity and stride length) occurred in HD (16,20). Notably, cadence was reduced in HD to 100.6 steps/min compared with 111.7 steps/min in the control subjects [$F(1,35) = 8.4$, $P = 0.006$] (Fig. 37.2). Of note, the variability of velocity, stride length, and cadence in HD was markedly increased. The standard deviation of each gait parameter was in excess of twice that of the control subjects. The duration of DS was unaffected by HD.

The UHDRS motor score correlated with velocity ($R = -0.53$, $P < 0.05$) and stride length ($R = -0.60$, $P < 0.05$), but not cadence ($R = -0.31$, $P > 0.05$) or double stance ($R = 0.20$, $P > 0.05$). The duration of symptomatic disease did not correlate with any of velocity, stride length, cadence, or double stance (data not shown).

In summary, the preferred gait velocity was slowed in HD because both the rhythmical stepping rate (cadence) and stride length were reduced in comparison to control subjects. Moreover, step-by-step variability of cadence and stride length were increased, indicating a disturbance of both timing and amplitude regulation of gait.

Fast and Slow Walking

When instructed to walk either quickly or slowly, HD patients could modify velocity and stride length, but each remained less than for the control subjects in both conditions (Fig. 37.1; Table 37.2). Velocity at fast walking was 84.6 m/min for those with HD versus

TABLE 37.2. *Mean (SD) velocity, stride length, cadence, and duration of double stance in Huntington's disease (HD) and control subjects during all gait conditions*

	Normal walking		Fast walking		Slow walking		Digits backward		Metronome (80 bpm)	
	HD	Control	HD	Control	HD	Control	HD	Control	HD	Control
Velocity (m/min)	59.7 (21.3)	84.5[a] (8.1)	84.6 (26.4)	109.7[a] (12.0)	45.5 (18.2)	59.1[a] (10.0)	57.7 (18.2)	65.4 (13.7)	49.4 (13.2)	53.9 (4.9)
Stride length (m)	1.16 (0.32)	1.51[a] (0.11)	1.43 (0.34)	1.74[a] (0.15)	1.00 (0.31)	1.28[a] (0.12)	1.16 (0.31)	1.36[a] (0.14)	1.11 (0.17)	1.32[a] (0.07)
Cadence (step/min)	100.6 (13.6)	111.7[a] (7.7)	120.6 (15.0)	126.5 (11.4)	89.1 (15.4)	91.8 (10.4)	90.4 (17.1)	95.2 (13.1)	88.1 (11.5)	81.6[a] (2.2)
Duration of double limb support (%)	34.8 (8.1)	31.0 (2.9)	30.3 (5.7)	29.9 (4.2)	36.2 (6.1)	34.1 (3.4)	35.0 (7.7)	32.9 (3.0)	33.0 (6.5)	32.2 (3.3)

Velocity, stride length and cadence were reduced in HD in all gait conditions. Duration of double stance was the same in the HD and control subjects. Variability of all gait parameters was markedly greater in the HD subjects than in the controls.

[a] $P < 0.05$.

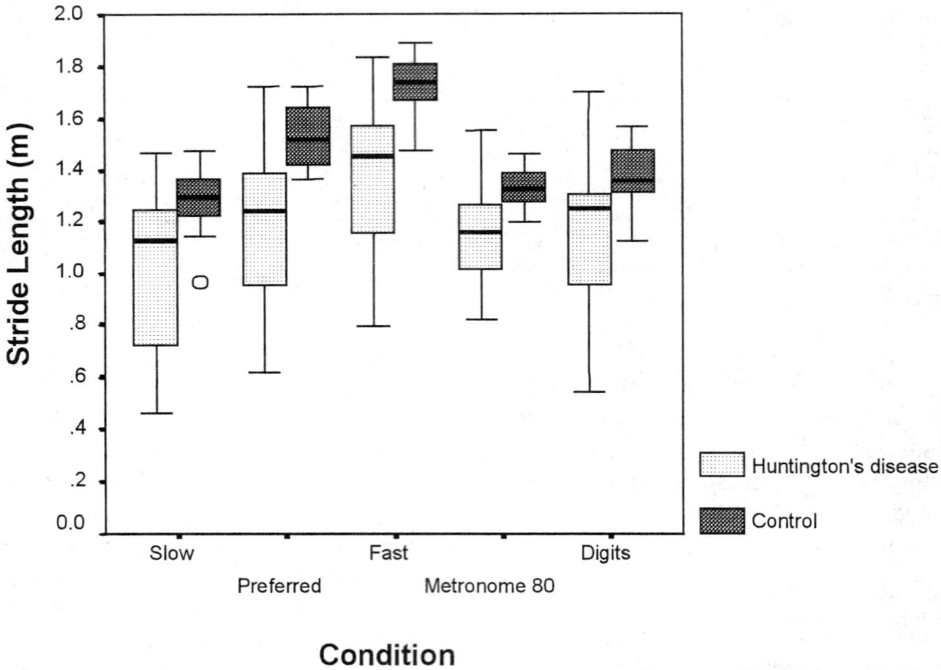

FIG. 37.1. Stride length (m) in Huntington's disease (HD) and control subjects. Stride length was reduced in HD in all the conditions, indicating hypokinesia (parkinsonism) of gait. Variability of stride length was markedly increased in all conditions in the subjects with HD.

109.7 m/min in the controls [$F(1,35) = 12.3$, $P < 0.005$] and stride length was 1.43 and 1.74 m [$F(1,35) = 11.7$, $P < 0.005$], respectively, in the HD and control subjects. In the slow walking condition, velocity was only 45.5 m/min for those with HD compared with 59.1 m/min for the control subjects [$F(1,35) = 8.2$, $P = 0.007$]. Stride length was 1.00 and 1.28 m [$F(1,35) = 11.9$, $P < 0.005$] in the HD and control subjects, respectively. Cadence in both groups varied according to the demands of the task, but was not significantly different in HD from the controls (Fig. 37.2). The duration of double stance was similar for the two groups. As with free walking, there was markedly more variability in velocity, stride length, and cadence in the HD subjects than the control subjects, with standard deviations in the former being generally twice that of the latter.

Metronome Gait

When walking in time to a metronome set at 80 bpm, velocity remained less in those with HD than for the control subjects, but this difference was not statistically significant [HD 49.4 m/min versus controls 53.9 m/min; $F(1,35) = 1.8$, $P = 0.183$]. Stride length remained less in those with HD [HD 1.11 m versus controls 1.32; $F(1,35) = 17.7$, $P < 0.005$] (Fig. 37.1). Cadence was modulated in response to the beat of the metronome to 88.1 steps/min in HD and 81.6 steps/min in the controls. However, cadence was different in the two groups [$F(1,35) = 5.1$, $P = 0.031$], implying that its regulation in response to an external cue is impaired in HD. Neither group was able to perfectly entrain foot step rates to the metronome as cadence in each was significantly greater than 80 bpm ($P < 0.05$ student's t-test for each group versus test value of 80). The duration of double stance remained the same in the two groups. Notably, there was markedly more variability in velocity, stride length, and cadence in the HD subjects than the control subjects with standard deviations in the former being invariably twice or more than that of the latter (Table 37.2; Fig. 37.2).

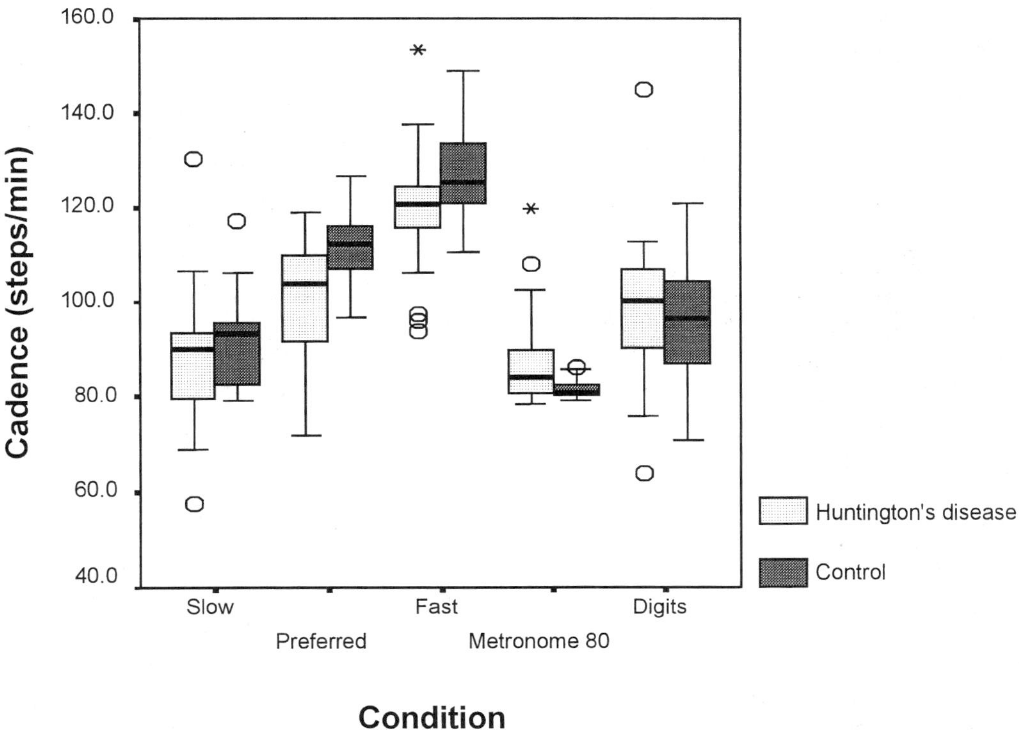

FIG. 37.2. Cadence (steps/min) in Huntington's disease (HD) and control subjects. Cadence was reduced in patients with HD in all the conditions. Variability of cadence was markedly increased in the subjects with HD. This variabilty was particularly prominent when walking in time to a metronome striking at 80 bpm. The abnormality of cadence is consistent with a disorder of timing of gait.

Digits Backward Task

When walking while counting backward, velocity [HD 57.7 m/min versus controls 65.4 m/min; $F(1,35) = 2.6$, $P = 0.119$] and cadence [HD 90.4 steps/min versus controls 95.2 steps/min; $F(1,35) = 0.5$, $P = 0.488$] remained less in those with HD than for the control subjects, but this difference was not statistically significant. Stride length remained less in those with HD [HD 1.16 m versus controls 1.36; $F(1,35) = 5.8$, $P < 0.05$]. The duration of double stance remained the same in the two groups. The variability in each gait parameter was greater in the HD subjects than the control subjects, but was most marked for stride length. Overall, reduced attention to walking (distraction) had little or no effect on stride length or duration of double stance, but reduced velocity and cadence when compared to free walking (Figs. 37.1 and 37.2; Table 37.2).

Movement and Reaction Times

Only 10 of the 20 HD subjects could perform the MT and RT tasks. Analysis is therefore confined to these patients, who were the least severely affected with respect to both motor and cognitive function. Only one of these patients was receiving a major tranquilizer and he was not overtly parkinsonian (Webster score 5). In this relatively mildly impaired group, both MT and RT were significantly increased (Table 37.3). Thus, MT and RT were 299 and 858 msec, respectively, in the HD group and 177 and 584 msec, respectively, in the controls [MT: $t(18) = 3.58$, $P < 0.01$ and RT: $t(18) = 2.13$, $P < 0.05$].

RT failed to correlate with any gait parameter (velocity, stride length, cadence, and duration of double stance; $P > 0.05$ all). In contrast, MT correlated with velocity ($R = -0.73$, $P < 0.05$), cadence ($R = -0.68$, $P < 0.05$), and stride length ($R = -0.73$, $P < 0.05$), but not

TABLE 37.3. *Mean (SD) reaction time (RT), movement time (MT) and scores for tests of frontostriatal cognitive function (Stroop, Trails A and B, Controlled Oral Word Association [COWA])*

	RT (N = 10)	MT (N = 10)	Stroop Interference (N = 12)	Trails A and B (switching component) (N = 12)	COWA (N = 12)
Huntington's disease	858 msec[a] (393)	299 msec[a] (106)	77 (37)	72 msec[a] (34)	33[a] (12)
Controls (N = 16)	584 msec (103)	177 msec (21)	73 (27)	43 msec (20)	50 (16)

RT and MT (examined in 10 Huntington's disease [HD] subjects) were slowed and the variability of each was increased in HD. Performance on the Trails A and B and Controlled Oral Word Association was impaired in HD, but the Stroop test score was unaffected (12 HD subjects examined).

[a] $P < 0.05$.

duration of double stance ($R = 0.11$, $P > 0.05$). RT and MT did not correlate with duration of disease or the UHDRS motor score (data not shown, $P > 0.05$ both).

Neuropsychological Studies

Only 12 of the 20 HD subjects were able to perform the neuropsychologial tasks (Stroop, Trails A and B, Controlled Oral Word Association) and therefore could be analyzed. The remaining eight cases were too cognitively impaired (MMSE < 22) to successfully complete these tasks. HD and control subjects were matched for age [HD: 54 ± 10 versus controls: 53 ± 10, $t(22) = 0.39$, $P > 0.05$] and years of education [HD: 13 ± 2 versus controls: 14 ± 3, $t(22) = -1.57$, $P > 0.05$]. However, the HD subjects were more depressed as measured by the Montgomery-Asberg Depression Scale [HD: 9.8 ± 6.4 versus controls: 1.4 ± 1.7, $t(22) = 4.42$, $P < 0.001$] and their MMSE was lower [HD: 27.0 ± 1.7 versus controls: 29.4 ± 0.8, $t(22) = -4.48$, $P < 0.001$].

The HD patients took longer to switch between tasks on the Trail Making test [HD: 72 msec $\pm$ 34 versus controls: 43 msec $\pm$ 20, $t(16) = 2.21$, $P < 0.05$] and achieved a lower score on the Controlled Oral Word Association test than the controls [HD: 33 ± 12 versus controls: 50 ± 16, $t(22) = -2.88$, $P < 0.01$] (Table 37.3). However, performance of the Stroop task was similar in both groups [Interference score: HD 77 ± 37 versus controls 73 ± 27, $t(22) = 0.29$, $P > 0.05$]. There was no correlation between either the Trail Making test score or the Controlled Oral Word Association test score and any of velocity, stride length, cadence, and duration of double stance (data not shown).

The UHDRS score correlated with the Controlled Oral Word Association test score ($R = -0.62$, $P < 0.05$), but not the Trail Making test score ($R = -0.11$, $P > 0.05$) or the MMSE for all 20 HD subjects ($R = -0.39$, $P > 0.05$). The MMSE score correlated with the Controlled Oral Word Association test score ($R = 0.55$, $P < 0.05$), but not the Trail Making test score ($R = 0.33$, $P > 0.05$). The MMSE score did not correlate with the duration of disease in the full sample of 20 HD patients ($R = -0.43$, $P > 0.05$). Correlations were not attempted for the Stroop test scores.

DISCUSSION

The major finding of this study is that locomotion in HD is abnormal because of a combination of hypokinesia, evidenced by reduced stride length, and disordered regulation of rhythmic stepping manifest as reduced stepping rates, poorly modulated cadence, and increased variability of velocity, stride length, and cadence.

The gait velocity of the HD subjects was very slow for free (preferred speed) walking (Table 37.2). Patients with HD could voluntarily vary their speed of walking yet remained significantly slower during the fast and slow walking tasks than the control subjects. The velocity of walking in time to an external auditory cue and in a distraction task was also less than for controls. That is, although HD patients could vary the velocity of locomotion, it was invariably slowed. Similarly, stride length was decreased relative to the control subjects in all the gait tasks and again could not be "normalized" in reponse to varying requirements. Reduced velocity in association with a shortened stride length and impaired capacity to change either according to the requirements of different gait tasks is characteristic of PD and is indicative of gait hypokinesia (16–20). Reduced velocity of gait and stride length has previously been described in HD (21–23). Upper limb RT and MT were decreased in HD as in previous studies (Table 37.3) (3,4). MT, but not RT, correlated with velocity, stride length, and cadence. These findings are consistent with current concepts that MT, which comprises most of the gait cycle as distinct from the brief RT of each step, is a long-duration preprogrammed motor act.

The pathophysiologic substrate of hypokinesia in HD appears likely to be basal ganglia degeneration, which is centered on the caudate nucleus (Cd) and subsequently putamen (Pu) (24). Initially, GABAergic striatal projection neurones are selectively destroyed, but as the disease progresses other striatal neurones degenerate and involvement of the globus pallidus (GP) is invariable in advanced HD (24,25). Marked loss of neurones in the substantia nigra pars compacta occurs rarely. Gross parkinsonism may occur without severe loss of dopaminergic nigral neurones, and striatal dopamine receptors are equally affected in the choreic and rigid variants (24,26,27). Current theories suggest that the basal ganglia form part of partially segregated, parallel functional loops that run from cortex to striatum to GP to thalamus to cortex (28). Because the associative loop includes the Cd, and the motor loop the Pu, both are likely to be dysfunctional in HD. Functional positron emission tomography studies have related upper limb bradykinesia in HD to reduced activation of the striatum and key frontal premotor cortices that comprise the corticobasal ganglia-thalamocortical motor circuit (24,28,29). Rigid HD has been associated with a greater loss of GABA in the internal GP and more severe destruction of GABAergic striatal neurones projecting to this nucleus than the choreic form (26,30). Thus, it appears that hypokinesia in HD is caused by destruction of the striatal neurones that project to the GP and causes disinhibition of inhibitory pallidal outflow. Chorea is thought to be a consequence of overactivity of the subthalamic nucleus as a result of reduced inhibition of the lateral GP.

The symptomatic severity of HD has been shown to correlate with the degree of striatal and pallidal destruction (24). We found that the UHDRS motor score correlated well with stride length and velocity of free walking. That is, the severity of gait hypokinesia correlated with the overall degree of motor disability and, by implication, the extent of basal ganglia damage, as would be predicted by the hypothesis that hypokinesia in HD is caused by loss of inhibitory striatal neurones projecting to the GPi. We found no relationship between the UHDRS motor score and the two objective indices of upper limb hypokinesia (RT and MT) studied; however, the numbers of cases studied was small (N = 10). Larger studies with adequate power are required to determine if upper limb hypokinesia correlates with UHDRS score.

Cadence of free walking was reduced in HD as previously described (Table 37.2) (21,23,32). The proportion of the gait cycle spent in double stance was unaffected (32). Thus, the abnormalities of locomotion in HD differ from those of PD, where the proportion of the gait cycle spent in double stance is increased and cadence is unaffected (18). The deficits in cadence were more profound than a simple reduction of the rate of stepping alone. HD patients could vary cadence crudely in keeping with the requirement to voluntarily increase or decrease the speed of walking. However, since gait velocity and stride length were reduced in all tasks, by implication the HD patients were unable to increase the rate of stepping in compensation. The HD patients were less able to entrain steppage in time with an external auditory cue (metronome chiming at 80 bpm) than the control subjects as evidenced by a grossly inaccurate mean of 88.1 steps/min versus 81.6 steps/min, respectively, but also by the remarkable variability in the rate of steppage [standard deviation of 11.5 (13.1%) in HD versus 2.2 (2.6%) in controls] associated with this task. Moreover, there was a striking variability of stride length, velocity, and cadence in all the gait tasks and of RT and MT. The marked variability observed by us has been described in the gait and upper limb movements in HD (21–23,33). That is, there is excessive variability of amplitude and timing of movement in HD.

The basis of the excessive variability of both the amplitude and timing of movement in HD is unknown. Postural instability, which is common in HD, is a potential cause of excess variabilty of gait amplitudes and timing (34). We have not, thus far, quantified postural instability in the HD subjects, although it was impaired on the retropulsion test (UHDRS item 20) in 16 of 20 (mean score 1.7 ± 1.0). Because the duration of double stance was not increased in HD, postural stability might be thought to be intact in HD. However, it appears more likely that failure to increase the duration of double stance in the presence of postural instability represents another example of the inability of HD patients to appropriately adapt motor behavior to need. At the current level of understanding, the contribution of postural instability to the increased variabilty of gait parameters is unknown.

Timing of serial movements is thought to be a product of a distributed network which comprises many structures, including the basal ganglia, prefrontal and frontal cortices, brainstem premotor nuclei, and cerebellum (35–39). The basal ganglia are thought to regulate switching between learned motor acts, whereas the cerebellum controls timing and processes sensory feedback to optimize movement (35–39). Abnormal regulation of amplitude and timing of gait and upper limb movements occur in PD (21,32,40,41). However, such marked variability in velocity, stride length, and cadence in the different conditions studied and RT and MT is not found in PD and cannot be attributed to hypokinesia (16–19,21). Chorea appears unlikely to account for the observed variability because cadence did not correlate with the UHDRS score in this study or with the severity of chorea when examined by others (21). In this study, cadence during free walking could not be correlated with the UHDRS score in contrast to stride length. Since clinical disease severity is related to the extent of striopallidal degeneration, the deficits in timing and regulation of amplitude of gait parameters in HD observed by us might be unrelated to basal ganglia degeneration (24).

Cerebellar ataxia is associated with reduced stride length and increased variability of stride length and duration of stride with free walking, whereas cadence is only mildly reduced (40,42). Studies of postural control in cerebellar disease have also found increased variability of movement latencies (43,44). Cerebellar atrophy, unlike PD, results in increased variability of intertap intervals in a task requiring serial tapping (38). Increased variabilty of the timing and amplitude of movement is a fundamental consequence of cerebellar dysfunction. Mild to moderate destruction of cerebellar Purkinje cells has been detected in many HD patients even in the absence of gross degeneration and may be severe in a minority (24,45). We suggest that, although unproven, the deficits in the regulation of timing and amplitude of movement observed in HD might result from degeneration of cerebellar Purkinje cells.

The HD subjects were impaired in their ability to switch between tasks on the Trail Making test, achieved a lower score on Controlled Word Association test and showed a slower RT in a task that required discrimination between irrelevant and relevant stimuli (Simon effect, which depends on maintenance of attention) (Table 37.3) (7). Performance of these tasks is impaired with frontostriatal cognitive dysfunction (7,9,10). Surprisingly, another test of frontostriatal function, the Stroop test, was unaffected, and impaired attention while walking (counting digits backward) had a similar effect on gait in both the HD and control subjects. Nonetheless, this and many other studies demonstrate that frontostriatal cognitive impairment is an extremely common, if not invariable, result of even mild HD (46–48).

It is noteworthy that the neuropsychology tasks did not correlate with gait parameters, but that the score on Controlled Word Association test correlated with both the MMSE and the UHDRS motor score. There are three possible reasons to account for our failure to correlate frontostriatal cogitive impairment and motor dysfunction. First, the correlational studies were confined to a small subset of mildly affected subjects selected because they were able to complete the tasks; therefore, failure to detect any correlation might be an artefact attributable to limited statistical power. Second, no correlation between cognitive impairment might be expected in this mildly affected patient group because the corticobasal ganglia associative loop, which is centered on the Cd, regulates the direction and maintenance of attention, whereas the motor loop is centered on the Pu, and because the Cd is the focus of neuronal degeneration in early HD (24,28). This possibility is consistent with the repeated observation that cognitive impairment precedes overt motor dysfunction in HD and by the correlation of behavioral and cognitive abnormalities with the severity of metabolic changes in the Cd, but is difficult to reconcile with the correlation of the score on Controlled Word Association test with both the MMSE and the UHDRS motor score (46–49). Third, frontostriatal cognitive impairment may not contribute to gait dysfunction in HD.

MOVEMENT REHABILITATION IN PATIENTS WITH HUNTINGTON'S DISEASE

Although movement disorders are arguably the most common and disabling outcome of HD, little is known about the effects of movement rehabilitation strategies for people with this progressive basal ganglia disorder. To date there have been no randomized clinical trials (RCTs), comparative group outcome studies, or controlled single case studies investigating the effects of physical therapy treatment on movement disorders in HD. Apart from the data on external cues and dual task performance presented in this chapter, there is no information on the response of those with HD to interventions such as external cuing, attentional strategies, falls prevention programs, or even strengthening programs. Although physical therapists and occupational therapists play a role in educating people with HD and their caregivers on how to manage movement disorders and prevent falls, this has been done on a case-by-case basis without a theoretical framework from which to predict the likely effects of treatment. Currently, clinicians rely on general clinical decision-making strategies in order to determine the goals, priorities, and methods of movement rehabilitation for each individual, rather than a general paradigm of management suitable for the population of people with HD.

Working from first principles, as well as the findings on movement rehabilitation in PD, we suggest a model of movement rehabilitation for those with HD based on the following assumptions, which still need to be validated with RCTs.

1. Activity, participation, and independence in people with HD are compromised by movement disorders, postural instability, secondary adaptations to reduced activity, and cognitive impairment.
2. Physical therapy strategies can enable people with HD to retain their levels of activity, participation, and independence for longer periods compared with no therapy.
3. Physical therapy strategies can assist people with HD to reduce the number of falls and the severity of injuries from falls.
4. Physical therapy strategies can train people with HD to manage movement disorders such as hypokinesia, chorea, other forms of dyskinesia, weakness, and postural instability; and enhance independence and quality of life.

Given that hypokinesia is common in HD, it may be useful for therapists to teach people with HD strategies for overcoming hypokinesia that have been found to be useful in PD (3,4,16–19). These include attentional strategies such as focusing on walking with long steps, writing with large strokes, or reaching forward with a large movement of the hand (50). Avoiding dual-task performance or using external cues either in the form of visual markers or auditory stimuli can be effective in minimizing hypokinesia (50,51). Where postural instability and a history of falls are prominent, basic falls prevention strategies can be utilized (52,53). These strategies include modifications of the residential environment to make it safer as well as educating the person and their caregivers about the risk factors for falls. Moreover, general exercise programs to assist people with HD to maintain strength, endurance, and cardiopulmonary fitness may prove to be useful in minimizing the secondary effects on the musculoskeletal and cardiovascular systems that seem to appear as a consequence of reduced activity and disuse (53). Clearly, these suggestions need to be validated with controlled clinical trials. In addition, the capacity for people with HD to learn new ways to cope with their movement disorders and postural instability needs close scrutiny, given that the majority of people with HD will eventually develop significant cognitive impairment that may limit their capacity for new learning.

The role of allied health professionals in reducing severe or distressing chorea is uncertain. Although attentional strategies, such as thinking of keeping the part still or weight bearing through the affected part, appear to be effective in reducing dyskinetic movements in PD, the benefit is rarely prolonged (18). This is particularly the case when the person attempts to perform a second motor or cognitive task (50). In the absence of RCTs, neurolepts remain the mainstay of the treatment of chorea despite the risk that these drugs will worsen hypokinesia.

ACKNOWLEDGMENTS

We would like to thank HD patients and their caregivers and the control subjects for giving up their time and, in some cases, traveling large distances to be examined. The Huntington's Disease Association of Victoria actively supported us by assisting recruitment and also made a generous donation at a crucial time. The John Cockayne Memorial Trust supported the employment of RC. Judy Bradshaw and Robyn Gardiner capably performed some of the neuropsychological and gait assessments.

REFERENCES

1. Gusella J, MacDonald ME, Ambrose C, et al. Molecular genetics of Huntington's disease. *Arch Neurol* 1993;50:1157–1163.
2. Bruyn GW, Went LN. Huntington's chorea. In: Vinken PJ, Bruyn GW, Klawans HL, eds. *Handbook of clinical neurology*, vol. 5. Amsterdam: Elsevier, 1986:298–378.
3. Hefter H, Homberg V, Lange LW, et al. Impairment of rapid movement in Huntington's disease. *Brain* 1987;110:585–612.
4. Thompson PD, Beradelli P, Rothwell J, et al. The coexistence of bradykinesia and chorea in Huntington's disease and its implications for theories of basal ganglia control of movement. *Brain* 1988;111:223–244.
5. Bradshaw J, Phillips J, Dennis C, et al. Initiation and control of movement sequences in those suffering from and at risk of Huntington's disease. *J Clin Exp Neuropsychol* 1992;14:179–192.
6. Garnett ES, Firnau G, Nahmias C, et al. Reduced striatal glucose consumption and prolonged reaction time are early features of Huntington's disease. *J Neurol Sci* 1984;65:231–237.
7. Georgiou N, Bradshaw J, Phillips J, et al. The Simon effect and attention deficits in Gilles de la Tourette's syndrome and Huntington's disease. *Brain* 1995;118:1305–1318.
8. Girotti F, Marano R, Soliveri P, et al. Relationship between motor and cognitive disorders in Huntington's disease. *J Neurol* 1988;253:454–457.
9. Georgiou N, Bradshaw J, Pillips J, et al. Reliance on advanced information and movement sequencing in Huntington's disease. *Mov Disord* 1995;10:477–481.
10. Georgiou N, Bradshaw JL, Phillips JG, et al. Effect of directed attention in Huntington's. *J Clin Exp Neuropsychol* 1997;19:367–377.
11. Folstein M, Folstein S, McHugh P. Mini-mental State: a method for gathering cognitive state of patients. *J Psych Res* 1975;12:189–198.
12. Stroop JR. Studies of interference in serial verbal reactions. *J Exp Psychol* 1935;18:643–662.
13. Reitan RM. Validity of the trail making test as an indication of organic brain damage. *Percept Motor Skills* 1958;8:271–276.
14. Benton AL, Eslinger PJ, Damasio AR. Normative observations on neuropsychological performance. *J Clin Neuropsychol* 1981;3:33–42.
15. Montgomery S, Asberg M. A depression scale sensitive to change. *Br J Psych* 1979;134:382–389.
16. Morris M, Iansek R, Matyas TA, et al. The pathogenesis of gait hypokinesia in Parkinson's disease. *Brain* 1994a;117:1169–1181.
17. Morris M, Iansek R, Matyas TA, et al. Ability to modulate walking cadence remains intact in Parkinson's disease. *J Neurol Neurosurg Psych* 1994b;57:1532–1534.
18. Morris M, Iansek R, Matyas TA, et al. Stride length regulation in Parkinson's disease. Normalization strategies and underlying mechanisms. *Brain* 1996;119:551–568.
19. Morris M, Iansek R, Matyas TA, et al. Abnormalities in stride length– cadence relation in parkinsonian gait. *Mov Disord* 1998;13:61–69.
20. Blin O, Ferrandez A, Serratice G. Quantitative analysis of gait in Parkinson patients: increased variability of stride length. *J Neurol Sci* 1990;98:91–97.
21. Hausdorff JM, Mitchell SN, Firtion R, et al. Altered fractal dynamics of gait: reduced stride-interval dynamics with Huntington's disease. *J Appl Physiol* 1997;82:262–269.
22. Koller WC, Trimble J. The gait abnormality of Huntington's disease. *Neurol* 1985;35:1450–1454.
23. Reynolds NC, Myklebust J, Prieto T, et al. Analysis of gait abnormalities in Huntington disease. *Arch Phys Med Rehabil* 1999;80:59–65.
24. Vonsattel J-P, Myers R, Stevens T, et al. Neuropathological classification of Huntington's. *J Neuropathol Exp Neurol* 1985;44:559–577.

25. Albin R, Reiner A, Anderson K, et al. Preferential loss striato-pallidal projection neurons Huntington's. *Ann Neurol* 1992;31:425–430.
26. Albin RL, Reiner A, Anderson K, et al. Striatal and nigral neuron subpopulations in rigid Huntington's. *Ann Neurol* 1990;27:357–365.
27. Turjanski N, Weeks R, Dolan R, et al. Striatal D1 and D2 receptor binding in patients with Huntington's. *Brain* 1995;118:689–696.
28. Alexander G, Crutcher M. Functional architecture of basal ganglia circuits. *TINS* 1990;13:266–271.
29. Bartenstein P, Weind A, Speingel S, et al. Central motor processing in Huntington's disease. *Brain* 1997;120:1553–1567.
30. Storey E, Beal C. Neurochemical substrates of rigidity and chorea in Huntington's. *Brain* 1993;116:1201–1222.
31. Ebersbach G, Sojer M, Valldeoriola F, et al. Comparative analysis of gait in Parkinson's disease, cerebellar ataxia and subcortical arteriosclerotic encephalopathy. *Brain* 1999;122:1349–1355.
32. Hausdorff JM, Cudkowicz ME, Firtion R, et al. Gait variability and basal ganglia disorders: stride-to-stride variations of gait cycle in Parkinson's disease and Huntington's disease. *Mov Disord* 1998;13:428–437.
33. Phillips JG, Bradshaw J, Chiu E, et al. Bradykinesia and movement precision in Huntington's disease. *Neuropsychologia* 1996;34:1241–1245.
34. Tian J, Herdman S, Zee D, et al. Postural stability in patients with Huntington's disease. *Neurol* 1992;42:1232–1238.
35. Ivry R. Cerebellar timing systems. *Int Rev Neurobiol* 1997;41:555–573.
36. Jeuptner M, Rijntjes M, Weiller C, et al. Localization of a cerebellar timing process using PET. *Neurology* 1995;45:1540–1545.
37. Jeuptner M, Weiller C. A review of differences between basal ganglia and cerebellar control of movements as revealed by functional imaging studies. *Brain* 1998;121:1437–1449.
38. Keele SW, Ivry R. Does the cerebellum provide a common computation for diverse tasks? *Ann NY Acad Sci* 1990;608:179–211.
39. Rao SM, Harrington D, Haaland K, et al. Distributed neural systems underlying the timing of movements. *J Neurosci* 1997;17:5528–5535.
40. Ebersbach G, Heijmenberg M, Kindermann L, et al. Interference of rhythmic constraint on gait in healthy subjects and patients with early Parkinson's disease. *Mov Disord* 1998;14:619–625.
41. Pastor M, Artieda J, Jahanshahi M, et al. Performance of repetitive wrist movements in Parkinson's disease. *Brain* 1992;115:211–225.
42. Palliyath S, Hallett M, Thomas SL, et al. Gait in patients with cerebellar ataxia. *Mov Disord* 1998;13:958–964.
43. Diener HC, Dichgans J, Guschlbauer B, et al. The coordination of posture and voluntary movement in patients with cerebellar dysfunction. *Move Dis* 1992;7:14–22.
44. Timmann D, Horak FB. Perturbed step initiation in cerebellar subjects. I. *Exp Brain Res* 1998;119:73–84.
45. Jeste D, Barban L, Parisi J. Reduced Purkinje cell density in Huntington's disease. *Exp Neurol* 1984;85:78–86.
46. Jason GW, Suchowersky O, Pajurkova E, et al. Cognitive manifestations of Huntington's disease in relation to genetic structure and clinical onset. *Arch Neurol* 1997;54:1081–1088.
47. Kirkwood S, Siemers E, Stout J, et al. Longitudinal cognitive and motor changes among presymptomatic Huntington disease gene carriers. *Arch Neurol* 1999;56:563–568.
48. Lawrence AD, Weeks R, Brooks D, et al. Evidence for specific cognitive deficits in preclinical Huntington's disease. *Brain* 1998;121:1329–1355.
49. Mazziota JC. PET and Huntington's disease. In: Martin W, ed. *Functional imaging in movement disorders.* Boca Raton, FL: CRC Press, 1990.
50. Bond J, Morris M. Goal-directed secondary motor tasks: their effects on gait in subjects with Parkinson disease. *Arch Phys Med Rehab* 2000;81:110–116.
51. McIntosh GC, Brown SH, Rice RR, et al. Rhythmic auditory–motor facilitation of gait patterns in patients with Parkinson's disease. *J Neurol Neurosurg Psychol* 1998;62:22–26.
52. Morris ME, Huxham F, McGinley J. Strategies to prevent falls in people with Parkinson's disease. *Physiotherapy Singapore* 1999;2:135–141.
53. Morris ME, Iansek R. An interprofessional team approach to rehabilitation in Parkinson's disease. *Eur J Phys Med Rehabil* 1997;7:166–170.

Subject Index

Page numbers followed by *f* indicate figures. Page numbers followed by *t* indicate tabular material.

D

G

H

I

J

K

W